A set of 35 mm. slides including many of the illustrations in this book is available from the publisher.

SYNOPSIS
OF
RADIOLOGIC
ANATOMY

with Computed Tomography
Revised Reprint

ISADORE MESCHAN, M.A., M.D.

Professor and Director until July, 1977, of the Department of Radiology,
The Bowman Gray School of Medicine of Wake Forest University,
Winston-Salem, North Carolina; Consultant in Radiology,
Department of Radiology, Walter Reed Army Hospital, Washington, D.C.

W. B. SAUNDERS COMPANY

Philadelphia   London   Toronto   Mexico City   Rio de Janeiro   Sydney   Tokyo

W. B. Saunders Company: West Washington Square
Philadelphia, PA 19105

1 St. Anne's Road
Eastbourne, East Sussex BN21 3UN, England

1 Goldthorne Avenue
Toronto, Ontario M8Z 5T9, Canada

Apartado 26370 — Cedro 512
Mexico 4, D.F., Mexico

Rua Coronel Cabrita, 8
Sao Cristovao Caixa Postal 21176
Rio de Janeiro, Brazil

9 Waltham Street
Artarmon, N.S.W. 2064, Australia

Ichibancho, Central Bldg., 22-1 Ichibancho
Chiyoda-Ku, Tokyo 102, Japan

Library of Congress Cataloging in Publication Data

Meschan, Isadore.

Synopsis of radiologic anatomy.

1. Anatomy, Human.   2. Radiography, Medical.
   I. Title.

QM23.2.M47   611   80–5042

ISBN 0-7216-6275-1

Synopsis of Radiologic Anatomy with Computed Tomography   ISBN 0-7216-6296-X
Revised Reprint

Last digit is the print number: 9   8   7   6

To my wife,
RACHEL M. F. FARRER-MESCHAN, M.B., B.S., M.D.,
who collaborated on several of our previous books.

PREFACE

The purpose of this text is to present a *Synopsis* of our previous text, published as both a one- and two-volume version, entitled *An Atlas of Anatomy Basic to Radiology* (1975).

Small sections on Computed Tomography have been added, since these represent new applications of anatomy to radiology. This revised reprint includes material on recent engineering developments in computed tomography and makes use of CT scans produced by new equipment.

The present *Synopsis* has been written to fill the needs of medical students and technologists who must know considerable anatomy in their increasingly sophisticated daily practice; the larger text, *An Atlas of Anatomy Basic to Radiology,* is available for the practicing radiologist.

It is possible that even in this *Synopsis* there is more detail than is essential for the junior student technologists, and for those individuals who would prefer a more abbreviated manual, the second edition of *Radiographic Positioning and Related Anatomy* is also available from W. B. Saunders.

As was the case with *An Atlas of Anatomy Basic to Radiology,* the subject is so broad that decisions had to be made as to omissions and inclusions. I accept full responsibility for all these decisions based upon my experience in the practice and teaching of radiology. At the same time, however, I wish to acknowledge the very extensive help given me in the choice of material, as indicated in the acknowledgments section.

In order to keep the book compact, I have not repeated those references that are all available in the larger text—*An Atlas of Anatomy Basic to Radiology*—and in medical libraries and offices.

As with all publications of this type, I would certainly welcome any suggestions from teachers, students, or readers which in their opinion may enhance the timeless value of this text for a field as rapidly advancing and exciting as is Diagnostic Radiology.

ISADORE MESCHAN, M.D.

CREDITS AND ACKNOWLEDGMENTS

Material presented in this text is a *Synopsis* of the larger text in every detail, with the exception of the addition of sections related to Computed Tomography, which have been co-authored by Dr. Neil T. Wolfman and Mr. George Lynch, medical artist. Their generous cooperation at this particular time made the inclusion of this material possible.

The larger volume has been condensed with respect to both page size and number of pages. Because of this change in format, there has been considerable deletion of text material and number of illustrations.

Since this *Synopsis* is intended particularly for radiologic technologists and medical students, the author sought consultation with individuals well suited by background to judge the requirements for these purposes. These individuals are:

Dr. Richard J. Kelly, at present a resident in Radiology and Nuclear Medicine in the Department of Radiology of the Bowman Gray School of Medicine of Wake Forest University, Winston-Salem, North Carolina. Prior to being a medical student he was a radiologic technologist for several years. His applications of medicine to radiology were timely and extremely helpful.

Three senior faculty technologists from the Forsyth Technological Institute, Winston-Salem, North Carolina, were of great assistance in selection of materials and replacement of a number of radiographs from the original text. These individuals are:

Mr. Clyde Ritchie, B.S., senior instructor, Forsyth Technical Institute, Radiologic Technology Program.

Mrs. Rachel Clanton, A.A.S., R.T., Clinical Instructor, Forsyth Technical Institute, Radiologic Technology Program.

Miss Bonita Compton, A.A.S., R.T., Instructor, Forsyth Technical Institute, Radiologic Technology Program.

I would also like to thank *Mrs. Helen Matthews,* B.S., R.T., Assistant Professor, Radiologic Technology, University of Arkansas for Medical Sciences, and *Ms. Judith Gardner,* B.S., R.T., Instructor, Acting Director, School of Radiologic Technology, University of Arkansas for Medical Sciences, for their help in providing me with the completed manual that we had jointly prepared for use of technology students at the University of Arkansas. I am also indebted to Dr. W. Martin Dinn for the use of body scans in Chapter 16. These have been retouched by an artist.

Mr. Dale Trudo, Department of X-ray Technology, Middlesex Community College, Bedford, Massachusetts, provided assistance with more recent terminology that has been adopted by radiologic technologists. Since Mr. Trudo represents technologists from another area, he was helpful in reviewing this text from another perspective.

As always, the various editors and members of W. B. Saunders Company have been extremely helpful in every detail and unstinting in their support of this *Synopsis.*

Our Department of Audiovisual Aids deserves a debt of gratitude for its continued support and excellence. *Mr. Jack Bodenhamer,* head of the photography section, was most meticulous in executing a difficult task.

Mr. George Lynch, medical artist and head of the Audiovisual Department, has already been mentioned as a co-author of those sections dealing with Computed Tomography of the head and body. He has also been helpful in other areas of this text in which improved versions of diagrams were desirable, and in developing new overlay techniques for labeling.

Last, but not least, once again I wish to mention my very conscientious secretary, *Mrs. Betty Stimson,* who has often been called upon in the course of this text, as in others, to help with the manuscript preparation. *Mrs. Jean Wilson* and *Mrs. Carolyn Ezzell* also entered extensively into the clerical work connected with this book.

CONTENTS

1

ROUTINE PROCEDURES
OUTLINE

ROUTINE PROCEDURES*†
Comparison views: Made on all patients through age 15 on initial examination

Examination	Point of Interest or Special Situation	Projections	Number and Size of Film	Page
	Upper Extremity			
Hand	Trauma	PA	1/2–10 × 12 RPM	88–91
		Oblique	1/2–10 × 12 RPM	
		Lateral	1– 8 × 10 RPM	
	Pathologic condition	PA	1/2–10 × 12 M	
		Oblique	1/2–10 × 12 M	
		Lateral	1– 8 × 10 M	
	Arthritis	PA—both hands	1–10 × 12 M	
		"Ball catcher's" views	1–10 × 12	
Finger	Injury or pathologic condition	AP	1/3–8 × 10 cb	92–93
		Oblique	1/3–8 × 10 cb	
		Lateral	1/3–8 × 10 cb	
Thumb	Injury or pathologic condition	AP	1/2–8 × 10 cb	92
		Lateral	1/2–8 × 10 cb	
Wrist	Injury or pathologic condition	PA or AP	1/3–10 × 12 cb	82–87
		Oblique	1/3–10 × 12 cb	
		Lateral	1/3–10 × 12 cb	
	Navicular injury or disease	Routine wrist	1–10 × 12 cb	
	Pisiform injury or disease	Special navicular view	1–8 × 10 cb	
		AP oblique	1–8 × 10 cb	
Forearm	Injury or pathologic condition	AP	1/2–11 × 14 cb	80
		Lateral	1/2–11 × 14 cb	
	NOTE: Both joints must be demonstrated on both views			

*Courtesy of Mrs. Helen Matthews, R. T., University of Arkansas School of Medicine, Little Rock, Arkansas.
†Abbreviations:
AP: Anteroposterior
PA: Posteroanterior
RPM: Rapid processing mode; par speed screens
cb: Cardboard or plastic film holder without intensifying screens
s: Screen containing cassette
g: Grid cassette (or oscillating grid)
b: Bucky (film in cassette in Potter-Bucky diaphragm)
B: Tomogram with oscillating Bucky

ROUTINE PROCEDURES
Comparison views: Made on all patients through age 15 on initial examination

Examination	Point of Interest or Special Situation	Projections	Number and Size of Film	Page
Elbow	Injury or pathologic condition	AP	1/2–8 × 10 cb	74–77
		Lateral	1/2–8 × 10 cb	
	When elbow cannot be flexed or fully extended	AP with tip of olecranon centered.	1/2–8 × 10 cb	
		Lateral	1/2–8 × 10 cb	
	Alternate films	AP – two films		
		Forearm flat	1/2–8 × 10 cb	
		Humerus flat	1/2–8 × 10 cb	
	Acute flexion	Inferior-superior	1/2–8 × 10 s	
		Lateral	1/2–8 × 10 s	
Humerus	Injury or pathologic condition	AP	1/2–10 × 12 s	
		Lateral (elbow flexed)	1/2–10 × 12 s	
	With hanging cast, allow to hang free	AP erect	1–10 × 12 s or g	71–72
		Transthoracic lateral	1–10 × 12 g	
		AP shoulder	1–10 × 12 s or g	
		Transthoracic lateral	1–10 × 12 g	
	Entire humerus for disease or survey	AP recumbent	1–7 × 17 s	
Shoulder	Injury	AP	1–10 × 12 s or g	58–64
		Transthoracic lateral	1–10 × 12 g	
	Pathologic condition (use direction indicator)	Rotations:		
		Neutral	1–10 × 12 s or g	
		External	1–10 × 12 s or g	
		Internal	1–10 × 12 s or g	
Clavicle	Injury or pathologic condition	PA with 10′ caudad angle	1–7 × 17 s	65–66
		AP with 10′ cephalad angle	1–7 × 17 s	
Scapula	Injury or pathologic condition	AP	1–10 × 12 b	65–67
		Lateral	1–10 × 12 b	
Acromioclavicular Region		AP – erect, weight bearing of both shoulders	1–7 × 17 s	62–65
Sternoclavicular Region	Injury or pathologic condition	PA	1–8 × 10 b	413–414
		Both obliques	2–8 × 10 b	

ROUTINE PROCEDURES
Comparison views: Made on all patients through age 15 on initial examination

Examination	Point of Interest or Special Situation	Projections	Number and Size of Film	Page
		Lower Extremity		
Toes	Injury or pathologic condition	Dorsoplantar	1/2–8 × 10 c	140
		Oblique–distal 1/3 of foot	1/2–8 × 10 c	
Foot	Injury	AP	1/2–10 × 12 RPM	137–139
		Oblique	1/2–10 × 12 RPM	
		Lateral	1–8 × 10 RPM	
	Pathologic condition	AP	1/2–10 × 12 M	
		Oblique	1/2–10 × 12 M	
		Lateral	1–8 × 10 M	
	Flat feet (Pes planus)	AP – erect (both feet)	1–10 × 12 c	140
		Lateral – erect	2–10 × 12 c	
Heel (Os Calcis)	Injury or pathologic condition	Lateral	1–6-1/2 × 8-1/2 c	135
		Inferior-superior tangential	1–6-1/2 × 8-1/2 s	136
Ankle	Injury or pathologic condition	AP	1/3–11 × 14 c	133; 134; 135
		Oblique	1/3–11 × 14 c	
		Lateral	1/3–11 × 14 c	
Leg (Tibia and Fibula)	Injury or pathologic condition	AP	1–7 × 17 c or s	129
		Lateral	1–7 × 17 c or s	
	NOTE: Include both joints in both views in cases of trauma; use 14 × 17 film if necessary (diagonal)			
Knee	Injury or pathologic condition	AP	1–8 × 10 s or b	118–120
		Lateral	1–8 × 10 s or b	
		Oblique	1–8 × 10 s or b	
	Loose bodies, osteochondritis	Tunnel view (semiaxial view)	1–8 × 10 s	
Patella	Injury or pathologic condition	PA	1–8 × 10 s	121–122
		Lateral	1–8 × 10 s	
		Skyline or axial	1–8 × 10 s	

ROUTINE PROCEDURES
Comparison views: Made on all patients through age 15 on initial examination

Examination	Point of Interest or Special Situation	Projections	Number and Size of Film	Page
Femur	Injury or pathologic condition	AP	1–7 × 17 b	115
		Lateral	1–7 × 17 b	
		NOTE: Include joint nearest area of interest		
	Intramedullary nail	AP	1–7 × 17 b	
		Lateral	1–7 × 17 b	
		AP hip	1–10 × 12 b	
Hip Pelvis	Injury (initial exam)	AP pelvis	1–14 × 17 b	99–103
		Lateral hip (horizontal beam)	1–10 × 12 g	
	(Return visit)	AP hip	1–10 × 12 b	111–114 (hip)
		Lateral	1–10 × 12 g	
		NOTE: If fracture, AP recumbent chest (to avoid bedside film later)		
	Pathologic condition	AP pelvis	1–14 × 17 b	
		Frog lateral	1–14 × 17 b	
		Vertebral Column		
Neck	Pathologic condition	AP moving mandible	1–8 × 10 b	339–343
		Lateral	1–10 × 12 g	
		Both oblique	2–10 × 12 g	
		Flexion, extension lateral	2–10 × 12 g	
	Fracture	AP		
		Lateral (transthoracic)		
		Obliques		
		Pillars		350
		NOTE: AP and lateral should be checked with radiologist before proceeding with obliques, pillars, flexion, or extension views		
Chest	Injury or pathologic condition	AP	1–7 × 17 b	423
		Right lateral	1–7 × 17 b	420
Lumbar Region	Injury or pathologic condition	AP	1–14 × 17 b	354–357
		Both obliques	2–11 × 14 b	
		Lateral	1–7 × 17 b	
		Cone down	1–8 × 10 b	
		L-5, S-1		
		Flexion, extension, lateral standing*		

*Spondylolisthesis.

ROUTINE PROCEDURES
Comparison views: Made on all patients through age 15 on initial examination

Examination	Point of Interest or Special Situation	Projections	Number and Size of Film	Page
Sacrum	Injury or pathologic condition	AP	1–10 × 12 b	356
		Lateral	1–10 × 12 b	
Coccyx	Injury or pathologic condition	AP } Do laterals first to determine configuration	1–8 × 10 b	
		Lateral	1–8 × 10 b	
Sacroiliac Joints		Right posterior oblique	1–10 × 12 b	101
		Left posterior oblique	1–10 × 12 b	
		Bony Thorax		
Sternum	Injury or pathologic condition	Right lateral	1–10 × 12 b	411–413
		Right anterior oblique	1–10 × 12 b	
Ribs	Injury or pathologic condition (Place lead marker on point of pain)	PA chest	1–14 × 17	418–419
		AP	1–10 × 12 b	423
		Posterior oblique or anterior oblique (affected side down if possible; if painful, affected side may be turned up)	1–10 × 12 b	413
Cervical Ribs		PA chest	1–14 × 17	418–419
		Skull		
Skull	Injury or pathologic condition	Caldwell	1–10 × 12 b	186–190
		Town's	1–10 × 12 b	
		Basilar	1–10 × 12 b	
		Both laterals	2–10 × 12 b	
Orbit*	Routine	Water's (closed mouth)	1–8 × 10 b	191; 206–207
		Lateral	1–8 × 10 b	193
	If fracture is suspected, add:	Blowout views: stereo Water's†	2–8 × 10 b	216–218
Optic Foramina*		Right and left parieto-orbital (12′–15′ caudad)	2–8 × 10 b	208

*Use cylinder.
†Body section radiography where indicated

ROUTINE PROCEDURES
Comparison views: Made on all patients through age 15 on initial examination

Examination	Point of Interest or Special Situation	Projections	Number and Size of Film	Page

Eye—Opaque Foreign Body*	Survey	Lateral-double exposure
		  Eye straight
		  Eye down
		Water's
		Bone-free
			1–6-1/2 × 8-1/2 cb
			200 × 7/10 × 94
			200 × 1-1/2 + 100 kvp cb
			200 × 1-1/2 × 100 kvp cp
			Dental film
			100 × 7/10 × 42
				216–218
				
				191

	Sweet's method of foreign body localization, radiologist present			
Mastoid Process		Routine skulls may precede Modified stenver's* (right and left) AP polytome cuts	5–10 × 12 b 2–8 × 10 b	220–225 161–167
Sinus		Submental-vertex Water's (open mouth)* Caldwell* Lateral* Water's *only**	1–10 × 12 b 1–8 × 10 b 1–8 × 10 b 1–8 × 10 b 1–8 × 10 b	191–193
	Children			
Facial Bones		Submentovertical Water's (closed mouth)* Lateral* Caldwell*	1–10 × 12 b 1–8 × 10 b 1–8 × 10 b 1–8 × 10 b	191–193
Nasal Bones*		Water's Caldwell Lateral facial bones Lateral nose Axial	1–8 × 10 b 1–8 × 10 b 1–8 × 10 b 1–6-1/2 × 8-1/2 b Occusal film	191–193 203
Mandible		PA semiaxial* Both obliques* Towne's (center between angle and symphysis)	1–8 × 10 b 2–8 × 10 b 1–10 × 12 b	194–195; 197–198; 199 188
	Initial visit, add:			
Temporomandibular Joints*		Routine mandible Polytome cuts, usually in lateral (or Law's) (open and closed mouth)		194–195 196

*Use cylinder: May add Schüller's, Mayer's, Law's, Rönstrom's or mastoid "tip" views, as required.

ROUTINE PROCEDURES
Comparison views: Made on all patients through age 15 on initial examination

Examination	Point of Interest or Special Situation	Projections	Number and Size of Film	Page
		Films made: Erect with 72-inch focal-film distance inspiratory, unless stated otherwise		
		Thorax		
Heart (with barium paste)	Full cardiac series (initial visit)	PA Right anterior oblique Left anterior oblique Left lateral	Smallest Film adequate to cover chest	
	Children (1–15 years)	Left anterior oblique (do first without barium) PA Right anterior oblique Left lateral		418–422
Chest		PA Right lateral		418–419 420
Goiter or Thyroid (with barium paste)		PA chest Lateral chest Lateral neck		1–10 × 12
Foreign Body or Atelectasis		Routine chest PA expiratory chest (use lead indicator)		
		Digestive System		
Esophagus (esophagram)		Fluoroscopy Right anterior oblique Left lateral	1–14 × 17 b 1–14 × 17 b	592–595

ROUTINE PROCEDURES
Comparison views: Made on all patients through age 15 on initial examination

Examination	Point of Interest or Special Situation	Projections	Number and Size of Film	Page
Upper Gastrointestinal Tract		Fluoroscopy		616–619
		Right anterior oblique—cone down of duodenal bulb*	1–8 × 10 b	620–624
		Right anterior oblique—stomach	1–10 × 12 b	
		Right lateral	1–10 × 12 b	
		Left posterior oblique	1–10 × 12 b	
		PA	1–14 × 17 b	

NOTE: In machines permitting, use 11 × 14 for PA and omit right anterior oblique cone down

Examination	Point of Interest or Special Situation	Projections	Number and Size of Film	Page
Duodenum hypotonic duodenography	Have patient empty his bladder before starting study. Barium (GI) room temperature. 45 mg. propantheline bromide. Radiologist should check on possible contraindications			625; 628
		Fluoroscopy: Patient drinks barium mixture to demonstrate loop; fluoroscopy is then done. Injection of propantheline bromide given I.M. Fluoroscope and make spot films. Caution patient and/or family or call ward if person is house patient: Restrict fluids until after patient empties bladder once again. If patient has any difficulty in voiding, have him report to physician.		
Small Bowel (add 10 cc. gastrografin to barium)		PA—15-minute film. Sequential films (as directed by radiologist). Fluoroscope spot at terminal ileum		659–662

*Use spot-film compression studies under fluoroscopic control.

ROUTINE PROCEDURES
Comparison views: Made on all patients through age 15 on initial examination

Examination	Point of Interest or Special Situation	Projections	Number and Size of Film	Page
Colon		AP abdominal survey	1–14 × 17 b	663–673
		PA	1–14 × 17 b	
		Right anterior oblique	1–14 × 17 b	
		Left anterior oblique	1–14 × 17 b	
		PA postevacuation	1–14 × 17 b	
Gall Bladder	Survey:	PA of right upper quadrant	1–10 × 12 b	696; 700–701
	Visualization series	PA of right upper quadrant	1–10 × 12 b	
		Left anterior oblique	1–10 × 12 b	
		Right lateral decubitus	1–8 × 10 b	
		or		
		Erect fluoro spots		
	NOTE: If visualization does not occur on 12-hour film, take abdominal film 14 × 17 b			

Abdomen and Urinary System

Examination	Point of Interest or Special Situation	Projections	Number and Size of Film	Page
Abdomen	Survey	AP recumbent	1–14 × 17 b	477
Acute Abdomen	Obstruction, ruptured viscus	Routine chest	2–14 × 17	476
		AP recumbent	1–14 × 17 b	
		AP erect abdomen	1–14 × 17 b	
	NOTE: If patient is unable to stand, take a left lateral decubitus abdomen			
Liver, Spleen, Pancreas and Sinus Tract Injection				631–636 (pancreas)
			1–14 × 17	477; 492–493
Urinary Tract (excretory urography—intravenous pyelogram)	Adult	AP survey	1–14 × 17 b	517–518
		5-minute AP	1–14 × 17 b	
		10-minute right posterior oblique and left posterior oblique	1–14 × 17 b	
		20-minute PA	1–14 × 17 b	
	NOTE: If hypertension is indicated, make a 2-minute AP in addition			
	Infants and young children	AP survey	Smallest film necessary	519
		3-minute AP		
		8-minute PA		
	NOTE: Additional films may be necessary			

ROUTINE PROCEDURES
Comparison views: Made for all patients through age 15 on initial examination

Examination	Point of Interest or Special Situation	Projections	Number and Size of Film	Page
Gall Bladder and Bile Ducts (Cholangiogram, postoperative)	Diatrizoate meglumine (Reno-M-60)	Make spot films and drainage films		702–703
	Fluoroscopy and spot films by radiologist			
Kidney and Ureter (rapid-sequence intravenous pyelogram)	Survey films (Renografin 60) injected according to body weight by radiologist:	Abdomen	1–14 × 17	519
		30 sec.	1–14 × 17	
		2 min.	1–14 × 17	
		3 min.	1–14 × 17	
		5 min.	1–14 × 17	
	Obliques	10 min.	1–14 × 17	
		20 min.	1–14 × 17	
	NOTE: Check films with radiologist			
Kidney (urea or mannitol washout)	Survey films	Abdomen	1–14 × 17 1/2–14 × 17 centered over kidney	519–520
	50 cc (Renografin 76)	Injected by radiologist:		
		30 sec.	1/2–14 × 17	
		2 min.	1/2–14 × 17	
		3 min.	1/2–14 × 17	
		5 min.	1/2–14 × 17	
		8 min.	1–14 × 17	
	NOTE: Make baseline film (1–14 × 17) just before infusion of urea or mannitol; after beginning of infusion take these films:			
		3 min.	1/2–14 × 17	
		6 min.	1/2–14 × 17	
		9 min.	1/2–14 × 17	
		12 min.	1/2–14 × 17	
		15 min.	1/2–14 × 17	
		18 min.	1/2–14 × 17	
	Allow patient to void before 21-minute film			
		21 min.	1–14 × 17	
	Check with radiologist for addition films			

ROUTINE PROCEDURES
Comparison views: Made on all patients through age 15 on initial examination

Examination	Point of Interest or Special Situation	Projections	Number and Size of Film	Page
Kidney drip infusion pyelogram	300 cc. meglumine diatrizoate (Reno-M-Dip) or Sodium diatrizoate (Hypaque 25)	AP survey AP midinfusion Postinfusion, as requested by radiologist	1–14 × 17 b 1–14 × 17 b	519
	NOTE: Additional films and/or tomograms may be indicated			
Pregnancy Detection		AP Abdomen* (with added filtration and 63″ focal film distance)	1–14 × 17 b	549; 552–553 554–555
	*NOTE: Check with radiologist to see if an oblique is necessary			
	Usually used in detection of dead fetus; ultrasonography used in detection of live fetus and for measurement of fetal head			

SPECIAL EXAMINATIONS

Examination	Point of Interest or Special Situation	Projections	Number and Size of Film	Page
Cerebral Blood Vessels (cerebral angiogram; carotid arteriogram)	*As ordered by the radiologist*			274–304
Pneumography of Brain				250–266
Computed Tomography Brain and Orbits				305–327
Face and Remainder of Body				710–745
Biliary Ducts (infusion intravenous cholangiography)	Survey films		1. 10 × 12 of right upper quadrant 702–703 1. Tomographic cuts at presumed level of common bile duct	

Infusion: Mix 40 cc of iodipamide (Cholografin) and 50 cc of sterile isotonic saline. Take a film immediately after the end of the infusion and thereafter at 30 min., 45 min., 1 hour, and 1-1/2 hour time intervals. Expose one film 15 min. after completion of infusion. If common duct is visualized, take appropriate tomographic cuts. If not, repeat film at 30 min.

NOTE: 60-minute, 90-minute, and 24-hour films should be obtained for time-density evaluation

ROUTINE PROCEDURES

Examination for Special Purposes	Point of Interest or Special Situation	Projections
Bone Age	The following is the routine to be carried out for determination of bone age at various chronological ages: Birth to 5 years: 1. AP left* shoulder 2. Left hand and wrist 3. AP left elbow 4. AP left hip 5. Lateral left knee 6. Oblique left foot and ankle 5 years to adult: PA left wrist and hand 1, 2, and 3 may be combined if child is small; 4 and 5 may be combined if child is small.	
Bone Survey		Lateral cervical spine Lateral skull AP and lateral lumbar spine AP pelvis AP ribs (if no chest available within 1 month) AP upper and lower extremities (omit below knees and below elbows if looking for metastatic disease) PA hands (omit for metastatic disease)
Lead Lines (any age)		1. AP hands 2. AP wrists 3. AP knees 4. AP abdomen
Scurvy or Rickets		AP of both wrists and knees
Long Bone Survey		AP of entire upper and lower extremities
Retrograde Pyelogram, Cystogram, and Urethrogram	*As ordered by the urologist* Children: Urethrograms; fluoroscoped by the radiologist	

*Taken for uniformity in follow-up.

SPECIAL EXAMINATIONS

Examination	Point of Interest or Special Situation	Projections
Heart and Great Vessels (angiocardiogram)	As ordered by the radiologist	
Aorta (aortogram)	As ordered by the radiologist	
Arteries (arteriogram)		AP survey film AP film after injection Other films, as ordered by the radiologist
Veins (venogram)		Same procedure as arteriogram
Peritoneal Cavity; Perirenal Area; Sacral Area (pneumoperitoneum; perirenal insufflation; pneumoretroperitoneum and presacral air)		1. Dorsal decubitus 2. Ventral decubitus 3. Right and left lateral decubitus 4. AP erect — if subphrenic abscess is suspected
Pelvis; Peritoneal Cavity (gynogram; pelvic intra-pneumoperitoneum)		PA; table tilted 45° Trendelenburg Central ray vertical PA; table tilted 45° Trendelenburg Central ray 15° caudad Patient prone; Transtabular lateral (ventral decubitus) with table tilted 30° Trendelenburg
Uterus (hysterosalpingogram)		1. AP survey film 2. Fluoroscopy and spots by radiologist* 3. AP film 20 min. after injection 4. Check with radiologist for additional films

*Sinografin recommended at this writing

SPECIAL EXAMINATIONS

Examination	Point of Interest or Special Situation	Projections	Number and Size of Film
Lymphatic Vessels (lymphangiogram)*	Survey	AP pelvis AP abdomen PA and lateral chest	1–14 × 17
	Film immediately after injection	AP and both obliques of abdomen AP pelvis PA and lateral chest AP and lateral legs and thighs	
	24-hour films	AP and both obliques of abdomen AP pelvis PA and lateral chest Lateral abdomen	
Spinal Cord (myelogram)	Films of questionable area if patient does not have recent study Fluoroscopy for position and direction of needle After injection of iophendylate (Pantopaque)	1. PA 2. Patient prone; transtabular lateral (ventral decubitus) 3. Other films as requested by radiologist	
Lungs (bronchial brushing)	Fluoroscopy: Films as ordered by radiologist		
Lungs (bronchogram)	Survey films	1. AP chest 2. Lateral chest	1–14 × 17 1–14 × 17
	First side injected	1. AP 2. Posterior oblique 3. Lateral	1–14 × 17 1–14 × 17 1–14 × 17
	Second side injected	1. Posterior oblique 2. AP	1–14 × 17 1–14 × 17
		NOTE: Check with radiologist for additional film	

*May be combined with excretory urogram on the 24-hour films.

SPECIAL EXAMINATIONS

Examination	Point of Interest or Special Situation	Projections	Number and Size of Film
Fluid-Containing Structures of Brain (pneumoenceph- alogram)	Routine chest film before or after examination. Film used to determine if a primary lung tumor is present; a significant number of brain lesions are secondary to bronchogenic carcinoma. The chest film may also reveal other evidence of tumor metastases.		

Cerebral Ventricles (ventriculogram)	Routine Views	A. Supine
		  1. Towne's
		  2. AP
		  3. Brow-up lateral
		B. Prone
		  1. Caldwell
		  2. PA
		  3. Brow-down lateral
		C. Right side down
		  1. Transtabular AP (PA)
		  2. Stereo right lateral
		D. Left side down
		  1. Transtabular PA (AP)
		  2. Left Lateral
		E. Erect
		  1. AP
		  2. Towne's
		  3. Left lateral
		F. Special 4th ventricle view
		G. Tomograms if requested
			1–10 × 12

Salivary Ducts (sialogram)		1. Lateral skull centering over gland with neck hyperextended 2. Oblique mandible 3. Tangential view of gland region in either AP or PA position 4. Intraoral	
Spine (scoliosis series— initial study)		1. AP erect film to include all of neck 2. Erect AP bending to right 3. Erect AP bending to left 4. Recumbent lateral 5. Erect lateral	1–14 × 36 1–14 × 17 b 1–14 × 17 b 1–14 × 17 b 1–14 × 17 b #2–5 with Bucky

2

BACKGROUND FUNDAMENTALS FOR DIAGNOSTIC RADIOLOGY

INTRODUCTION

X-rays are produced when fast-moving electrons with sufficient energy strike a target. Most of the electron energy is converted to heat, but a very minute amount—less than 1 per cent—is converted to x-ray.

NATURE OF X-RAYS

Spectrum of Electromagnetic Radiations. X-rays resemble visible light rays very closely but have the distinguishing feature that their wave lengths are very short—only about 1/10,000 the wave length of visible light. It is this characteristic that permits x-rays to penetrate materials which otherwise would absorb or reflect light. X-rays form a part of the spectrum of electromagnetic radiations, of which the long electric and radio waves are found at one end; the infrared, visible, and ultraviolet light waves in the middle; and the short wave x-rays, gamma rays, and cosmic rays at the other end (Fig. 2–1).

There are three properties of x-rays that become particularly useful in diagnostic radiology. Apart from their property to penetrate matter, these are their *fluorescent* and *photosensitization* effects and their ability to cause a *phosphorescence* or *fluorescence* in certain cystalline materials.

The radiographer, however, must also be familiar with other fundamental properties of x-rays, particularly from the standpoint of radiation protection. When x-rays strike matter, particles are ionized, and this ionization produces various phenomena in biological material. In practically all instances this is a destructive effect, at least to some degree. Some reparative processes do occur, but in any case *the utilization of x-rays must be carried forward extremely judiciously* and with every care taken to ensure protection. These protective measures are briefly summarized in Chapter 3.

X-RAY TUBE

The device which produces the fast-moving electrons is the x-ray tube (Fig. 2–2). The electrons are produced when a filament within the tube is heated. A large electrical force drives these electrons onto a target or focal spot. Upon impact with this focal spot, the electrons give rise to a stream of x-rays which are emitted over a 180-degree hemispherical angle surrounding the focal spot.

A lead-shielded window, along with a lead tube casing, is provided as part of the housing of the x-ray tube, so that only a small fraction of these x-rays pass through the portal of the tube.

The intricate details of the tube and the circuitry responsible for producing the electrons are outside the scope of this text.

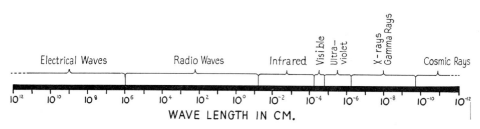

FIGURE 2–1   Spectrum of electromagnetic radiations.

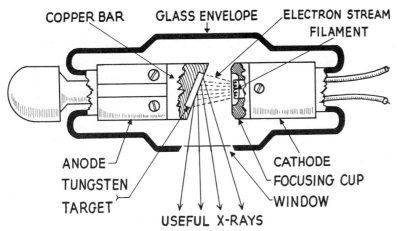

COPPER BAR   GLASS ENVELOPE   ELECTRON STREAM
FILAMENT

ANODE
TUNGSTEN
TARGET
USEFUL X-RAYS
CATHODE
FOCUSING CUP
WINDOW

FIGURE 2–2   Diagram of standard stationary anode x-ray tube.

the better the detail, since there is less "shadow effect" (penumbra) around the image. (See the later section on the geometry of the x-ray image.)

Most x-ray tubes come equipped with two filaments, each of a different size; since small targets present a greater problem of heat dissipation, the larger target may be necessary when an abundance of x-rays is required to penetrate the large anatomic parts.

The focusing cup helps direct the stream of electrons. Additionally, special grid devices introduced in the x-ray tube facilitate extremely short exposure times when rapid sequential films are necessary.

ADVANTAGES AND LIMITATIONS OF SMALL FOCAL SPOT. As in all instances of light emission, the smaller the light source, the sharper the image produced; just so in radiography, *as the focal spot diminishes, the radiographic image becomes sharper*. However, the *smaller the focal spot, the lower the amount of energy that can be applied without producing damage to the target*, so that heat dissipation and

Focal Spot Size. Surrounding the filament is a focusing cup (Fig. 2–3) which focuses the electron stream upon the so-called focal spot on the anode. Upon impact with this focal spot, the electrons give rise to a stream of x-rays which are emitted over a 180 degree hemispherical angle surrounding the focal spot. A lead-shielded window (Fig. 2–2) is provided, along with a lead tube casing, so that only a small fraction of these x-rays passes through the portal of the tube.

The actual target is a small rectangular plate of tungsten fused into the beveled end of a large copper bar, causing an angulation of the target of about 20 degrees. This angulation affects the size of the "effective" focal spot. The copper bar acts to dissipate the heat from the target.

The cross-sectional area at the site of origin of the rays (Fig. 2–3) is called the "effective focal spot size" and usually ranges between 0.5 mm. and 2.0 mm., although some special tubes are now made with effective focal spot sizes of 0.12 mm. which are useful in magnification techniques.

The size of the effective focal spot is responsible for the detail of the roentgen image produced. The smaller the effective focal spot

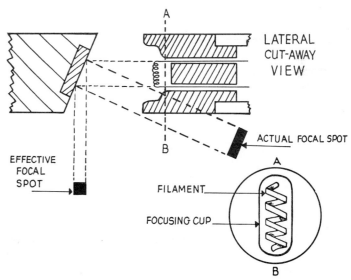

LATERAL
CUT-AWAY
VIEW

ACTUAL FOCAL SPOT

EFFECTIVE
FOCAL
SPOT

FILAMENT

FOCUSING CUP

FIGURE 2–3   Diagram of focusing cup and filament.

mechanical design of the x-ray tube are of fundamental importance in radiography.

The Rotating Anode. A much more efficient anode is provided if the anode is made to rotate (Fig. 2–4) while the electrons strike the target, so that the electrons never strike a single rectangular area but rather the rim of a wheel which is angled at about 15 degrees. In this type of "rotating anode" tube the effective focal spot can be very small, and yet because the actual target is the rim of a wheel it does not heat up as readily as it would in a "stationary anode" type tube.

SPECIAL PROPERTIES OF X-RAYS IN DIAGNOSTIC RADIOLOGY

The special properties of x-rays which make them so useful in diagnostic radiology are: (1) their *ability to penetrate* organic matter, (2) their ability to produce a *photographic effect* on photosensitive film surfaces, and (3) their ability to produce a *phosphorescence* (fluorescence) in certain crystalline materials.

Penetrability of Tissues and Other Substances by X-rays. Tissues and other substances with medical applications may be classified as indicated in Figure 2–5 on the basis of their density and atomic structure. At one end of the spectrum are the *radiolucent* materials, through which the x-rays pass readily; at the other end are the *radiopaque* substances in which the x-rays are absorbed to a considerable degree in their passage so that little radiation escapes.

Until recently, x-ray film was the modality of choice for recording the "remnant radiation" leaving the body part, and it is still used predominantly for conventional radiography. Special computerized devices now available for recording x-ray images have opened up an entire new field of radiography known as *computed tomography,* which will be described in special sections of this text. Briefly, this new modality has allowed the radiation leaving the body part to be recorded on an extremely broad scale of shades of gray (or color), thereby increasing tremendously the potential to separate the above-described categories into many more than just the five mentioned. This separation will be described in greater detail later.

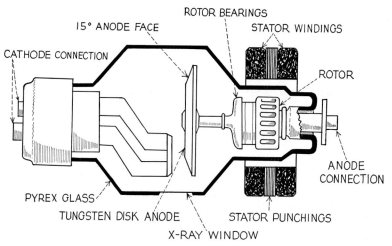

FIGURE 2–4 Diagram of rotating anode x-ray tube.

VERY RADIOLUCENT	MODERATELY RADIOLUCENT	INTERMEDIATE	MODERATELY RADIOPAQUE	VERY RADIOPAQUE
Gas	Fatty tissue	Connective tissue Muscle tissue Blood Cartilage Epithelium Cholesterol stones Uric acid stones	Bone Calcium salts	Heavy metals

FIGURE 2–5 Classification of tissues and other substances with medical application in accordance with five general categories of radiopacity and radiolucency. This tabulation relates to conventional, but not computerized, tomographic radiography. An entirely different scale of densities will be shown for computed tomography (formerly called "computerized" tomography).

Photographic Effect of X-rays. Just as visible or ultraviolet rays alter light-sensitive photographic emulsion, so do roentgen rays, so that when appropriately "developed," "fixed," and "washed," a permanent image is produced. The film employed for this purpose is ordinarily made with a thicker emulsion, although this is not absolutely necessary. The utilization of intensifying fluorescent screens (to be described below) has largely replaced such direct radiography, since less x-irradiation is necessary for radiography by intensification techniques. However, when the body part under study (such as an extremity) is not large, and when optimum detail is required, direct radiography may be preferable. Direct radiography is also preferable when it is necessary to be certain that no dust or other similar artefacts may be interposed or projected on the x-ray image.

Fluorescent Effects of X-rays (Fig. 2–6). When roentgen rays strike certain crystalline materials, phosphorescence results. The spectrum of light so produced will vary with the crystalline substance; at times, it is mostly ultraviolet, at other times, mostly visible, light. Ultraviolet light has proved to be most advantageous in respect to x-ray

film emulsion. An intensifying screen consists mostly of a thin coating of crystals on a cardboard surface (Fig. 2–7). Its function is to provide a brighter image than would result from the direct photographic effects of the x-rays alone. Intensifying screens are categorized according to brightness (called "speed") and detail, each being inverse to the other and thus requiring some compromise.

Prior to the advent of image amplification, which has replaced conventional fluoroscopy, the crystalline substance chosen for its fluorescence produced light in the visible light range. In image amplification requiring electromagnetic enhancement, the "input phosphorescent" and "output phosphorescent" screens are similarly constructed.

Other Fundamental Properties of X-rays. Other fundamental properties of x-rays to be briefly mentioned here are: (1) ionization, (2) chemical effects, (3) heat production, and (4) biologic effects.

Ionization is a primary effect of x-rays whenever these photons strike matter with sufficient energy. It produces various observable phenomena, depending upon the matter affected. Ionization of air by x-rays has been used in the quantitative measurement of radiation.

Chemical effects are produced by x-rays by altering atomic structure. Salt, for example, ordinarily turns yellow from liberation of chlorine.

Heat production is a phenomenon whenever electrons strike matter and only a very small number of x-rays are produced. The heat produced in the x-ray tube target is so great that special cooling devices have to be provided. On the other hand, heat production in organic matter may be infinitesimally small—so small that is is difficult to measure.

Biologic effects may be among the most important changes wrought by x-rays, and they are utilized constantly in x-ray therapy. Radiation in diagnostic radiology, however, seldom produces detectable or measureable biologic effects and, hence, further discussion falls outside the scope of this text, except as pertains to radiologic protection (Chapter 3).

ACCESSORIES NECESSARY FOR THE RECORDING OF THE X-RAY IMAGE

The accessories which make radiography and fluoroscopy possible are:

1. The x-ray film.

2. The x-ray cassette, with its enclosed intensifying screens.

3. The x-ray film not requiring an intensifying screen or conventional cassette but placed in a plastic or cardboard folder.

4. The stationary and moving grids, such as the Potter-Bucky diaphragm.

5. Various cones, apertures, and adjustable diaphragms for delimiting the x-ray beam to the body part in question.

6. Body section radiographic equipment.

7. Stereoscopic radiographic accessories.

8. The fluoroscopic screen and the fluoroscope.

9. Image amplifiers used in conjunction with fluoroscopy and radiography.

10. Equipment for television fluoroscopy and radiography with television tape recording.

11. Accessories for spot film radiography.

12. Devices for photographing the output phosphor of an image amplifier; the radiographs may be miniature in size, such as 16 mm., 35 mm., 70 mm., 90 mm., or 100 mm., or 105 mm., or cineradiographic sequences.

13. Rapid sequence film changers for either roll film or cut film, or rapid sequence cassette changers for recording rapidly changing x-ray images.

14. Magnification accessories.

15. Contrast media.

16. Computed tomography (to be discussed in Chapters 7 and 16).

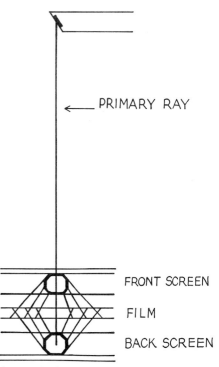

PRIMARY RAY

FRONT SCREEN

FILM

BACK SCREEN

FIGURE 2–6   Diagram illustrating fluorescence from intensifying screen.

Each of these devices will now be briefly illustrated and discussed.

X-ray Film. X-ray film consists of a transparent cellulose acetate or plastic base coated on each side with a photosensitive emulsion such as silver bromide crystals. Rarely, single emulsion films are employed. The emulsion is designed to be most efficiently photosensitized in an ultraviolet radiation range by the light rays emitted by the intensifying screens, when these latter structures are activated by x-rays. X-ray film, with a somewhat different emulsion, is utilized when the film is contained in a light-proof folder without intensifying screens, in which case the film is photosensitized by the x-rays directly. X-ray film is developed in a special developing solution which precipitates the exposed crystals; the unused developing solution clinging to the film is rapidly washed away, and the precipitated silver halide crystals are "fixed" in "hypo" solution. The film is then washed and dried prior to viewing and interpretation. Film processing from start to finish may now be carried out very efficiently in 90 seconds, or even less with appropriate automated equipment.

The X-ray Cassette (Fig. 2–7). The x-ray cassette is a lightproof container for the film, designed to permit easy loading and unloading, while near perfect contact is maintained with the intensifying screens. When the x-ray beam strikes the intensifying screen, ultraviolet and visible light rays are produced and the film is photosensitized. A suitable "x-ray" image is thereby produced, employing fewer x-rays than are necessary when no intensifying screens are used. Unfortunately, any external particles upon the film or intensifying screen, or defects in either film or screen will also produced an image on the film, so that the x-ray cassette must be cleaned and handled with extreme care.

X-ray Film in a Cardboard or Plastic Holder. When minute foreign bodies are to be detected by x-ray examination, x-ray film in a cardboard or plastic holder is used whenever possible because it eliminates potential artefacts. This film, of course, requires greater radiation exposure for adequate imaging.

The Stationary and Moving Grids (Fig. 2–8). X-rays are scattered in all directions when they strike an object. The grid is a device for collimating the x-rays after transmission through the patient so that the image on the film is formed by "orderly" rays which have penetrated the body part. The grid is composed of alternating strips of lead with intervening pieces of wood, bakelite, or plastic. The grid is placed between the part to be radiographed and the film, usually under the table top.

When a focused grid is employed, only the rays in direct radial alignment with the target can pass through the grid, since the scattered rays are absorbed by the lead strips. The lead strips are placed so that the plane of each is parallel to the ray projections from the x-ray focal spot. Thus, a special grid must be employed for each major change in grid-to-tube target distance; this is called the "grid radius." The wood-filled slots between the lead strips are usually about 6 to 32 times as deep as they are wide; this ratio of the height to the width of the wood slot is the "grid ratio." The strips of lead have the function of absorbing the scattered rays as they come from the body part before they can strike the beam, so that the image is formed by the primary parallel radiation that has penetrated the body part. The greater the grid ratio, the more efficient is the grid in absorbing scattered radiation—but the greater is the amount of radiation necessary to obtain a given suitable exposure.

If the grid is stationary, the lead lines are reproduced on the radiograph and are objectionable unless the lead strips are extremely fine; but if the grid is placed in motion by a spring or motor device while the exposure is being made, the grid lines are not seen and the efficiency of the grid is improved. This moving grid is called the "Potter-Bucky diaphragm." In the Camp grid cassette, a stationary grid of special design has been incorporated into the cover of the cassette. Although such cassettes are expensive, they delimit scattered radiation very efficiently, and the grid lines are visible only on closest inspection. Great care must be exercised in the handling of these wafer-thin grids, since the slightest bending of the grid will distort the relationship of the lead strips to the primary beam and diminish the efficiency of the grid.

It is also important to recognize that a focused grid has a "tube side" and a "film side." These must not be reversed or a virtually blank radiograph will result. If the lead strips are all perpendicular to the grid surface (an unfocused grid) either side may be used as the tube side, but a sufficient target-to-grid distance (usually in excess of 48 inches) must be employed.

A focused grid must be carefully centered with respect to the x-ray tube. Otherwise more radiation will be absorbed on one side of the grid than on the other, and an uneven radiograph will result.

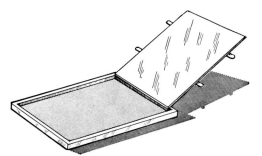

1. AVOID INJURY OR DROPPING.
2. AVOID CHEMICAL CONTACT WITH SCREENS.
3. HANDLE ON DRY BENCH.
4. AVOID STORAGE OF ITEMS ABOVE LOADING BENCH.

5. DO NOT LEAVE CASSETTE OPEN.
6. INSPECT FREQUENTLY TO DETECT WEARING OF FELT OR BENDING OF HINGES.
7. TEST SCREEN FILM CONTACT WITH FLAT WIRE MESH.

A

Cassette Front	Bakelite
Intensifying Screen	Cardboard Backing / Calcium Tungstate
X-ray Film	Silver Bromide Crystals / Cellulose Acetate Base / Silver Bromide Crystals
Intensifying Screen	Calcium Tungstate / Cardboard Backing
Backing	Felt Cushion Back
Cassette Back	Steel Back

SPRING STEEL

B

FIGURE 2–7 *A.* The cassette and its care. *B.* Diagrammatic cross section of x-ray cassette.

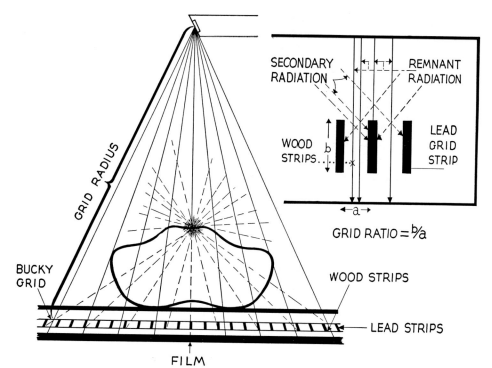

GRID RADIUS

SECONDARY RADIATION

REMNANT RADIATION

WOOD STRIPS

LEAD GRID STRIP

GRID RATIO = b/a

BUCKY GRID

WOOD STRIPS

LEAD STRIPS

FILM

FIGURE 2–8 Diagram of a Potter-Bucky diaphragm and how it is used.

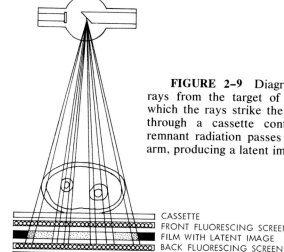

FIGURE 2–9 Diagram illustrating x-rays from the target of an x-ray tube in which the rays strike the forearm and pass through a cassette containing film. The remnant radiation passes through the forearm, producing a latent image upon the film.

CASSETTE
FRONT FLUORESCING SCREEN
FILM WITH LATENT IMAGE
BACK FLUORESCING SCREEN
CASSETTE

The grid method of eliminating the major portion of secondary radiation requires considerably more exposure; therefore, intensifying screens are usually employed along with the grid. These devices increase the distance of the part to be radiographed from the film and thereby increase the distortion of the image unless a long tube target-to-skin distance is employed with a small focal spot.

Cones and Aperture Diaphragms (Fig. 2–10). Cones and aperture diaphragms are applied to the tube window to delimit the x-ray beam and thus reduce the secondary radiation. There are various designs of these coning devices, but it is generally desirable to choose the cone best suited to the anatomical part and to the size of the film being exposed. Adjustable cones are also available for this purpose. In these devices a reflected visible light source contained within it will give the radiographer the cone's exact field of visualization. Cones have the additional advantage of reducing the stray radiation toward the operator, and thus they furnish a very important protective mechanism as well.

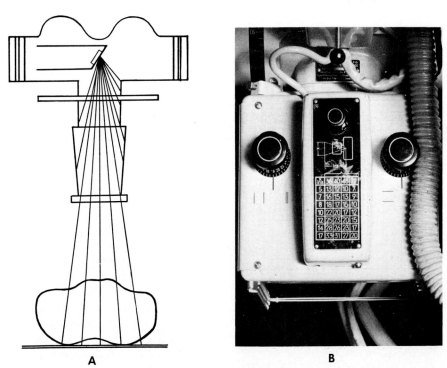

A   B

FIGURE 2–10 *A.* Diagram illustrating effect of cone in delimiting scattered radiation. *B.* Photograph of an adjustable collimator.

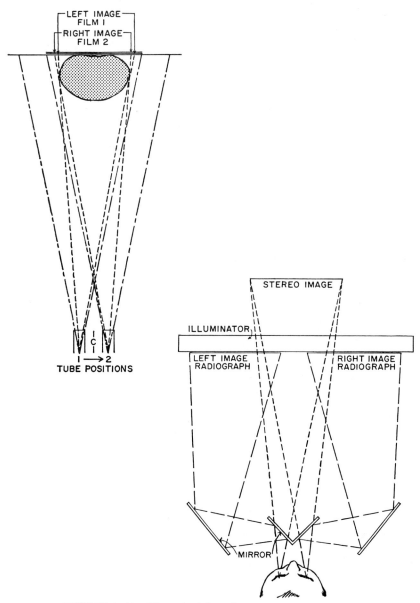

FIGURE 2–11 The principles of roentgen stereoscopy.

Stereoscopic Radiographic Accessories (Fig. 2–11). To obtain radiographs that can give a true stereoscopic effect, two slightly different views are obtained—first the view as seen by one eye, and second, that seen by the other eye. This is done by taking two radiographs from two separate tube positions; the amount of tube shift is based on a definite ratio of the normal interpupillary distance. These two radiographs are then placed in a stereoscope or viewed with special prismatic lenses or mirrors so that each eye will see the separate image. The brain fuses the two images into one and the correct spatial, three-dimensional relationship is reconstructed.

The Fluoroscopic Screen and the Fluoroscope; Electronic Amplification of the Fluoroscopic Image (Fig. 2–12). Fluoroscopy is the study of the x-ray image after its transformation into visible light. By this means the physician may study an anatomic part in motion. After passing through the patient, the remnant rays strike a special screen composed of fluorescent crystals that transform the x-rays.

Instead of the image appearing directly after it strikes the fluoroscopic screen, it is electronically amplified and directed toward an "output phosphor," which may then be viewed through appropriate lens and mirror systems, or by a television camera.

Television Camera. The image may thus be projected by closed circuit television systems to appropriately placed monitors.

Spot Film Radiography. This refers to instantaneous radiography while the patient is being examined by fluoroscopy. Spot film radiography is accomplished by storing a cassette in a lead-protected frame on the fluoroscopic screen, or on the frame support of the image tube. When radiography is desired, a rapid spring release brings the cassette over the patient, and the x-ray technique selector switch rapidly and automatically switches from fluoroscopic exposure values to radiographic factors, and the exposure is made. Often photoelectric ion chambers (or cells) are interposed, so that the exposure is automatically timed to produce an optimum radiographic image.

Radiography with the Image Amplifier. When the image amplifier is used, a movie camera or any other suitable still camera may be focused on the output phosphor of the image tube, and the image may be totally or in part transmitted to the camera, even while it is being viewed by the television camera system. It is also possible to photograph the television monitor (called *kineradiography*).

Rapid Sequence Film Changers for Roll Film or Cut Film, or Rapid Sequence Cassette Changers. Rapid sequence film changers allow x-ray films to be interposed between two intensifying screens in rapid sequence, and rapid sequence cassette changers allow cassettes to be changed rapidly and mechanically. Films may be changed as rapidly as 12 per second, and cassettes as fast as two per second, simultaneously in each of two planes if desired. Programmers are provided with changers so that appropriate sequences may be chosen. Long films (as long as three 14- by 17-inch films in tandem) may thus be exposed in one

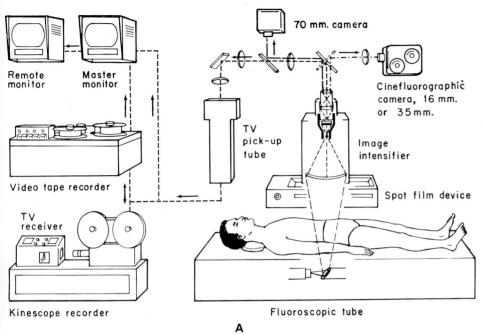

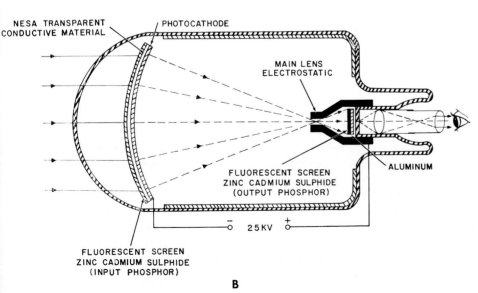

FIGURE 2–12 *A*. Diagram of currently available fluoroscopic equipment, containing image amplification, cinefluoroscopy, cineradiography, and kineradiography. The amplified image from the output phosphor may be conducted through a lens and mirror system directly to the human eye, directly to a stationary or movie camera device, through a television camera to a television receiver, or through a television camera to a television tape recorder. The image on the television screen may be viewed by the human eye or by an additional camera. *B*. Diagram of image intensifier tube. X-rays which pass through an object form an image on the input phosphor screen emitting visible light proportional to the impinging radiation. The photocathode in contact with this screen is an alkali metal layer that emits electrons proportional to the brightness of the fluorescing screen. This electron image is focused by electrostatic lenses on the output phosphor screen. The electrons are also accelerated by a potential difference of 25,000 volts, and a further increase in brightness results. The proper optical system permits the eye to view the brilliant image. To obtain cineradiography or television fluoroscopy one needs only to substitute a movie or television camera for the eye, or a mirror system, to obtain simultaneous viewing and filming.

apparatus, and may include, for example, the lower aorta and an entire lower extremity simultaneously and in rapid sequence.

Magnification (Fig. 2–13). Magnification of an anatomic part results when the film is placed at a considerable distance from the part. The degree of magnification is directly related to the square of the distance between the film and the focal spot of the x-ray tube, as compared with the distance between the anatomic part and the x-ray tube. When the film-to-focal spot distance is equal to the film-to-anatomic part distance, a magnification of 4 times will result. The limiting factor in this procedure is the size of the focal spot of the x-ray tube, which must be virtually pinpoint in size for optimum detail with magnification. Special high-speed fractional focal spot tubes have been manufactured for this purpose, with effective focal spots approaching 0.1 mm. Heat dissipation must be very efficient for x-ray tubes of this design. Magnification of small anatomic parts with films in rapid sequence is becoming available.

Magnification of the x-ray film itself is limited by the grain size of the x-ray film emulsion; usually 6 to 8 times is the maximum magnification possible.

Contrast Media. A body part may be visualized radiographically in the following ways:

> 1. By its delineation by a naturally occurring fatty envelope or fascia.
> 2. By its naturally occurring gaseous content, such as lungs and gastrointestinal tract.
> 3. By its naturally occurring mineral salts, such as the calcium salts of bone.
> 4. By abnormally occurring gas, fat, or calcium salts in certain pathologic processes.
> 5. By the introduction of a contrast agent, which may be either *radiolucent* or *radiopaque,* into or around the body part. Such contrast agents should be physiologically inert and harmless. The addition of contrast agents has permitted great strides in anatomic depiction.

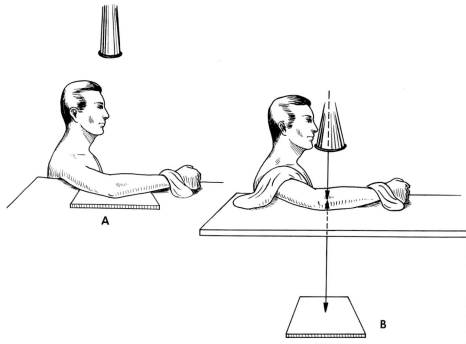

FIGURE 2–13 *A.* When the film is in close contact with the part being radiographed, and the x-ray tube target is 36 to 40 inches from the film, very little magnification of the part ensues. *B.* When the film is at a considerable distance from the part being radiographed, and the target-to-film distance is 24 to 30 inches, considerable magnification results. To avoid blurring of the image, the effective focal spot size must be 0.6 mm. or less.

COMMONLY USED RADIOPAQUE CONTRAST MEDIA. *Barium sulfate* is particularly useful in studies of the gastrointestinal tract. It is inert, is not absorbed, and does not alter the normal physiologic function. It is used in colloidal suspension and in high density, weight/volume to obtain a particular type of mucosa coating, which is most effective for demonstration of small filling defects.

Organic iodides, which are *predominantly excreted by the liver or secreted selectively by the kidneys,* include Hypaque (sodium diatrizoate), Renografin (meglumine diatrizoate), and iothalamates, such as Conray or Angioconray. These compounds are also widely favored for visualization of blood vessels. In low concentrations they may be used for visualization of hepatic and biliary radicles by T-tube and operative cholangiography.

Organic iodides in suspension may be particularly useful in visualization of oviducts (hysterosalpingography) or the urethra (Salpix, Skiodan Acacia, Cystokon, and Thixokon).

Iodized oils, slowly absorbable, are used in myelography (Pantopaque) or bronchography (Dionosil oily).

Radiolucent contrast substances are *gases:* air, oxygen, helium, carbon dioxide, nitrous oxide, and nitrogen. These are commonly used for visualization of the brain (pneumoencephalograms and ventriculograms), joints (arthrograms), and occasionally, the subarachnoid space surrounding the spinal cord (air myelograms). Air may also be used in the pleural space, peritoneal cavity, and pericardial space. Carbon dioxide is of particular value since it is well tolerated and very rapidly absorbed.

OTHER ANCILLARY ITEMS OF X-RAY EQUIPMENT

Shutter Mechanism Over X-ray Tube. Immediately in front of the x-ray tube under the table is a lead shutter mechanism which may be opened and closed in both the vertical and horizontal directions. The shutter is controlled either electrically or by cables connected to knobs on the fluoroscopic screen. The lead is sufficiently thick to prevent any primary radiation from escaping in a forward direction and is so constructed that secondary emanations are also largely absorbed. Thus, the field of vision of the fluoroscopic screen is delimited by these controls beside the screen. This field should always be no larger than is absolutely necessary for visualization of the part in question, and the margins of the shutter itself should always be visible on the screen. The smaller the field, the better the detail—an added inducement for maintaining this standard.

Filtration. Additional filters should always be added in front of the fluoroscopic tube to the extent of 4 mm. of aluminum or more. Only the more highly penetrating rays are effective in radiography and fluoroscopy, and the addition of such filters removes a higher percentage of the less penetrating rays than of the more penetrating. Moreover, the patient's skin has a higher tolerance for the more penetrating rays (this will be more fully described in Chapter 3).

Physical Factors. Ordinarily, 2 milliamperes of current or less are adequate for fluoroscopy. It is common practice to use 85 kilovolts peak for abdominal fluoroscopy, 70 kilovolts for chest, and 60 kilovolts for the extremities. In examining children with the fluoroscope, 0.5 milliamperes and 60 kilovolts need never be exceeded. A small field is imperative for protection of the gonads since a much greater proportion of the entire body of a child is covered by radiation when any single part is radiographed.

Use of X-ray Protective Devices. X-ray protective devices such as lead-lined gloves, lead rubber, or lead glass fiber aprons, and small lead rubber shields dangling beneath the fluoroscopic screen are imperative (see Chapter 3). The operator should never permit his unprotected hands, wrists, or other parts to be exposed to the x-ray beam. Palpation with the hand or other manipulation under the fluoroscope, setting fractures, localizing foreign bodies, or other procedures should be avoided. Intermittent and serial radiography is much to be preferred to such dangerous exposure.

Roentgen Xeroradiography. In xeroradiography, an x-ray image is produced using a photoconductive surface of selenium on an aluminum plate as a substitute for x-ray film. The plate is contained in a cassette to protect it from casual damage or ambient light (Fig. 2–14). With the cassette open, an electrostatic charge is first placed on the surface of the selenium in darkness. The plate is then exposed to an x-ray beam in conventional fashion. The selenium photoconductor is discharged thereby in amounts corresponding to the remnant radiation passing through the patient's anatomic part. The remnant radiation produces an electrostatic charge pattern depicting the anatomic part being examined. To make this pattern visible the plate is then developed in a closed chamber into which a blue, finely divided charged plastic powder, called "toner," is sprayed. A powder image on the plate surface is produced in this way (Fig. 2–14 B).

A permanent record of the image may be obtained by transferring the image from the plate to paper or plastic. This may be done by bringing the paper into contact with the toner image and applying pressure, or by charging the back of the paper during the moment of contact. The transferred powder image is then fixed, typically by heating or momentarily softening the plastic layer encapsulating the toner. The residual toner is then removed by brushing the plate appropriately. Actually, the original selenium plate may be reused by heating the photoconductor to about 135 degrees for 30 seconds.

The xeroradiographic image resembles a film image except that (1) there is a greater resolution, (2) small point densities appear to be easier to recognize by virtue of their high contrast, and (3) there is good detail on the image.

This process is gaining application in radiography of the extremities (orthopedic radiology) and in soft tissue roentgenography such as mammography, where it has shown excellent results (Fig. 2–14 C) (Wolfe).

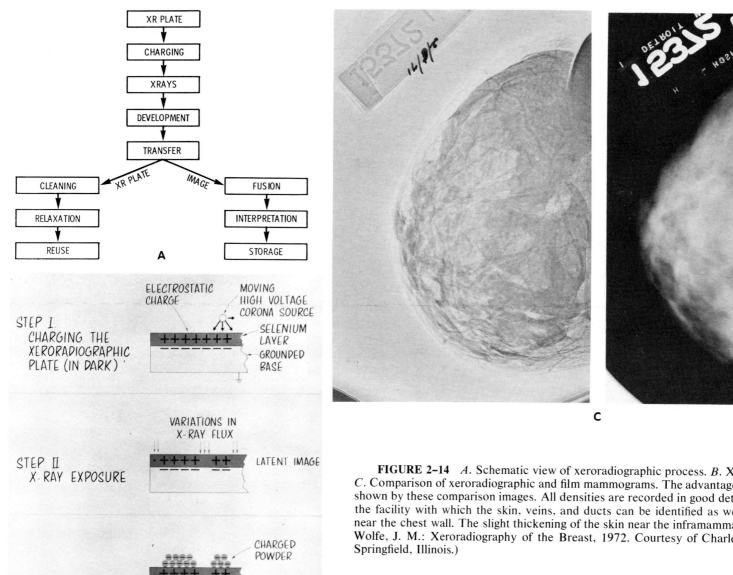

A

XR PLATE → CHARGING → XRAYS → DEVELOPMENT → TRANSFER

XR PLATE → CLEANING → RELAXATION → REUSE

IMAGE → FUSION → INTERPRETATION → STORAGE

B

STEP I. CHARGING THE XERORADIOGRAPHIC PLATE (IN DARK)

ELECTROSTATIC CHARGE
MOVING HIGH VOLTAGE CORONA SOURCE
SELENIUM LAYER
GROUNDED BASE
+++++++

STEP II X-RAY EXPOSURE

VARIATIONS IN X-RAY FLUX
LATENT IMAGE
++++ ++

STEP III DEVELOPMENT

CHARGED POWDER
++++ ++

C

FIGURE 2–14 *A*. Schematic view of xeroradiographic process. *B*. Xeroradiographic process. *C*. Comparison of xeroradiographic and film mammograms. The advantages of xeroradiography are shown by these comparison images. All densities are recorded in good detail on the XR (*left*). Note the facility with which the skin, veins, and ducts can be identified as well as the deep structures near the chest wall. The slight thickening of the skin near the inframammary fold is normal. (From Wolfe, J. M.: Xeroradiography of the Breast, 1972. Courtesy of Charles C Thomas, Publisher, Springfield, Illinois.)

Subtraction Techniques. The principle of subtraction technique has been carefully elucidated by DesPlantes. He demonstrated that in radiographs obtained prior to and after the introduction of a contrast agent, the appearance of the contrast agent can be intensified more clearly by removing interfering bony shadows in the following manner (Fig. 2–15). A negative transparent "diapositive" is obtained from the control radiograph, and this negative is superimposed on the radiograph containing the contrast agent. Since in a negative diapositive the bony structures appear black, this blackness will ordinarily neutralize the bony structures as visualized on the second film when light is transmitted through the two films superimposed over one another. In a third film obtained from the first two, this neutralization process results in virtual obliteration of the bony shadows and a clear demonstration of the contrast agent.

A further modification of this technique has been suggested by Oldendorf. In this modification, a second order diapositive is introduced to subtract more of the detail not subtracted by the first. The initial contrast agent–free control film is contact-printed onto a Dupont commercial S film or Eastman commercial film. These two diapositives combined are then superimposed over the succeeding films in an angiographic series to obtain the final subtracted film.

In each instance the control film prior to the introduction of the contrast agent must be obtained in exactly the same position as the later films with the contrast agent in order to get ideal subtraction.

Television subtraction that accomplishes a subtracted image instantaneously is also available.

Rapid Automatic Film Processing. After a latent image is deposited on the film by the x-rays, the cassette or film holder is taken to the darkroom where the film is carefully removed under light conditions that do not allow fogging of the film. The film is loaded directly into automated apparatus (Fig. 2–16 A) and a completely dried and processed film is available for viewing at the end of 90 seconds. During this process the film is transported through developing, fixing, washing, and drying operations. Exposure factors must be optimum and control conditions ideal to produce a good radiograph with such automatic film processors.

Wet film processing may still be employed and requires that the film be allowed to remain in a developing solution for a definite period of time, depending upon the temperature and degree of exhaustion of the developer. The film is then removed from the developer and inserted into a stop bath, where it is quickly rinsed and transferred to a fixing solution for approximately 10 minutes. It is allowed to fix in hypo solution for at least twice the developing time and then transferred to the "wash" for at least one-half hour, after which it is dried. The rapid processing of film is, however, almost universal now, except with industrial and some thick emulsion films.

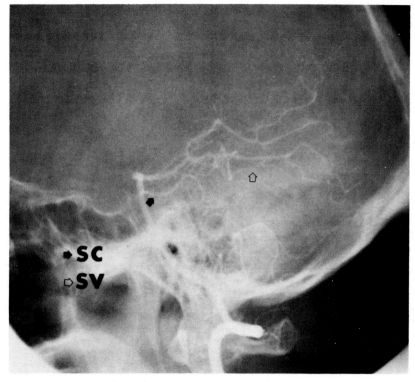

A

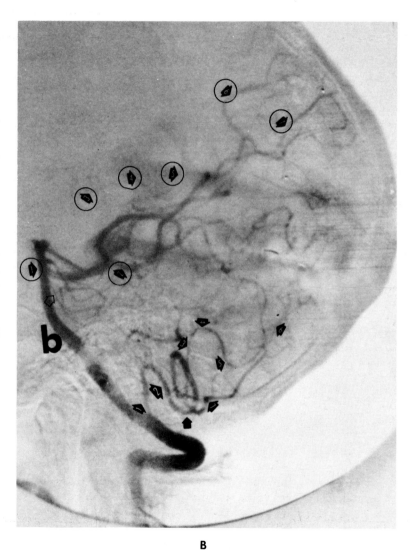

B

FIGURE 2–15 *A*. Lateral vertebral arteriogram: (*SC*) superior cerebellar, (*SV*) superior vermian. The detail is considerably enhanced by the "subtraction technique," as shown in *B*. *B*, Subtraction study of *A*. Open arrow, posterior inferior cerebellar; circled arrows: (1) posterior cerebral, (2) temporal occipital, (3) medial branch of posterior choroidal, (4) lateral branch of posterior choroidal, (5) dorsal callosal, (6) occipital branch, (7) calcarine artery; plain arrows: (1) anterior medullary segment of posterior inferior cerebellar artery (PICA); (2) lateral medullary segment of PICA, (3) posterior medullary segment of PICA, (4) choroidal point, (5) retrotonsillar segment, (6) inferior vermian branch, (7) tonsillohemispheric branch; black arrow, caudal loop; b, basilar artery.

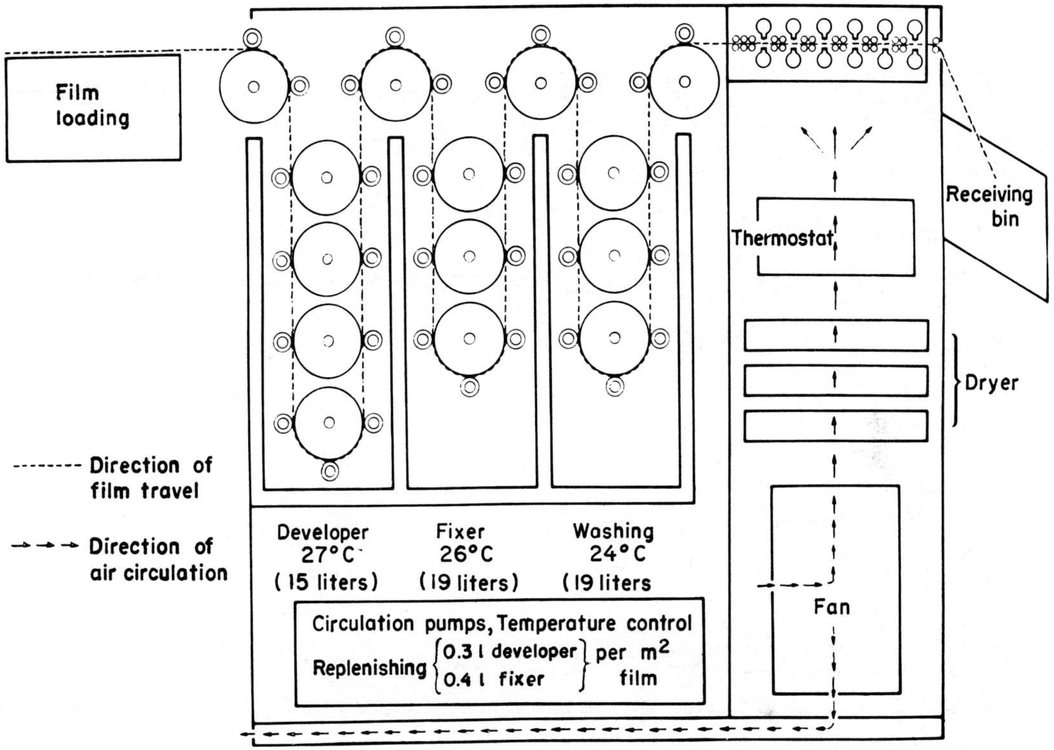

FIGURE 2–16 Diagram of an automatic film processor. (From Schinz, H. R., et al. (eds.): Roentgen Diagnosis. Vol. 1, General Principles and Methods, 2nd Ed. New York, Grune & Stratton, Inc., 1968. Reprinted by permission.)

THE FUNDAMENTAL GEOMETRY OF X-RAY IMAGE FORMATION AND INTERPRETATION

Image Sharpness. X-rays obey most common laws of light. The manner in which any object placed in the path of the x-ray beam is projected depends on: (1) the size of the light source (focal spot), i.e., whether pinpoint or a larger surface, (2) the alignment of the object with respect to the light source (focal spot) and the screen or film, (3) the distance of the object from the light source, (4) the distance of the object from the screen or film, and (5) the plane of the object with respect to the screen or film.

When the image is projected from a pinpoint light source, the borders of the image are sharp, but if the light source is a larger surface, as in the case of the focal spot of an x-ray tube, the image is ill-defined at its periphery owing to penumbra formation (Fig. 2–17). Measures must be taken to reduce the penumbra as much as possible. To accomplish this the focal spot must be as small as possible, and the object-to-film distance as short as possible. The object-to-focal spot distance should be as long as possible (Fig. 2–18). Also, the film should be perpendicular to the central ray arising from the focal spot.

Image Distortion. When the object is not centrally placed with respect to the central ray its image will be distorted, and this distortion may be considerable (Fig. 2–19). Sometimes this distortion is unavoidable if one is to visualize a part, and in some of the radiographic positions, this distortion brings a part into view which otherwise would be

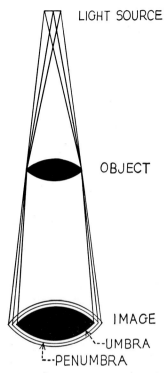

FIGURE 2–17   Diagram of penumbra formation from surface light source.

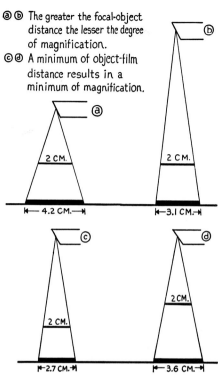

FIGURE 2–18   Diagram illustrating effect of focal-object distance and object-film distance on magnification.

hidden (Fig. 2–20). Thus, the phenomenon of projection may be utilized to good advantage.

Image Magnification.   The farther an object is from the light source and the closer it is to the film, the less will be the magnification (Fig. 2–18). The magnification of an object as much as 15 cm. from the film when a relatively usual focal spot-film distance is employed (such as 36 inches) is approximately 20 per cent. Such magnification must be considered in interpreting the size of the heart, the pelvis or any other structure which is to be measured.

These various phenomena of magnification, projection, distortion, and penumbra formation must be constantly borne in mind in viewing radiographic images.

STEPS IN THE PRODUCTION OF A RADIOGRAPH

There are many steps in the production and final interpretation of a radiograph, and it is well to have some concept of all of them. Given the problem of the radiography of an anatomic part, the following steps are pursued:

1. The patient is placed in a position with respect to the central ray of the x-ray tube in full accordance with our knowledge of the gross anatomy.

2. The most suitable method of eliminating secondary radia-

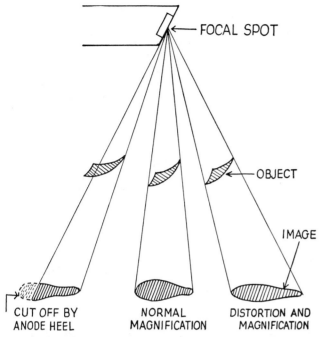

FIGURE 2–19 Diagram illustrating effect of position of object with respect to central ray on distortion, magnification, and anode-heel effect.

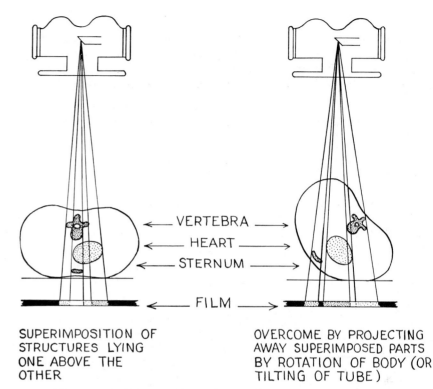

FIGURE 2–20 Diagram illustrating utilization of projection to overcome superimposition of anatomic parts.

tion is chosen, whether it be a diaphragm, cone, grid, or all three. In some types of movable grids, a grid movement time must be chosen depending upon the exposure time, and the moving mechanism must be cocked.

3. The proper type of film and the film holder or cassette are placed in position with respect to the central ray, either directly under the anatomic part, or under the grid in a special carriage.

4. Optimum exposure factors are chosen: (a) milliamperage; (b) kilovoltage; (c) time; (d) distance; and (e) focal spot after the anatomic part has been measured as to its relative size.

5. A latent image is obtained on the film by the x-rays.

6. The cassette or film holder is taken to the darkroom where the film is carefully removed, and allowed to remain in the developing solution for a definite time depending upon the temperature and degree of exhaustion of the developer.

7. The film is removed from the developer and inserted into a stop bath or it is quickly rinsed and transferred to a fixing solution.

8. The film is then allowed to fix in hypo solution and then transferred to the "wash."

9. The film is then dried.

10. The finished radiograph is then attached to the original film consultation request, and other pertinent records of the patient in the office, and the entire folder on the patient is brought to the radiologist (physician) for interpretation in the light of all information on the patient.

FILM IDENTIFICATION

Various methods of film identification include: (1) lead markers; (2) photographic transfer in the darkroom from a card to a previously unexposed corner of the film; or (3) the insertion of a special data card into the cassette in the lighted room just prior to radiographic exposure.

The following data are essential: (1) name and address of the radiologist or institution; (2) name and identification number of the patient; (3) the date of the examination; (4) the side of the body being examined, or a clear label of one side; (5) stereoradiography, if employed; (6) time intervals between films, if films are obtained in sequence; (7) distances of laminographic cuts, if body-section studies are done.

GENERAL TERMS AND CONCEPTS IN DIAGNOSTIC RADIOLOGY

1. *Increased subject density* denotes a lighter or whiter shadow on the x-ray film or a darker shadow on the fluoroscopic screen, as produced by substances of greater density or thickness.

2. *Decreased subject density* denotes a darker or blacker shadow on the x-ray film or a lighter one on the fluoroscopic screen. It is produced by substances of low density or slight thickness.

3. *Increased radiolucency (hyperlucency)* implies greater penetrability by the x-rays and has the same connotation as decreased density.

4. *Increased radiopacity* implies diminished penetrability by the x-rays and has the same connotation as increased density.

5. *Anteroposterior projection* (Fig. 2–21) indicates that the x-ray

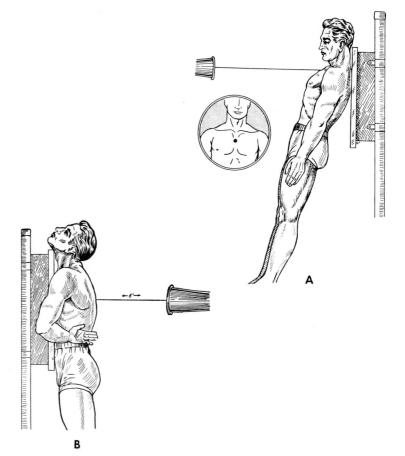

FIGURE 2–21 *A.* Anteroposterior (apical lordotic) projection of the chest. *B.* Posteroanterior projection of the chest.

beam strikes the anterior aspect of the patient first; *posteroanterior* indicates that the x-ray beam strikes the posterior aspect first.

6. In describing the *laterality* of the patient relative to the x-ray beam, the lateral or oblique projection is always named according to the *side of the patient closer to the film.* Thus, a *right lateral projection* (Fig. 2–22) is taken with the right side of the patient next to the film. A *left lateral* is the reverse.

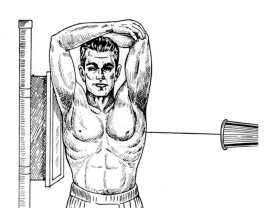

FIGURE 2–22   Right lateral projection of the chest.

7. The *oblique* projections are likewise named according to the side of the patient closer to the film. Thus, a *right posteroanterior oblique projection* is taken with the patient's right anterior aspect closer to the film. A *right anteroposterior oblique projection* is taken with the patient's posterior aspect near the film. When viewed by the radiologist, these films are often turned so that the patient "faces" the doctor, and

hence the "view" or "film" is seen by the doctor in a *view* opposite to the actual projection. In this text, the position of the patient is shown in the actual *projection* employed; often, the film is shown as the doctor conventionally *views* the film. These opposite relationships of *projection* and *view* must be borne in mind in the anatomic interpretations.

8. *Recumbency* indicates that the patient is lying down when the film is taken. He may either be *supine* (on his back) or *prone* (on his abdomen). The beam in these cases is vertical with respect to the patient.

9. The patient is in the *decubitus position* when he is lying down and the beam in these cases is always horizontal. Thus, right lateral decubitus means that the right side of the patient is down. Left lateral decubitus is the reverse. A more accurate terminology is desirable as follows: (1) *horizontal beam study, anteroposterior, with the patient on right (or left) side;* (2) *horizontal beam study, posteroanterior, with the patient on right (or left) side;* (3) *horizontal beam study, with patient supine (or prone) and right (or left) side nearest the film;* (4) *erect position*—with the patient or the anatomic part upright and the beam horizontal. An erect chest film may be obtained with the patient standing or sitting; (5) *semirecumbent, also called semi-erect*—this term implies that this vertical axis of the part being radiographed is at an angle of approximately 45 degrees to the horizontal.

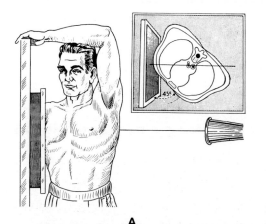

A

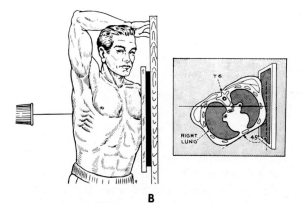

B

FIGURE 2–23   *A. Right posteroanterior oblique projection of the chest. B. Left posteroanterior oblique projection of the chest. The radiologist usually* views *the films so obtained as though he were facing the patient; hence, by common acceptance, the word "view" connotes the opposite of the word "projection."*

10. *Artefacts* (Fig. 2–24 *A, B*) are changes on the film which do not have an anatomic basis directly related to the part being radiographed but are introduced by some technical fault, such as dirt in the cassette or static electrical charge. Occasionally, artefacts are produced by items of clothing, immobilization devices, or even hair braids projected over the film.

11. *Comparison films* are taken of the opposite side for comparison with a suspected abnormal side. These are very useful, particularly in children, and should be taken whenever possible.

12. *Serial films* are films taken in sequence either during a single study or after longer intervals of time (days or weeks).

13. *Trendelenburg* refers to a recumbent position with the body plane tilted so that the head is lower than the feet. An angle of tilt is usually indicated.

14. *Sagittal* refers to that plane of the body which is in line with the sagittal suture of the skull (see Chapter 7, on the skull).

15. *Coronal* refers to that plane of the body which is in line with the coronal suture of the skull.

16. *Abduction* indicates a movement away from the sagittal plane of the body.

17. *Adduction* indicates a movement toward the sagittal plane of the body.

18. *Caudad* refers to the central ray pointing toward the feet (or an object distal in the body).

19. *Cephalad* refers to a central ray of the x-ray tube pointing toward the head, or an object pertaining to the head.

20. *Varus deformity* refers to one in which the vertex of the angle of the deformity points toward the sagittal plane.

21. *Valgus deformity* refers to one in which the vertex of the angle of the deformity points away from the sagittal plane.

22. *Eversion* indicates a turning outward of an anatomic part.

23. *Inversion* indicates a turning inward of an anatomic part.

24. *Distal* is away from the head or origin of an anatomic part.

25. *Proximal* is toward the head or origin of an anatomic part.

26. *Medial* pertains to the center of the body, or its sagittal plane.

27. *Cross-sectional plane* is one which is perpendicular to the longitudinal axis of the body. The *perpendicular* forms an angle of 90 degrees.

28. *Pronation* is medial rotation.

29. *Supination* is lateral rotation.

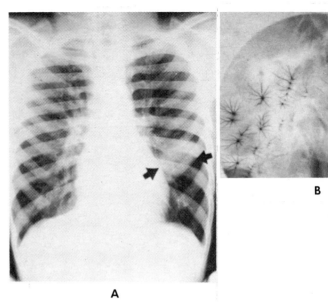

A

FIGURE 2–24 *A.* "Kissing" artefact caused by two films being in contact with each other during developing process. *B.* Static electricity artefacts.

30 *Computed Axial Tomography* (CAT, or CT). Computer-assisted tomography with special equipment designed for this purpose, in which the plane of tomography with respect to the transverse or cross-sectional plane is specified at a particular angle with respect to a specified reference line in the body part being so examined. (See Chapter 16.)

GENERAL RULES IN RADIOGRAPHY

Usually, two views of an anatomic part are taken at 90 degrees to one another.

With joints, however, an oblique view is usually added.

Projection refers to the path of the x-ray beam, describing its point of entrance and exit in sequence. Posteroanterior (PA) projection means that the beam has traveled from the posterior side of the patient through to the anterior.

Position refers to the specific body position employed (e.g., supine, prone).

View describes the body part as seen on the x-ray film. The "view" is opposite to the "projection." The radiologist usually *views* a film as though he were looking at the patient. In the case of the chest, for example, the projection is posteroanterior even though the radiologist is viewing the film as an anteroposterior view.

3

PROTECTIVE MEASURES IN X-RAY DIAGNOSIS

DEFINITION OF PHYSICAL TERMS

Quality of Ionizing Radiation. The quality of ionizing radiation depends in great part on the *kilovoltage* applied and the so-called *"filters"* inserted in the beam.

X-rays produced by low voltage cathode ray tubes are ordinarily referred to as *"soft"* and do not penetrate the body part for great distances. X-rays produced by high voltage (*"hard"*) cathode rays penetrate more deeply.

The term "filters" with respect to radiation refers to a layer of absorbing medium, usually a metal such as aluminum, copper, tin, or lead. This absorbing medium *diminishes* the soft rays relative to the hard ones, but, unlike chemical filters, does not eliminate all soft rays.

Generally, radiation produced by kilovoltages below 60 is considered soft, whereas 120 to 150 kilovolts are moderately penetrating. Hard radiation derived from kilovoltages higher than 150 Kv, is seldom used in conventional diagnostic radiology.

In diagnostic radiology, at least 2 to 4 mm. of aluminum are ordinarily added as filtration at the open diaphragm of the tube to produce an optimum quality of radiation.

Quantification of Ionizing Radiation. Ionizing radiations are radiations such as alpha, beta, gamma, neutron rays (or particles) and x-rays which produce biological effects because they ionize, or separate, electrons from their parent atoms in compounds in the body. The *roentgen* (Fig. 3–1) is the internationally accepted unit for quantity of ionizing radiation. It is illustrated in Figure 3–1 and defined as *"The quantity of x— or gamma radiation such that the associated corpuscular emission per 0.001293 gram of air produces in air, ions carrying one electrostatic unit of electric charge of either sign."* The *rad* and the *rem* are similarly illustrated in Figure 3–2. (Newer definitions, but exactly equivalent to these, may evolve as the result of committee actions.)

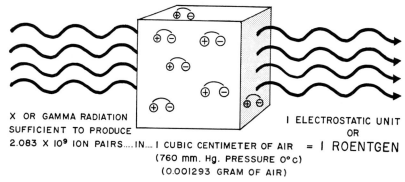

X OR GAMMA RADIATION SUFFICIENT TO PRODUCE 2.083 X 10^9 ION PAIRS....IN.... I CUBIC CENTIMETER OF AIR (760 mm. Hg. PRESSURE 0°C) (0.001293 GRAM OF AIR) = I ELECTROSTATIC UNIT OR I ROENTGEN

FIGURE 3–1 Definition of the roentgen in diagrammatic form.

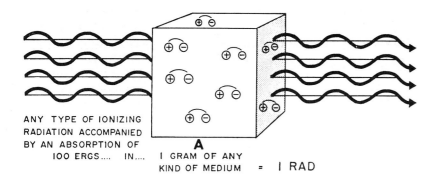

ANY TYPE OF IONIZING
RADIATION ACCOMPANIED
BY AN ABSORPTION OF
100 ERGS.... IN....   I GRAM OF ANY
KIND OF MEDIUM = I RAD

A

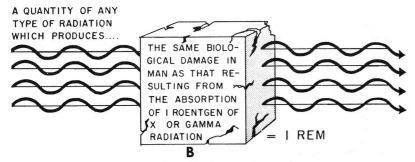

A QUANTITY OF ANY
TYPE OF RADIATION
WHICH PRODUCES....

THE SAME BIOLO-
GICAL DAMAGE IN
MAN AS THAT RE-
SULTING FROM
THE ABSORPTION
OF I ROENTGEN OF
X OR GAMMA
RADIATION = I REM

B

FIGURE 3–2 *A*. Diagram of the rad. *B*. Diagram of the rem.

TABLE 3–1. Radiation Dose from Roentgenography and Fluoroscopy*

Examination Site	kvp.	mas.	Focus Film Distance (in.)	Added Filtration (mm. Al)	Skin Dose (mrad)	Gonadal Dose (mrad) MALE	FEMALE
Skull (5 views)	74–90	20	36	3.0	635.6	2.32	.72
Paranasal sinuses (3 views)	66–86	20	36	3.0	327.2	<0.03	<0.03
Hand and wrist (3 views)	54	5	40	2.5	–	<0.01	<0.01
Chest, PA	100	5	72	2.5	9.21	0.02	0.04
Chest, lat.	110	15	72	2.5	37	0.03	0.08
Chest, obl.	100	10	72	2.5	17	0.02	0.04
Thoracic spine, AP	100	30	40	2.5	249	0.19	0.26
Thoracic spine, lat.	110	60	40	2.5	707	0.17	0.54
Lumbar spine, AP	100	30	40	2.5	221	14.7	70.4
Lumbar spine, lat.	120	60	40	2.5	820	9.77	61.5
Lumbar spine, obl.	120	40	40	2.5	290 (×2)	20 (×2)	94 (×2)
Lumbosacral spine, lat.	120	70	40	2.5	1100	55	82
Pelvis, AP	100	30	40	2.5	219	83.0	79.0
Abdomen, AP	100	20	40	2.5	159	11.6	51.1
Upper GI series							
Fluoroscopy	90	–	–	3.0	328/min.	.348/min.	12.8/min.
Spot film	90	PHT	–	3.0	101/film	.07/film	2.68/film
4 routine films	100–120	20–40	40	2.5	1237	25.99	138.5
Barium enema							
Fluoroscopy	90	–	–	3.0	480/min.	11/min.	140/min.
Spot film	90	PHT	–	3.0	110/film	3.20/film	28.0/film
Gallbladder series							
Fluoroscopy	90	–	–	3.0	400/min.	0.1/min.	0.6/min.
3 views	90–120	20–30	36–40	2.5–3.0	684	17.39	82.59
Spot film	90	PHT	–	3.0	173/film	1.0/film	7.1/film
IVP, AP abdomen	120	30	40	2.5	675/film	60.2/film	132/film
IVP, bladder, AP	120	30	40	2.5	659/film	181/film	105/film
IVP, Tomo, Kidneys	120	20	40	2.5	450/film	12/film	80/film
Arm, AP and lat.	70	5	40	2.5	–	<0.01	<0.01
Thigh, AP and lat.	100	20	40	2.5	328	124.7	73.9
Fluoroscopy, chest	90	–	–	3.0	150/min.	.03/min.	0.38/min.
Myelogram							
Fluoroscopy	90	–	–	3.0	360/min.	3.0/min.	45/min.
Spot films	90	PHT	–	3.0	820/film	16/film	94/film

*Extracted from: Antoku Shigetoshi, and Walter J. Russell: Dose to the active bone marrow, gonads, and skin from roentgenography and fluoroscopy. Radiology, *101*:669–678, 1971.

PROTECTIVE MEASURES IN X-RAY DIAGNOSIS

For the Patient

In x-ray diagnosis, exposure of the patient may be considered from the standpoint of protection against the acute effects and the chronic effects of overexposure, each being dealt with in relation to fluoroscopy on the one hand and radiography on the other. The acute effects are epilation and erythema; the chronic effects may be reflected in the blood-forming organs, may cause induction of malignant tumors or cataracts, impaired fertility, reduction of the life span, and genetic changes.

The methods of diminishing x-ray exposure of the patient may be outlined as follows.

Maximum Filtration of the Primary Beam. The inherent filtration of the tube structure is ordinarily equivalent to 0.5 mm. of aluminum. The addition of 2.0 to 4.0 mm. of aluminum is highly desirable. In the usually employed voltage range (40 kvp to 120 kvp), 1 mm. of aluminum will reduce the dose to the skin about 60 per cent; 2 mm. of aluminum about 80 per cent at 50 kvp and 60 per cent at 130 kvp; and 3 mm. of aluminum about 80 to 85 per cent.

It is also interesting that added filtration of this order has very little effect on the resulting roentgenograms. The effective radiation is that which is transmitted through the part being radiographed and hence is the more penetrating, hard type. The addition of a filter increases the transmission by a large factor, at the same time reducing the percentage of soft radiations. The quality of the resulting radiograph is not materially altered by the additional filtration, and the necessary increase in the exposure time is relatively small.

It is concluded that it is advisable to use 2 mm. of aluminum filter for voltages of 50 to 70 kvp and 4 mm. of aluminum for voltages above 70 kvp. If voltages above 100 kvp are employed, use 0.25 mm. of copper added filtration.

Higher Voltages. Whenever possible without significantly altering the quality of the radiograph, higher voltages should be used. This expedient also increases the penetration of the beam, thereby relatively diminishing the total quanta of rays which must strike the skin of the patient to produce a satisfactory radiograph.

This, of course, is of particular importance in pregnancy examinations.

Increased Target-to-skin Distance. As far as this is practicable, on the basis of the inverse square law, it increases the intensity of the remnant radiation (producing the radiographic or fluoroscopic image) for a given entry dose. In fluoroscopy a minimum target-to-skin distance of 18 inches should be used. In radiography, a minimum target-to-film distance of 40 inches is recommended.

Small Field of Radiation. The use of as small a field of radiation as is necessary to achieve the desired diagnostic result may be achieved with cones or an adjustable diaphragm.

Diminished Fluoroscopic Exposure. Using an 18-inch target-to-table-top distance, 80 kvp, and 2 ma., with 3 mm. of aluminum filtration added, fluoroscopy adds 2 to 4 roentgens per minute to the skin of the irradiated area. Five minutes of fluoroscopy to one area must be considered maximum.

Calculation of Dosage to Patients in Diagnostic Examinations. Various tables and nomograms have been provided which permit ready calculation of dose delivered. Table 3–1 is representative.

Needless to say, these are representative values and will vary with the technique employed. It is advised that each radiologist become familiar with the dosages obtained by his techniques.

Although maximum tolerance doses for workers with radiation are established at 0.1 rem per week (3 rems not be exceeded in 13 weeks), the maximum permissible dose to patients is not established.

We do not actually know the limitation to impose on diagnostic procedures except to avoid untoward reaction or visible reactions of any kind. Radiation hazards to the embryo and fetus are particularly important to bear in mind. The developing embryos of a great variety of animals, including several mammals, are highly susceptible to the induction of malformations by radiation. These occur in a well-defined critical period for each genus. There is no reason to doubt that this also applies to human embryos. In man this would correspond to the second to the sixth week of gestation for the majority of characters, when doses of less than 10 roentgens may be detrimental. Beyond this period, the effects are less obvious or possibly delayed with such doses. *Certainly, if pregnancy is known, radiation should at all costs be avoided in the first trimester and as much as possible thereafter.*

For the Physician and Technician

Protection Against Radiation Hazard. Most local injuries sustained by the physician or technician are of the hands. Such injuries can be avoided by certain protective measures:

1. Personnel working near an x-ray machine (who are not behind a proper screen) should at all times wear protective lead gloves of at least 0.5 mm. lead equivalent, as well as a lead-lined apron or its equivalent. Roentgenoscopic screens with lead-rubber drapes also diminish radiation exposure.

2. The physician's or technician's unprotected hands, wrists, arms or other parts should never be exposed to the x-ray beam.

3. Suitable kilovoltage and milliamperage settings at fluoroscopy should be adopted, as follows:

Abdomen	95–110 Kvp.	2 Ma or less
Chest	70 Kvp.	2 Ma. or less
Thick extremities	60 Kvp.	2 Ma. or less
Thin extremities	50 Kvp.	1/2–1 Ma.
Children	50–60 Kvp.	1/2–1 Ma.

4. The following general principles of fluoroscope use should be adhered to:

(a) Shutters must be closed down to no more than 30 to 40 square centimeters.

(b) The fluoroscope should be used intermittently, and should be avoided when the patient is not intercepting the beam.

(c) The examination should be concluded as quickly as possible, usually within five minutes. It is well to have a special timing device in the circuit to turn off the machine automatically when this time is exceeded.

(d) When fractures are being set or foreign bodies located, alternating radiography with intermittent manipulation should be used, if possible, rather than fluoroscopy.

Metabolic changes are perhaps incurred by physicians even though sufficient protection is worn. There is a high incidence of leukemia in radiologists, and even among nonradiologists; it is possible that when certain susceptible individuals receive even the minimal exposure allowed for in the foregoing methods, they ultimately develop leukemia.

TABLE 3–2. Methods to Insure Adequate Protection

For Patient	*For Physician*
1. Avoid examination in the first trimester of pregnancy.	1. Wear lead impregnated gloves and apron.
2. Work with a minimum of 2 to 4 mm. of aluminum filter over aperture of tube.	2. Never expose unprotected areas to x-ray beam.
3. Use as high a kilovoltage as possible.	3. Always use repeated x-ray film examination rather than fluoroscopic unit in the setting of fractures.
4. Increase target-skin distance as much as possible.	
5. Use narrow shutter for fluoroscopy screen and use unit intermittently with limitation of time.	4. Avoid head fluoroscopy.

PROTECTION AGAINST ELECTRICAL HAZARDS

A potential electrical hazard may exist within any radiology department due to any of the following factors: the high energy side of the x-ray equipment, the presence of explosive anesthetic gases, and hazards caused by sources of low voltages and low currents which may induce ventricular fibrillation in the patient.

1. All exposed cables should be protected against mechanical damage and these should be periodically inspected for defects or abrasions to prevent high energy electrical shock.

2. Explosive anesthetic gases should not be used in the presence of x-ray equipment, if possible. If these are absolutely essential, however, it is well to employ only explosion-proof procedures and apparatus. No switch devices should be permitted below 5 feet from the floor and all switches should be explosion-proof.

All exposed noncurrent-carrying parts of the apparatus should be permanently grounded in acceptable fashion with excellent ground leads.

3. Low voltage and low currents, with their potential of inducing ventricular fibrillation, have become a more frequent hazard in radiology. It has been demonstrated that currents as low as 20 microamperes with voltages as low as 60 millivolts can induce ventricular fibrillation in dogs.

When electrodes are applied directly to the human heart, currents as low as 180 microamperes with voltages as low as 100 millivolts will produce ventricular fibrillation.

An intracardiac catheter filled with blood or a conducting solution offers an excellent current path directly to the heart, making ventricular fibrillation feasible. A similar hazard exists when there are electrodes from an electrocardiographic monitor in contact with the patient. Grids, when they are dampened, are likewise potentially hazardous. Power injectors connected to catheters are particularly hazardous if they do not have a good separate grounding system, or if they are incorrectly plugged into the wall socket and inadequately grounded.

In general, the majority of problems associated with electric shock hazards of this type can be solved by providing adequate grounding systems in the angiographic room and connecting them to each item of apparatus that has contact with either the x-ray machine or the patient.

First aid practices such as artificial respiration and emergency treatment for burns should be thoroughly familiar to personnel in case they are needed.

Although the dangers of electric shock are not as extreme in the darkroom, they do exist. Lighting fixtures are the greatest potential hazard in this regard and they must be carefully installed with every attention to proper insulation and grounding.

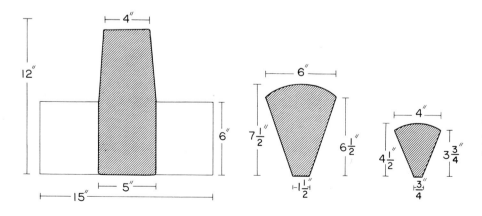

Male   Female   Infant

FIGURE 3–3 Design of lead gonad shields used in radiography. These should be ⅛ inch lead (or equivalent) in thickness. They should be placed over the patient's gonads whenever such exposure is not required as part of the diagnostic test.

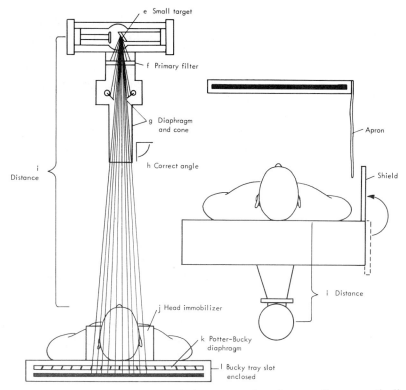

FIGURE 3–4 Additional radiation protection factors diagrammatically illustrated.

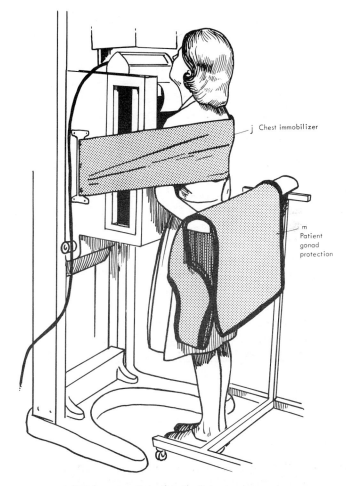

FIGURE 3–5 Other radiation protection factors.

PROTECTION OF PERSONS OCCUPATIONALLY EXPOSED TO RADIATION

In this discussion special emphasis is placed on the protection of physicians and radiologic technicians.

The International Commission on Radiological Protection (ICRP). This agency has made separate regulations for three types of personnel:

(1) those occupationally exposed, (2) those near controlled areas or atomic energy establishments, and (3) the population at large. The ICRP has also made separate regulations for different tissues of the body (Johns).*

---

*Johns, H. E.: The Physics of Radiology. 2nd Ed. Springfield, Ill., Charles C Thomas, Publisher, 1964.

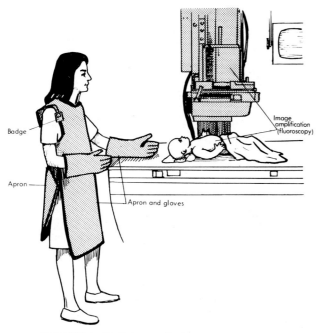

FIGURE 3–6   Other radiation protection factors.

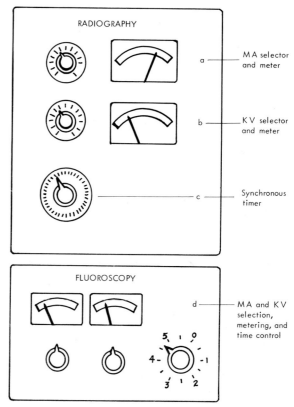

FIGURE 3–7   Diagram of x-ray control panel to emphasize control of physical factors in radiation protection.

PERSONS OCCUPATIONALLY EXPOSED

1. The blood-forming organs, gonads, and lenses of the eyes:

The maximum permissible total dose (D) accumulated in these tissues shall be governed by the formula:

$$D = 5 (N - 18) \text{ rems}$$
$$N = \text{age in years}$$

This formula implies a dose not exceeding 5 rems per year or 0.1 rem per week. However, in any period of 13 weeks, a dose of 3 rems may be accumulated.

The ICRP allows for an accidental exposure of 25 rems once in a lifetime, and this accidental dose may be added to that allowed by the above formula

2. For single organs other than the gonads, blood-forming organs, and eyes:

A higher yearly dose for these other organs is permitted as follows: skin: 30 rems; hands, forearms, feet, and ankles: 75 rems; other internal organs not mentioned above: 5 rems.

3. For whole body exposure from the uptake of several isotopes:

The same limitations are applied as for blood-forming organs, gonads, and lenses of the eyes.

It is well for the physician and his personnel to have frequent blood counts (at least at 6 month intervals), and if there is any opportunity for absorption of internal emitters, frequent urinary assays should also be performed. *A radiation monitoring device should be worn at all times and frequent assays noted in a permanent record.* The film badge or pocket chamber measurement device is ordinarily considered adequate for this purpose, unless there is a single opportunity for excessive exposure, in which case an accurately calibrated milliroentgen pocket chamber would be more accurate and should be employed.

PUBLIC AT LARGE

The limits for members of the public exclude the radiation dose contributed by background and medical radiation and are one tenth of the maximum permissible dose for occupational exposure (0.5 rem per year).

A major concern in the irradiation of large numbers of people is the genetic hazard. The total accumulated genetic dose for those up to age 30 must not exceed 5 rems plus the lowest possible contribution from medical procedures. Since the background varies in different parts of the country, this is excluded from consideration. Also, the dose of 5 rems is actually an average figure which includes those who are occupationally exposed—and thus the average for the rest of the population is less. It is estimated that the general population is exposed to about 3 rems from background radiation and about 3 rems from diagnostic procedures.

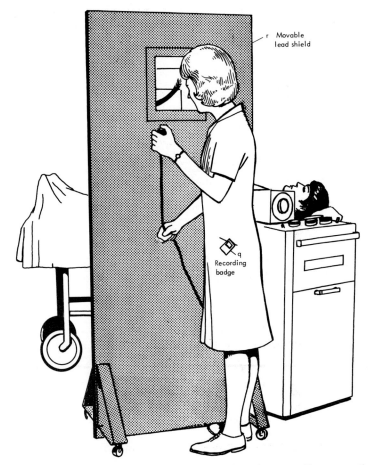

r Movable
lead shield

q
Recording
badge

FIGURE 3–8 Further radiation protection factors diagrammatically illustrated.

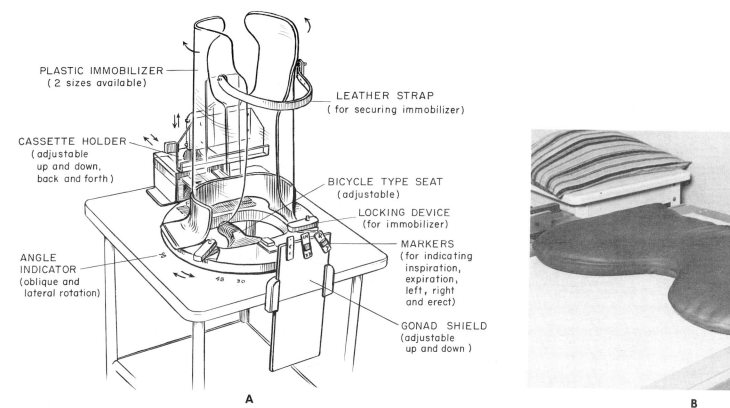

PLASTIC IMMOBILIZER
(2 sizes available)

LEATHER STRAP
(for securing immobilizer)

CASSETTE HOLDER
(adjustable
up and down,
back and forth)

BICYCLE TYPE SEAT
(adjustable)

LOCKING DEVICE
(for immobilizer)

MARKERS
(for indicating
inspiration,
expiration,
left, right
and erect)

ANGLE
INDICATOR
(oblique and
lateral rotation)

GONAD SHIELD
(adjustable
up and down)

A

B

FIGURE 3-9 *A.* Pigg-O-Stat infant immobilization device for erect radiography (manufactured by Modern Way Immobilizers, Memphis, Tennessee). *B.* Photograph of immobilization apparatus useful in pediatric radiology. This device consists of a radiolucent bag shaped as shown and containing innumerable plastic beads. When this bag is evacuated and placed around the patient, it forms a firm immobilization device around the individual so wrapped (obtainable from Picker X-Ray Corporation, Cleveland, Ohio).

Safety Recommendations for Radiography

1. Whenever possible, *fast film–screen combinations* should be used if they are suitable for a given purpose *without sacrifice of detail.*

2. *Added filtration,* up to 3 or 4 mm. of aluminum, should almost invariably be used. A minimum of 0.5 mm. of aluminum must be added for beryllium window x-ray tubes for mammography.

3. An adequate range of *adjustable or fixed cones* and *diaphragms* for limiting the useful beam to the smallest dimension necessary in any given examination ought to be available and used.

4. Tests should be made to *insure that leakage of radiation from the tube housing to cones is limited to the degree recommended* by the National Bureau of Standards Handbook 60.

5. For diagnostic examinations in general: (a) *Gonadal exposure must be minimized.* With suitable cones and diaphragms and special lead protective devices, the gonads can be kept out of the direct beam in most cases. In particular, shielding of the testes can be practiced without much difficulty or inconvenience. (b) *Expert assistance and calibration should be sought for every x-ray machine installation.* Dosage factors should be established at tabletop, and the maximum permissible fluoroscopic time posted; tests must ascertain that there is no radiation leakage from the x-ray tube housing. The equipment should be designed to afford a maximum of shielding for the operator.

6. There are *three basic factors* to consider always: (a) *time of exposure,* (b) *distance from the radiation source,* and (c) *shielding provided.*

7. It is recommended that, prior to the examination of all females *under 45 years of age* who could conceivably be pregnant, a brief *menstrual history be obtained.* Rapid immunologic type tests are now available which may, if desired, be performed in minutes prior to radiation exposure. Where impregnation is a possibility, radiation exposure of the embryo should be avoided except in dire emergencies. If pregnancy is known to exist, radiation should be avoided in the first trimester and as much as possible in pregnancy thereafter.

8. Patients should be immobilized as much as is comfortably possible to avoid movement during the radiographic exposure. (For chest immobilizer in children see Figure 3–9.)

4

THE UPPER EXTREMITY

BASIC ANATOMY

Shoulder Girdle and Humerus

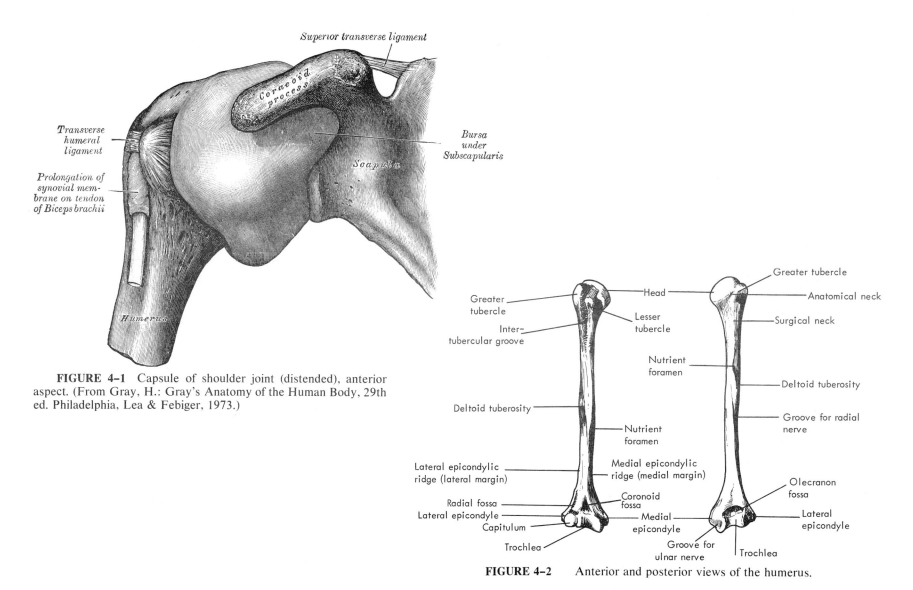

FIGURE 4–1 Capsule of shoulder joint (distended), anterior aspect. (From Gray, H.: Gray's Anatomy of the Human Body, 29th ed. Philadelphia, Lea & Febiger, 1973.)

FIGURE 4–2 Anterior and posterior views of the humerus.

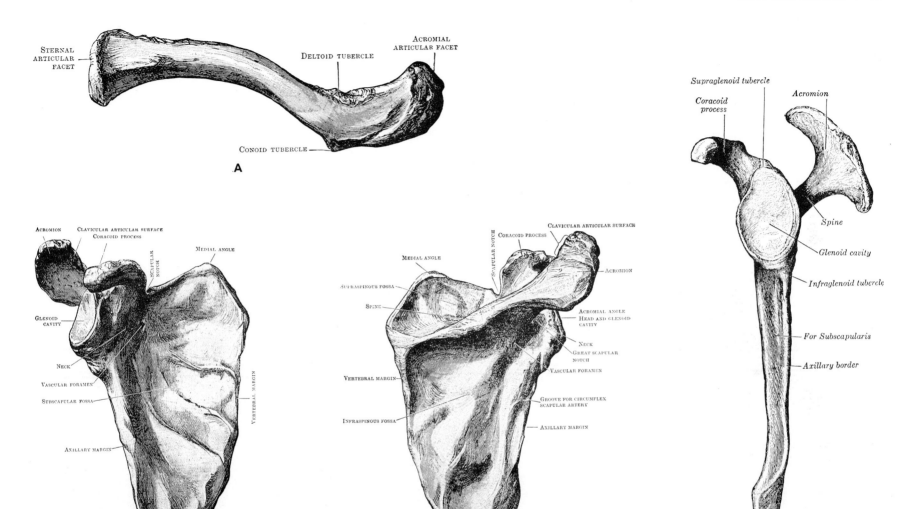

FIGURE 4–3 *A.* Clavicle viewed from above. (From Cunningham, D. J. in Robinson, A. (ed.): Textbook of Anatomy. London, Oxford University Press.) *B, C, D,* Anterior, posterior, and lateral views of the scapula. (*B* and *C.* From Cunningham, D. J. *in* Robinson, A. (ed.): Textbook of Anatomy. London, Oxford University Press. *D.* From Gray, H. *in* Goss, C. W. (ed.): Gray's Anatomy of the Human Body. Philadelphia, Lea & Febiger, 1973.)

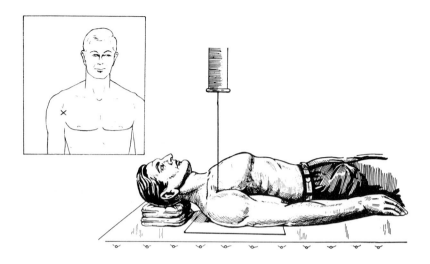

ROUTINE RADIOGRAPHIC STUDIES OF THE SHOULDER REGION

The Shoulder with the Arm in Rotation (Figs. 4–4, 4–5, and 4–6)

NEUTRAL ANTEROPOSTERIOR PROJECTION OF THE SHOULDER (FIG. 4–4)

POINTS OF PRACTICAL INTEREST ABOUT FIGURE 4–4

1. The patient may be examined either in the erect position or supine as shown, and centered so that the central ray passes midway between the summit of the shoulder and lower margin of the anterior axillary fold.

2. Better contact of the affected shoulder with the film is produced by rotating the opposite shoulder away from the table top approximately 15 to 20 degrees, and supporting the elevated shoulder and hip on sandbags.

3. When looking for faint flecks of calcium in the soft tissues, nonscreen film and technique should be employed unless the shoulder is very muscular, in which case the Potter-Bucky apparatus may be employed in addition. When using the Potter-Bucky diaphragm (or grid cassette) it is best to position the cassette so that the central ray will pass through the center of the cassette and the coracoid process.

4. Intercondylar axis is internally rotated approximately 45 degrees.

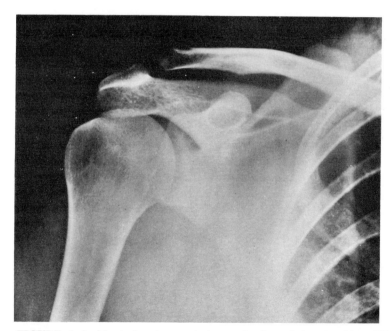

FIGURE 4–4 Neutral anteroposterior projection of the shoulder. (ITS) intertubercular sulcus. (The right shoulder is *viewed* in this manner also.)

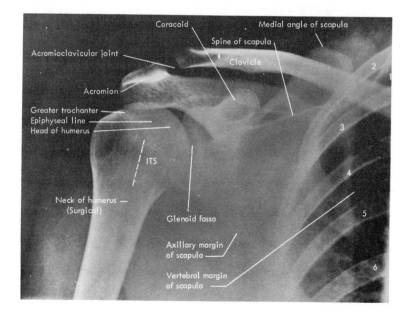

ANTEROPOSTERIOR PROJECTION OF THE SHOULDER WITH INTERNAL ROTATION OF THE HUMERUS (FIG. 4–5)

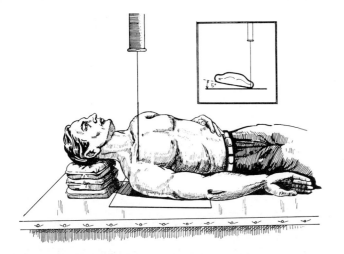

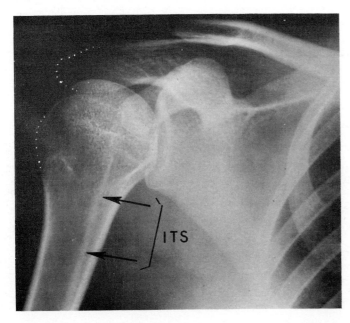

POINTS OF PRACTICAL INTEREST ABOUT FIGURE 4–5

1. One must make certain in this position that the entire humerus is rotated inward in addition to merely the forearm and hand.

2. The central ray may pass through the region of the coracoid process.

3. The angle of rotation of the body may be increased to 15 to 20 degrees instead of 5 degrees as shown. This will produce a slightly better profile view of the glenoid process.

4. It is most important that sandbags be used on the hand and forearm to immobilize the patient. (These have been omitted from the illustration for clarity.)

5. *The intercondylar axis of the humerus is approximately perpendicular to the film.*

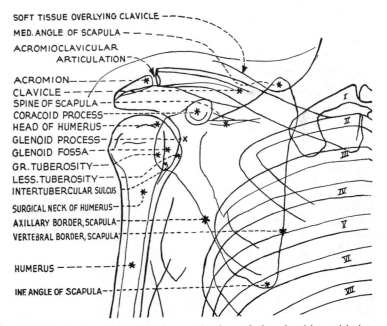

SOFT TISSUE OVERLYING CLAVICLE
MED. ANGLE OF SCAPULA
ACROMIOCLAVICULAR ARTICULATION
ACROMION
CLAVICLE
SPINE OF SCAPULA
CORACOID PROCESS
HEAD OF HUMERUS
GLENOID PROCESS
GLENOID FOSSA
GR. TUBEROSITY
LESS. TUBEROSITY
INTERTUBERCULAR SULCUS
SURGICAL NECK OF HUMERUS
AXILLARY BORDER, SCAPULA
VERTEBRAL BORDER, SCAPULA
HUMERUS
INF. ANGLE OF SCAPULA

FIGURE 4–5 Anteroposterior projection of the shoulder with internal rotation of the humerus. (The right shoulder is *viewed* in this manner also.)

ANTEROPOSTERIOR PROJECTION OF THE SHOULDER WITH EXTERNAL ROTATION OF THE HUMERUS (FIG. 4–6)

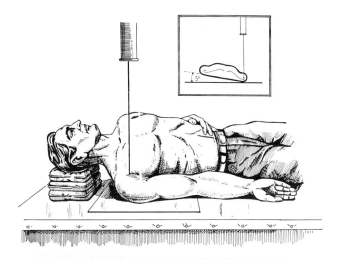

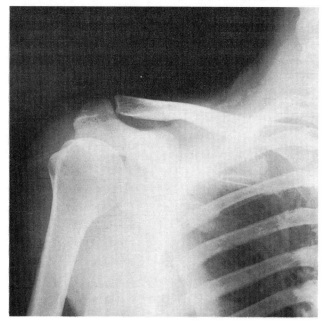

POINTS OF PRACTICAL INTEREST ABOUT FIGURE 4–6

1. One must make certain to rotate the entire arm externally in addition to the forearm and hand. (Sandbags as indicated for Fig. 4–5.)

2. In order to obtain a slightly better profile view of the glenoid process of the scapula, the angle of rotation may be increased from 5 degrees as shown to 15 or 20 degrees.

3. When looking particularly for small flakes of calcium deposit in the soft tissues of the shoulder, one must use a nonscreen technique with or without the Potter-Bucky diaphragm. The central ray may be directed through the coracoid process rather than as shown in the centering diagram.

4. *The intercondylar axis is rotated externally as much as possible.*

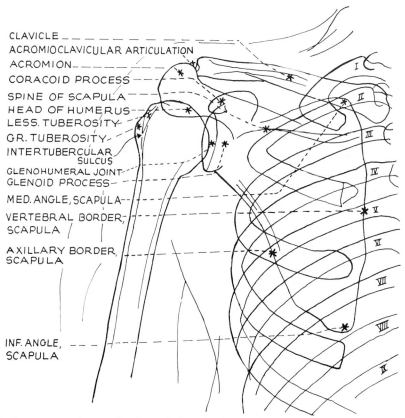

CLAVICLE
ACROMIOCLAVICULAR ARTICULATION
ACROMION
CORACOID PROCESS
SPINE OF SCAPULA
HEAD OF HUMERUS
LESS. TUBEROSITY
GR. TUBEROSITY
INTERTUBERCULAR SULCUS
GLENOHUMERAL JOINT
GLENOID PROCESS
MED. ANGLE, SCAPULA
VERTEBRAL BORDER, SCAPULA
AXILLARY BORDER, SCAPULA
INF. ANGLE, SCAPULA

FIGURE 4-6 Anteroposterior projection of the shoulder with external rotation of the humerus. (The right shoulder is *viewed* in this manner also.)

Projection of the Shoulder for Greater Detail in Reference to the Glenoid Process (Fig. 4–7)

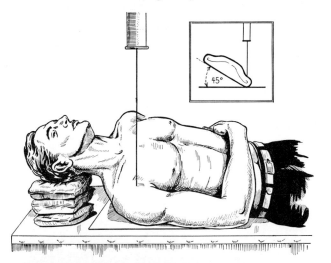

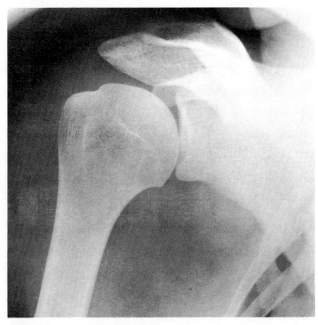

POINTS OF PRACTICAL INTEREST ABOUT FIGURE 4–7

1. Adjust the degree of rotation to place the scapula parallel with the plane of the film, and the head of the humerus in contact with it. This will usually come to an angle of 45 degrees as shown.

2. The arm is very slightly abducted and internally rotated, and the forearm is rested against the side of the body.

3. For a more uniform density, respiration is suspended in the expiratory phase.

4. The central ray is directed to a point 2 inches medial and 2 inches distal to the upper-outer border of the shoulder.

5. This view is particularly valuable in cases of suspected chronic dislocation of the shoulder, since in such instances the inferior margin of the glenoid process is frequently eroded or contains spurs rather than having the smooth contour shown.

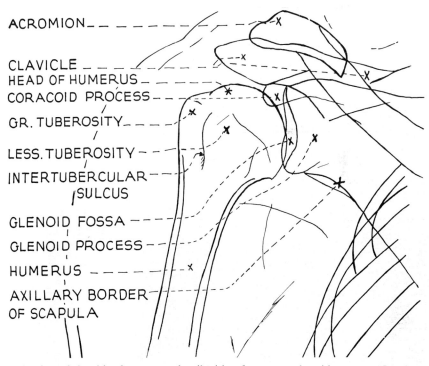

ACROMION

CLAVICLE
HEAD OF HUMERUS
CORACOID PROCESS

GR. TUBEROSITY

LESS. TUBEROSITY

INTERTUBERCULAR
SULCUS

GLENOID FOSSA

GLENOID PROCESS

HUMERUS

AXILLARY BORDER
OF SCAPULA

FIGURE 4–7 Projection of shoulder for greater detail with reference to glenoid process (Grashey position). (The right shoulder is *viewed* in this manner also.)

Projection of the Shoulder for Testing the Integrity and Degree of Separation of the Acromioclavicular Joint (Fig. 4–8)

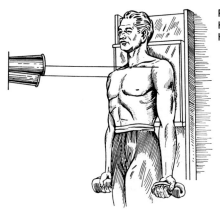

PATIENT *ERECT* HOLDING HEAVY OBJECTS IN HIS HANDS

POINTS OF PRACTICAL INTEREST ABOUT FIGURE 4–8

1. When there is a tear in the acromioclavicular joint capsule, there is a tendency for the distal end of the clavicle to rise above the level of the adjoining acromion process. The two films must be so equivalent in the projection as to make it possible to measure not only the joint space between the clavicle and the acromion process, but also the difference in relation to a horizontal line which would connect the superior margins of the acromion processes.

2. The technique employed should be such as to demonstrate the acromioclavicular joint capsule on each side by soft tissue contrast. Hemorrhage and swelling of the joint capsule may thereby be detected as well.

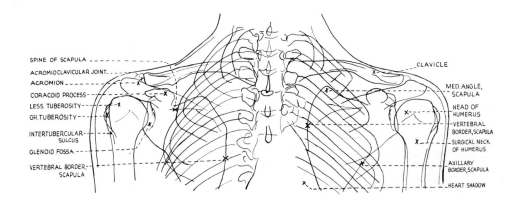

SPINE OF SCAPULA

ACROMIOCLAVICULAR JOINT

ACROMION

CORACOID PROCESS

LESS. TUBEROSITY

GR. TUBEROSITY

INTERTUBERCULAR SULCUS

GLENOID FOSSA

VERTEBRAL BORDER, SCAPULA

CLAVICLE

MED. ANGLE, SCAPULA

HEAD OF HUMERUS

VERTEBRAL BORDER, SCAPULA

SURGICAL NECK OF HUMERUS

AXILLARY BORDER, SCAPULA

HEART SHADOW

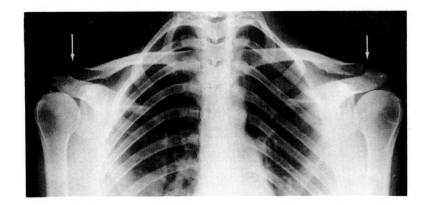

FIGURE 4–8 Projection of the shoulder for testing integrity and degree of separation of the acromioclavicular joint. In small individuals, a single exposure may be sufficient; in larger individuals, two separate exposures may be required with the cone centered over each joint separately and without moving the patient. (Pearson position, when projection is posteroanterior, instead of anteroposterior as shown.) (This film is *viewed* as though the radiologist is facing the patient.)

Inferosuperior Axial Projection of the Shoulder through the Axilla (Fig. 4–9)

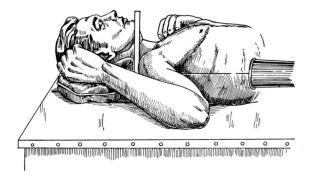

POINTS OF PRACTICAL INTEREST ABOUT FIGURE 4–9

1. The arm is kept in external rotation, while the forearm and hand are adjusted and supported in a comfortable position.

2. The central ray is directed through the axilla to the region of the acromioclavicular joint.

3. The arm should be abducted as nearly as possible to a right angle with respect to the long axis of the body.

4. It is important to push the cassette against the patient's neck as far as possible to obtain maximal visualization of the scapula.

5. The coracoid process is projected anteriorly, and the acromion process is projected posteriorly.

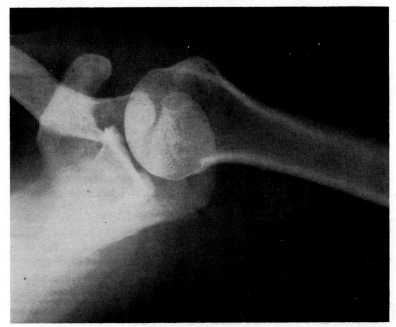

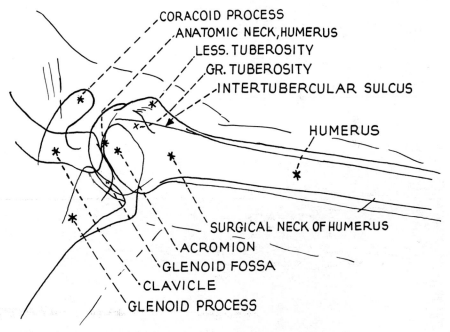

FIGURE 4–9 Inferosuperior axial projection of shoulder with the central horizontal ray projected through the axilla (Lawrence position). (Although the *position* drawing is of the right shoulder, the *film* shown happens to be a *left* shoulder.)

Lateral Projection of the Shoulder Projected through the Body (Fig. 4–10)

POINTS OF PRACTICAL INTEREST ABOUT FIGURE 4–10

1. For best results one must employ a screen film, with a vertical Potter-Bucky diaphragm, or grid-front cassette.

2. The cassette is centered to the region of the surgical neck of the affected humerus, as is the central ray. The central ray may be angled cephalad 5 to 15 degrees.

3. The patient stands perfectly perpendicular to the film as shown, with the opposite shoulder raised out of the way by resting his forearm upon his head and elevating the opposite scapula.

4. It is best to suspend respiration in full inspiration in this instance so that the air in the lungs will improve the contrast of the bone and decrease the exposure necessary to penetrate the body.

5. This may be the only method of obtaining a lateral view of the upper humerus in the event of a fracture in this location, when the patient is unable to abduct the arm.

6. While the erect position is shown, the recumbent position may also be employed, although it is less desirable.

7. The thoracic vertebrae technique is used.

8. The body may be rotated slightly if it is desired to project the humerus away from the spine.

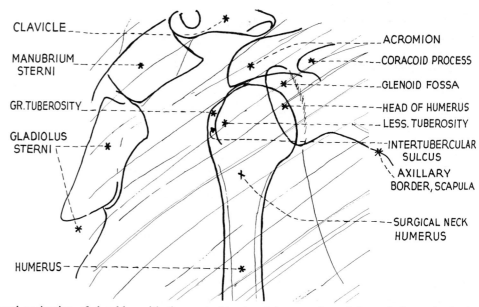

CLAVICLE

MANUBRIUM STERNI

GR. TUBEROSITY

GLADIOLUS STERNI

HUMERUS

ACROMION

CORACOID PROCESS

GLENOID FOSSA

HEAD OF HUMERUS

LESS. TUBEROSITY

INTERTUBERCULAR SULCUS

AXILLARY BORDER, SCAPULA

SURGICAL NECK HUMERUS

FIGURE 4–10 Lateral projection of shoulder with the central horizontal ray projected through the entire body (Lawrence position). (The right shoulder in the example above is closest to the film; therefore, this is a *right lateral projection.*)

Special Projection of the Clavicle (Fig. 4–11)

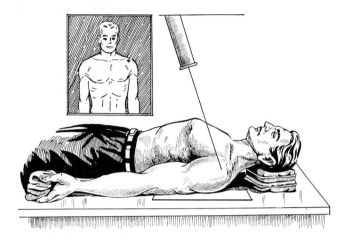

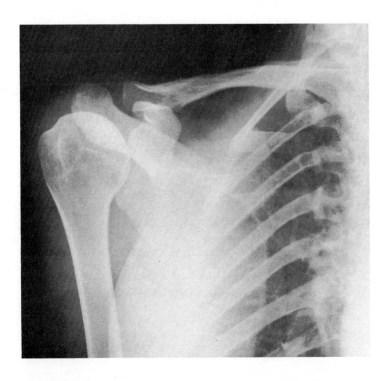

POINTS OF PRACTICAL INTEREST ABOUT FIGURE 4–11

1. A 15-degree angulation of the tube is usually adequate to project the clavicle away from the rest of the thoracic cage in this view.

2. When interpreting this film, the physician must take into account a considerable element of projection and distortion, since the clavicle is a fair distance from the film.

3. The central ray should pass through the middle of the clavicle in this projection, or through the acromioclavicular articulation as shown.

4. An anomalous articulation between the coracoid process and the conoid tubercle may occur.

5. The sternoclavicular joint is not well shown in this view.

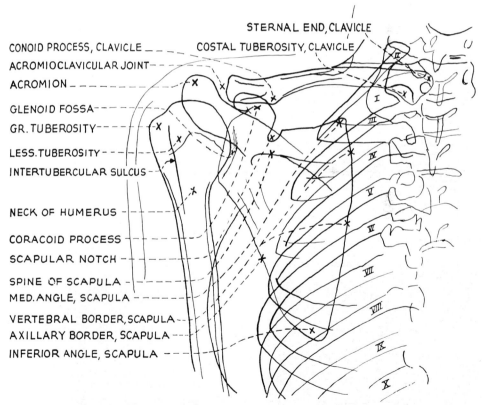

CONOID PROCESS, CLAVICLE
ACROMIOCLAVICULAR JOINT
ACROMION
GLENOID FOSSA
GR. TUBEROSITY
LESS. TUBEROSITY
INTERTUBERCULAR SULCUS
NECK OF HUMERUS
CORACOID PROCESS
SCAPULAR NOTCH
SPINE OF SCAPULA
MED. ANGLE, SCAPULA
VERTEBRAL BORDER, SCAPULA
AXILLARY BORDER, SCAPULA
INFERIOR ANGLE, SCAPULA

STERNAL END, CLAVICLE
COSTAL TUBEROSITY, CLAVICLE

FIGURE 4–11 Special anteroposterior projection of the clavicle and coracoid process of the scapula. (The *position* drawing is that of a *left* shoulder; the film is that of a *right* anteroposterior projection.)

Special Erect Projection of the Clavicle (Fig. 4–12)

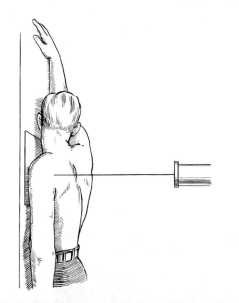

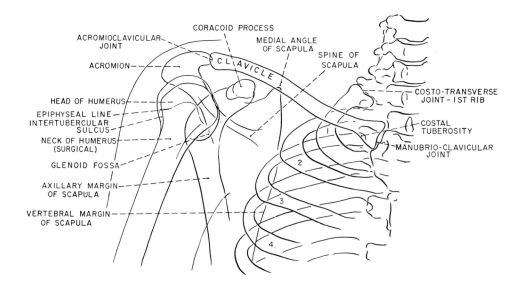

ACROMIOCLAVICULAR JOINT

CORACOID PROCESS

MEDIAL ANGLE OF SCAPULA

SPINE OF SCAPULA

ACROMION

CLAVICLE

HEAD OF HUMERUS

EPIPHYSEAL LINE
INTERTUBERCULAR SULCUS

NECK OF HUMERUS (SURGICAL)

GLENOID FOSSA

AXILLARY MARGIN OF SCAPULA

VERTEBRAL MARGIN OF SCAPULA

COSTO-TRANSVERSE JOINT - 1ST RIB

COSTAL TUBEROSITY

MANUBRIO-CLAVICULAR JOINT

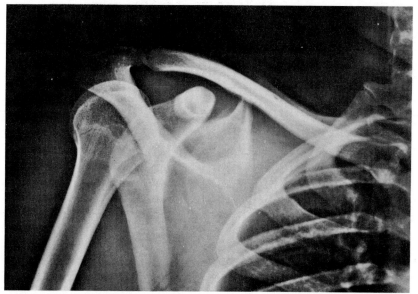

FIGURE 4–12 Special posteroanterior erect projection of clavicle. (The *position* drawing is that of a *left* shoulder; the *film* is that of a right shoulder.)

POINTS OF PRACTICAL INTEREST ABOUT FIGURE 4–12

1. This view may be employed with either the erect or the prone position. The erect position is probably more readily obtained in the event of injury to the clavicle.

2. The central ray passes through the center of the clavicle in this instance; an angulation of 10 degrees toward the feet may be employed.

3. Approximately one half of the clavicle is projected over the bony thorax as shown, but there is less distortion and magnification in this view than in Figure 4–11, and hence it is more desirable in some instances.

Lateral Projection of the Scapula (Fig. 4–13)

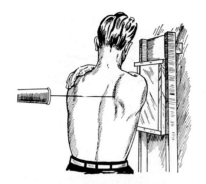

POINTS OF PRACTICAL INTEREST ABOUT FIGURE 4–13

1. The Potter-Bucky diaphragm is necessary to obtain best results with this projection.

2. The scapula is placed perpendicular to the film, rotating the opposite shoulder out of view. After palpating it, one centers over the spine of the scapula.

3. To rotate the wing of the scapula outward to its maximum it is best to rest the forearm of the affected side on the opposite shoulder, bringing the arm as close to the anterior chest wall as possible. Although the erect position is preferable, the recumbent position may also be employed in this instance.

4. The forearm of the injured shoulder lies across the chest and grasps the opposite shoulder with the hand.

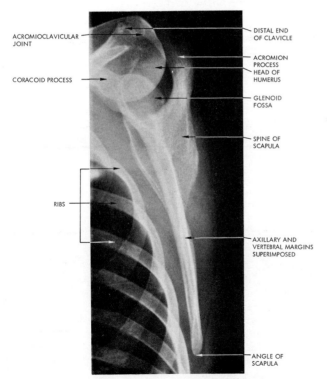

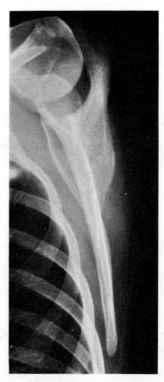

FIGURE 4–13 Lateral projection of scapula (modification of Lilienfeld position). (The *position* drawing is that of a *left* scapula. The film in this instance is a view of the *left scapula*.)

Special Views of the Bursae of the Shoulder Joint

Sodium or meglumine diatrizoate (6 to 10 ml.) is injected beneath the coracoid process or beneath the acromion, under fluoroscopic control (Fig. 4–14 *B*).

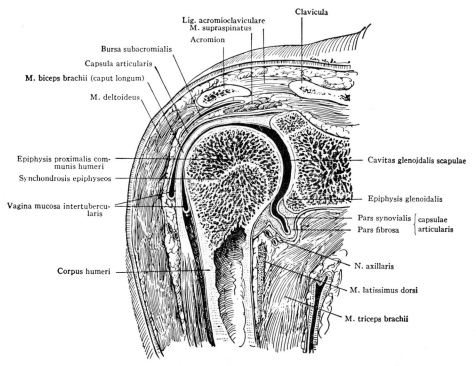

FIGURE 4–14 *A*. Subdeltoid bursa and its anatomic relationships. (From Anson, B. J., and McVay, C. B.: Surgical Anatomy, 5th Ed., Philadelphia, W. B. Saunders Co., 1971.)

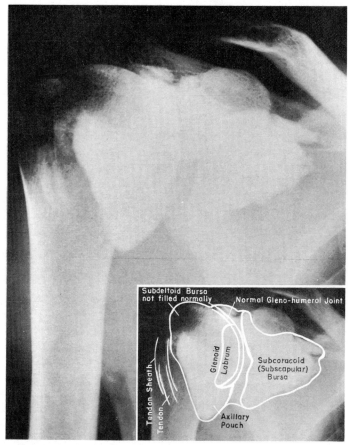

FIGURE 4–14 *B*. Normal Hypaque arthrogram of an adult's shoulder, demonstrating the normal joint, subscapular bursa, and dependent axillary pouch. The capsule cannot extend on the lesser and greater tubercles of the humerus because of the four short muscles (subscapularis, supraspinatus, infraspinatus, and teres minor) inserted there. It can—and does—extend on to the surgical neck via the synovial sheath of the biceps. In some patients, the subcoracoid bursa does not communicate with the rest of the joint.

VARIATIONS OF NORMAL RADIOGRAPHIC APPEARANCES IN THE SHOULDER

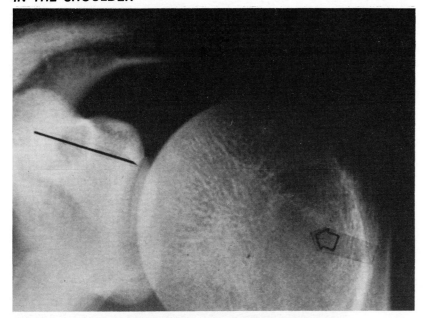

A

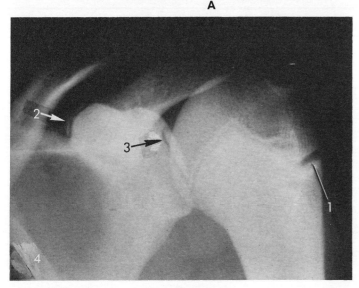

B

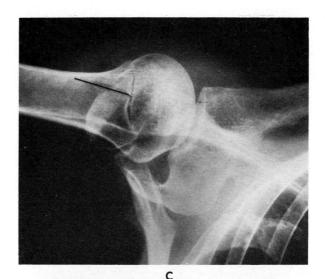

C

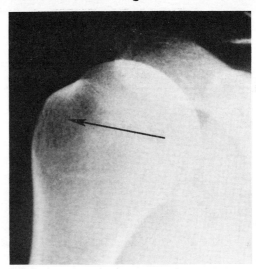

D

FIGURE 4–15 *A*. The "in vacuo" stripe in the shoulder joint upon first stretching the joint. *B*. Radiograph of the shoulder in an adolescent, showing the epiphyses of the shoulder region: (1) Epiphyseal plate beneath the head of the humerus. (2) Epiphysis of the coracoid process. (3) Epiphysis of the glenoid process or rim. *C*. Another view of the curvilinear nature of the epiphyseal plate between the head and metaphysis of the upper shaft of the humerus. *D*. Normal lucency found in the greater tuberosity of the humerus in shoulder films.

Axial Relationships at the Upper Part of the Humerus. The axial relationships at the head of the humerus to the anatomic neck and shaft are illustrated in Figure 4–16. The original axes as defined by Toldt have been reinvestigated by Keats et al., who showed that the values in males range from 52 to 70 degrees in the angle shown and in females from 50 to 70 degrees. The average for the entire group was 60 degrees with no significant sex variation in the axial relationships (Keats et al.).

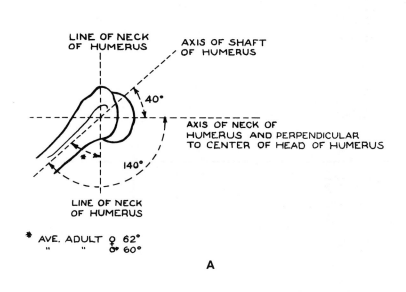

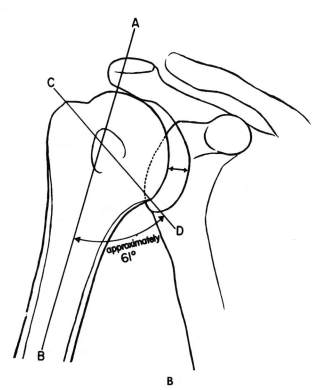

FIGURE 4–16 *A.* Axial relationships at the upper part of the humerus. (Modified from Toldt, C.: An Atlas of Anatomy for Students and Physicians. New York, Macmillan Co., © 1926; and Keats, T. E., et al.: Radiology, *87*:904–907, 1966.) *B,* Axial relationships of the shoulder and measurement of the joint space. The width of the joint space in adults is 0 to 6.0 mm., depending on the degree of rotation of the humerus. More than 6 mm. is significant and is particularly useful in the diagnosis of dislocation of the humeral head. (From Lusted, L. B., and Keats, T. E.: Atlas of Roentgenographic Measurement, 3rd ed. Copyright © 1972 by Year Book Medical Publishers, Inc., Chicago. Used by permission.)

Anteroposterior Projection of the Arm (Fig. 4-17)

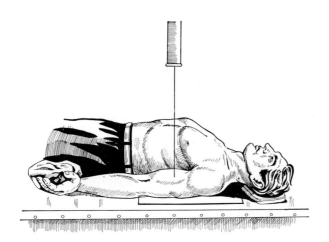

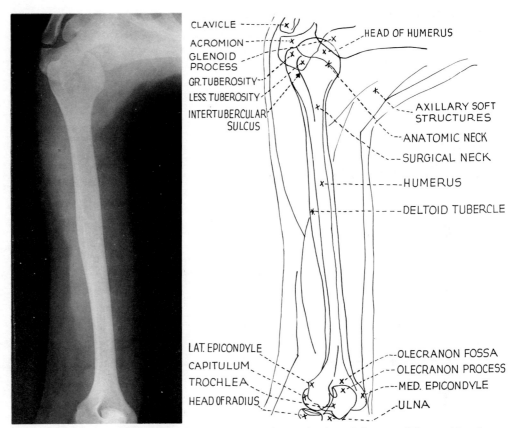

FIGURE 4-17 Anteroposterior projection of the arm. (The *position* drawing is that of the *left* arm; the film shown is that of an anteroposterior *projection* of the *right* arm.)

POINTS OF PRACTICAL INTEREST ABOUT FIGURE 4-17

1. The entire humerus from head to epicondyle should be included if at at all possible.

2. One must make certain to supinate the hand sufficiently so that the epicondyles both lie flat on the film.

3. The central ray is directed through the mid-shaft of the humerus.

4. The opposite shoulder may be rotated up and supported by sandbags in order to facilitate placing the humerus in better contact with the film.

5. The important landmarks for identification are the intertubercular sulcus lying between the greater and lesser tuberosity, the deltoid tubercle, which forms a landmark for the position of the radial nerve; and the anatomic parts labeled around the distal shaft near the elbow.

Lateral Projection of the Arm (Fig. 4–18)

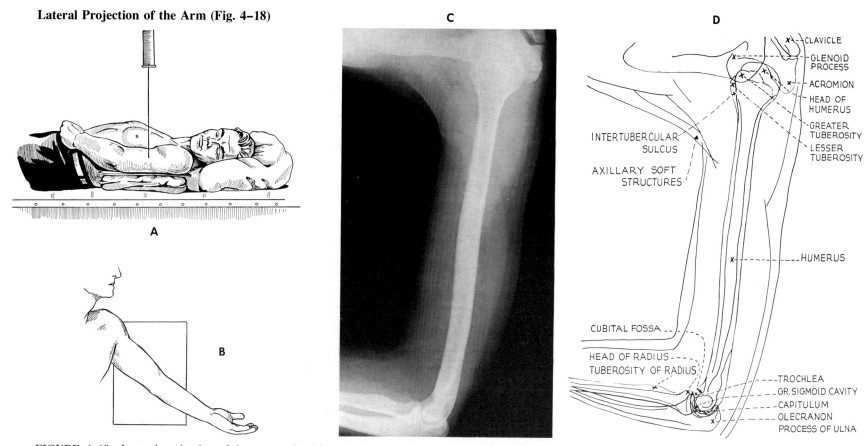

FIGURE 4–18 Lateral projection of the arm. *A.* Position of patient in recumbency. *B.* Position of patient when erect. *C.* Radiograph so obtained. *D.* Labeled line drawing of *C.*

POINTS OF PRACTICAL INTEREST ABOUT FIGURE 4–18

1. One must make certain that the film size chosen is adequate to include the entire shaft of the humerus from head to elbow joint.

2. The two epicondyles must be perfectly superimposed over one another and perpendicular to the film surface. To accomplish this, the technologist may have to elevate the film on a sandbag as shown, and flex the forearm, resting the forearm upon the abdomen.

3. An alternative technique allows the patient to sit in a chair and extend the arm across the table. The arm, particularly its lower two-thirds, must be in perfect contact with the film.

4. The central ray is directed through the midshaft of the humerus.

5. An alternative view for positioning is shown in position B. The patient is turned with the affected side against the film and bends from the waist slightly so that his body is posterior to the arm and is not superimposed over the arm. The unaffected hand may assist in maintaining this position. The upper shaft of the humerus is not clearly identified in this alternate position.

6. When the patient is unable to abduct the arm, the previously described view of the arm taken through the body must be obtained (Fig. 4–10).

The Elbow

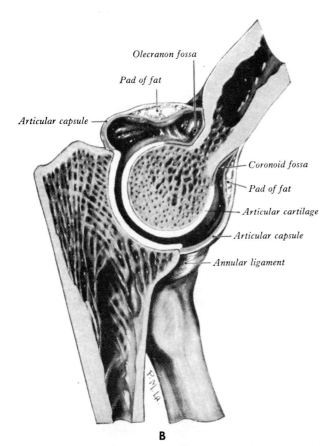

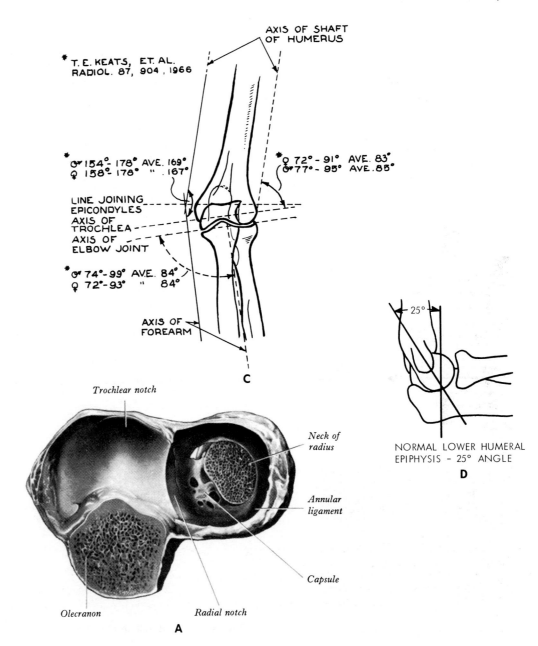

FIGURE 4-19 *A.* The annular ligament of the right radius, superior aspect. The head of the radius has been sawed off, and the bone dislodged from the ligament. *B.* A sagittal section through the left elbow joint, medial aspect. *C.* Axial relationships of the elbow. *D.* Normal lower humeral angle. (*B* and *D,* from Warwick, R., and Williams, P. L.: Gray's Anatomy. 35th British edition. London, Longman [for Churchill Livingstone], 1973.)

Anteroposterior Projection of the Elbow (Fig. 4–20)

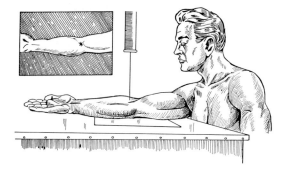

POINTS OF PRACTICAL INTEREST ABOUT FIGURE 4–20

1. Note that the patient is seated low enough to place the shoulder joint and the elbow in approximately the same plane. This assures a good contact between the distal humerus and the film.

2. The anterior surface of the elbow and the plane passing through the epicondyles must be perfectly parallel with the film. To accomplish this the hand must be completely supinated and usually supported in this position by means of a sandbag. Occasionally also the patient must lean somewhat laterally.

3. The olecranon and coronoid fossae of the humerus, being superimposed and merely being a very thin plate of bone, will frequently appear as a foramen rather than as a bony plate, which may be misleading. A foramen in lieu of this bony plate does occur very rarely in anomalous conditions.

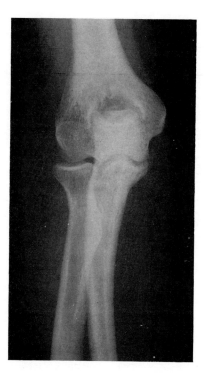

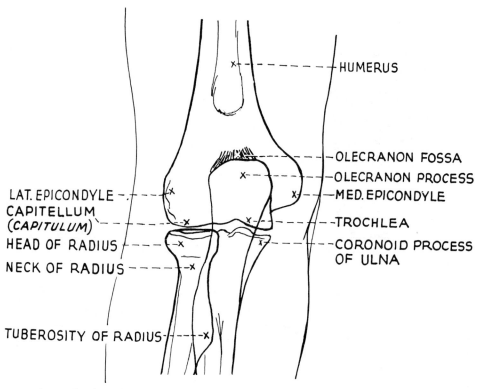

FIGURE 4–20 Anteroposterior projection of the right elbow.

Anteroposterior Projection of the Elbow When the Patient Cannot Extend It (Figs. 4–21 and 4–22)

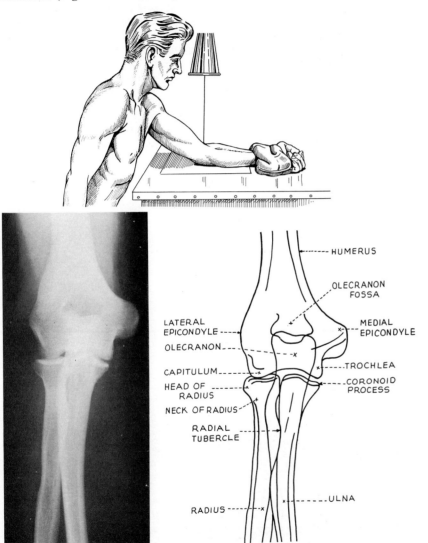

FIGURE 4–21 Projections of the elbow region when the elbow cannot be fully extended. Projections of the proximal forearm, with a distorted view of the distal humerus. (The *position* drawings are of the left elbow in both Figure 4–21 and Figure 4–22. The *projections* portrayed on the films are those of the *right* elbow.)

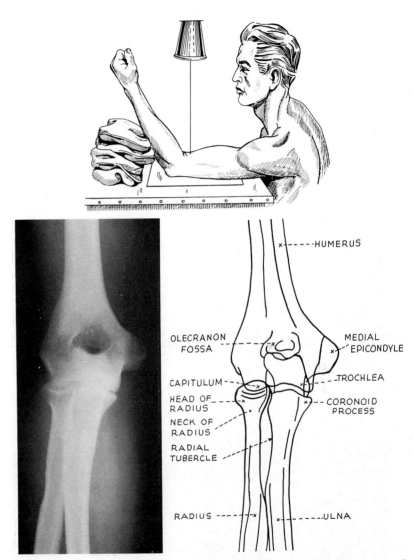

FIGURE 4–22 Projections of the elbow region when the elbow cannot be fully extended. Projection of the distal humerus, with a distorted view of the proximal forearm.

Tangential Projection of Olecranon Process (Fig. 4–23)

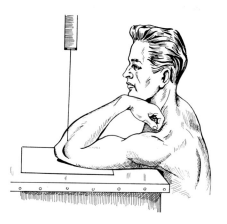

POINTS OF PRACTICAL INTEREST ABOUT FIGURE 4–23

1. The patient must be seated in such a way as to allow the entire humerus to be placed in good contact with the table top and film.

2. The elbow is flexed as acutely as possible and the hand pronated.

3. It is important in this instance also to obtain a visualization of the soft tissues immediately outside the olecranon process in view of their frequent involvement by inflammatory process and calcium deposit.

4. *Note that the long axis of the humerus is placed flat on the film.* After positioning, the KvP is determined by measuring through the flexed arm at about 3 inches above the elbow joint.

5. Immobilization is obtained by holding the hand against the shoulder.

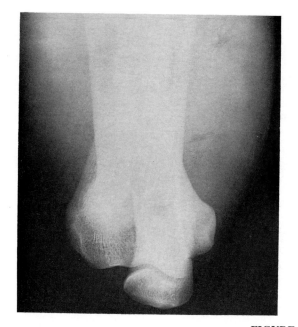

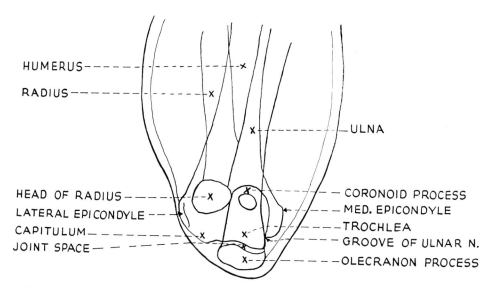

FIGURE 4–23   Special tangential projection of the left olecranon process.

Routine Lateral Projection of the Elbow (Fig. 4–24)

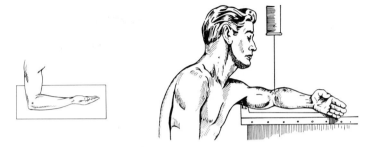

POINTS OF PRACTICAL INTEREST ABOUT FIGURE 4–24

1. The patient is so placed with respect to the table that the arm is at the same levels as the shoulder. Unless this is done the elbow joint proper will not be visualized clearly, and a rather oblique view of the head and neck of the radius will be obtained.

2. The elbow is ordinarily flexed approximately 90 degrees. The center of the film is placed immediately beneath the elbow joint and the central ray passes through the joint and center of the film, *the epicondyles of the humerus being superimposed and perpendicular to the latter.* The forearm is placed so that the thumb points directly upward and the palm of the hand is perpendicular to the table top surface. The fist may be clenched to facilitate maintenance of position. It is best to immobilize the forearm in this position by means of sandbags.

3. Since fractures of the head and neck of the radius are among those most frequently missed in radiography, one must examine the contour and structure of these regions with extreme care to avoid such an error.

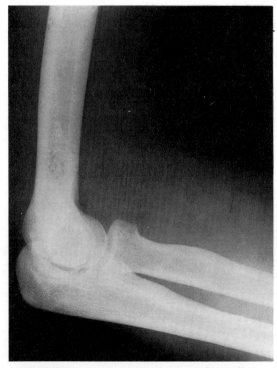

FIGURE 4–24 Lateral projection of the elbow.

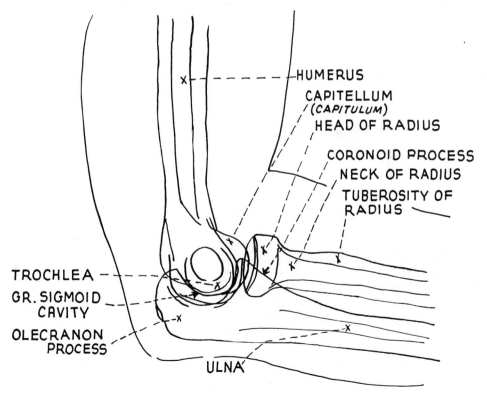

The Elbow and Forearm

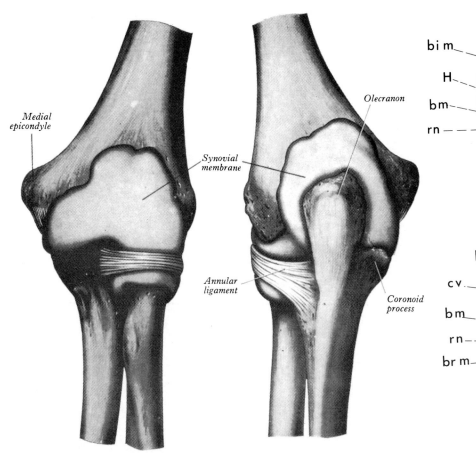

FIGURE 4–25 The synovial cavity of the left elbow joint (*left*), partially distended; anterior aspect. The fibrous capsule of the elbow joint has been removed, but the annular ligament has been left in situ. Note that the synovial membrane descends below the lower border of the annular ligament. The synovial cavity of the left elbow (*right*), partially distended. (*Right*) The same elbow as seen on its posterior aspect.

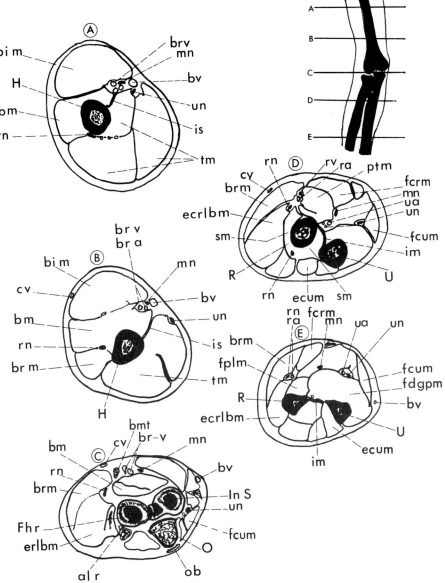

FIGURE 4–26 Diagrams demonstrating the cross-sectional anatomy in and around the elbow. *A, B, C, D,* and *E* are shown in relation to the orientation diagram in the upper right. The meanings of the abbreviations are as follows: (alr) annular ligament of radius; (bi m) biceps muscle; (bm) brachialis muscle; (bmt) biceps muscle tendon; (br m) brachioradialis muscle; (br v) brachial vein; (br a) brachial artery; (bv) basilic vein; (cv) cephalic vein; (ecrlbm) extensor carpi radialis longus and brevis muscle; (ecum) extensor carpi ulnaris muscle; (fcrm) flexor carpi radialis muscle; (fcum) flexor carpi ulnaris muscle; (Fhr) fovea for head of radius; (fplm) flexor pollicis longus muscle; (H) humerus; (In S) incisura semilunaris; (im) interosseous membrane; (is) intermuscular septum; (mn) median nerve; (O) olecranon; (ob) olecranon bursa; (ptm) pronator teres muscle; (R) radius; (ra) radial artery; (rn) radial nerve; (rv) radial vein; (sm) supinator muscle; (tm) triceps muscle; (U) ulna; (ua) ulnar artery; (un) ulnar nerve; (uv) ulnar vein.

The Radius and Ulna

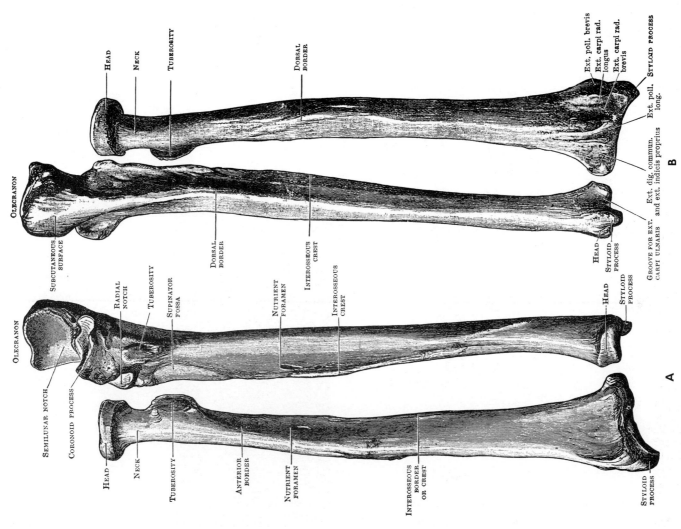

FIGURE 4-27 A. Volar aspect of the radius and ulna. B. Dorsal aspect of radius and ulna. (From Cunningham, D. J.: In Robinson, A. (ed.): Textbook of Anatomy. London, Oxford University Press.)

Routine Anteroposterior Projection of the Forearm (Fig. 4–28)

Routine Lateral Projection of the Forearm (Fig. 4–29)

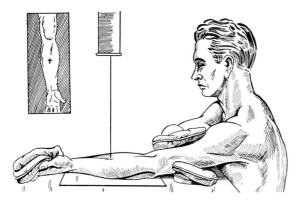

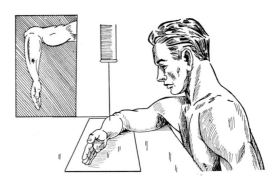

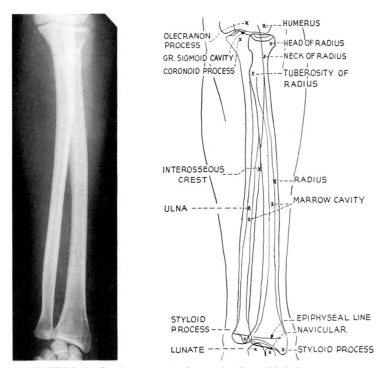

FIGURE 4–28 Anteroposterior projection of left forearm.

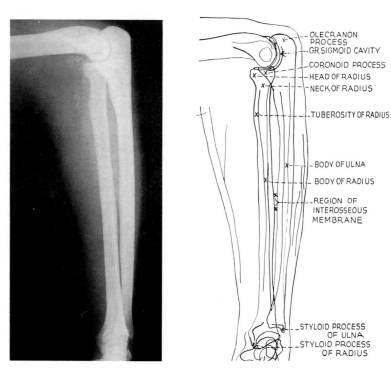

FIGURE 4–29 Lateral projection of forearm.

The Wrist

POINTS OF PRACTICAL INTEREST ABOUT FIGURES 4–28 and 4–29

1. The forearm is always in a supinated position with the volar aspect uppermost in these views.

In any case, it is well to seat the patient low enough to place the shoulder and the elbow in approximately the same plane, to assure good contact between the distal humerus and the film. A platform on the table top, with the patient's arm and the film on the platform, can achieve the same purpose.

2. In both these views, it is important to obtain an accurate concept of the integrity of the interosseous membrane. The ability of the patient to pronate and supinate his forearm depends in greatest measure upon an adequacy of this membrane and the space between the two bones of the forearm throughout their lengths. With injury to the bones of the forearm, there is a tendency for the fragments of the radius and ulna to contact one another and form a bony bridge between them across the interosseous membrane. This bridging must be recognized early and prevented.

3. Both the elbow and wrist joints should be included wherever possible.

4. Sandbags should be utilized to immobilize the arm and hand.

5. The central ray passes through the center of the forearm.

Axial Relationships at the Wrist (Fig. 4–30). The axis of flexion of the hand is perpendicular to the axis of the forearm, and forms an angle of 10 to 15 degrees with the line connecting the styloid processes of the radius and ulna. Keats et al. measured 25 normal males and 25 normal females in the posteroanterior projection with the results shown in Figure 4–30. The average measurement of the angle formed on the ulnar side between the shaft of the radius and the line drawn between the styloid processes of the radius and ulna was 83 degrees. In the lateral perspective the angle shown measured an average of 85.5 degrees, with ranges as indicated between 79 and 94 degrees in the two groups.

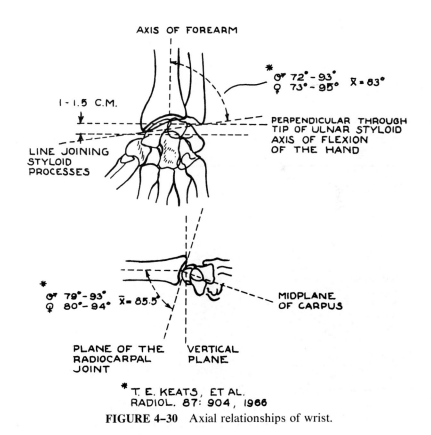

FIGURE 4–30 Axial relationships of wrist.

Routine Posteroanterior Projection of the Wrist (Fig. 4–31)

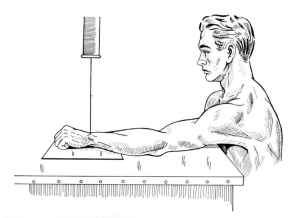

POINTS OF PRACTICAL INTEREST ABOUT FIGURE 4–31

1. The posteroanterior projection of the wrist is usually preferable because it permits better contact between the carpus and the film than is obtained in the reverse projection. In contrast to this, however, the anteroposterior projection of the forearm is the more desirable since pronation of the hand would cause the two bones of the forearm to cross one another.

2. The central ray is projected immediately over the navicular carpal bone, midway between the styloid processes.

3. The clenched fist as shown places the wrist at a very slight angulation but the navicular carpal bone is at right angles to the central ray, so that it is usually projected without any superimposition either by itself or by adjoining structures.

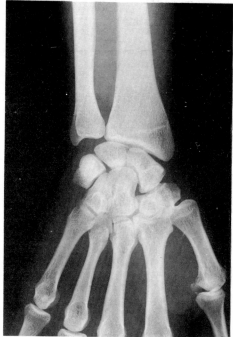

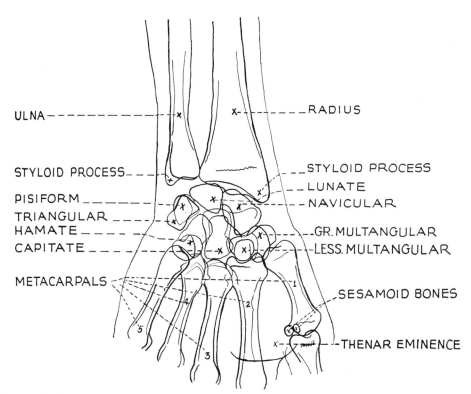

FIGURE 4–31 Posteroanterior projection of right wrist. (Left wrist is shown in position drawing.)

Routine Lateral Projection of the Wrist (Fig. 4–32)

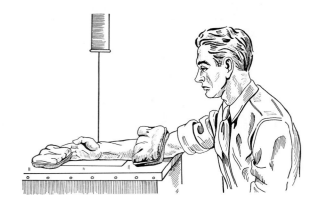

Chart of Related Terminology for Carpal Bones

Scaphoid = Navicular
Lunate
Triquetrum = Triangular Carpal
Pisiform
Multangular majus = Trapezium
Multangular minus = Trapezoid
Capitate
Hamate
Dorsal = posterior
Palmar = anterior (or volar)

The carpal tunnel is filled with tendons and the median nerve passing from the forearm into the palm of the hand. The ulnar vessels and nerve lie on the lateral side of the pisiform bone. The trapezium and part of the scaphoid bone lie in the floor of the "anatomic snuff box."

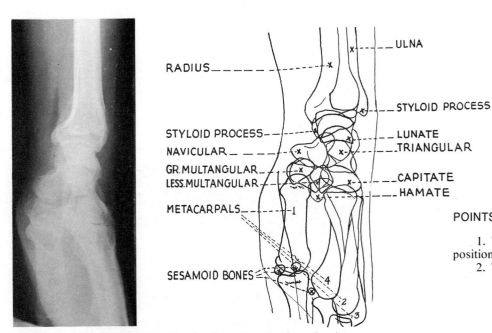

FIGURE 4–32 Routine lateral projection of wrist.

POINTS OF PRACTICAL INTEREST ABOUT FIGURE 4–32

1. The elbow should be flexed to 90 degrees to rotate the ulna to the lateral position. *Immobilize.*
2. The central ray is directed vertically to the styloid process of the radius.

Carpal Tunnel Projection of the Wrist (Fig. 4–33)

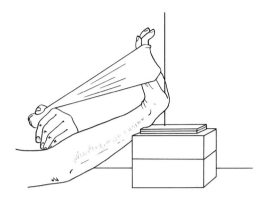

POINT OF PRACTICAL INTEREST ABOUT FIGURE 4–33

If hyperextension of the wrist cannot be maintained as shown, the central ray is directed at an angle of 20 to 30 degrees to the long axis of the hand.

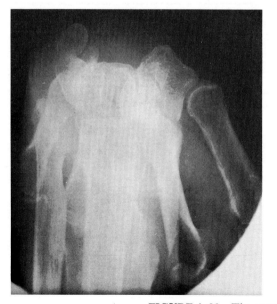

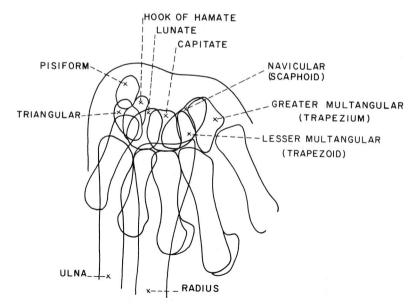

FIGURE 4–33   The carpal tunnel projection of the right wrist (modification of Gaynor-Hart position, and Templeton and Zim carpal tunnel projection).

Special Projection for Demonstration of the Midsection of the Navicular Carpal Bone (Fig. 4–34)

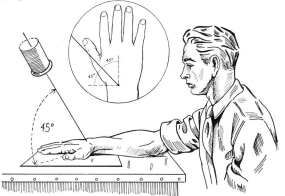

POINTS OF PRACTICAL INTEREST ABOUT FIGURE 4–34

1. This projection is an application of the principle of distortion in order to provide increased clarity of a pathologic process within a bony structure. Actually a rather distorted and elongated view of the navicular carpal bone is obtained, but it will be noted that it is completely clear of adjoining structures, for the most part, particularly in the area that is most prone to be fractured, namely its midsection. Also its own structure is not superimposed upon itself.

2. This projection is also of some value with reference to the base of the first metacarpal, but is of very little value with reference to the rest of the carpus.

3. The palm is outstretched, spreading the thumb and index finger, with the central ray bisecting the angle between the thumb and index finger directed at the scaphoid.

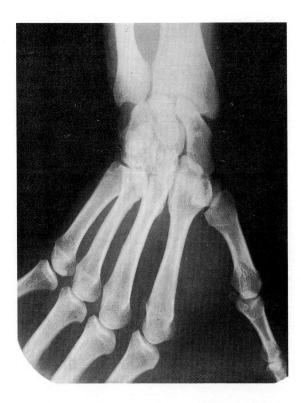

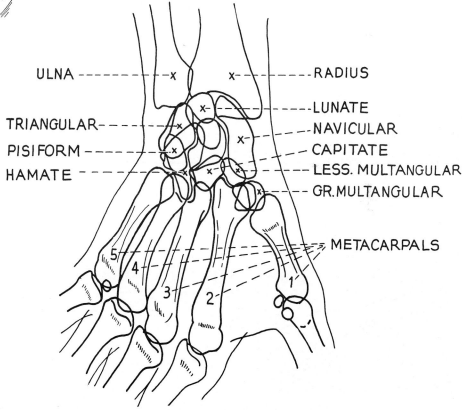

FIGURE 4–34 Special projection for demonstrating the right navicular carpal bone (scaphoid).

Special Navicular Projection of the Wrist (Fig. 4–35)

POINTS OF PRACTICAL INTEREST ABOUT FIGURE 4–35

1. Place the film holder on a 15-degree angle board opening away from the hand. Adjust the wrist in the P.A. position and center the carpus approximately ½ inch above the midpoint of the film. Immobilize.

2. Direct the central ray vertically to the navicular bone.

3. If an angle board is not available, place the film flat on the table, positioning the same. Immobilize.

4. Direct the central ray at an angle of 15 degrees toward the forearm. Centering is the same.

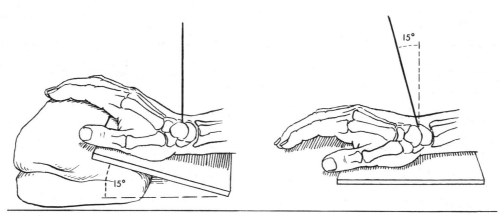

FIGURE 4–35 Alternate special navicular (scaphoid) projections (position drawings only).

Oblique Projection of the Carpus (Fig. 4–36)

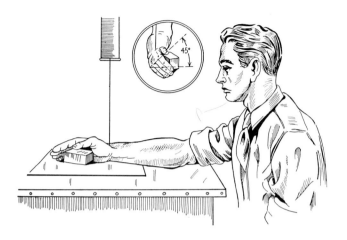

POINTS OF PRACTICAL INTEREST ABOUT FIGURE 4–36)

1. The film is placed under the wrist so that the center of the film is approximately 3 to 4 cm. anterior to the carpal bones. This will place it immediately under the navicular carpal bone when the wrist is slightly pronated to about 45 degrees from the lateral position. The hand is supported on a balsa wood block or sandbag as shown, and the forearm may be immobilized by an additional sandbag.

2. The central ray is directed immediately over the navicular carpal bone.

3. This projection is also particularly valuable in obtaining a clear perspective of the joint between the greater multangular and the first metacarpal.

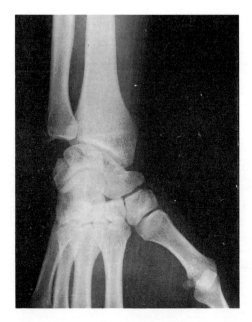

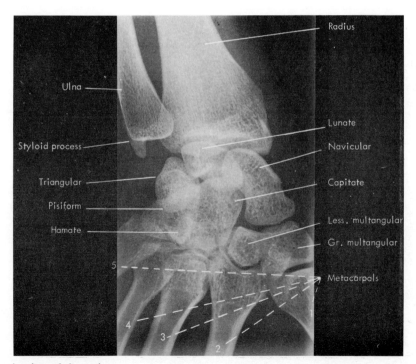

FIGURE 4–36 Oblique projection of the wrist.

The Hand

Routine Posteroanterior Projection of the Hand (Fig. 4–37)

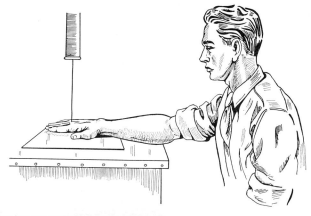

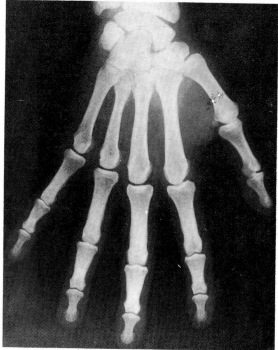

POINTS OF PRACTICAL INTEREST ABOUT FIGURE 4–37

1. The fingers should be spread slightly, and completely extended and in good contact with the film.

2. The central ray should pass through the third metacarpophalangeal joint.

3. It is well to immobilize the forearm just above the wrist by means of a sandbag.

4. The greatest care must be exercised to obtain a clear view, particularly of the tufted ends of the distal phalanges as well as the shafts of the phalanges, since many pathologic processes of a systemic type will produce minute and very important changes in these structures. The student should obtain a very clear mental concept of the normal appearance of the phalanges and metacarpals.

5. If a single finger is in question, a lighter exposure technique is employed and usually four views of that finger from all perspectives are taken.

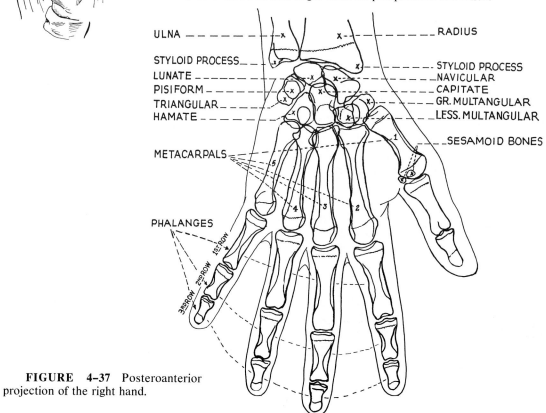

FIGURE 4–37 Posteroanterior projection of the right hand.

Routine Oblique Projection of the Hand (Fig. 4-38)

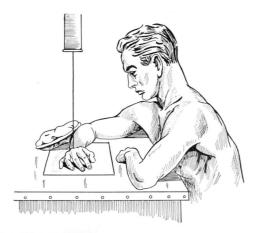

1. One should adjust the obliquity of the hands so that the metacarpophalangeal joints form an angle of approximately 45 degrees with the film.

2. The central ray is directed vertically through the third metacarpophalangeal joint.

3. Cotton pledgets may be employed to spread the fingers. A 2 inch square of balsa wood placed under the thumb makes an excellent immobilization device.

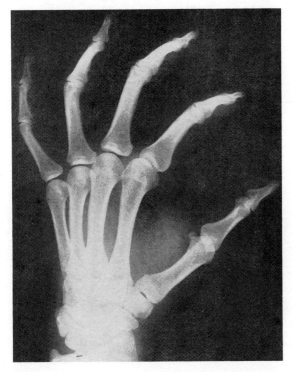

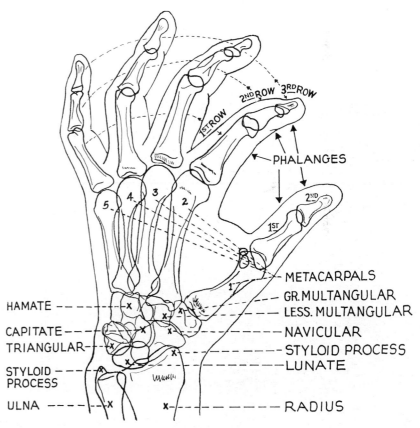

FIGURE 4-38 Oblique projection of the left hand. (The right hand is shown in the position drawing.)

Oblique Projection of the Carpus

Ball-Catcher's Projection (Fig. 4–39)

POINT OF PRACTICAL INTEREST ABOUT FIGURE 4–39

This projection has its greatest application in the study of early manifestations of arthritides.

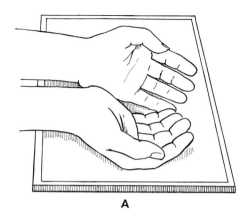

A

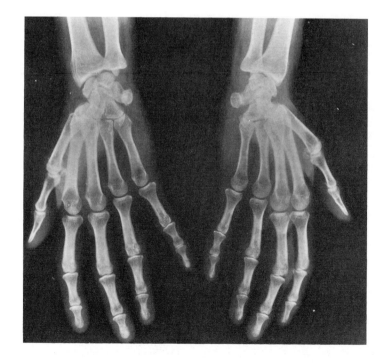

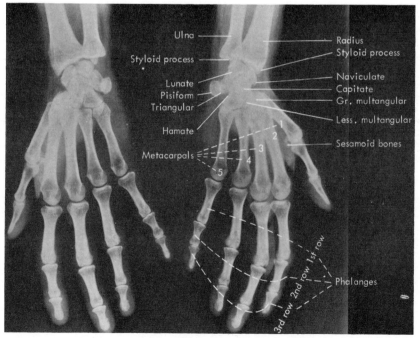

B

FIGURE 4–39 "Ball-catcher's" projection of the hands. *A.* Position of the hands. *B.* Unlabeled and labeled radiograph of same.

Straight Lateral Projection of the Hand (Fig. 4–40)

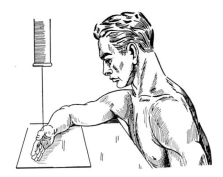

POINTS OF PRACTICAL INTEREST ABOUT FIGURE 4–40

1. The hand is placed perpendicular to the film contained within a cardboard or plastic holder, with the thumb pointing upward. (Fingers are often flexed as shown in the radiograph.)

2. The central ray is made to pass through the line of the heads of the metacarpals.

3. Note the normal curvature of the metacarpals in this projection with their concavity on the palmar aspect of the hand.

4. Various sesamoid bones will also be demonstrated clearly in this view as well.

5. The fingers may be fully extended, as shown in the unlabeled film on the *left*, or they may be partially flexed, as shown in the labeled film on the *right*.

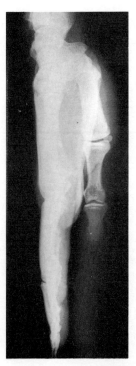

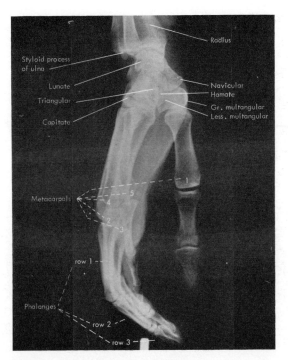

FIGURE 4–40 Lateral projection of the hand. The labeled radiograph shows the fingers flexed, a comfortable position for the patient.

Various Positions for Projections of Fingers and Thumb (Fig. 4–41)

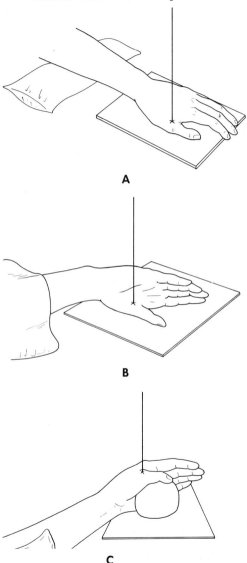

FIGURE 4–41 *A, B,* and *C.* Various positions for projections of the thumb and metacarpophalangeal joints, especially for patients with rheumatoid arthritis.

The patient is seated on a stool by the table; the hand and forearm rest on the table. The hand is placed palm down with the center phalanx of the affected finger centered to the film.

Direct the central ray vertically to the film. Immobilize with a sandbag across the wrist.

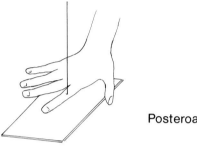

Posteroanterior

FIGURE 4–41 *Continued D.* Posteroanterior projection of the index finger.

The hand is placed palm up with the middle phalanx of the affected finger centered to the film. Immobilize.

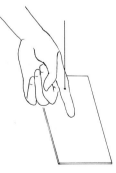

Anteroposterior

FIGURE 4–41 *Continued E.* Anteroposterior projection of the index finger.

With the affected finger extended and the other fingers folded into a fist, the middle phalanx is centered to the film.

It is necessary to elevate the finger to place its long axis parallel to the plane of the film. Both laterals are done in this way. Immobilize.

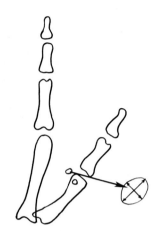

Sesamoid Index

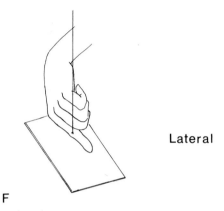

Lateral

F

FIGURE 4–41 *Continued* *F*. Lateral projection of the index finger.

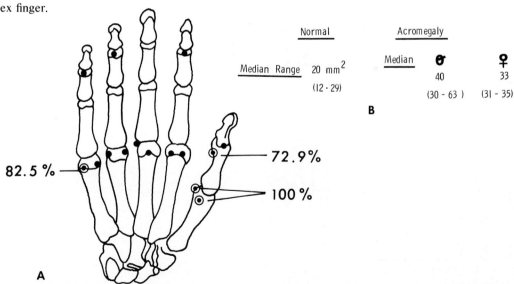

82.5 %

72.9%

100 %

Normal		Acromegaly	
Median Range	20 mm^2	Median	♂	♀
	(12 · 29)		40	33
			(30 - 63)	(31 - 35)

B

A

FIGURE 4–42 *A*. Schematic drawing (after Degen) of the sesamoids of the adult human hand. The most common are indicated by percentage occurrence. (Degen, St.: Med. Klin., *46*:1330, 1959.) *B*. Diagram of the sesamoid index (Kleinberg, et al.)

VASCULAR ANATOMY OF THE UPPER EXTREMITIES

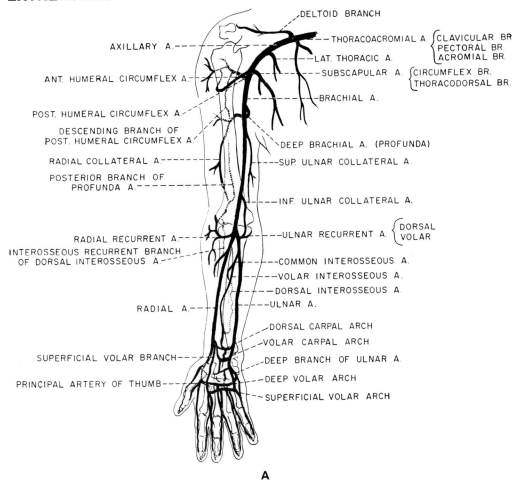

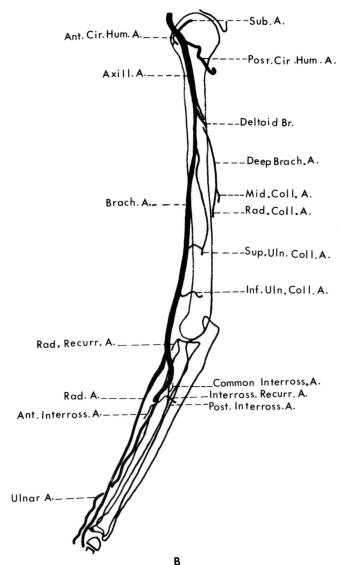

Figure 4–43 Diagram of arterial circulation of upper extremity. *A.* Frontal projection. *B.* Lateral projection.

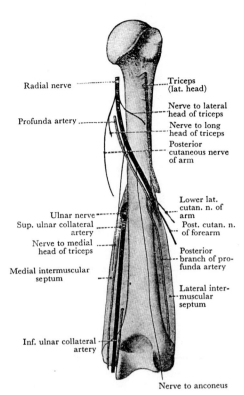

Radial nerve

Profunda artery

Ulnar nerve
Sup. ulnar collateral
artery
Nerve to medial
head of triceps

Medial intermuscular
septum

Inf. ulnar collateral
artery

Triceps
(lat. head)

Nerve to lateral
head of triceps
Nerve to long
head of triceps
Posterior
cutaneous nerve
of arm

Lower lat.
cutan. n. of
arm
Post. cutan. n.
of forearm

Posterior
branch of pro-
funda artery

Lateral inter-
muscular
septum

Nerve to anconeus

FIGURE 4–44 Diagram showing relation of the radial nerve to the posterior aspect of the humerus, and of vessels and nerves to the intermuscular septa. (From Cunningham, D. J.: Manual of Practical Anatomy, Vol. I, 12th ed., London, Oxford University Press, 1959.)

FIGURE 4–45 Superficial veins of the upper limb (dissected and drawn by Miss Nancy Joy). The arrows indicate where perforating veins pierce the deep fascia and bring the superficial and deep veins of the limb into communication with each other. For obvious mechanical reasons the palmar veins are few and small, and the dorsal veins are large. (Reproduced by permission from Grant, J. C. B.: An Atlas of Anatomy, 5th ed., Baltimore, The Williams & Wilkins Co. © 1962, The Williams & Wilkins Co.)

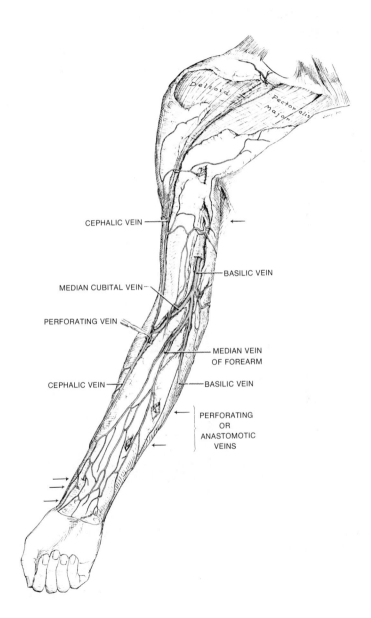

CEPHALIC VEIN

MEDIAN CUBITAL VEIN

PERFORATING VEIN

CEPHALIC VEIN

BASILIC VEIN

MEDIAN VEIN
OF FOREARM

BASILIC VEIN

PERFORATING
OR
ANASTOMOTIC
VEINS

5

THE PELVIS AND
LOWER EXTREMITY

Diagrams of Basic Anatomy (Fig. 5–1)

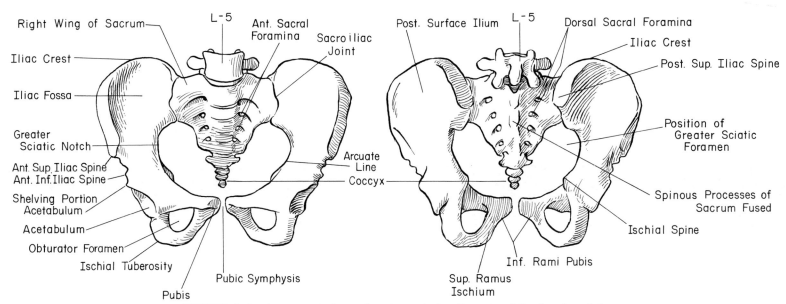

Right Wing of Sacrum

L-5

Ant. Sacral Foramina

Sacroiliac Joint

Iliac Crest

Iliac Fossa

Greater Sciatic Notch

Ant. Sup. Iliac Spine
Ant. Inf. Iliac Spine

Shelving Portion Acetabulum

Acetabulum

Obturator Foramen

Ischial Tuberosity

Pubis

Pubic Symphysis

Arcuate Line

Coccyx

Post. Surface Ilium

L-5

Dorsal Sacral Foramina

Iliac Crest

Post. Sup. Iliac Spine

Position of Greater Sciatic Foramen

Spinous Processes of Sacrum Fused

Ischial Spine

Inf. Rami Pubis

Sup. Ramus Ischium

FIGURE 5–1 Anteroposterior and posteroanterior diagrams of the female pelvis.

The Pelvis

Anteroposterior Projection of the Pelvis (Fig. 5-2)

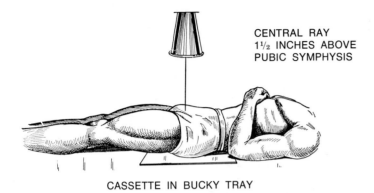

CENTRAL RAY
1½ INCHES ABOVE
PUBIC SYMPHYSIS

CASSETTE IN BUCKY TRAY

POINTS OF PRACTICAL INTEREST ABOUT FIGURE 5-2

1. Center the patient to the median line of the table with the center of a 14 × 17 inch cassette placed crosswise 1½ inches above the superior margin of the pubic symphysis. This will place the upper border of the film above the iliac crest and the lower border of the film well below the lesser trochanters of the femurs.

2. In order to project the necks of the femurs in their full length it is well to invert the feet about 15 degrees and immobilize them with sandbags in this position.

3. The entire pelvis must be symmetrical. This may necessitate placing a folded sheet or balsa wood block under one side.

4. There are various special views for the ilium, the acetabulum, the anterior pelvic bones and the pubes which have not been included in this text. These special views need be employed only on rare occasions.

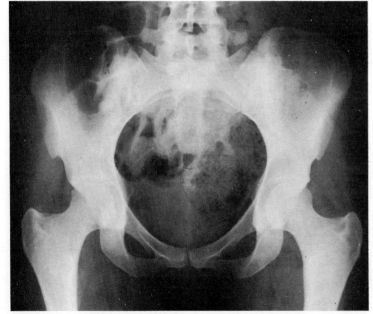

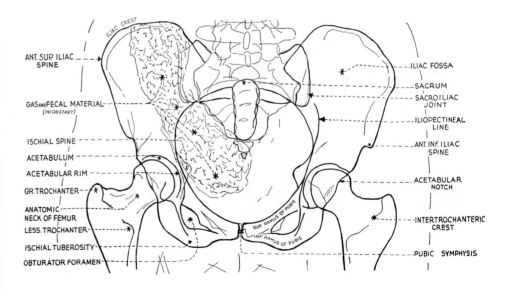

FIGURE 5-2 Anteroposterior projection of the pelvis.

Lateral Projection of the Pelvis for Visualization of the Sacrum (Fig. 5–3)

POINTS OF PRACTICAL INTEREST ABOUT FIGURE 5–3

1. The patient is placed in the lateral position, either erect or recumbent, and the film is placed in the Potter-Bucky diaphragm. The knees and hips are slightly flexed to facilitate maintenance of position.

2. The gluteal cleft is placed parallel with the film.

3. Immobilization with a compression band is frequently very helpful. This is applied across the trochanteric region of the pelvis.

4. Center in the midaxillary plane over the depression between the iliac crest and the greater trochanter of the femur.

5. There should be almost perfect superposition of the ischial spines as well as the acetabula in this projection.

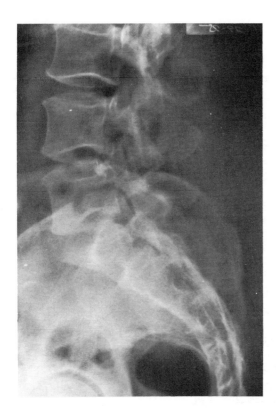

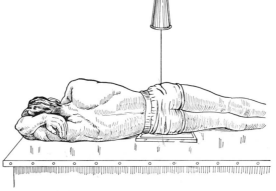

FIGURE 5–3 Lateral projection of pelvis for visualization primarily of the sacrum. (Film shown is left lateral projection, or right lateral view.)

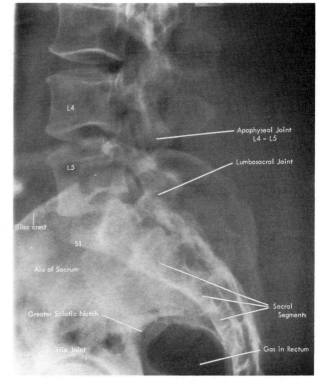

Oblique Projection of the Sacroiliac Joints (Fig. 5-4)

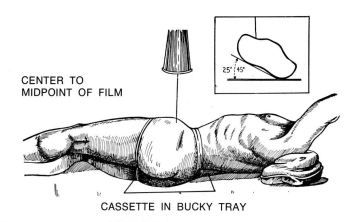

CENTER TO
MIDPOINT OF FILM

CASSETTE IN BUCKY TRAY

POINTS OF PRACTICAL INTEREST ABOUT FIGURE 5-4

1. Elevate the side being examined approximately 45 degrees and support the shoulder and the upper thigh on sandbags, making certain that the sandbags do not appear on the radiograph (25 degrees for sacroiliac joints; 45 degrees for lower lumbar).

2. The sacroiliac joint which is farthest from the film will appear most clearly and this is the one which is being examined. The two articular surfaces of the sacroiliac joint closest to the film are superimposed over one another, and hence this area is not shown to best advantage.

3. A somewhat similar oblique view of the sacroiliac joints may be obtained in the posteroanterior projection by placing the patient obliquely prone instead of supine as just noted.

4. Oblique views of both sacroiliac joints are always obtained because one joint offers some comparison for analysis of the other.

5. The central ray may be angled 5 degrees cephalad. In some patients this improves visualization of the sacroiliac and lumbar apophyseal joints.

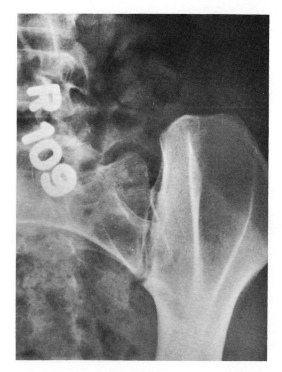

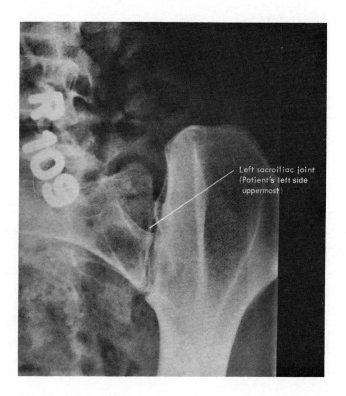

FIGURE 5-4 Oblique projection of the left sacroiliac joint with the patient lying on his right side obliquely, as shown. This is the right anteroposterior oblique projection. The opposite projection is made in the same manner. (For labeled parts of the adjoining lumbar spine, see Chapter 8, on the spine.)

Left sacroiliac joint
(Patient's left side uppermost)

Distorted Projection of the Sacrum (Fig. 5–5)

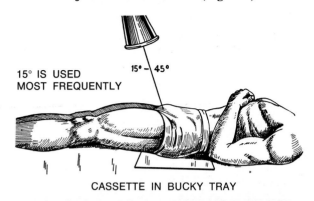

15° IS USED
MOST FREQUENTLY

15° – 45°

CASSETTE IN BUCKY TRAY

POINTS OF PRACTICAL INTEREST ABOUT FIGURE 5–5

1. For more marked distortion, angulation up to 45 degrees of the tube cephalad may be employed.

2. The central ray is adjusted so that it enters the body just above the pubic symphysis and so that it will leave the body at approximately the upper margin of the sacrum or at the level of the fifth lumbar segment. Care is exercised to center the x-ray film to the central ray of the x-ray tube, otherwise one will not obtain the anatomic structures depicted.

3. This view is particularly valuable for demonstrating sacralization of the last lumbar transverse processes as is indicated in the accompanying diagram. Also defects in the neural arch of the fifth lumbar vertebra are well demonstrated in this view.

4. Immobilize with a compression band.

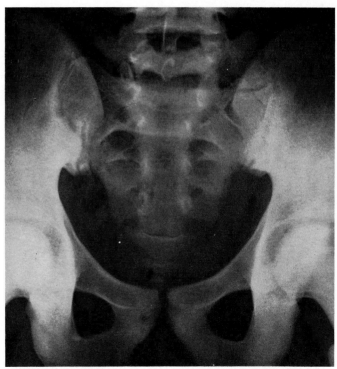

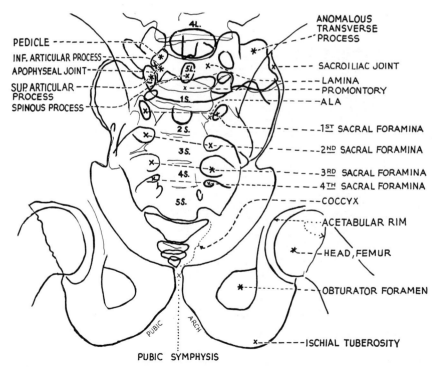

FIGURE 5–5 Distorted projection of the sacrum (Taylor, or Meese, position). Note the anomalous transverse process on the patient's left.

Anteroposterior Projection of the Coccyx (Fig. 5–6)

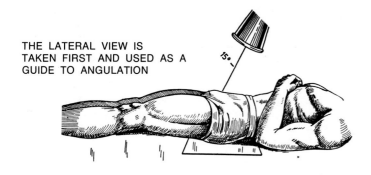

THE LATERAL VIEW IS
TAKEN FIRST AND USED AS A
GUIDE TO ANGULATION

15°

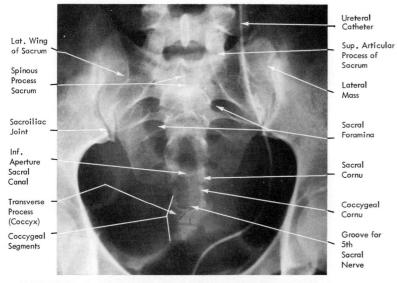

Lat. Wing of Sacrum

Spinous Process Sacrum

Sacroiliac Joint

Inf. Aperture Sacral Canal

Transverse Process (Coccyx)

Coccygeal Segments

Ureteral Catheter

Sup. Articular Process of Sacrum

Lateral Mass

Sacral Foramina

Sacral Cornu

Coccygeal Cornu

Groove for 5th Sacral Nerve

FIGURE 5–6 Anteroposterior projection of the coccyx. The cassette is placed in the Bucky tray, and the central ray is centered at the level of the soft tissue depression just above the greater trochanters, in the midline, 10 to 15 degrees, angled caudad, as shown.

Lateral Projection of the Coccyx (Fig. 5–7)

This projection lies about 5 inches posterior to the midaxillary plane of the body. Place sandbags between knees and ankles, and a folded sheet or sponges under the lower thorax. Immobilize with a compression band.

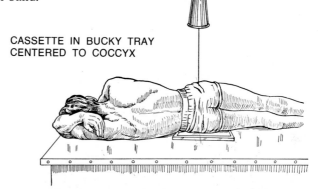

CASSETTE IN BUCKY TRAY
CENTERED TO COCCYX

FIGURE 5–7 Lateral projection of the coccyx.

Projection of the Symphysis Pubis (Fig. 5–8)

The patient is placed prone with the symphysis over the center of the table. A 10″ × 12″ film in the Bucky tray is centered to the symphysis. The central beam is centered perpendicular to the film. Immobilize with a compression band.

The greater trochanters lie in the same transverse plane as the symphysis pubis.

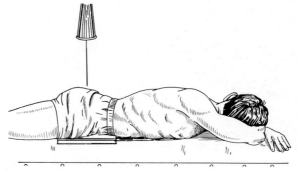

FIGURE 5–8 Posteroanterior projection of the pubic symphysis.

The Femur and Hip Joints

TABLE 5–1. Normal Degrees of Anteversion of the Femoral Neck*

Age	Anteversion (in degrees)
Birth to 1 year	30–50
2 years	30
3–5	25
6–12	20
13–15	17
16–20	11
Greater than 20	8

*Averages adapted from Billing, L.: Acta Radiol. Supp. *110*:1–80, 1954; and Budin, E., and Chandler, E.: Radiology *69*:209–213, 1951.

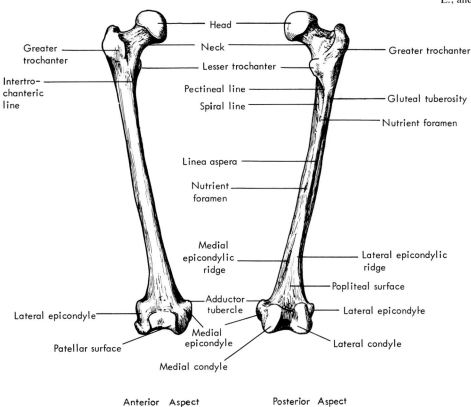

Anterior Aspect   Posterior Aspect

FIGURE 5–9 Diagram of anterior and posterior aspects of femur; anatomic parts are labeled.

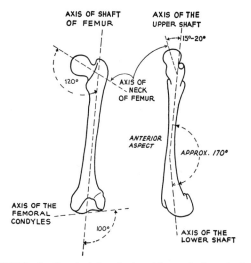

FIGURE 5–10 Axial relationships of the shaft of the femur. (Angles are approximations and not invariable.)

POINTS OF PRACTICAL INTEREST ABOUT FIGURE 5–11

1. The hip joint capsule is largely the ileofemoral ligament attached to the intertrochanteric line anteriorly, and to the ischial femoral ligament posteriorly. The "joint capsule" seen radiographically is largely the fatty sheath encompassing the muscles around the joint.

2. There may be 4 or more bursae adjoining the greater trochanter and one adjoining the ischial tuberosity.

3. The "os acetabuli" forms an extra ossicle that often adjoins the superior margin of the acetabulum.

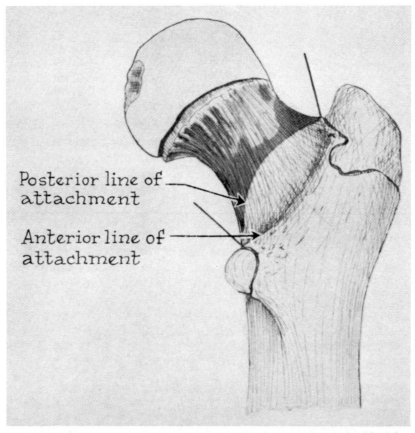

FIGURE 5–11 The line of attachment of the capsule of the hip joint. (Modified from Perry, in Morris' Human Anatomy, The Blakiston Co. Publishers.)

Special Projection to Measure Degree of Anteversion of the Hip (See Table 5–1 for Normal Values)

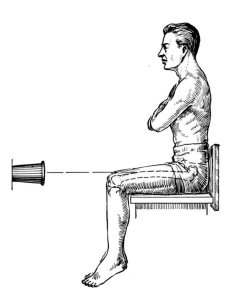

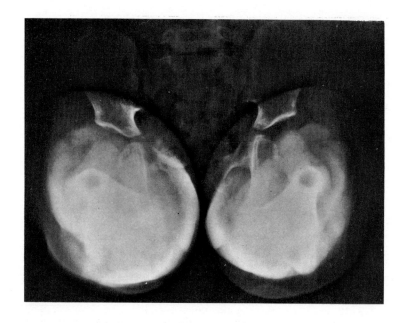

FIGURE 5–12 Special projection designed to measure the degree of anteversion of the neck of the femur with respect to the shaft. Note that the patient is positioned so that the central ray strikes the middle of the shaft of the femur, and not the knee joint proper. The shaft of the femur arches posteriorly. It is the *proximal* one-half of the femoral shaft which is horizontal and actually the distal one-half of the femur dips downward toward the floor slightly. It is this expedient which will permit a diagnostic film to be obtained using lumbosacral spine technical factors. Otherwise, the detail procured will be inadequate for measurement. In the film so obtained (shown intensified), the detail is poor, but adequate to draw the angle of anteversion as indicated in the tracing. One line is drawn along the inferior margins of the femoral condyles; the other is drawn through the axis of the neck of the femur. The angle between may then be measured.

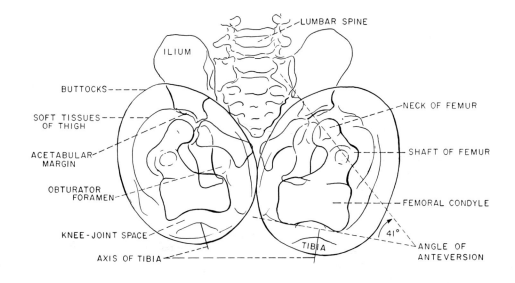

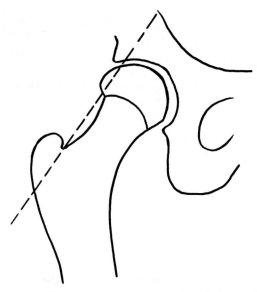

FIGURE 5–13 Line along the outer margin of the neck of the femur demonstrating the proper relationship of the head of the femur to the neck. This line should intersect the head in both the anteroposterior and lateral projections.

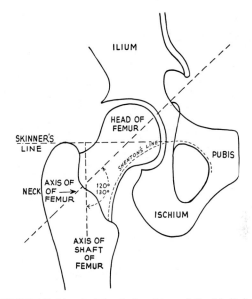

FIGURE 5–14 Axial relationships of the hip joint.

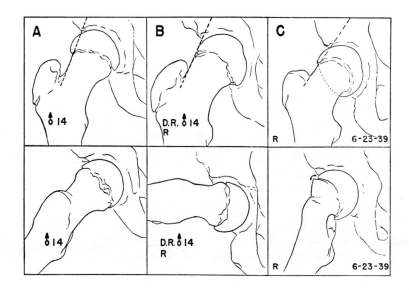

FIGURE 5–15 Medial and posterior slipping. *A*. Normal hip for comparison. *B*. Medial slipping. In this case, slipping is detectable only in the anteroposterior view where the head is not transected by the prolongation of the superior neck line. *C*. Posterior slipping. In the anteroposterior view the posteriorly displaced head is projected through the proximal portion of the neck. In the lateral view the amount of posterior slipping is denoted by the curved arrow. (From Klein, A., et al.: Am. J. Roentgenol., *66*, 1951.)

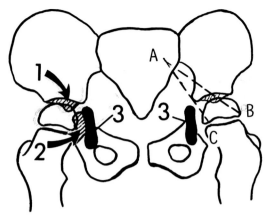

FIGURE 5–16 Areas to study for asymmetry in the growing hip. *1* and *2*. Overlap of posterior rim of acetabulum. *3*. Tear drops are symmetrical. Lines *AC* and *AB*: The heads of the femurs appear symmetrical when a triangle is drawn as shown. (After Martin, H. E.: Radiology, *56*:842, 1951.)

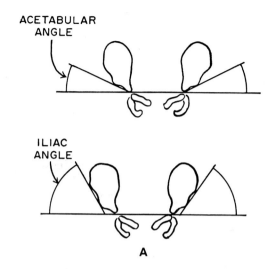

A

TABLE 5–2. Acetabular and Iliac Angles.

Category	Mean Acetabular Angle	Actual Range	SD	± 2 SD
Young normal infants less than 3 months of age	28°	44–12	4.7	37–18
Normal infants 3–12 months of age	22°	34–8	4.2	30–14
	Mean Iliac Angle			
Less than 3 months	81°	97–68	8.0	97–65
3–12 months	79°	101–62	9.0	96–60

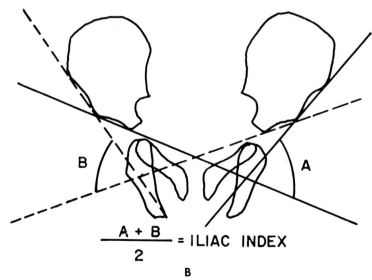

$$\frac{A + B}{2} = \text{ILIAC INDEX}$$

B

FIGURE 5–17 *A*. Acetabular and iliac angles. *B*. Tong's method for measuring the iliac index.

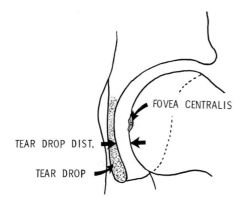

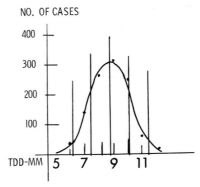

WHEN>11mm or 2mm>OPPOSITE HIP=ABNORMAL

A

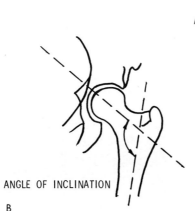

ANGLE OF ANTEVERSION

ANGLE OF INCLINATION

B

FIGURE 5–18 *A,* Line diagram showing the tear drop distance and the distribution of normal tear drop distances as measured in a large series of normal hips. Note that when the tear drop distance is greater than 11 mm. or when it is 2 mm. greater on one side than on the opposite side, the hip joint may be considered abnormal. This sign is one of the early indicators of osteochondrosis of the hip. (After Eyring, E. J., Bjornson, D. R., and Peterson, C. A.: Am. J. Roentgenol., *104*:851, 1968.) *B.* Diagrams illustrating methods of measurement of "angle of inclination" and "angle of anteversion" of head and neck of femur.

GENERAL COMMENTS REGARDING HIP JOINT RADIOGRAPHY

To provide accurate radiographs extreme care should be exercised in positioning the patient. The patient must be properly aligned, and no rotation of the pelvis may occur. A folded sheet or a piece of balsa wood placed under one side of the pelvis will compensate for any tilt that may be present.

Three degrees of rotation of the femur are commonly employed, each has a purpose in projection. The first rotation is made in the true anatomic position with the medial edge of the foot vertical. This position will permit visualization of both trochanters, with the image of the neck foreshortened because the axis of the neck is oblique to the plane of the film. This position is preferred by some, because it shows the anatomic relation between the femoral head and the acetabulum. It is easy to obtain and it is easy to reproduce.

The next rotation is with the femur rotated internally 20 degrees. With this position the axis of the neck becomes parallel to the plane of the film and thus more nearly projects the neck into its proportion. Orthopedic surgeons frequently request this method, since it permits more accurate measurement of the neck and the angle of inclination. This is the view generally preferred.

In the third rotation the lower extremity is rotated externally. The image of the head and neck is foreshortened, but the full profile of the lesser trochanter is brought into view.

In making both AP and lateral projections of the hips, one must utilize the same degree of rotation of the lower extremity for both projections so that the lateral projection will be a true 90 degrees perpendicular to the AP.

Routine Anteroposterior Projection of the Hip (Fig. 5–19)

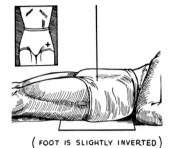

(FOOT IS SLIGHTLY INVERTED)

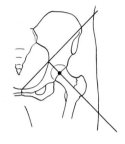

POINTS OF PRACTICAL INTEREST ABOUT FIGURE 5–19

1. The patient is placed in the perfectly supine position. The entire pelvis must be symmetrical even though only one side is considered.

2. *For maximum elongation and detail of the femoral neck, the foot is inverted approximately 15 to 20 degrees and immobilized in that position by means of a small sandbag.*

3. A line is drawn between the anterior-superior iliac spine and the superior margin of the pubic symphysis. The centering point is 1 inch distal to the midpoint of this line. Ordinarily, this will fall immediately over the hip joint proper.

4. If the foot is everted instead of inverted, the lesser trochanter will be shown in maximum detail and the neck of the femur will be completely foreshortened.

5. For maximum detail of both the greater and the lesser trochanter the foot should point directly upward and remain perpendicular to the table top at the time the film is obtained.

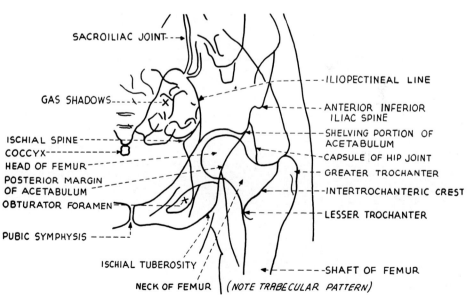

FIGURE 5–19 Routine anteroposterior projection of the hip.

Routine Lateral (Inferosuperior) Projection of Hips Employing a Horizontal X-ray Beam (Fig. 5–20)

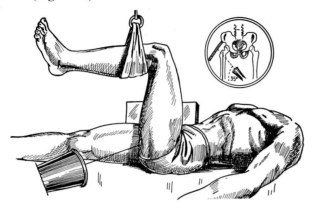

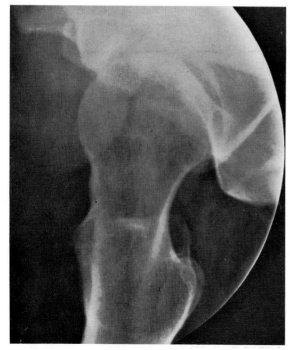

POINTS OF PRACTICAL INTEREST ABOUT FIGURE 5–20

1. The patient is placed in a supine position and the pelvis is elevated on a firm pillow or folded sheets, sufficiently to raise the ischial tuberosity approximately 3 cm. from the table top. This support of the gluteus must not extend beyond the lateral margin of the body so that it will not interfere with the placement of the cassette directly on the table top.

2. To localize the long axis of the femoral neck: (a) Draw a line between the anterior-superior iliac spine and the upper border of the pubic symphysis and mark its center point. (b) Next draw a line approximately 4 inches long perpendicular to this midpoint, extending down to the anterior surface of the thigh. This latter line represents the long axis of the femoral neck.

3. Adjust the central ray so that it is perpendicular to the midpoint of this long axis and adjust the film perpendicular to the table top so that the projection of this long axis will fall entirely upon the film. The plane of the film must be parallel to the axis of the neck of the femur.

4. If the foot is maintained in a vertical position the anteversion of the neck with respect to the shaft of the femur will be demonstrated. If the foot of the affected side is inverted approximately 15 degrees the plane of the neck will be parallel with the film and form a straight line with the axis of the shaft of the femur.

5. The unaffected side may be supported over the x-ray tube or by a sling from above as shown.

6. The thickness of the part traversed by the central ray is comparable with that of a lateral lumbar spine, and the same technical factors as for a lateral lumbar spine film should ordinarily be employed.

7. A grid cassette is a very desirable adjunct for this projection.

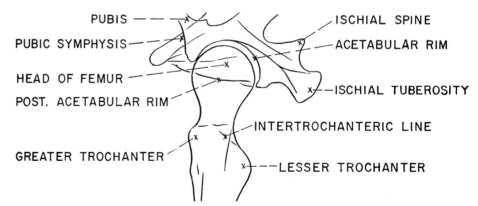

PUBIS — — — — — — ISCHIAL SPINE

PUBIC SYMPHYSIS — — — — ACETABULAR RIM

HEAD OF FEMUR — —

POST. ACETABULAR RIM — — — ISCHIAL TUBEROSITY

— INTERTROCHANTERIC LINE

GREATER TROCHANTER — — — — LESSER TROCHANTER

FIGURE 5–20 Routine lateral projection of hip, employing a horizontal x-ray beam. (Danelius-Miller modification of Lorenz position).

Lateral Projection of the Hip Employing the Frog-leg Position (Fig. 5–21)

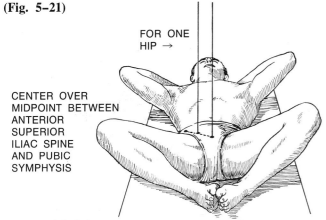

FOR ONE HIP →

CENTER OVER MIDPOINT BETWEEN ANTERIOR SUPERIOR ILIAC SPINE AND PUBIC SYMPHYSIS

POINTS OF PRACTICAL INTEREST ABOUT FIGURE 5–21

1. The "frog-leg" lateral projection of the hip is actually a useful but imperfect lateral perspective of the head, neck and upper shaft of the femur. The acetabulum remains in an anteroposterior relationship, and the normal anteversion of the neck of the femur with respect to the shaft is not shown. Moreover, this technique cannot be employed following most injuries in which the hip joint motion is very limited and painful. Nevertheless, it is particularly useful in analysis of suspected hip abnormalities in children, and when acetabular lateral perspectives are unnecessary. Technically, this view is easier to obtain than is the true lateral shown in Figure 5–20.

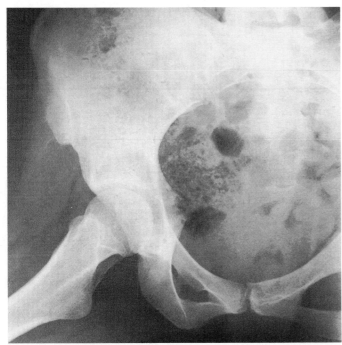

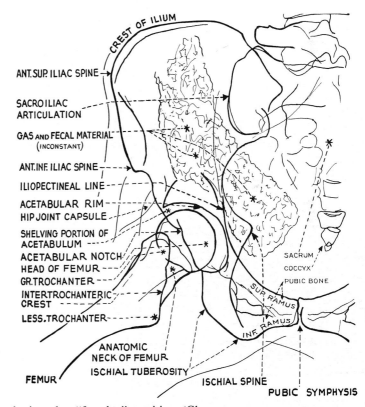

CREST OF ILIUM

ANT. SUP. ILIAC SPINE →

SACROILIAC ARTICULATION

GAS AND FECAL MATERIAL (INCONSTANT)

ANT. INF. ILIAC SPINE

ILIOPECTINEAL LINE

ACETABULAR RIM

HIP JOINT CAPSULE

SHELVING PORTION OF ACETABULUM

ACETABULAR NOTCH

HEAD OF FEMUR

GR. TROCHANTER

INTERTROCHANTERIC CREST

LESS. TROCHANTER

ANATOMIC NECK OF FEMUR

ISCHIAL TUBEROSITY

FEMUR

ISCHIAL SPINE

SACRUM

COCCYX

PUBIC BONE

SUP. RAMUS

INF. RAMUS

PUBIC SYMPHYSIS

FIGURE 5–21 Lateral projection of one hip, employing the "frog-leg" position (Cleaves position).

Frog-leg Lateral View of the Hip in an Adolescent (Fig. 5–22)

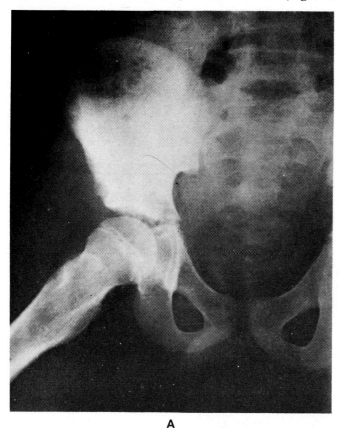

A

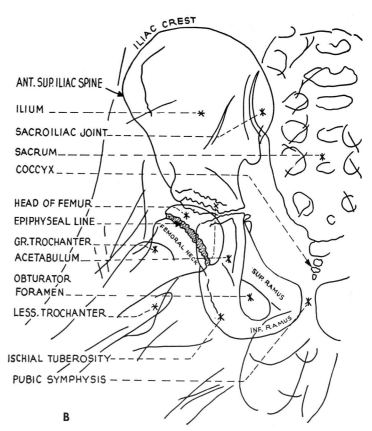

ANT. SUP. ILIAC SPINE

ILIUM

SACROILIAC JOINT

SACRUM

COCCYX

HEAD OF FEMUR

EPIPHYSEAL LINE

GR. TROCHANTER

ACETABULUM

OBTURATOR FORAMEN

LESS. TROCHANTER

ISCHIAL TUBEROSITY

PUBIC SYMPHYSIS

ILIAC CREST

FEMORAL NECK

SUP. RAMUS

INF. RAMUS

B

FIGURE 5–22 *A*. "Frog-leg" view in an adolescent, showing the relationship of the epiphyses. *B*. Labeled line tracing of *A*.

Hip Arthrography with Opaque Contrast Media (Barnett and Arcomano;* Laage et al.†). Methylglucamine diatrizoate in 20 per cent solution has been employed for definition of the following anatomic detail: the limbus of the joint; the thickness of the ligamentum teres; the fixation of the capsule to the ilium; the relationship of the uncalcified femoral head to the uncalcified limbus in children; the presence or ab-

sence of complete or partial dislocation, especially in children; and the degree of "hour-glassing" of the capsule.

This procedure is performed in selected cases, particularly prior to surgery. A needle is inserted anteriorly into the hip joint, usually just beneath the head of the femur, and 5 to 10 ml. of the methylglucamine diatrizoate solution are injected under fluoroscopic control. Appropriate films are obtained after moving the hip about for approximately 1 minute. Ideally, the films should be obtained with a 0.6 mm. focal spot, either by spot-film fluoroscopic techniques or by vertical x-ray beam and Bucky grid.

---

*Barnett, J. C., and Arcomano, J. P.: Hip arthrography in children with Renografin. Radiology, *73*:245–249, 1959.

†Laage, H. et al.: Horizontal lateral roentgenography of the hip in children. A preliminary report. J. Bone Joint Surg., *35–A*:387–389, 1953.

The Femur

Anteroposterior Projection of the Femur (Fig. 5-23)

1. The knee is adjusted to the true AP position and is included in the film.

2. The central ray is adjusted so that it is distal to the film, usually in a Bucky tray for the thicker thigh.

Routine Lateral Projection of the Thigh (Fig. 5-24)

1. The patient is placed on affected side and the knee is flexed, with the opposite thigh usually posterior.

2. The central ray is just distal to the midsection of the thigh. The knee joint is included.

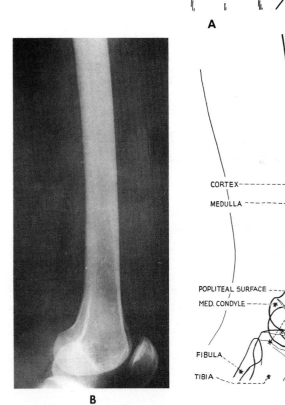

A

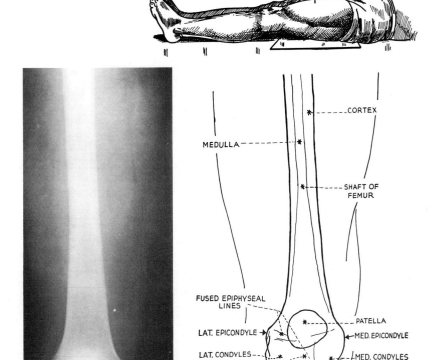

FIGURE 5-23 Routine anteroposterior projection of femur (adjudged accurately when condyles are equidistant from film).

B

C

FIGURE 5-24 Routine lateral projection of the thigh. *A.* Position of patient. *B.* Radiograph so obtained. *C.* Labeled line tracing of *B.* (Condyles should be almost perfectly superimposed for absolute excellence in radiographic technique.)

The Knee

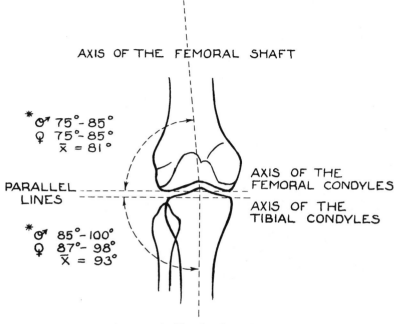

AXIS OF THE FEMORAL SHAFT

♂ 75°- 85°
♀ 75°- 85°
$\bar{x}$ = 81°

PARALLEL LINES

AXIS OF THE FEMORAL CONDYLES

AXIS OF THE TIBIAL CONDYLES

♂ 85°-100°
♀ 87°- 98°
$\bar{x}$ = 93°

AXIS OF THE TIBIAL SHAFT

* KEATS, T. E., ET AL. RADIOLOGY 87: 904, 1966

TABLE 5–3. Distance from the Lower Pole of the Patella to Blumensaat's Line in 44 Knees

Distance (cm)	No. of Knees
0.0	0
0.5	3
1.0	15
1.5	12
2.0	9
2.5	3
3.0	2
TOTAL	44

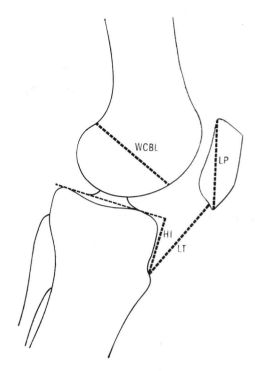

FIGURE 5–25 *A.* Axial relationships of the knee joint. *B.* Tracing of a radiograph of a normal knee showing the relationship of the patella to the femur and the tibia. Four measurements are obtained: LT (length of tendon), length of patellar tendon on its deep or posterior surface; LP (length of patella), greatest diagonal length of patella; WCBL (width of the femoral condyle at Blumensaat's line), both condyles measured at the level of Blumensaat's line and an average obtained; and HI (height of insertion), perpendicular distance from level of tibial condylar surface to the point of insertion of the patellar tendon. The point of insertion is represented on the radiograph by a clearly defined notch.

$$\frac{LT}{LP} = 1.02 \pm 0.13$$

$$\frac{LP}{WCBL} = 0.95 \pm 0.07 \text{ (in each instance, one standard deviation)}$$

$$\frac{LT}{HI} = 1.85 \pm 0.24$$

The length of the patellar tendon does not differ from that of the patella by more than 20 per cent.

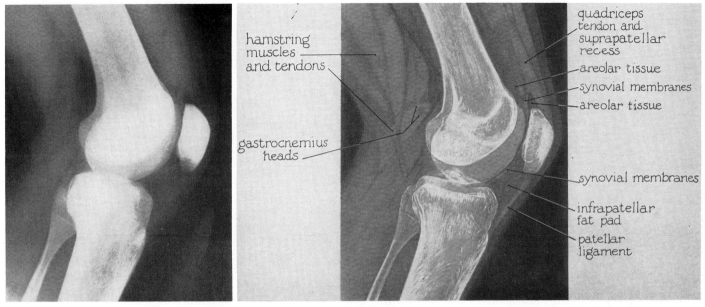

FIGURE 5–26   A normal lateral view of the knee with the associated soft tissue anatomy that can sometimes be identified either by routine views or by viewing the film with a bright light. (From Lewis, R. W.: Am. J. Roentgenol., *65*:200–220, 1951.)

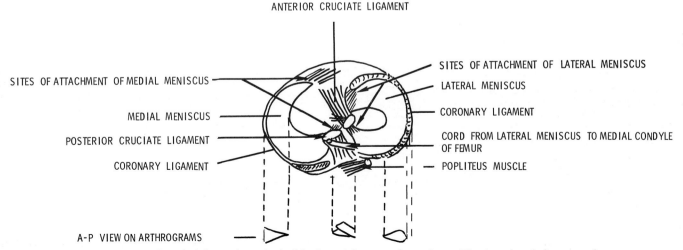

FIGURE 5–27   The condyles and menisci of the knee joint, seen from above. The correlated view on arthrograms is also shown.

Routine Anteroposterior Projection of the Knee (Fig. 5–28)

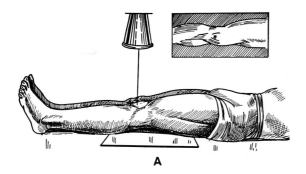

A

POINTS OF PRACTICAL INTEREST ABOUT FIGURE 5–28

1. The knee should be completely extended with the patient in the supine position. If the patient is unable to extend the knee completely, the postero-anterior projection is preferable.

2. Alternatively, if the knee cannot be fully extended the cassette may be elevated on sandbags to bring it into closer contact with the popliteal space. If the degree of flexion of the knee is great, a curved cassette or curved film holder should be employed.

3. The leg is adjusted in the true anteroposterior position and the distal apex of the patella is noted.

4. Center the cassette and the central ray of the x-ray tube approximately 1 cm. below the patellar apex.

5. When radiographing the joint space it may be helpful to tilt the tube approximately 5 degrees cephalad. This will help to give a clear view of the knee joint space because the superimposition of the anterior and posterior margins of the tibial plateau is somewhat more satisfactory.

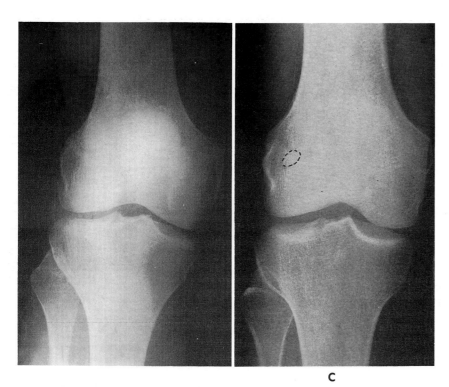

C

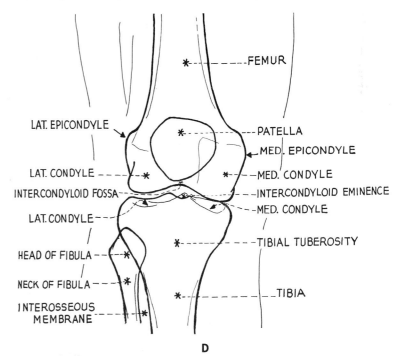

D

FIGURE 5–28   Routine anteroposterior projection of the knee. *A.* Method of positioning patient. *B.* Radiograph. *C.* Radiograph showing fabella. *D.* Labeled tracing of *B.* (The position drawing is of the left knee. The film shown is an antero-posterior projection of the right knee.)

Routine Lateral Projection of the Knee (Fig. 5–29)

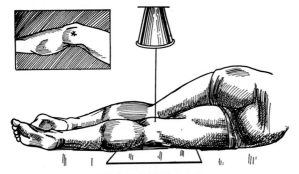

POINTS OF PRACTICAL INTEREST ABOUT FIGURE 5–29

1. The knee must be partially (20 to 30 degrees) flexed with its lateral aspect next to the film.

2. The central ray passes through the midcondylar plane and the knee joint space.

3. To superimpose the two tibial condyles, a 5 degree angulation cephalad may be employed.

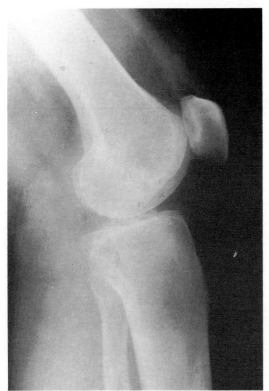

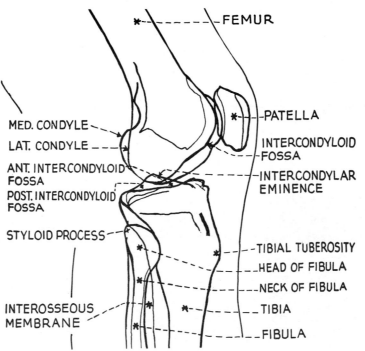

- FEMUR
- PATELLA
- MED. CONDYLE
- LAT. CONDYLE
- INTERCONDYLOID FOSSA
- ANT. INTERCONDYLOID FOSSA
- INTERCONDYLAR EMINENCE
- POST. INTERCONDYLOID FOSSA
- STYLOID PROCESS
- TIBIAL TUBEROSITY
- HEAD OF FIBULA
- NECK OF FIBULA
- TIBIA
- INTEROSSEOUS MEMBRANE
- FIBULA

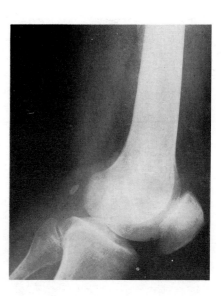

FIGURE 5–29 Routine lateral projection of knee. Radiograph at right demonstrates fabella on posterior aspect of femoral condyles.

Projection of the Intercondyloid Fossa of the Femur (Semiaxial or Tunnel Projection) (Fig. 5–30)

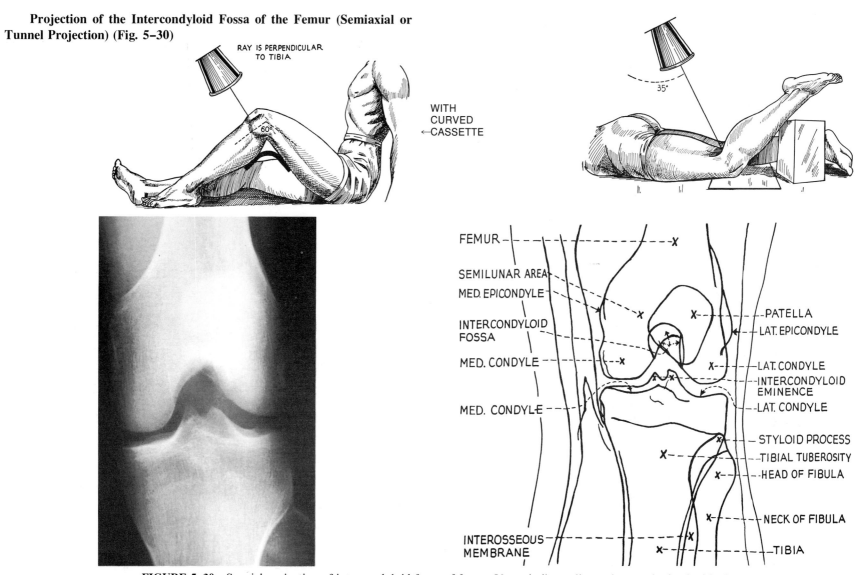

RAY IS PERPENDICULAR TO TIBIA

60°

WITH CURVED ←CASSETTE

35°

FEMUR ———————— x

SEMILUNAR AREA

MED. EPICONDYLE

INTERCONDYLOID FOSSA

MED. CONDYLE

MED. CONDYLE

INTEROSSEOUS MEMBRANE

PATELLA

LAT. EPICONDYLE

LAT. CONDYLE

INTERCONDYLOID EMINENCE

LAT. CONDYLE

STYLOID PROCESS

TIBIAL TUBEROSITY

HEAD OF FIBULA

NECK OF FIBULA

TIBIA

FIGURE 5–30 Special projection of intercondyloid fossa of femur. Very similar radiographs are obtained with alternate methods of positioning the patient (Camp-Coventry position with patient prone; Béclére position with patient sitting). These projections provide a clearer view of the knee joint space and may reveal a loose body within the joint when the other projections fail in this respect.

Posteroanterior Projection of the Patella (Fig. 5–31)

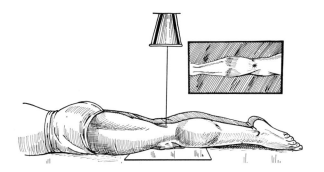

POINTS OF PRACTICAL INTEREST ABOUT FIGURE 5–31

1. The patient is placed in the prone position with the ankles and the feet usually supported by sandbags.

2. The film is centered to the patella and the central ray so adjusted as to pass through the center of the patella. The heel may have to be rotated outward slightly to accomplish this.

3. Ordinarily, it is desirable to use a telescopic cone and bring the cone fairly close to the knee in order to produce a distortion of the superimposed femoral condyles and a clearer concept of the patella, which lies next to the film.

4. This projection definitely gives better detail of the patella than can be obtained in the anteroposterior projection.

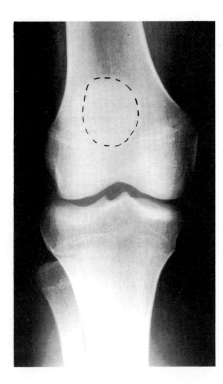

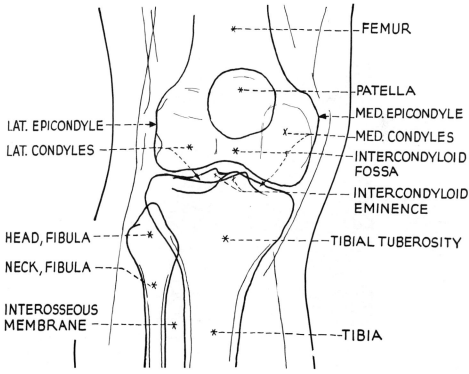

FIGURE 5–31 Posteroanterior projection of patella.

Tangential Projection of the Patella (Axial or "Sunrise" Projection) (Fig. 5–32)

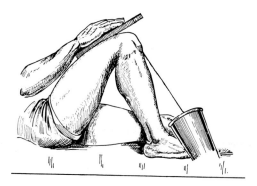

POINTS OF PRACTICAL INTEREST ABOUT FIGURE 5–32

1. This projection may be obtained with the patient either prone or supine. In the prone position, the thigh is placed flat against the table and the leg flexed by means of a band wrapped around the ankle and the ends held by the patient's hand. If the patient is supine, the film is placed along the distal aspect of the thigh as shown.

2. The central ray is directed at right angles to the joint space between the patella and the femoral condyles; the degree of central ray angulation depends upon the degree of flexion of the knee. Ordinarily the central ray should be parallel to the articular margin of the patella.

3. The outer margin of the patella as projected in this view frequently presents a rather serrated and irregular appearance which must not be interpreted as abnormal. This serrated appearance is due to points of tendinous attachments to the bony substance of the patella, as well as to penetration by nutrient vessels.

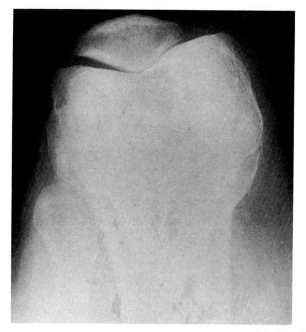

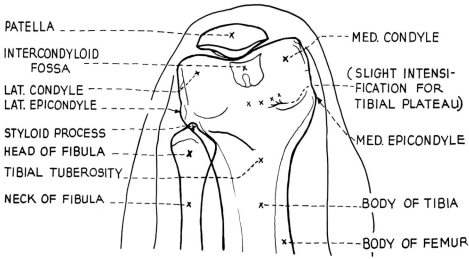

PATELLA

INTERCONDYLOID FOSSA

LAT. CONDYLE
LAT. EPICONDYLE

STYLOID PROCESS
HEAD OF FIBULA

TIBIAL TUBEROSITY

NECK OF FIBULA

MED. CONDYLE

(SLIGHT INTENSIFICATION FOR TIBIAL PLATEAU)

MED. EPICONDYLE

BODY OF TIBIA

BODY OF FEMUR

FIGURE 5–32 Special tangential projection of patella (Settegast position).

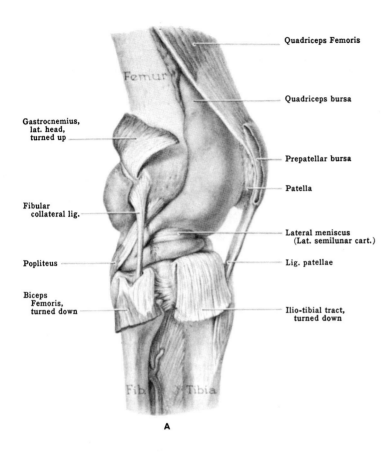

Quadriceps Femoris

Quadriceps bursa

Prepatellar bursa

Patella

Lateral meniscus
(Lat. semilunar cart.)

Lig. patellae

Ilio-tibial tract,
turned down

Gastrocnemius,
lat. head,
turned up

Fibular
collateral lig.

Popliteus

Biceps
Femoris,
turned down

A

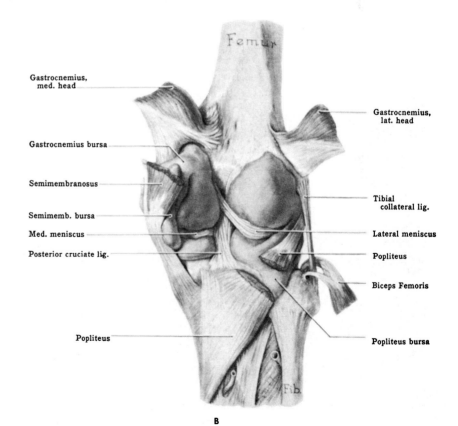

Gastrocnemius,
med. head

Gastrocnemius bursa

Semimembranosus

Semimemb. bursa

Med. meniscus

Posterior cruciate lig.

Popliteus

Gastrocnemius,
lat. head

Tibial
collateral lig.

Lateral meniscus

Popliteus

Biceps Femoris

Popliteus bursa

B

FIGURE 5–33 *A.* Distended knee joint, lateral view, demonstrating bursae. *B.* Distended knee joint, posterior view. (Reproduced by permission from Grant, J. C. B.: An Atlas of Anatomy, 5th ed. Copyright © 1962, The Williams & Wilkins Company.)

Arthrography of the Knee (Double Contrast)

1. Oblique views are also obtained in each position.

2. Modified simplified apparatus: A single board is used taped to the ankle and the thigh, but the "spreader" block is maintained as shown.

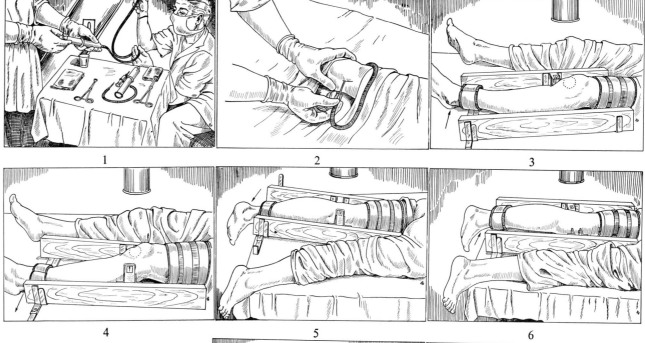

FIGURE 5–34 Routine technique of arthrography of the knee.

1. Method of loading syringe with contrast agent.

2. Method of inserting needle under the superior margin of the patella into the suprapatellar bursa where 10 to 15 ml. of meglumine diatrizoate is thereafter injected with about 10 ml. of air.

3. Method of positioning the patient for the anteroposterior view of the lateral meniscus. Note the lateral side of the knee joint is being spread by a special device for this purpose. Actually only one board is necessary, and the double board device is not needed.

4. Method of positioning patient for anteroposterior view of the medial meniscus, spreading the medial side of the knee joint. Again, only one board is necessary, not two.

5. Method of positioning for posteroanterior view of lateral meniscus.

6. Method of positioning patient for posteroanterior view of medial meniscus.

7. Method of positioning patient for a horizontal or decubitus view of the lateral meniscus in anteroposterior projection.

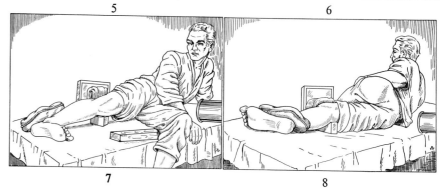

8. Method of positioning patient by employing a horizontal beam spreading the medial joint space. In both of these latter projections, air —if present in small amounts—rises to the top, whereas the contrast agent falls to the bottom by gravity, thereby providing a maximum double-contrast delineation of the top-most portion of the knee as well as the meniscus, still obtaining a spread visualization of the knee.

Arthrography of the Knee

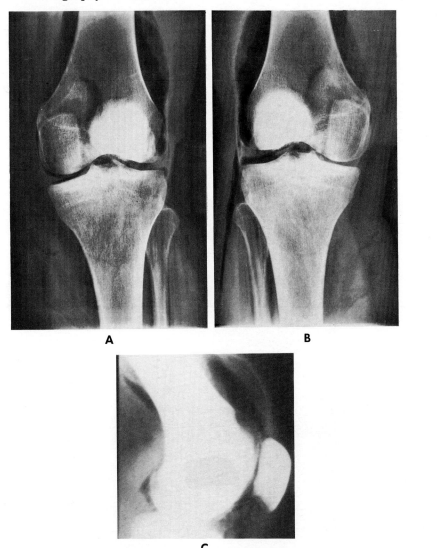

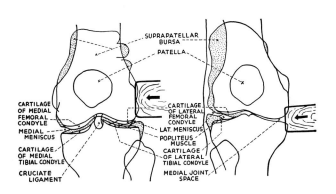

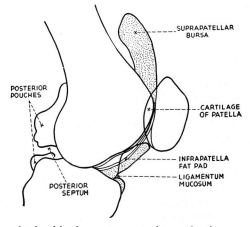

FIGURE 5–35 Pneumoarthrography of the knee. Radiographs *A* and *B* were obtained in the posteroanterior projection, first with the medial knee joint spread, and next with the lateral knee joint spread; *C* shows the knee in a straight lateral projection.

Arthrography of the Knee

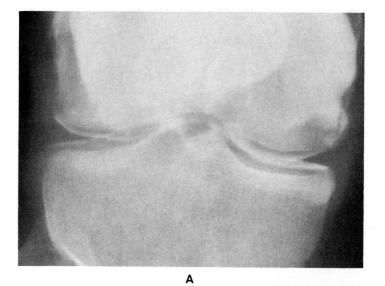

A

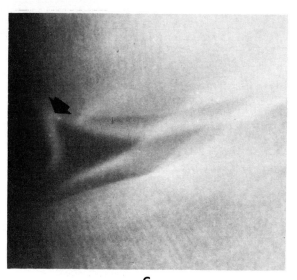

B

C

FIGURE 5–36 Opaque contrast arthrograms of the knee. *A* and *B* represent normal or variations of normal. The arrow in *B* points toward a normal undulation often found in the lateral meniscus. *C* shows a fracture through the medial meniscus and its appearance with opaque media.

The Patella

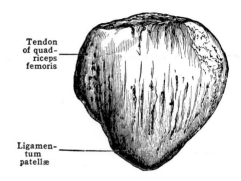

Anterior surface

Tendon
of quad-
riceps
femoris

Ligamen-
tum
patellæ

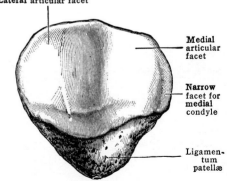

Posterior surface
Lateral articular facet

Medial
articular
facet

Narrow
facet for
medial
condyle

Ligamen-
tum
patellæ

FIGURE 5–37 The patella—anterior and posterior. (From Anson, B. J. (ed.): Morris' Human Anatomy, 12th ed. Copyright © 1966 by McGraw-Hill, Inc. Used by permission of McGraw-Hill Book Company.)

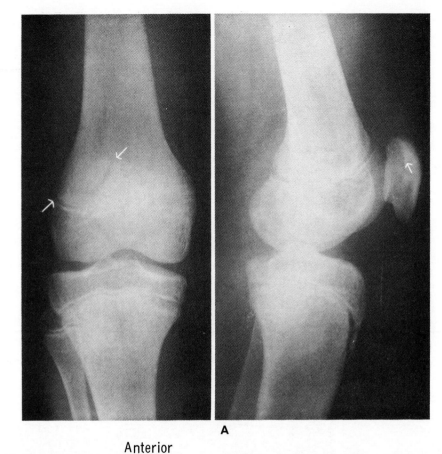

A

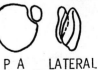

Medial

Anterior

P A   LATERAL

VARIOUS SHAPES OF PATELLA PARTITA

(MODIFIED FROM KÖHLER-ZIMMER
3rd AMERICAN EDITION, P. 436)

B

FIGURE 5–38 *A*. Bipartite patella. *B*. Various shapes of patella partita.

Correlated Anatomy of the Tibia and Fibula

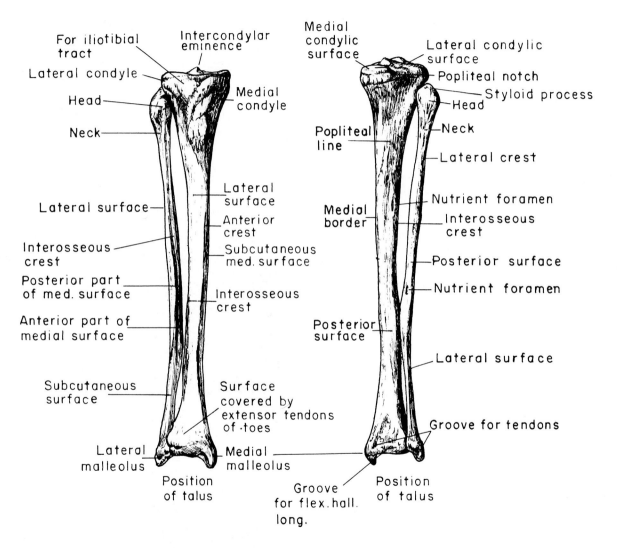

For iliotibial tract

Intercondylar eminence

Lateral condyle

Head

Neck

Medial condyle

Lateral surface

Lateral surface

Anterior crest

Subcutaneous med. surface

Interosseous crest

Posterior part of med. surface

Interosseous crest

Anterior part of medial surface

Subcutaneous surface

Surface covered by extensor tendons of toes

Lateral malleolus

Medial malleolus

Position of talus

Medial condylic surface

Lateral condylic surface

Popliteal notch

Styloid process

Head

Neck

Popliteal line

Lateral crest

Nutrient foramen

Medial border

Interosseous crest

Posterior surface

Nutrient foramen

Posterior surface

Lateral surface

Groove for tendons

Groove for flex. hall. long.

Position of talus

Anterior Aspect   Posterior Aspect

FIGURE 5–39 Tibia and fibula, anterior and posterior aspects.

Routine Anteroposterior Projection of the Leg (Fig. 5–40)

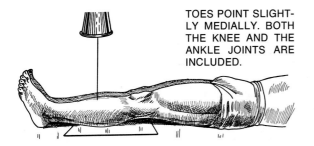

TOES POINT SLIGHT-
LY MEDIALLY. BOTH
THE KNEE AND THE
ANKLE JOINTS ARE
INCLUDED.

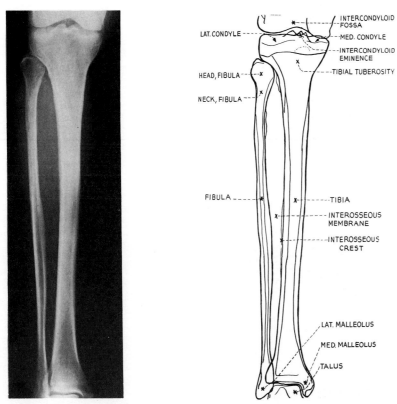

INTERCONDYLOID
FOSSA

LAT. CONDYLE

MED. CONDYLE

INTERCONDYLOID
EMINENCE

TIBIAL TUBEROSITY

HEAD, FIBULA

NECK, FIBULA

FIBULA — TIBIA

INTEROSSEOUS
MEMBRANE

INTEROSSEOUS
CREST

LAT. MALLEOLUS

MED. MALLEOLUS

TALUS

FIGURE 5–40 Routine anteroposterior projection of right leg. (Left leg is shown in diagram. Anteroposterior projection of right leg is shown in radiograph.)

Lateral Projection of the Leg (Fig. 5–41)

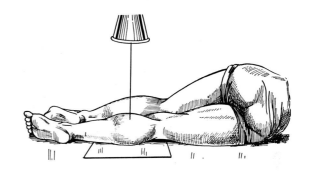

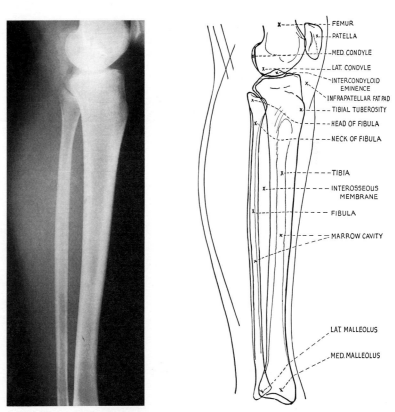

FEMUR

PATELLA

MED. CONDYLE

LAT. CONDYLE

INTERCONDYLOID
EMINENCE

INFRAPATELLAR FAT PAD

TIBIAL TUBEROSITY

HEAD OF FIBULA

NECK OF FIBULA

TIBIA

INTEROSSEOUS
MEMBRANE

FIBULA

MARROW CAVITY

LAT. MALLEOLUS

MED. MALLEOLUS

FIGURE 5–41 Routine lateral projection of leg.

The Foot and Ankle

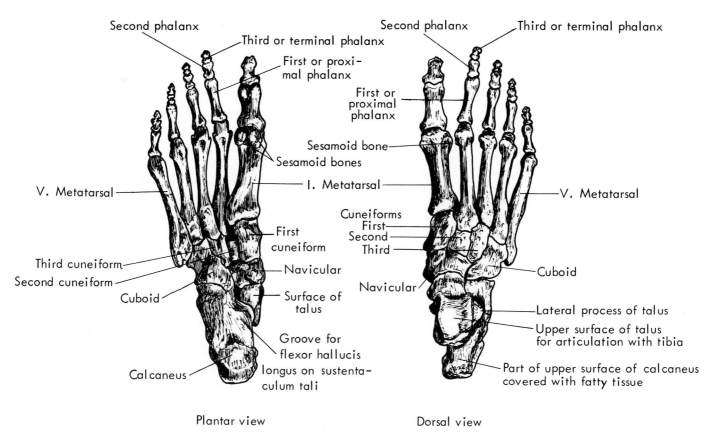

Second phalanx

Third or terminal phalanx

First or proxi-
mal phalanx

Second phalanx

Third or terminal phalanx

First or
proximal
phalanx

Sesamoid bone

Sesamoid bones

V. Metatarsal

I. Metatarsal

V. Metatarsal

Cuneiforms
First
Second
Third

First
cuneiform

Third cuneiform

Second cuneiform

Navicular

Navicular

Cuboid

Surface of
talus

Cuboid

Lateral process of talus

Calcaneus

Groove for
flexor hallucis
longus on sustenta-
culum tali

Upper surface of talus
for articulation with tibia

Part of upper surface of calcaneus
covered with fatty tissue

Plantar view

Dorsal view

FIGURE 5–42 Plantar and dorsal views of the foot.

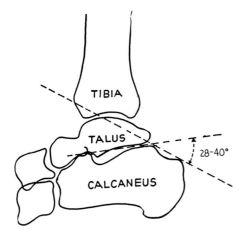

FIGURE 5–43 The criteria for a normal calcaneus (Boehler).

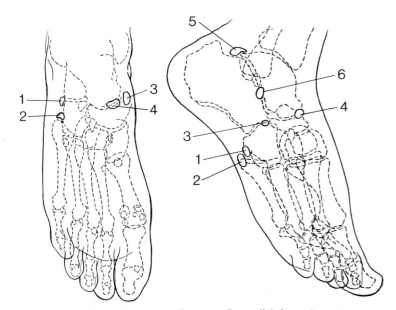

1, os peroneum; 2, os vesalianum; 3, os tibiale externum;
4, accessory navicular; 5, os trigonum; 6, os sustentaculum

FIGURE 5–44 Schematic diagram showing sesamoid bones and most frequently encountered supernumerary bones of the foot.

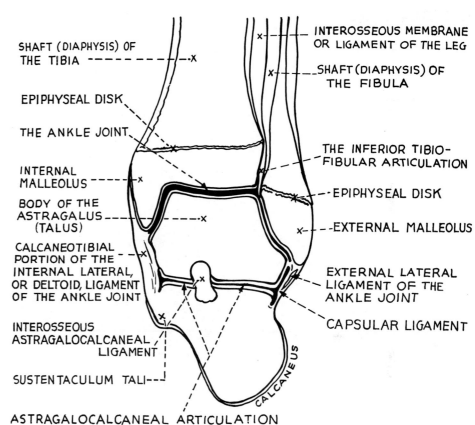

FIGURE 5–45 Coronal section through the ankle joint. (After Toldt, C.: An Atlas of Anatomy for Students and Physicians. New York, Macmillan Co., © 1926.)

Parallelism of the Articular Surfaces of the Ankle Joint

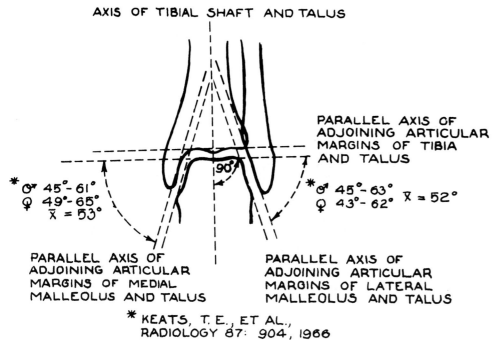

AXIS OF TIBIAL SHAFT AND TALUS

PARALLEL AXIS OF ADJOINING ARTICULAR MARGINS OF TIBIA AND TALUS

90°

* ♂ 45°- 61°
♀ 49°- 65°
X̄ = 53°

* ♂ 45°- 63°
♀ 43°- 62° X̄ = 52°

PARALLEL AXIS OF ADJOINING ARTICULAR MARGINS OF MEDIAL MALLEOLUS AND TALUS

PARALLEL AXIS OF ADJOINING ARTICULAR MARGINS OF LATERAL MALLEOLUS AND TALUS

* KEATS, T. E., ET AL., RADIOLOGY 87: 904, 1966

A

FIGURE 5–46 *A*. Diagram illustrating parallelism of articular surfaces of the ankle joint. *B*. Measurement of axial angles of the ankle. (From Lusted, L. B., and Keats, T. E.: Atlas of Roentgenographic Measurement, 3rd ed. Copyright © 1972 by Year Book Medical Publishers, Inc., Chicago. Used by permission.)

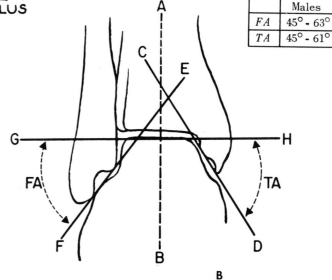

A

C

E

G ——————— H

FA

TA

F

B

D

B

	Males	Females	Av.
FA	45° - 63°	43° - 62°	52°
TA	45° - 61°	49° - 65°	53°

Routine Anteroposterior Projection of the Ankle (Fig. 5–47)

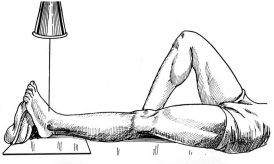

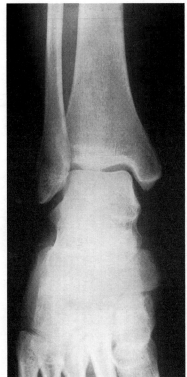

POINTS OF PRACTICAL INTEREST ABOUT FIGURE 5–47

1. If less overlapping of the distal tibia and fibula is desired, the foot should be inverted slightly. This expedient will increase the clarity of the lateral malleolus particularly, but will interfere with the measurement of the distance between the talal articular margin and the malleoli.

2. In young individuals, in whom the distal epiphyses of the tibia and fibula are not yet united to their respective shafts, it is particularly important to obtain comparison films of the opposite normal side. It may otherwise be very difficult to be certain of the absence of a slight fracture through the epiphyseal disk.

3. Although the ligaments around the ankle are not visualized radiographically, it is important to know their relationships accurately. Often the more important aspect of injury to the ankle concerns the ligamentous rather than the bony abnormality.

4. Center over midpoint between malleoli.

5. Immobilize at the knee and foot as shown.

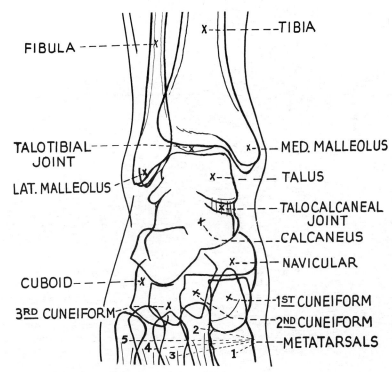

FIGURE 5–47 Routine anteroposterior projection of the right ankle. (Left ankle shown in projection drawing.)

Oblique Projection of the Ankle (Fig. 5–48)

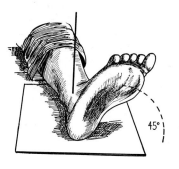

POINTS OF PRACTICAL INTEREST ABOUT FIGURE 5–48

1. As much as possible, keep the leg in the anteroposterior position while inverting the foot approximately 45 degrees. Immobilize with sandbags placed across the leg and against the plantar surface of the foot.

2. The central ray is directed to the middle of the talotibial joint.

3. This projection permits an unobstructed demonstration of the lateral malleolus and of the space between the talus and malleolus where so frequently injury may be manifest.

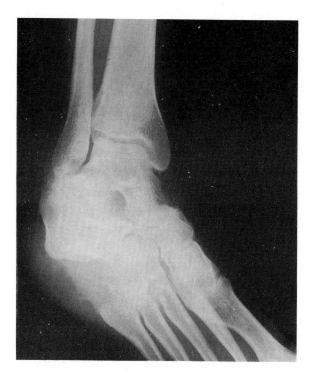

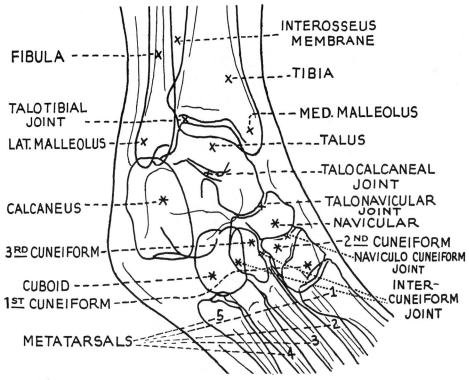

FIGURE 5–48 Oblique projection of ankle.

THE ANKLE / 135

Routine Lateral Projection of the Ankle (Fig. 5–49)

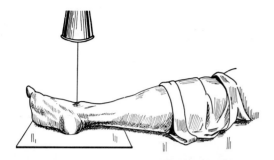

POINTS OF PRACTICAL INTEREST ABOUT FIGURE 5–49

1. The affected leg and ankle are so placed that the sagittal plane of the leg is perfectly parallel with the table top and film. The film holder and central ray are centered to a point approximately 2 cm. proximal to the tip of the lateral malleolus. A sandbag or balsa wood block placed under the distal one-third of the foot and under the knee facilitates true alignment.

2. The unaffected side is sharply flexed and placed in a comfortable position forward so that there will be no movement during the x-ray exposure.

3. The foot may be positioned perpendicular to the leg, if permissible.

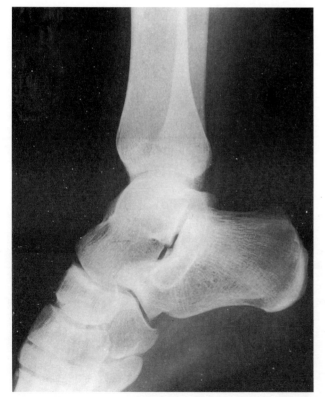

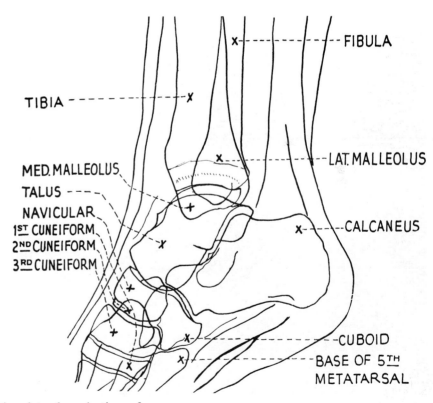

FIGURE 5–49 Routine lateral projection of ankle.

Special Tangential Projection of the Calcaneus (Os Calcis) (Fig. 5-50)

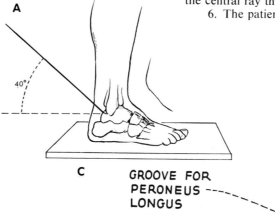

A

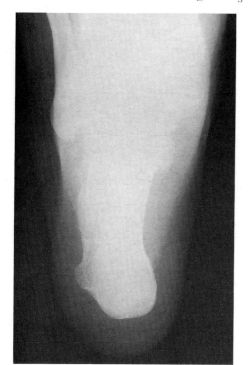

B

POINTS OF PRACTICAL INTEREST ABOUT FIGURE 5-50

1. The ankle is placed over the film so that the talotibial joint falls over the central portion of the film.

2. The plantar surface of the foot should be at as near to a right angle with the table top and film as possible in acute flexion.

3. The central ray should be centered to the midpoint of the film. It will usually enter the plantar surface at the level of the bases of the fifth metatarsals and emerge in the region of the upper tarsus.

4. Ordinarily all portions of the calcaneus are included between the tuberosity and the sustentaculum tali.

5. An alternate view may be obtained by placing the patient prone, film perpendicular to the table top in contact with the sole of the foot, and directing the central ray through the heel with 45 degree caudad angulation.

6. The patient may be standing in this alternate view.

C

GROOVE FOR PERONEUS LONGUS

TROCHLEAR PROCESS

LAT. PROCESS

SULCUS FOR FLEX. HALLUCIS LONGUS

SUSTENTACULUM TALI

TALOCALCANEAL ARTICULATION

MED. PROCESS

TUBEROSITY

D

FIGURE 5-50 Special tangential projection of the right calcaneus. *A* and *C* are alternate positioning diagrams for this projection. *B* is a radiograph so obtained, and *D* is a labeled tracing of *B*. In each instance a special tangential projection of the calcaneus is obtained. (*A* is a position drawing of the left calcaneus. *B*, *C* and *D* are the right.)

Anteroposterior Projection of the Foot (Fig. 5–51)

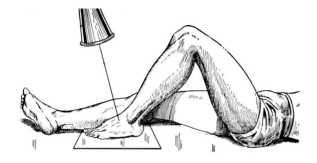

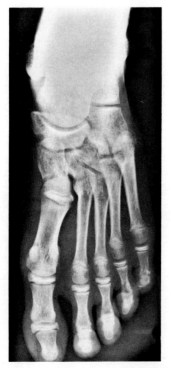

POINTS OF PRACTICAL INTEREST ABOUT FIGURE 5–51

1. It will be noted that for visualization of the entire tarsus, both this projection and the anteroposterior projection of the ankle (Fig. 5–47) are necessary. The talus is not shown to good advantage in this projection, whereas the more distal tarsal bones are not presented clearly in the anteroposterior projection of the ankle.

2. For special problems, this projection may also be required with the patient standing and bearing his weight.

3. The foot is flat on the film. The proximal end of the second metatarsal is centered to the film.

4. The tube is angled 10 degrees cephalad.

5. Sandbags are placed behind the middle third of the patient's leg.

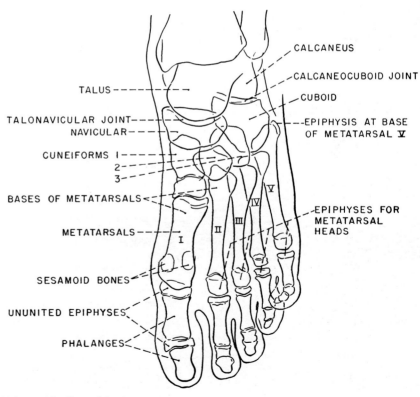

FIGURE 5–51 Anteroposterior projection of foot.

Oblique Projection of the Foot (Fig. 5–52)

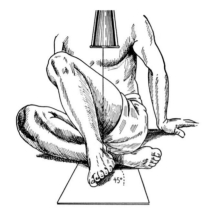

POINTS OF PRACTICAL INTEREST ABOUT FIGURE 5-52

1. This projection is particularly valuable (*a*) to demonstrate the intertarsal joints; (*b*) to outline the various tarsal bones more clearly; (*c*) to demonstrate the joint between the tarsus and the fourth and fifth metatarsals as well as the structural detail of the base of the fifth metatarsal.

2. This oblique projection is employed when structural detail of the bones of the foot is of paramount interest. It is ordinarily employed along with the anteroposterior projection of the foot. When, however, we desire to localize a foreign body accurately, it is the true lateral projection of the foot which is employed instead of this oblique projection.

3. The outer half of the foot is elevated as shown.

4. A point halfway between the ends of the foot is centered to the film.

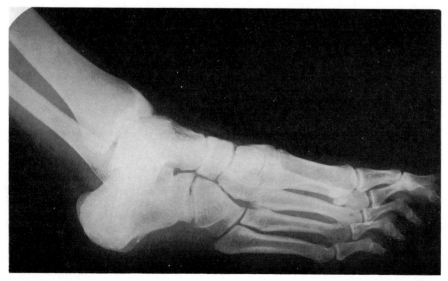

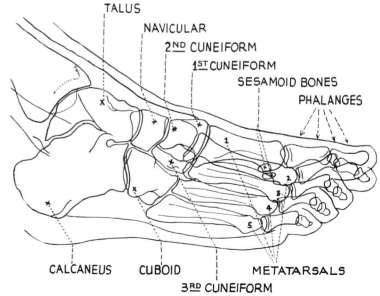

FIGURE 5–52 Oblique projection of foot.

Lateral Projection of the Foot (Fig. 5–53)

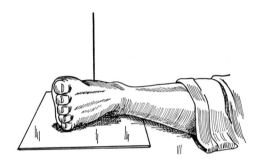

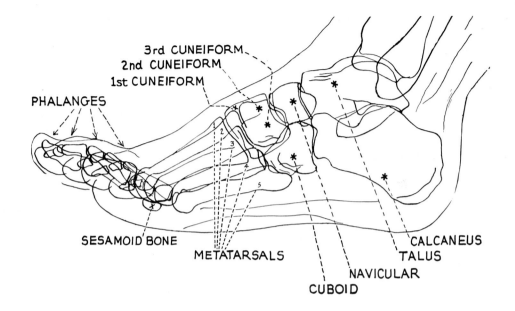

3rd CUNEIFORM
2nd CUNEIFORM
1st CUNEIFORM

PHALANGES

SESAMOID BONE

METATARSALS

CUBOID

NAVICULAR

TALUS

CALCANEUS

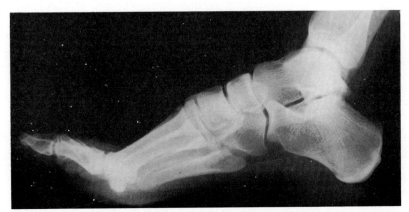

FIGURE 5–53 Lateral projection of foot.

POINTS OF PRACTICAL INTEREST ABOUT FIGURE 5–53

1. The knee may be elevated slightly on a sandbag so that the sagittal plane of the foot is perfectly parallel with the table top and film. The center of the tarsus is placed over the center of the film.

2. The ankle is immobilized by means of a sandbag.

3. The recumbent position is utilized to demonstrate the bony structure particularly. If one is desirous of showing the longitudinal arch under weight-bearing conditions, an erect film is obtained with the patient standing, but in rather similar fashion.

4. If a coned-down lateral view of the body of the calcaneus is desired, the foot is positioned similarly, but the central ray passes through the central portion of the calcaneus rather than through the center of the tarsus. The latter view of the calcaneus is particularly valuable for demonstration of Boehler's critical angle.

Standard Projections of the Foot

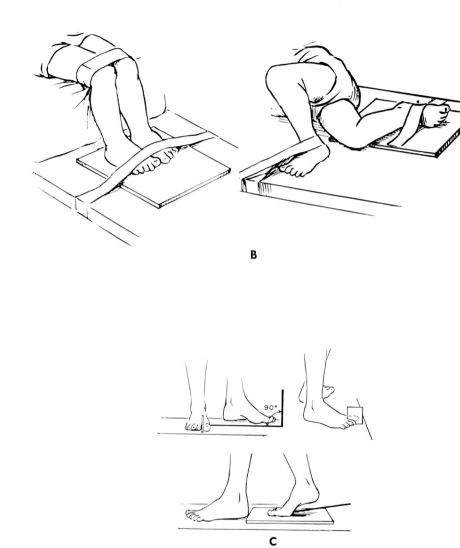

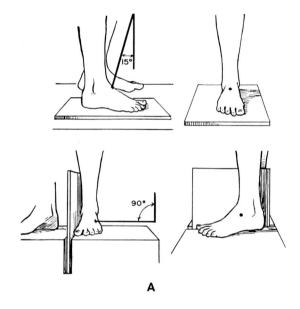

FIGURE 5–54 *A.* Standard projections of the foot. 1. Weight-supporting dorsoplantar projection: 2. weight-supporting lateral view (film support as devised by Gamble and Yale). *B.* Special technique for dorsoplantar and lateral projections of the feet in children (modified from Davis and Hatt). *C.* Special projections of the foot. *Upper.* Special lateral view of the great toe: *lower.* special axial projection for the ball of the foot and for the sesamoids (modified from Gamble and Yale). (*A, B,* and *C* from Meschan. I.: Sem. Roentgenol., 5:327–340, 1970. Reprinted by permission of Grune & Stratton, Inc.)

The Foot: Sesamoids; Talocalcaneal Angle: Growth and Development

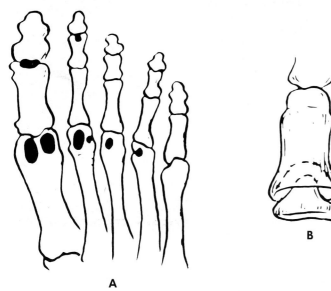

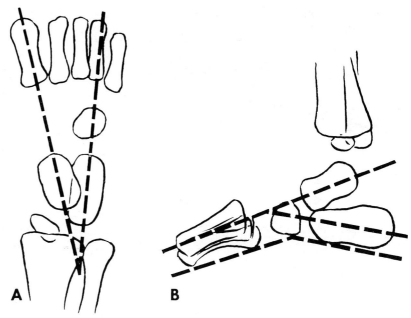

FIGURE 5–55 *A*. The most frequent sesamoids of the foot (modified from Köhler and Zimmer). *B*. Conical or bell-shaped epiphysis. According to Laurent and Brombart, they occur in the proximal phalanges of the second to the fourth toes. (From Meschan, I.: Sem. Roentgenol., *5*:327–340, 1970. Reprinted by permission of Grune & Stratton, Inc.)

FIGURE 5–56 Talocalcaneal angle in the dorsoplantar (*A*) and lateral (*B*) views in children. (From Davis, L. A., and Hatt, W. S.: Radiology, *64*:818, 1955.)

FIGURE 5–57 Changes in growth and development in the foot.

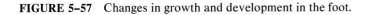

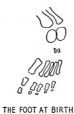

THE FOOT AT BIRTH

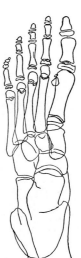

THE FOOT AT 5 YEARS

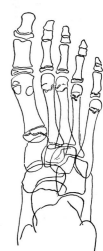

THE FOOT AT 8 YEARS   THE FOOT AT 16 YEARS

Calcaneal Pitch and Tarsometatarsal Relationships of the Foot

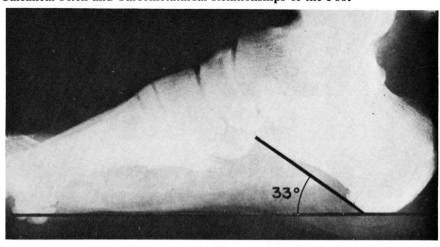

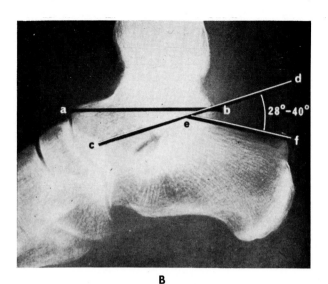

A   B

FIGURE 5–58 *A*. The calcaneal pitch is an index of the height of the foot framework. In this instance, the pitch is high since it exceeds 30 degrees. *B*. Boehler's critical angle of the os calcis; *cd* is drawn from the most superior anterior aspect of the os calcis to the joint space between the talus and the os calcis; *ef* is drawn from this joint to the most superior posterior point on the tuberosity of the os calcis. The diagonal axis of the talus (*ab*) is nearly horizontal. (From Meschan, I.: Sem. Roentgenol., 5:327–430, 1970. Reprinted by permission of Grune & Stratton, Inc.)

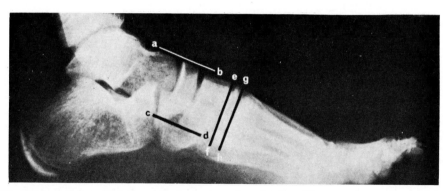

FIGURE 5–59 Tarsometatarsal relationships in the lateral projection. The superior surfaces of the talus, navicular, and first cuneiform tend to form a fairly straight line (*ab*). The inferior surfaces of the navicular and first cuneiform also tend to form a straight line, *cd*, parallel to *ab*. The cuneiform-metatarsal joints (*ef* and *gh*) are almost perpendicular to *ab* and *cd*. The degree of their obliquity with respect to the horizontal depends on the angular relationship of the long axis of the talus to the calcaneal pitch. (From Meschan, I.: Sem. Roentgenol., 5:327–340, 1970. Reprinted by permission of Grune & Stratton, Inc.)

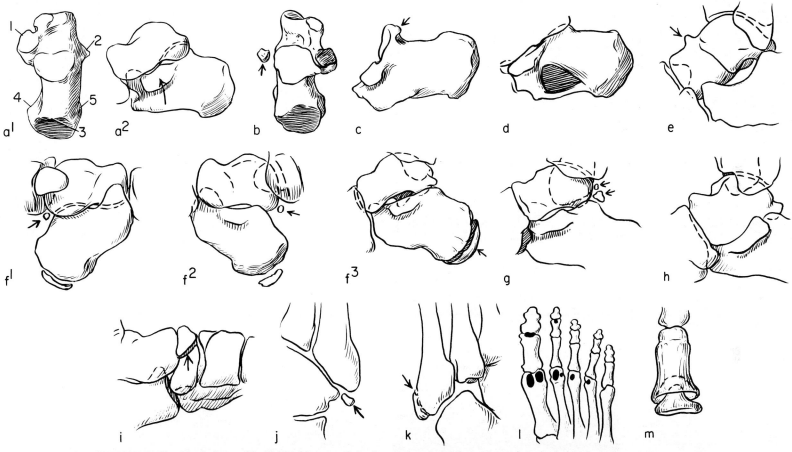

FIGURE 5–60 Variations of individual bones of the foot: a^1 and a^2. Normal os calcis: (1) sustentaculum tali; (2) trochlear process; (3) tuberosity; (4) medial process; and (5) lateral process. a^2. Unduly prominent sustentaculum tali on the medial border of the os calcis (arrow). *b*. The trochlear process of the os calcis as a separate ossicle, or apophysis. *c*. Secondary calcaneus fused with the anterior articular surface of the calcaneus and having a "swallow tail" prominence. This usually articulates with the talus and the cuboid. *d*. Cystlike appearance within the trabecular pattern of the os calcis due to locally increased spongy architecture, *e*, Spur on the anterior superior aspect of the talus near its anterior articular margin, producing a "turned up" appearance. f^1, f^2, and f^3. Variations in the appearance of the calcaneal epiphysis (arrow in f^3). The arrows in f^1 and f^2 point to a small os trigonum. *g*. Bipartite os trigonum (arrows). *h*. Spur on the anterior superior aspect of the talus near its anterior articular margin, producing a "turned-up" appearance. *i*. Bipartite navicular bone (arrow) may be mistaken for a fracture. *j*. Os vesalianum, located in the angle between the cuboid and the tuberosity of the fifth metatarsal (arrow) may be mistaken for a fracture. *k*. An apophysis at the base of the fifth metatarsal (arrow) may simulate a fracture. *l*. The most frequent sesamoids of the foot (modified from Köhler and Zimmer). *m*. Conical or bell-shaped epiphysis. According to Laurent and Brombart, they occur in the proximal phalanges of the second to the fourth toes. (From Meschan, I.: Sem. Roentgenol., 5:327–340, 1970. Reprinted by permission of Grune & Stratton, Inc.)

Relationships of the Midline of the Foot

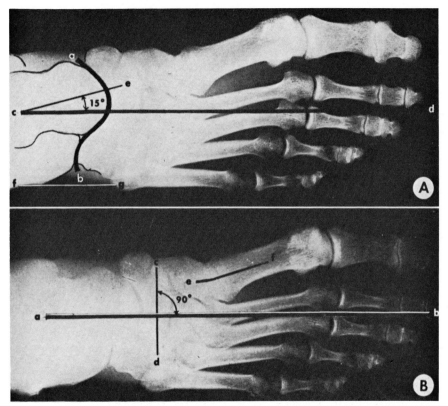

FIGURE 5–61 Relationships of the midline of the foot in the dorsoplantar view. *A.* The midline of the foot is represented by *cd* (see text); *dce* indicates a normal angle of approximately 15 degrees with the midaxis of the talus. The lateral border of the foot (*fg*) is parallel to *cd*. The partial sine wave curve formed by the midtarsal joint line (*ab*) is bisected by *cd*. *B.* The midline is represented by *ab*. There is a perpendicular relationship to the transverse axis of the navicular (*cd*), and an angle of approximately 15 degrees with the longitudinal axis of the first metatarsal (*ef*). (From Meschan, I.: Sem. Roentgenol., 5:327–340, 1970. Reprinted by permission of Grune & Stratton, Inc.)

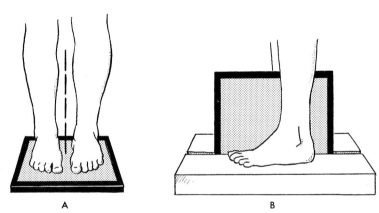

FIGURE 5–62 *A. Anteroposterior projection—weight-bearing:* Patient stands upright with equal weight on both feet, film beneath the feet on the floor. The feet are placed close together. The central ray is halfway between the two metacarpals at their proximal end, 10 degrees cephalad. *B. Lateral weight-bearing:* Patient stands on two balsa wood blocks, 3 inches high. The film is between the feet, perpendicular to the table top; central ray is midway between the heel and toes and is horizontal. *Patient should be carefully supported in this hazardous position.*

VASCULAR ANATOMY AND ANGIOLOGY

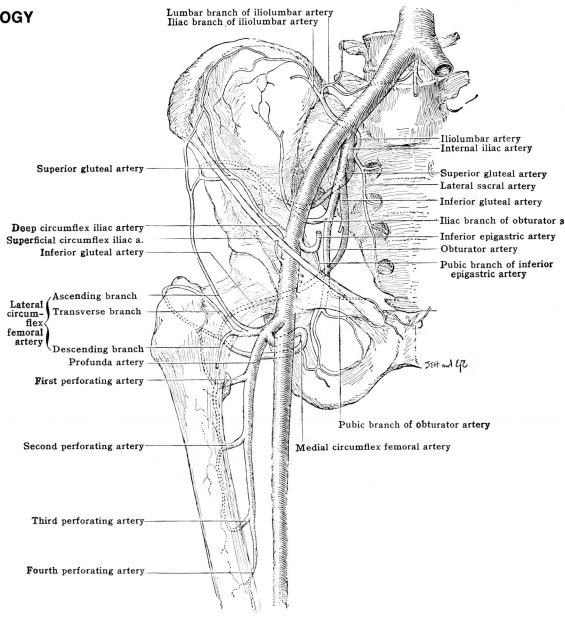

FIGURE 5-63 Major collateral channels connecting the arteries in the region of the hip. (From Anson, B. J. (ed.): Morris' Human Anatomy, 12th ed. Copyright © 1966 by McGraw-Hill, Inc. Used by permission of McGraw-Hill Book Company.)

Vascular Anatomy of the Leg and Hip (Figs. 5–64 and 5–65)

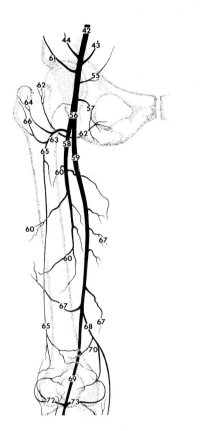

BLOOD SUPPLY OF THE FEMORAL CAPITAL EPIPHYSIS AND NECK OF THE FEMUR IN CHILDHOOD

EPIPHYSEAL PLATE - THIS PLATE PRECLUDES
ANASTOMOSIS OF EPIPHYSEAL AND METAPHYSEAL VESSELS

SUPERIOR METAPHYSEAL VESSELS

FEMORAL CAPITAL EPIPHYSIS

LATERAL EPIPHYSEAL VESSELS

NUTRIENT VESSELS

NOTE: BLOOD SUPPLY COMING THROUGH LIGAMENTUM TERES
AT THIS AGE IS VERY INADEQUATE AND CONFINED TO A SMALL
SEGMENT OF EPIPHYSIS

BLOOD SUPPLY OF THE FEMORAL HEAD

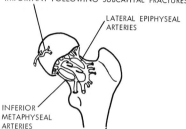

ARTERY OF LIGAMENTUM TERES, (NOT VERY
SIGNIFICANT ORDINARILY, BUT MOST
IMPORTANT FOLLOWING SUBCAPITAL FRACTURES)

LATERAL EPIPHYSEAL ARTERIES

INFERIOR METAPHYSEAL ARTERIES

FIGURE 5–65 Blood supply of the head and neck of the femur.

*Anatomic terms are based on Nomina Anatomica (N.A.), with one exception. The term *muscular branches of femoral and profunda femoris* (no. 67) has been included because these branches are often observed in arteriograms of the lower extremities. Commonly used synonyms are indicated parenthetically, and the N.A. term *fibular,* accepted by the Sixth International Congress of Anatomists as an alternative for *peroneal* (no. 79), is shown in brackets.

(From Muller, R. F., Figley, M. M., Rogoff, S. M., and DeWeese, V. A.: Arteries of the lower extremity. Published by Radiography Markets Division, Eastman Kodak Company. Used by permission of Eastman Kodak Company, Radiography Markets Division, Rochester, New York.)

Vascular Anatomy of the Leg and Foot (Figs. 5–66 and 5–67)

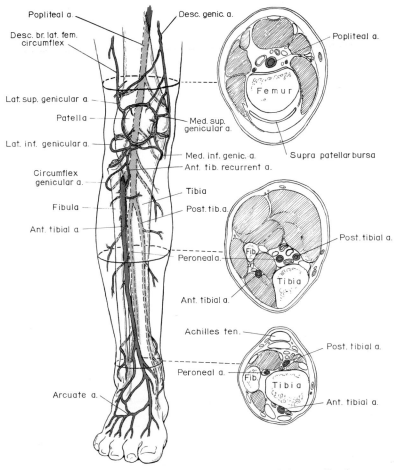

FIGURE 5–66 Three-dimensional perspective of the popliteal artery and its major branches, around the knee and terminally, as seen in arteriographic study.

FIGURE 5–67 Scheme of the distribution and anastomoses of the arteries of the right foot. *Dotted lines,* plantar arteries; *solid lines,* dorsal arteries. (After Walsham. Reprinted from Anson, B. J. (ed.): Morris' Human Anatomy. 12th ed. Copyright © 1966 by McGraw-Hill, Inc. Used by permission of McGraw-Hill Book Company.)

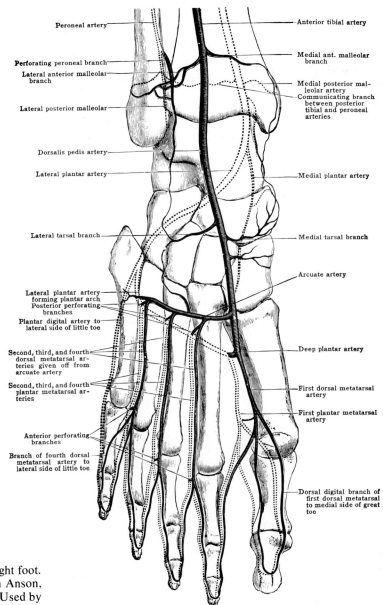

Vascular Anatomy of the Lower Extremity (Fig. 5–68)

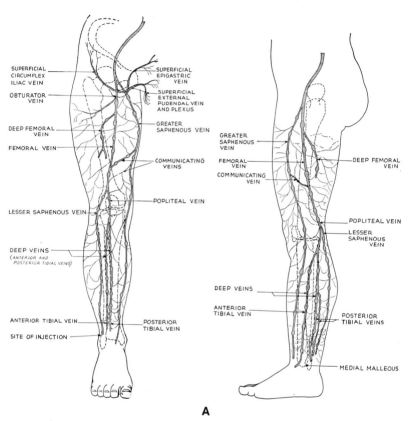

A

FIGURE 5–68 Diagram of the anatomy of conventional venograms of the leg. *Left*, anteroposterior projection. *Right*, lateral projection.
Legend continued on opposite page.

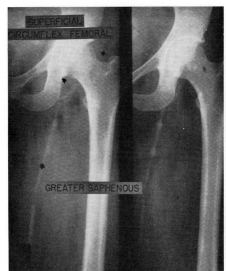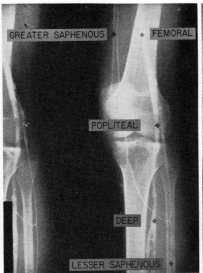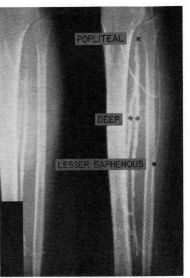

B

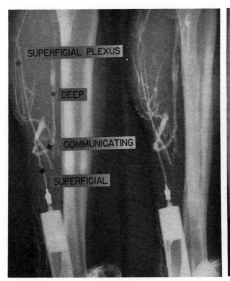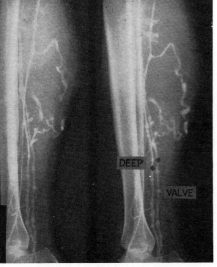

C   **D**

FIGURE 5–68 *Continued.* *B.* Representative conventional venograms of the lower extremity demonstrating primarily the lesser and greater saphenous veins and several deeper veins of leg and thigh. (Courtesy of Dr. E. C. Baker, Youngstown, Ohio.) *C.* Venograms of leg demonstrating the communicating veins joining superficial and deep veins. *D.* Venograms of deep veins of leg, showing their paired nature. (Courtesy of Dr. E. C. Baker, Youngstown, Ohio.)

Legend continued on following page.

Venograms of the Thigh and Leg (Figs. 5–68, 5–69, and 5–70)

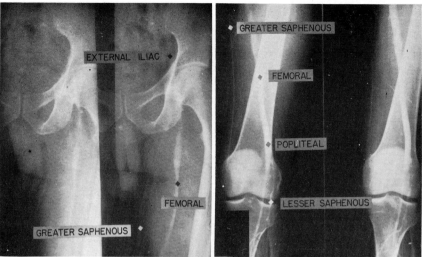

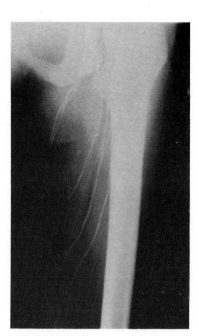

FIGURE 5–69 Radiograph demonstrating the superficial lymphatics of the upper thigh and deep lymphatics of pelvis.

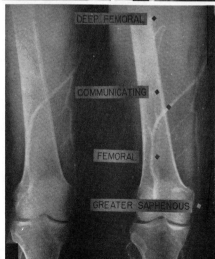

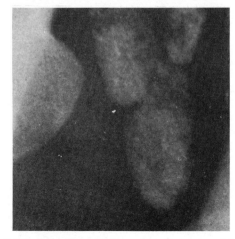

FIGURE 5–68 *Continued. E.* Venograms demonstrating the external iliac vein, and the femoral vein and its major tributaries. (Courtesy of Dr. E. C. Baker, Youngstown, Ohio.)

FIGURE 5–70 Magnified radiograph of a normal lymph node obtained after a lymphangiogram.

Lymphangiograms of the Leg, Thigh, and Pelvis (Figs. 5–71 and 5–72)

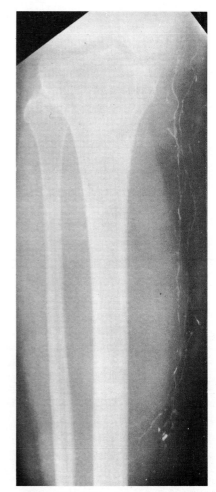

FIGURE 5–71 Lymphangiogram of the leg.

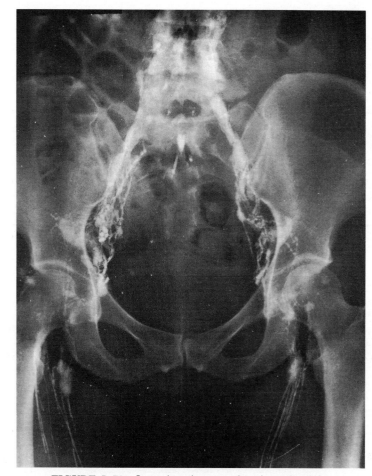

FIGURE 5–72 Lymphangiogram of groin and pelvis.

6

THE SKULL

BASIC ANATOMY AND RELATIONSHIPS

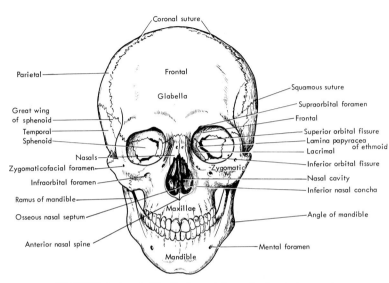

FIGURE 6–1 *A*. Skull viewed from its frontal aspect.

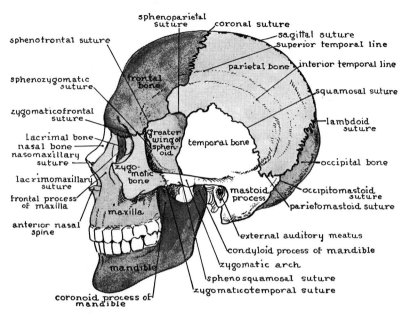

FIGURE 6–1 *B*. Lateral view of the skull showing the bones of the calvaria, face and mandible. (From Pendergrass, E. P., et al.: The Head and Neck in Roentgen Diagnosis. 2nd ed. Springfield, Ill., Charles C Thomas, Publisher, 1956. Courtesy of Charles C Thomas, Publisher.)

Introduction.* There are 22 bones in the skull, including the mandible, firmly bound together at immovable joints called sutures or primary cartilaginous joints (with the exception of the temporomandibular joints).

These are subdivided into the bones of the calvaria (or brain case) and the bones of the face and mandible (Fig. 6–1).

---

* In most cases the author has chosen to use the translated English equivalent to the Latin terms officially published in Nomina Anatomica, published by Excerpta Medical Foundation and printed in the Netherlands by Mouton and Company, The Hague, 1966. Students may refer to the Nomina Anatomica, if they so desire. Our experience in this country, however, indicates that the translated terms are preferred by both teachers and students.

The calvaria or cranium is composed of eight bones: the paired parietal and temporal bones, and the frontal, occipital, sphenoid, and ethmoid bones, which are single. The temporal bones contain the ossicles of the ear.

The cranial cavity lodges the brain and is formed by the frontal, parietal, occipital, temporal, sphenoid, and ethmoid bones. The roof of the cranial cavity is composed of the frontal, parietal, occipital, and squamous portions of the temporal bones, and the greater wings of the sphenoid bone. These bones are largely flat and are composed of a dense outer layer known as the outer table, a less dense middle zone known as the diploë, and another dense inner zone known as the inner table (lamina externa and interna).

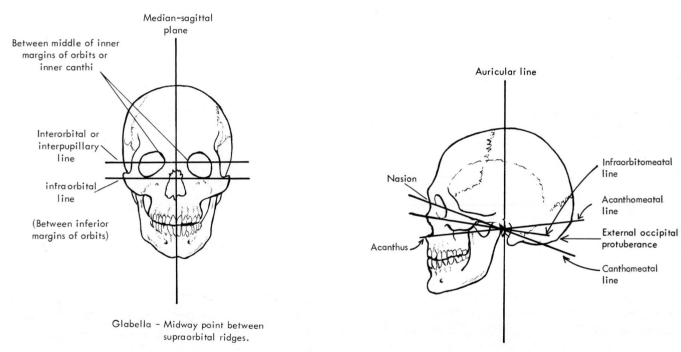

FIGURE 6-2 Commonly used reference points and lines on skull.

Definitions

Nasion: The point at the root of the nose where the frontal and two nasal bones meet.

Lambda: The point on the skull at the apex of the occipital bone.

Inion: The center of the external occipital protuberance.

Bregma: The point on the vault of the skull where the sagittal and coronal sutures meet.

Infraorbitomeatal Line: The line drawn between the infraorbital margin and the center of the external auditory meatus.

Acanthus: The anterior nasal spine.

Canthomeatal Line: Line drawn between the outer canthus of the eye and the external auditory meatus.

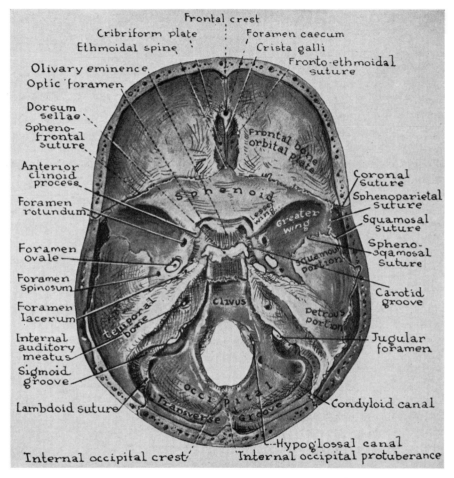

FIGURE 6–3 Internal aspect of the base of the skull. (From Pendergrass, E. P., et al.: The Head and Neck in Roentgen Diagnosis, 2nd ed., Springfield, Ill., Charles C Thomas, Publisher. 1956. Courtesy of Charles C Thomas, Publisher.)

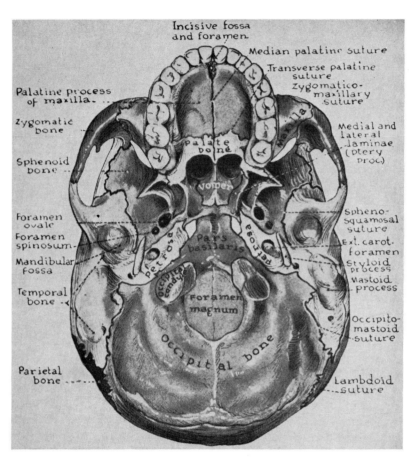

FIGURE 6–4 *A*. The skull viewed from below. (From Pendergrass, E. P., et al.: The Head and Neck in Roentgen Diagnosis, 2nd ed., Springfield, Ill., Charles C Thomas, Publisher, 1956. Courtesy of Charles C Thomas, Publisher.)

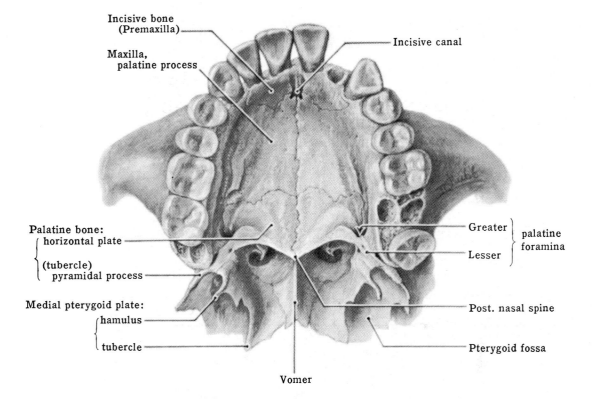

Incisive bone (Premaxilla)

Maxilla, palatine process

Incisive canal

Palatine bone:
horizontal plate

(tubercle) pyramidal process

Medial pterygoid plate:
hamulus

tubercle

Greater ⎫ palatine
Lesser ⎭ foramina

Post. nasal spine

Pterygoid fossa

Vomer

FIGURE 6–5 The bony palate. (Reproduced by permission from Grant, J. C. B.: An Atlas of Anatomy, 5th ed., Baltimore, The Williams & Wilkins Company, 1962. Copyright © 1962, The Williams & Wilkins Company.)

Comments Regarding the Foramina and Canals of the Skull

1. The *greater palatine foramen* usually measures about 2 mm. in diameter.

2. The *lesser palatine foramen* (there may be two) usually measures about 1 mm. in diameter.

3. The *foramen rotundum* connects the middle cranial fossa with the pterygopalatine fossa. Its average length is 3.4 mm. (with a range 2 to 5 mm.). It is best seen on Water's or Caldwell's projections.

4. The *foramen spinosum* is 2 to 3 mm. in diameter and transmits the middle meningeal artery.

5. The *foramen lacerum* is an aperture quite variable in size and is best seen on the submentovertical projection.

6. The *pterygoid canal* connects the foramen lacerum with the pterygopalatine fossa. Its length is 6 to 20 mm., and its width is 0 5 to 2.5 mm.

7. The *carotid canal* measures 5 to 6.5 mm. in width and 3 to 4 cm. in length, and transmits the internal carotid artery.

8. The *jugular foramen* connects the posterior fossa with the upper cervical region. It is divided into an anterior nervous part and posterior vascular part. Special radiographic views are necessary for its visualization.

9. The *foramen ovale* measures about 4 × 7 mm. (unmagnified).

10. The *foramen magnum* is 2.5 to 3.4 cm. in width and 3.2 to 3.6 cm. in length.

ANATOMY OF INDIVIDUAL BONES AND REGIONS

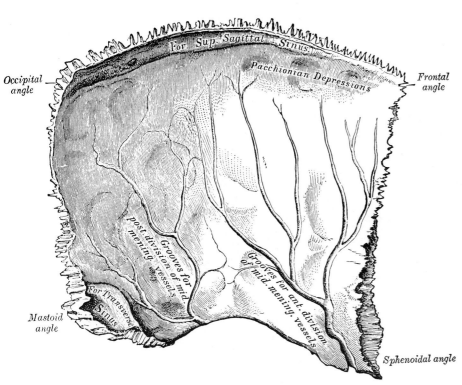

FIGURE 6–6 The left parietal bone, inner aspect, showing vascular grooves. (From Goss, C. M. (ed.): Gray's Anatomy of the Human Body. 29th ed., Philadelphia, Lea & Febiger, 1973.)

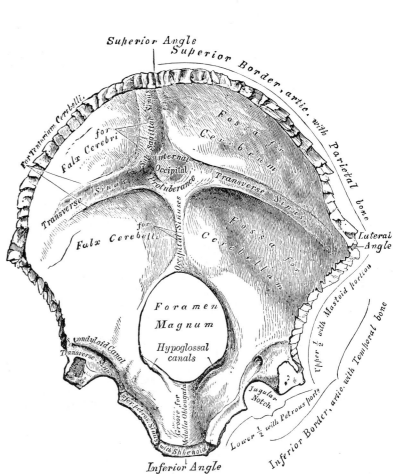

FIGURE 6–7 The occipital bone, inner surface (From Goss, C. M. (ed.): Gray's Anatomy of the Human Body. 29th ed., Philadelphia, Lea & Febiger, 1973.)

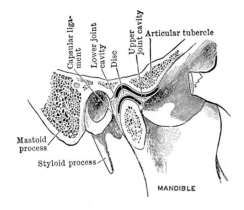

FIGURE 6–8 Anteroposterior section through the temporomandibular joint. (From Cunningham's Textbook of Anatomy, 6th ed., London, Oxford University Press, 1936.)

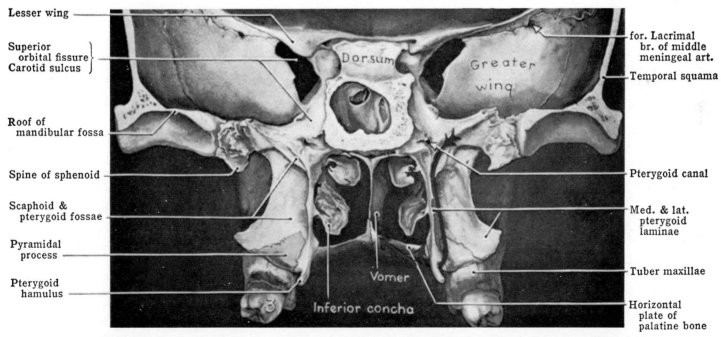

FIGURE 6–9 Coronal section of the skull at the sphenoid bone. (Reproduced by permission of Grant, J. C. B.: An Atlas of Anatomy. 5th ed., Baltimore, The Williams & Wilkins Co., 1962. Copyright © 1962. The Williams & Wilkins Co.)

The Internal Ear

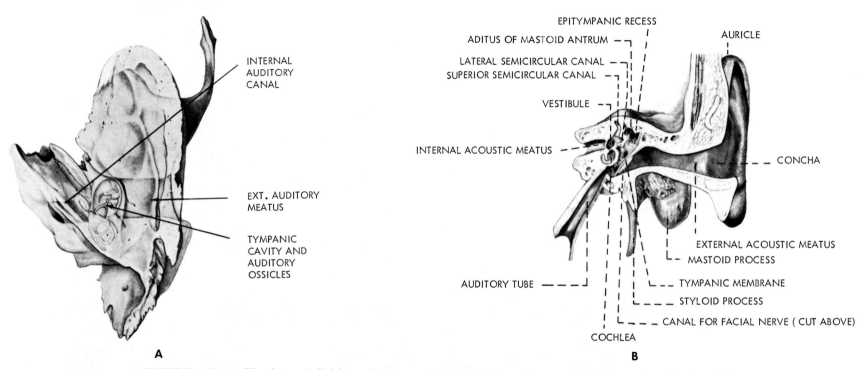

A

B

FIGURE 6–10   *A*. The three subdivisions of the ear projected on the bony framework. (Redrawn from Pernkopf, E.: Atlas of Topographical and Applied Human Anatomy. Vol. 1. Philadelphia, W. B. Saunders Co., 1963.) *B*. The parts of the ear (semi-diagrammatic). (Redrawn from Cunningham's Manual of Practical Anatomy, 12th ed., London, Oxford University Press, 1958.)

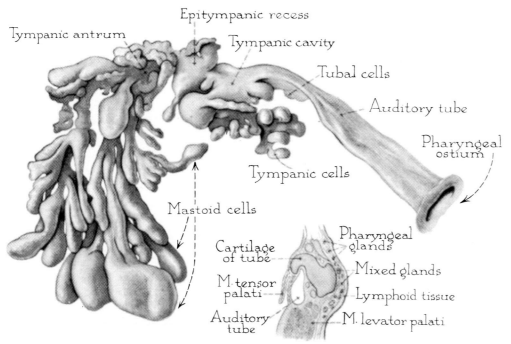

FIGURE 6–11 Cast of the tympanic cavity and communicating air cells, recess, and auditory tube (Siebenmann). (From Anson, B. J.: An Atlas of Human Anatomy. Philadelphia, W. B. Saunders Co., 1963.)

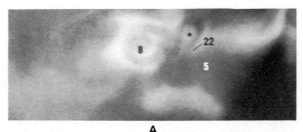

A

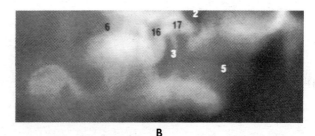

B

FIGURE 6–12 Anteroposterior tomograms of a normal left ear made in the "cochlear plane" and the "vestibular plane." *A*. Cochlear plane. The turns of the cochlea, the scutum (spur), the head and the handle of the malleus (*asterisk*), and the relation of the malleus to the epitympanic recess are clearly seen. *B*. Vestibular plane (2 mm. posterior to *A*). The vestibule, the internal auditory canal, two of the three semicircular canals, and the mastoid antrum are all clearly visible. (From Schaeffer, R. E.: Med. Radiogr. Photogr., *48(1)*:2-22, 1972. Published by Radiography Markets Division, Eastman Kodak Company.) (*8*) cochlea, (*22*) scutum or spur, (*5*) external auditory canal, (*6*) internal auditory meatus, (*16*) vestibule, (*17*) lateral semicircular canal, (*2*) mastoid antrum, and (*3*) middle ear (tympanic cavity).

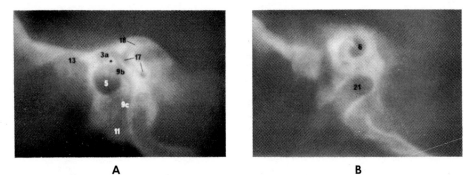

FIGURE 6–13 Lateral tomograms made in two levels, or planes, of a normal left ear. *A*. More superficial of the two levels. The facial nerve canal is visible all the way down to its point of exit at the stylomastoid foramen, and the ossicular mass (*asterisk*) can be seen in the epitympanic recess. The two limbs of the lateral semicircular canal are also visible. *B*. Deeper of the two levels (8 mm. deeper than *A*). A deep jugular fossa is visible, but the carotid canal is not shown to good advantage. The internal auditory canal is clearly visible. The thin, bony band that stretches across the diameter of the internal auditory canal is an edge-on view of the crista transversa (crista falciformis). (From Schaeffer, R. E.: Med. Radiogr. Photogr., *48(1)*:2–22, 1972. Published by Radiography Markets Division, Eastman Kodak Company.) (*13*) mandibular fossa, (*3a*) epitympanic recess, (*5*) external auditory canal, (*18*) superior semicircular canal, (*17*) lateral semicircular canal, (*9b*) 5th nerve canal, (*9c*) tympanic segment, (*11*) stylomastoid foramen, (*6*) internal auditory canal, and (*21*) jugular fossa.

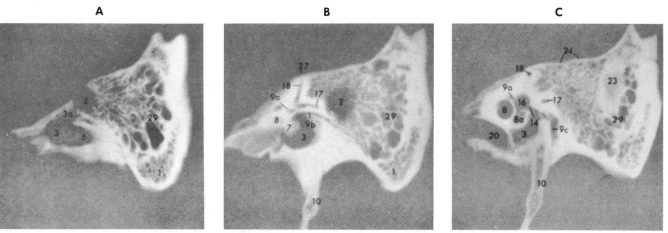

FIGURE 6–14 *See legend on opposite page.*

FIGURE 6–14 Stenver's (oblique posteroanterior) projection. Six pairs of radiographs (*top*) and tomograms (*bottom*) of a dried left temporal bone. Each pair represents a different level, or plane. The progression of levels from left to right is anterior to posterior. The anteromedian aspect of the bone is on the left; the posterolateral aspect is on the right. The jugular fossa, the labyrinth, the course of the facial nerve canal, and the relation of the jugular fossa to the middle ear (tympanic cavity) are shown particularly well in the Stenver's projection.

Legend: (*1*) Mastoid process. (*2*) mastoid antrum (*2a*) aditus of antrum, (*3*) middle ear (tympanic cavity), (*3a*) epitympanic recess (attic), (*4*) lateral wall of attic, (*5*) external auditory canal, (*6*) internal auditory canal, (*7*) promontory of middle ear, (*8*) cochlea, (*8a*) basal turn of cochlea, (*9a*) facial nerve canal, petrous segment, (*9b*) facial nerve canal, tympanic segment, (*9c*) facial nerve canal, mastoid (descending) segment, (*10*) styloid process, (*11*) stylomastoid foramen, (*12*) crista transversa (crista falciformis), (*13*) mandibular fossa, (*14*) oval window (fenestra vestibuli), (*15*) round window (fenestra cochleae), (*16*) vestibule, (*17*) lateral semicircular canal, (*18*) superior semicircular canal, (*19*) posterior semicircular canal, (*20*) carotid canal, (*21*) jugular fossa (*22*) scutum (spur), (*23*) sinus plate, (*24*) tegmen, (*25*) squamous portion of temporal bone, (*26*) crus commune (common limb), (*27*) arcuate eminence, (*28*) petrous apex, (*29*) mastoid air cells. (From Schaeffer, R. E.: Med. Radiogr. Photogr., *48(1)*:2–22, 1972. Published by Radiography Markets Division, Eastman Kodak Company.)

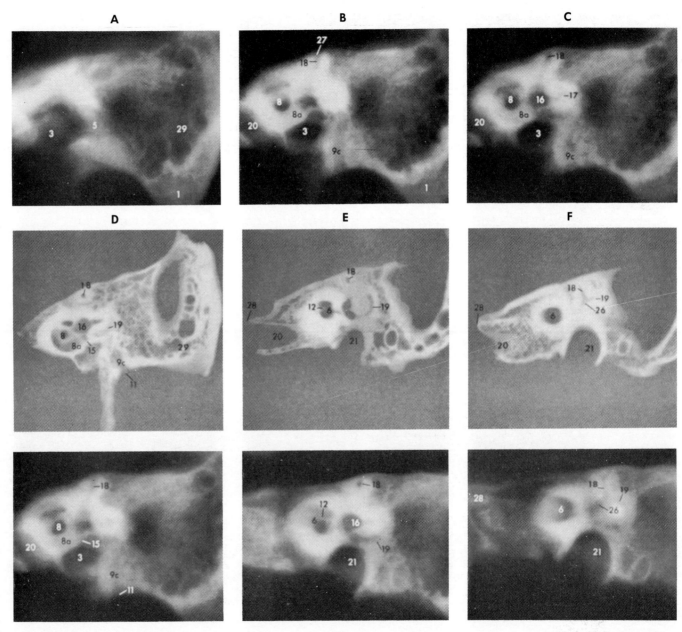

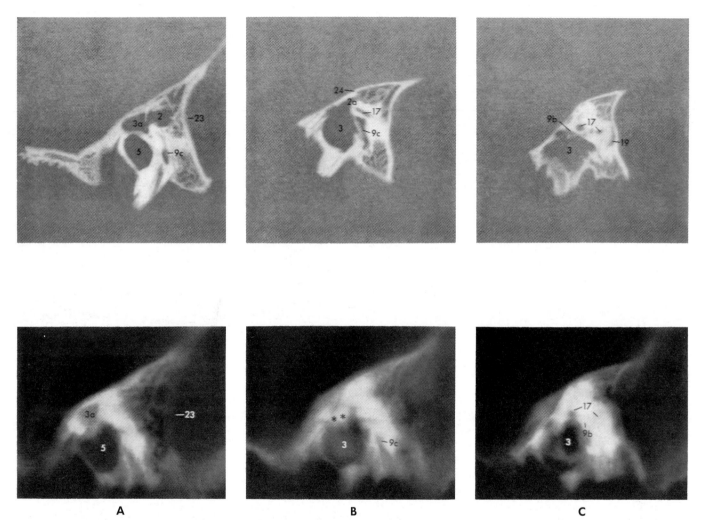

A **B** **C**

FIGURE 6–15 *A–F.* Lateral projection. Six pairs of radiographs (*top*) and tomograms (*bottom*) of a dried left temporal bone. Each pair represents a different level, or plane. From left to right, the levels progress from the lateral surface of the bone mediad. The posterior aspect of the bone is on the right. The lateral projection reveals the relation between the epitympanic recess and the mastoid antrum and shows the mastoid (descending) segment of the facial nerve canal. In the specimen used for this projection, the malleus and the incus happened to be present in their normal configuration. The tomogram made in the second level (*B, bottom*) clearly shows these ossicles (*asterisks*); the handle of the malleus is anterior, and the long process of the incus is posterior. (From Schaeffer, R. E.: Med. Radiogr. Photogr., *48*:1, 1972. Published by Radiography Markets Division, Eastman Kodak Company.)

Legend continued on opposite page.

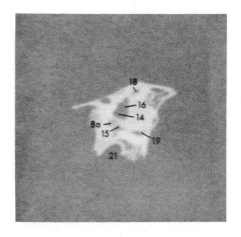
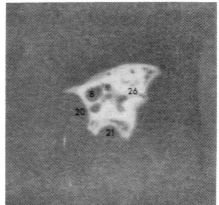
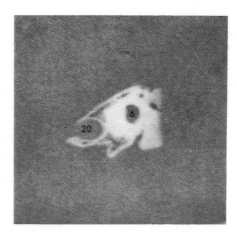

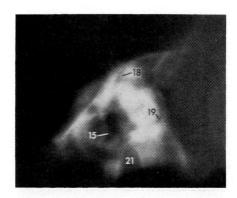
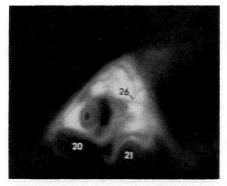
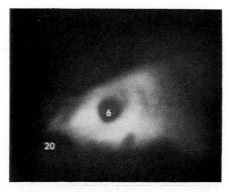

FIGURE 6–15 *Continued.*

D	**E**	**F**

Legend:

1   Mastoid process
2   Mastoid antrum
2a   Aditus of antrum
3   Middle ear (tympanic cavity)
3a   Epitympanic recess (attic)
4   Lateral wall of attic
5   External auditory canal
6   Internal auditory canal
7   Promontory of middle ear
8   Cochlea
8a   basal turn of cochlea
9a   Facial nerve canal, petrous segment

9b   Facial nerve canal, tympanic segment
9c   Facial nerve canal, mastoid (descending) segment
10   Styloid process
11   Stylomastoid foramen
12   Crista transversa (crista falciformis)
13   Mandibular fossa
14   Oval window (fenestra vestibuli)
15   Round window (fenestra cochleae)
16   Vestibule
17   Lateral semicircular canal
18   Superior semicircular canal
19   Posterior semicircular canal

20   Carotid canal
21   Jugular fossa
22   Scutum (spur)
23   Sinus plate
24   Tegmen
25   Squamous portion of temporal bone
26   Crus commune (common limb)
27   Arcuate eminence
28   Petrous apex
29   Mastoid air cells

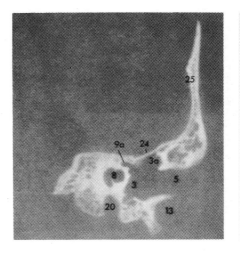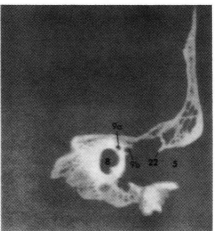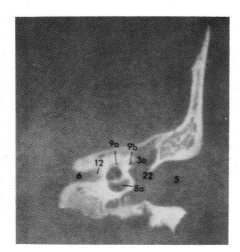

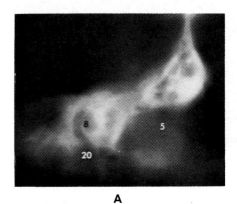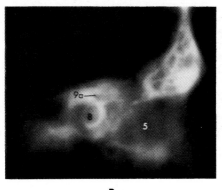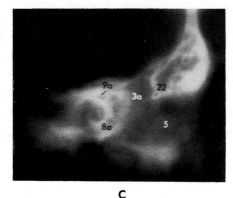

A **B** **C**

FIGURE 6–16 *A–F.* Anteroposterior (frontal) projection. Six pairs of radiographs (*top*) and tomograms (*bottom*) of a dried left temporal bone. Each pair represents a different level, or plane. The progression of levels from left to right is anterior to posterior, and there is about 1 mm. to 1.5 mm. between levels. The medial aspect of the bone is on the left; the lateral aspect, on the right. Structures seen particularly well in the anteroposterior projection including the internal auditory canal in its long axis and the epitympanic recess (attic).

Legend:

1	Mastoid process	*3*	Middle ear (tympanic cavity)
2	Mastoid antrum	*3a*	Epitympanic recess (attic)
2a	Aditus of antrum	*4*	Lateral wall of attic

5 External auditory canal
6 Internal auditory canal
7 Promontory of middle ear

Legend continued on opposite page.

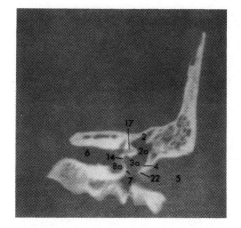
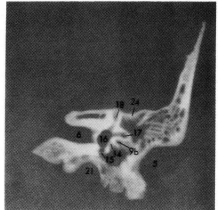
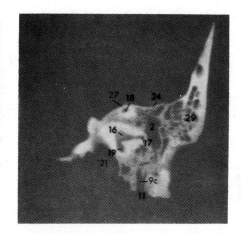

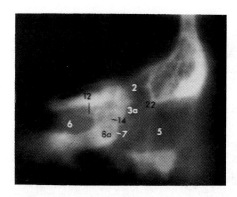
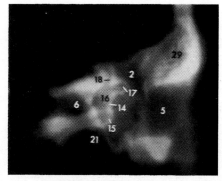
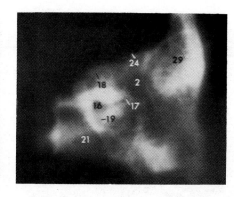

FIGURE 6–16 *Continued.*

D	E	F

8 Cochlea	*14* Oval window (fenestra vestibuli)	*23* Sinus plate
8a Basal turn of cochlea	*15* Round window (fenestra cochleae)	*24* Tegmen
9a Facial nerve canal, petrous segment	*16* Vestibule	*25* Squamous portion of temporal bone
9b Facial nerve canal, tympanic segment	*17* Lateral semicircular canal	*26* Crus commune (common limb)
9c Facial nerve canal, mastoid (descending) segment	*18* Superior semicircular canal	*27* Arcuate eminence
10 Styloid process	*19* Posterior semicircular canal	*28* Petrous apex
11 Stylomastoid foramen	*20* Carotid canal	*29* Mastoid air cells
12 Crista transversa (crista falciformis)	*21* Jugular fossa	
13 Mandibular fossa	*22* Scutum (spur)	

(From Schaeffer, R. E.: Med. Radiogr. Photogr., *48*:1, 1972. Published by Radiography Markets Division, Eastman Kodak Company.)

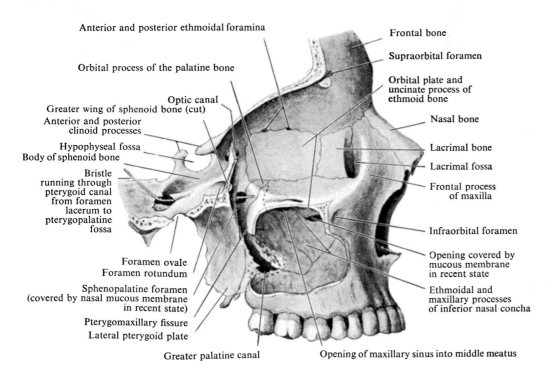

Anterior and posterior ethmoidal foramina

Orbital process of the palatine bone

Optic canal

Greater wing of sphenoid bone (cut)
Anterior and posterior clinoid processes

Hypophyseal fossa
Body of sphenoid bone

Bristle running through pterygoid canal from foramen lacerum to pterygopalatine fossa

Foramen ovale
Foramen rotundum

Sphenopalatine foramen (covered by nasal mucous membrane in recent state)

Pterygomaxillary fissure
Lateral pterygoid plate

Greater palatine canal

Frontal bone

Supraorbital foramen

Orbital plate and uncinate process of ethmoid bone

Nasal bone

Lacrimal bone

Lacrimal fossa

Frontal process of maxilla

Infraorbital foramen

Opening covered by mucous membrane in recent state

Ethmoidal and maxillary processes of inferior nasal concha

Opening of maxillary sinus into middle meatus

FIGURE 6–17 Sphenoid bone, medial wall of orbit (including ethmoid bone) and maxillary sinus. The lateral and posteromedial walls of the maxillary sinus have been partly removed to indicate the lateral relations of the palatine bone. Note how the medial wall of the maxillary sinus is completed by the palatine plate, the ethmoidal and maxillary processes of the inferior nasal concha, and the uncinate process of the ethmoid. (Reprinted by permission of Faber and Faber Ltd. from Anatomy of the Human Body, by Lockhardt, Hamilton, and Fyfe, Faber and Faber, London; J. B. Lippincott Company, Philadelphia.)

FIGURE 6–18 Vertical section of inferior canine tooth in situ.

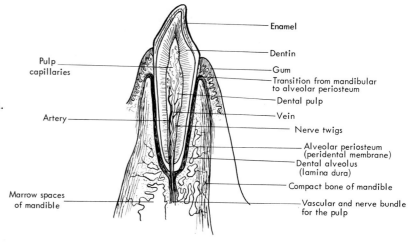

Pulp capillaries

Artery

Marrow spaces of mandible

Enamel

Dentin

Gum

Transition from mandibular to alveolar periosteum

Dental pulp

Vein

Nerve twigs

Alveolar periosteum (peridental membrane)

Dental alveolus (lamina dura)

Compact bone of mandible

Vascular and nerve bundle for the pulp

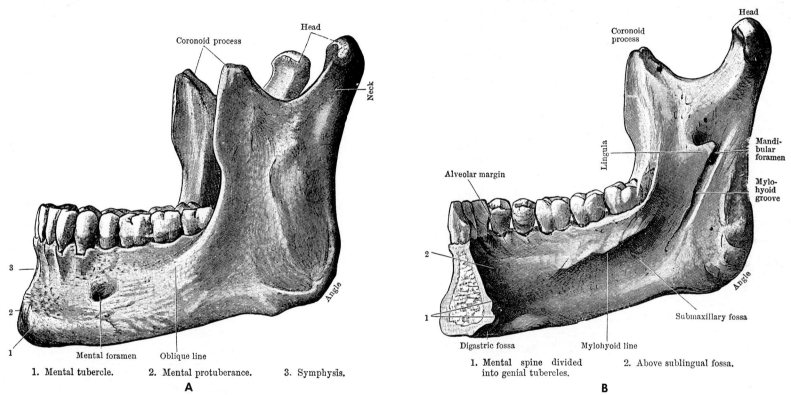

FIGURE 6–19 *A*. Mandible, seen from the left side. *B*. Medial surface of the right half of the mandible. (From Cunningham, D. J.: *in* Robinson, A. (ed.): Textbook of Anatomy. London, Oxford University Press.)

The Skull of Neonates and Children; Variations in Structure

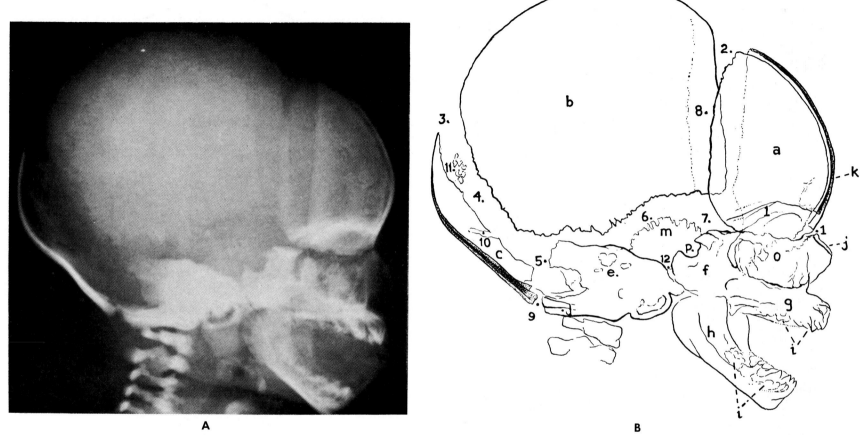

A

B

FIGURE 6–20 Normal neonatal skull. *A.* Roentgenogram, lateral view. *B.* Labeled tracing of *A.* (*a*) Frontal bone, (b) parietal bone, (c) squamous portion of occipital bone, (d) exoccipital portion of occipital bone, (e) superimposed petrous pyramids of temporal bone, (f) body of sphenoid, (g) upper maxilla, (h) mandible, (i) partially mineralized deciduous teeth, and dental crypts, (j) nasal bone, (k) squamosa of the frontal bone, (l) horizontal plates of the frontal bone, (m) squamosa of the temporal bone, (o) orbit, (p) pituitary fossa; (1) frontonasal suture, (2) anterior fontanelle, (3) posterior fontanelle, (4) lambdoidal suture, (5) posterolateral fontanelle, (6) squamosal suture, (7) anterolateral fontanelle, (8) coronal suture, (9) synchondrosis between exoccipitals and supraoccipital portions of occipital bone, (10) mendosal suture, (11) multiple ossification centers (wormian bones) in lambdoidal suture, (12) occipito-sphenoid synchondrosis. (From Caffey, J.: Pediatric X-ray Diagnosis, 6th ed. Chicago, Year Book Medical Publishers, 1972.)

Legend continued on opposite page.

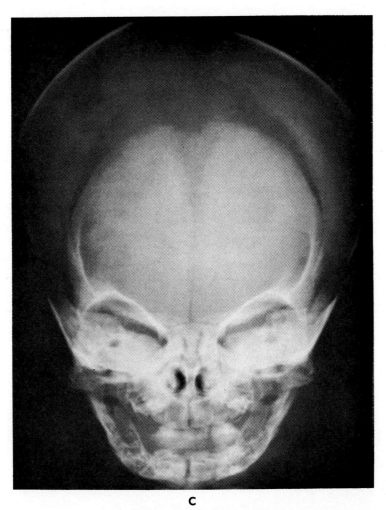

C

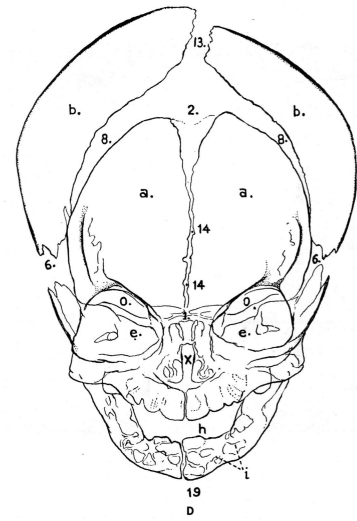

D

FIGURE 6–20 *Continued.* *C.* Roentgenogram, posteroanterior projection. *D.* Labeled tracing of *C.* (a) Frontal bone, (b) parietal bone, (e) superimposed petrous pyramids of temporal bone, (h) mandible, (i) partially mineralized deciduous teeth, and dental crypts, (o) orbit, (x) nasal septum, (2) anterior fontanelle, (6) squamosal suture, (8) coronal suture, (13) sagittal suture, (14) metopic suture dividing the frontal bone, (19) symphysis of mandible. (From Caffey, J.: Pediatric X-ray Diagnosis, 6th ed. Chicago, Year Book Medical Publishers, 1972.)

Legend continued on the following page.

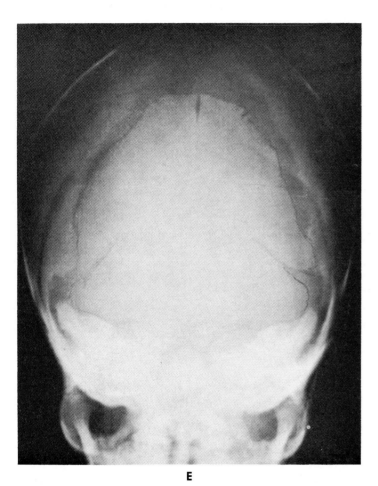

E

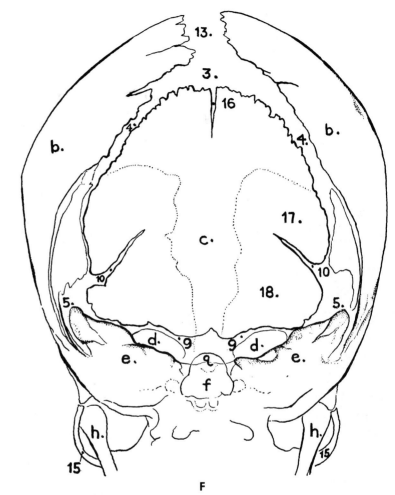

F

FIGURE 6–20 *Continued.* *E*. Roentgenogram, anteroposterior projection. Modified Towne's projection. *F*. Labeled tracing of *E*. (b) Parietal bone, (c) squamous portion of occipital bone, (d) exoccipital portion of occipital bone, (e) super-imposed petrous pyramids of temporal bone, (f) body of sphenoid, (h) mandible, (q) basioccipital portion of occipital bone, (3) posterior fontanelle, (4) lambdoidal suture, (5) posterolateral fontanelle, (9) synchondrosis between exoccipital and supraoccipital portions of occipital bone, (10) mendosal suture, (13) sagittal suture, (15) zygomatic arch, (16) superior median fissure of occipital bone, (17) interparietal portion of occipital bone, (18) supraoccipital portion of occipital bone. (From Caffey, J.: Pediatric X-ray Diagnosis, 6th ed. Chicago, Year Book Medical Publishers, 1972.)

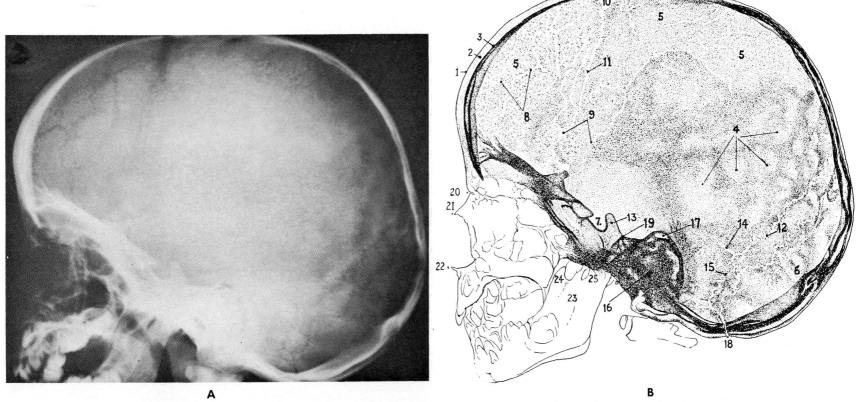

FIGURE 6–21 Normal skull at 2 years of age. *A.* Radiograph, lateral view. *B.* Labeled tracing of A. (1) Outer table, (2) diploic space, (3) inner table, (4) convolutional markings, (5) fine honeycomb of diploic structure, (6) internal occipital protuberance, (7) pituitary fossa, (8) diploic veins, (9) vascular grooves, (10) anterior fontanelle, (11) coronal suture, (12) lambdoidal suture, (13) dorsum sellae, (14) parietomastoid suture, (15) occipitomastoid suture, (16) petrous pyramids, (17) small temporal pneumatic cell, (18) synchondrosis between exoccipital and supraoccipital areas, (19) spheno-occipital synchondrosis, (20) nasofrontal suture, (21) nasal bone, (22) anterior nasal spine, (23) mandible, (24) coronoid process of mandible, (25) articular process of mandible. (From Caffey, J.: Pediatric X-ray Diagnosis, 6th ed. Chicago, Year Book Medical Publishers, 1972.)

LINES, IMPRESSIONS, CHANNELS, AND SUTURES OF THE CRANIAL VAULT

There are various lines and impressions on the cranial vault which are of great radiographic significance.

1. Granular Pits or Arachnoidal (Pacchionian) Granulation Impressions (Fig. 6–22).

2. Arterial and Venous Grooves. The arterial grooves (Fig. 6–23) are narrow branching grooves for the meningeal vessels—the middle meningeal being the largest.

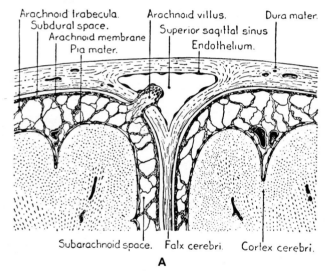

A

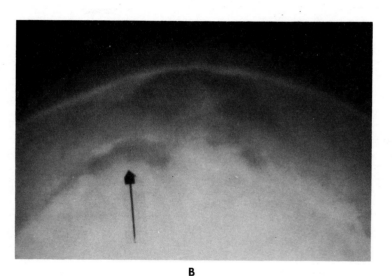

B

FIGURE 6–22 *A*. Diagram showing a pacchionian or arachnoidal granulation. (From Weed, Am. J. Anat., Courtesy of Wistar Institute); *B*. Close-up radiograph of arachnoidal granulation in Towne's projection.

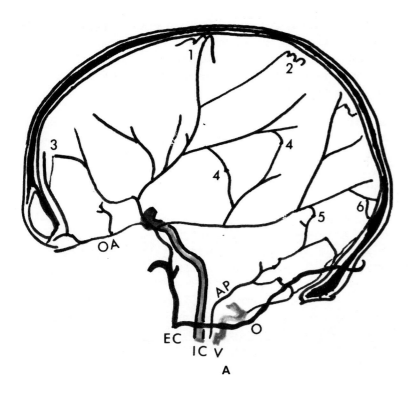

A

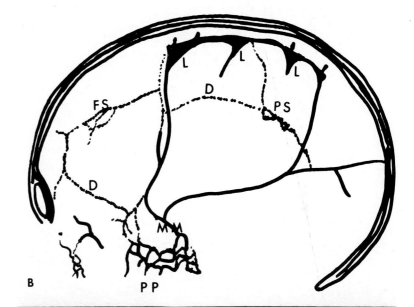

B

FIGURE 6–23 *A*. Diagrammatic and radiographic appearance of arterial and venous impressions on the bones of the calvarium. (*A* shows a diagram of the meningeal artery circulation. It has an anterior branch that crosses the great wing of the sphenoid; some branches, however, pass backward to the occipital region. The posterior branch supplies the posterior part of the dura mater and cranium. The various anastomoses of the branches of the middle meningeal are numbered. For specific details regarding these numbers the student is referred to the companion text, Meschan, I.: An Atlas of Anatomy Basic to Radiology. *B*. Diagram showing the main middle meningeal veins that generally accompany the middle meningeal arteries. Notice that the "frontal star" (*FS*) and the "parietal star" (*PS*) are collections of veins in the diploë. *C*. Lateral radiograph demonstrating vascular impressions: (*1*) parietal star, (*2*) middle meningeal artery and vein, anterior division; (*3*) parietal star; (*4*) middle meningeal vein, posterior branch; (*5*) lateral sinus; and (*6*) meningeal communications with the ophthalmic artery and vein. (From Meschan, I.: Sem. Roentgenol., *9*:125–136, 1974. Used by permission.)

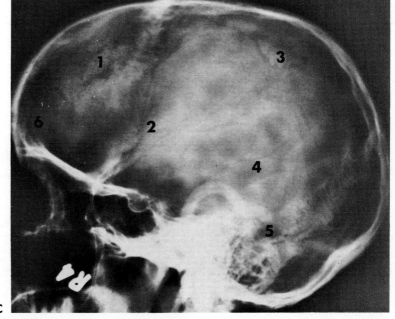

C

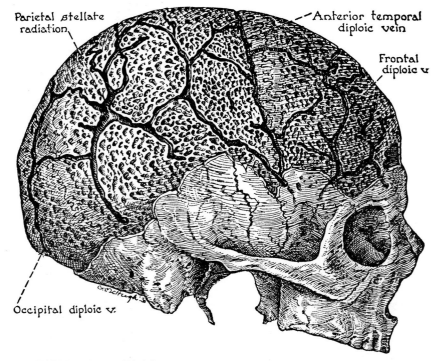

Parietal stellate radiation

Anterior temporal diploic vein

Frontal diploic v.

Occipital diploic v.

FIGURE 6–24 Diploic venous plexuses of the calvarium. (From Bailey, P.: Intracranial Tumors. Springfield, Ill., Charles C Thomas, Publisher. 1957. Courtesy of Charles C Thomas, Publisher.)

3. Venous Plexuses Within the Diploë. The venous plexuses within the diploë (Fig. 6–24) are impressions within the diploë found in each of the frontal, parietal, and occipital bones, giving the skull a mosaic appearance on the radiograph. In the parietal bones particularly, they have been referred to as the "parietal star" or "spider." At times these appear unusually accentuated. It is usually hazardous, however, to interpret any abnormality on the appearance of the venous diploë alone. Besides diploic veins there are diploic lakes that appear as irregular,

grossly oval or round areas of radiolucency and rarely exceed 2 cm. in widest diameter. They are most common in the parietal bones. They are well demarcated and the bone around them is intact.

4. Venous Sinuses. The venous sinuses (Fig. 6–25) produce their impression on the inner table of the skull so that they appear as radiolucent channels bounded by curved bony ridges. The lateral sinus (or transverse sinus) is the largest of these and has its origin near the internal occipital protuberance, passing forward around the occipital bone with a slightly upward convexity to the pneumatic portion of the mastoid bone. Here it curves downward to become the sigmoid sinus.

The sphenoparietal sinus is another commonly prominent venous sinus. It begins in connection with the anterior parietal diploic vein, just posterior to the coronal suture, and then courses along the inferior surface of the lesser wing of the sphenoid to become a tributary of the cavernous sinus.

The point of junction of the lateral sinuses and the superior sagittal sinus is virtually the point of confluence of all the major dural sinuses, and hence is called the *sinus confluens*. It has a variable appearance, resembling a crossroad with or without a bony island contained within it.

5. Emissary Veins. In the cranial vault, emissary veins are most frequent in the regions of the occipital protuberance and the parasagittal and posterior aspects of the parietal bone. These represent anastomotic channels between intracranial and extracranial vascular systems. Some of the emissary veins achieve considerable size. One of the most significant of these is the mastoid emissary vein, which is situated near the sigmoid sinus and can be identified posterior to the pneumatized portion of the mastoid. This may contain a small branch of the occipital artery, or it may be in a canal several centimeters in length and 1 to 10 millimeters in width.

Also, and quite distinct from the thinning-out of the parietal bones to be described, the parietal bone may contain enlarged *parietal foramina* (Fig. 6–26); this tendency toward enlarged foramina is apparently inherited. Ordinarily extremely small (not greater than 1 mm.), and transmitting an emissary vein, these are situated close to the sagittal suture, about 1 to 1½ inches above the lambdoid suture just medial to the parietal tuberosity.

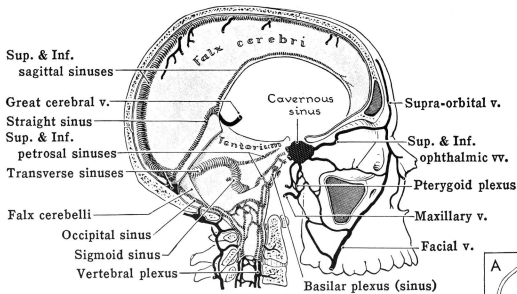

Sup. & Inf.
  sagittal sinuses

Great cerebral v.

Straight sinus

Sup. & Inf.
  petrosal sinuses

Transverse sinuses

Falx cerebelli

Occipital sinus

Sigmoid sinus

Vertebral plexus

Falx cerebri

Cavernous
sinus

Tentorium

Supra-orbital v.

Sup. & Inf.
  ophthalmic vv.

Pterygoid plexus

Maxillary v.

Facial v.

Basilar plexus (sinus)

FIGURE 6–25 Diagram of the venous sinuses of the dura mater. (Reproduced by permission from Grant, J. C. B.: An Atlas of Anatomy, 5th ed. Baltimore, The Williams & Wilkins Co., 1962. Copyright © 1962, The Williams & Wilkins Co.)

6. The Sutures. A number of important sutures mark the superior portion of the skull: the *sagittal suture* marks the junction of the two parietal bones superiorly, and extends from the bregma, which is its junction with the coronal suture, to the lambda, which is its junction with the lambdoid suture. The *coronal suture* is situated between the parietal bones posteriorly and the frontal bone anteriorly. It ends by joining the sphenoid bone laterally, and this point of union is known as the *pterion* on either side. The *lambdoid suture* is situated between the parietal bone anteriorly and the interparietal portion of the occipital bone posteriorly. Its point of junction with the squamosal suture is known as the *asterion*.

SUTURAL SCLEROSIS. Often a dense band of sclerosis occurs along sutures owing to a continuous bridging process across the suture. These bands vary in size and may be as large as 15 mm. Suture sclerosis is a normal physiologic process that becomes more apparent with advancing age.

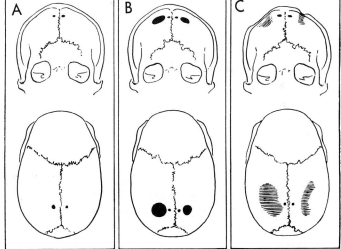

FIGURE 6–26 Three types of defects in parietal bone. (*1*) Normal defects in parietal bone containing veins; (*2*) Emissary foramina and fenestrae (enlarged parietal foramina) shown in same skull; (*3*) Two forms of thinness shown, quadrangular on left and grooved on right, in association with emissary foramina. (From Nashold, B. S., Jr., and Netsky, M. G.: J. Neuropathol. Exp. Neurol., *18*:432, 1959.)

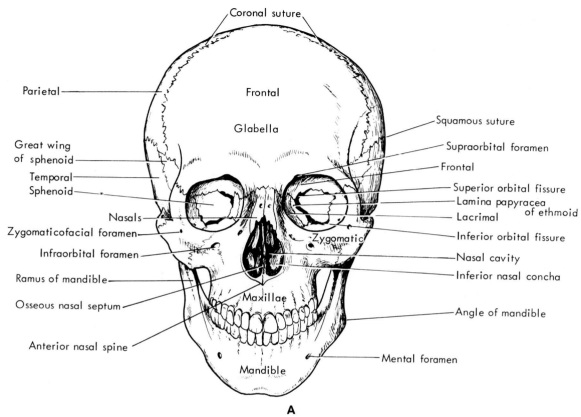

FIGURE 6–27 *A*. Skull viewed from the front.
Legend continued on opposite page.

7. The Digitate or Convolutional Markings (Fig. 6–28). These are irregular areas of increased and decreased density throughout the skull that are caused by thinning of the inner table from pressure produced by the convolutions or gyri of the brain. In persons under approximately 16 years of age, these may be readily detectable normally. Beyond this age, or when unduly accentuated in the younger age groups, they may indicate increased intracranial pressure and are of pathologic significance.

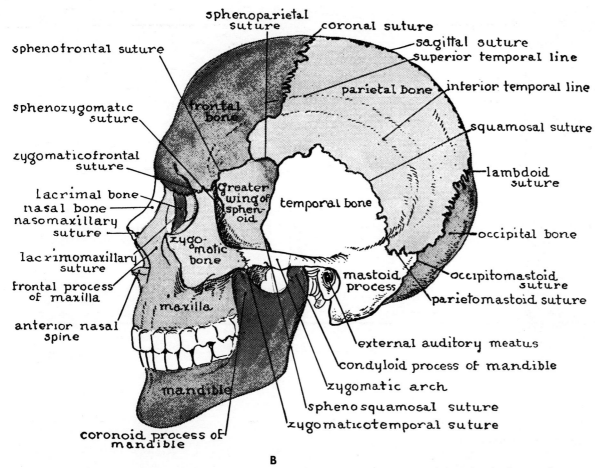

sphenoparietal suture

coronal suture

sphenofrontal suture

sagittal suture

superior temporal line

parietal bone

inferior temporal line

sphenozygomatic suture

squamosal suture

zygomaticofrontal suture

frontal bone

lambdoid suture

Greater wing of sphenoid

lacrimal bone

nasal bone

temporal bone

nasomaxillary suture

occipital bone

lacrimomaxillary suture

zygomatic bone

frontal process of maxilla

mastoid process

occipitomastoid suture

parietomastoid suture

anterior nasal spine

maxilla

external auditory meatus

condyloid process of mandible

mandible

zygomatic arch

sphenosquamosal suture

coronoid process of mandible

zygomaticotemporal suture

B

FIGURE 6–27 *Continued.* *B.* Lateral view of the skull showing the bones of the calvaria, face, and mandible. (From Pendergrass, E. P., et al.: The Head and Neck in Roentgen Diagnosis, 2nd ed., Springfield, Ill., Charles C Thomas, Publisher, 1956. Courtesy of Charles C Thomas, Publisher.)

8. Thinning of the Bones of the Calvaria. The parietal bone superiorly and laterally may on occasion be unusually thin owing to a lack of development of the diploë. There may be a bony dehiscence, the inner table being less affected than the outer. This thinning is usually bilateral, but may be unilateral, a variation that is usually normal but occasionally has pathologic significance.

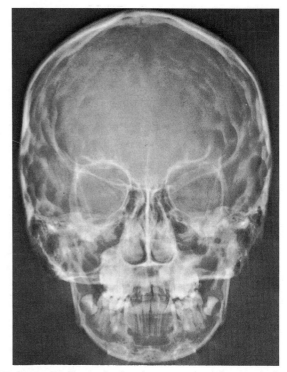

FIGURE 6–28 Radiograph showing accentuated convolutional markings in a normal young adolescent.

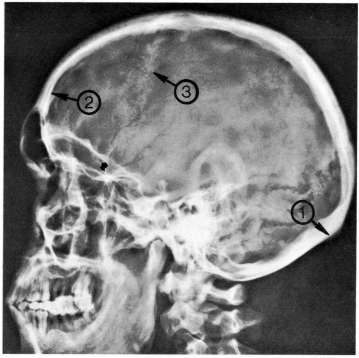

FIGURE 6–29 Some normal thickened areas of the calvaria. (*1*) Occipital protuberances; (*2*) thickening above the frontal sinuses; (*3*) sclerotic sutural margins.

9. Thickened Areas of the Calvaria (Fig. 6–29).

10. Depressions in the Contour of the Calvaria. There may be normal depressions in the contour of the calvaria in the region of the bregma or lambda. When greatly accentuated these may be an indication of developmental deficiency or abnormality, but otherwise may be considered a normal variant.

Intracranial Calcification

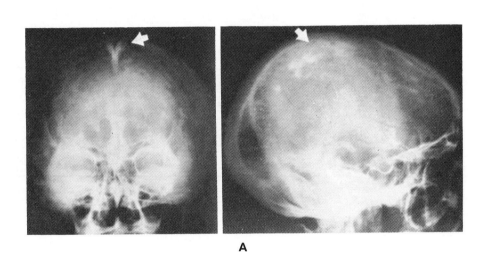

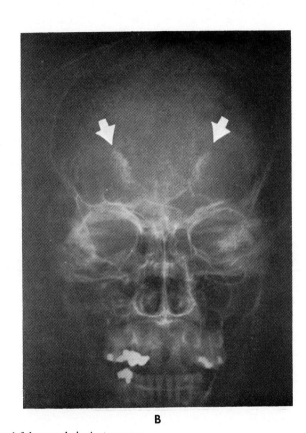

FIGURE 6–30 *A*. Calcium deposit in the dura mater and falx cerebri. Anteroposterior and lateral projections. (Courtesy of Chalmers S. Pool, M.D.) *B*. Calcification of the basal ganglia, posteroanterior projection.

Normal Intracranial Calcification

Pineal Gland. The incidence of pineal glandular calcification has varied in different studies from 33 per cent to 76 per cent (Kitay and Altschule). Vastine and Kinney reported an incidence of 80 per cent in Caucasian men and of 69 per cent in women over age 60. A considerably lower incidence has been reported in other racial groups—10 per cent in Japan, 8 per cent in India, 5 per cent in Nigeria—usually in somewhat younger age groups (Kieffer and Gold). Dyke reported an incidence of 5 per cent in Caucasian children under age 10, and of 55 per cent in patients over 20. Don's study was made with a group of Chinese, Indian, and Malay patients, both men and women.*

There are wide variations in the normal dimensions of the pineal, which normally averages about 5 mm. in length and 3 mm. in height and width. When the calcification is greater than 10 mm. in diameter, a pathologic process may be suspected, *especially in patients in the first two decades of life.*

In the frontal projection, a shift of the pineal of 3 mm. or more from the midline may be regarded as significant, unless the skull is markedly rotated. Slight rotations, even up to 15 per cent, may have no effect because of the remarkably central location in the vertical axis. Displacement of the pineal gland in the lateral view may be determined by a variety of methods which are illustrated in the following section.

*References may be obtained in Meschan, I.: An Atlas of Anatomy Basic to Radiology. Philadelphia, W. B. Saunders Co., 1975.

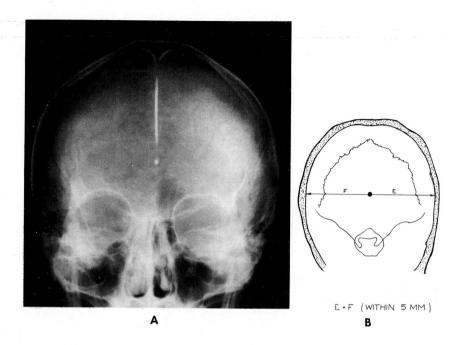

E = F (WITHIN 5 MM.)

A   B

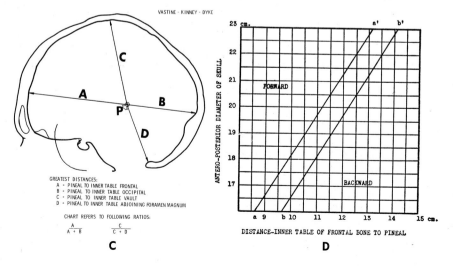

FIGURE 6–31 *A.* Radiograph demonstrating calcification in the pineal gland and falx cerebri in a posteroanterior projection. *B.* Line drawing of a skull, showing the pineal gland position equidistant from the inner tables of the parietal bones as projected in this view (within 5 mm.). It is basically a midline structure.
Legend continued on opposite page.

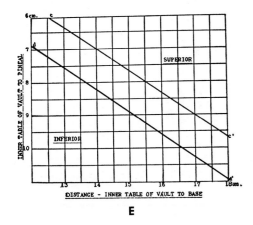

E

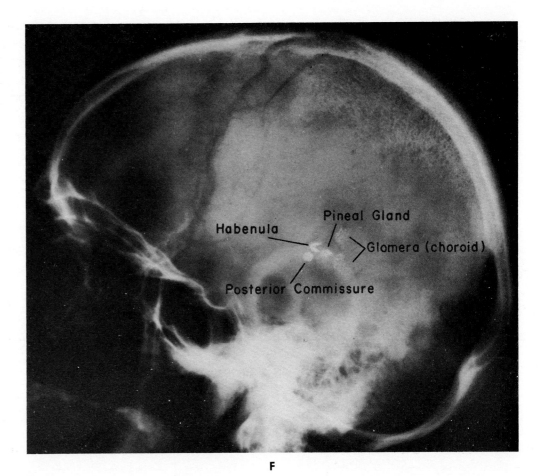

F

FIGURE 6–31 *Continued.* *C, D, E,* and *F.* Method of determination of the normal position of the pineal gland: method of Vastine-Kinney, as modified by Dyke. The measurement from line A–P is transposed to the graph indicated in *D* to demonstrate either forward or backward displacement of the pineal gland. The measurements of C + D are summated and transferred to the graph indicated in *E* to suggest either superior or inferior displacement of the pineal gland. *F.* Lateral view of the skull, indicating points from which measurements are made with surrounding areas of physiologic calcification such as occur in the posterior commissure, the habenular commissure, and the glomera of the choroid plexuses. (Graphs were obtained from Robbins, L. L. (ed.): Golden's Diagnostic Roentgenology. Baltimore, The Williams & Wilkins Co., Vol. 1, pp. 127, 128, 1968.)

Intracranial Areas of Calcification

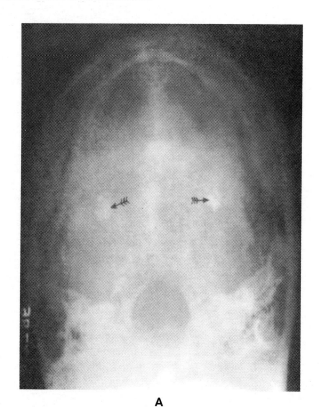

A

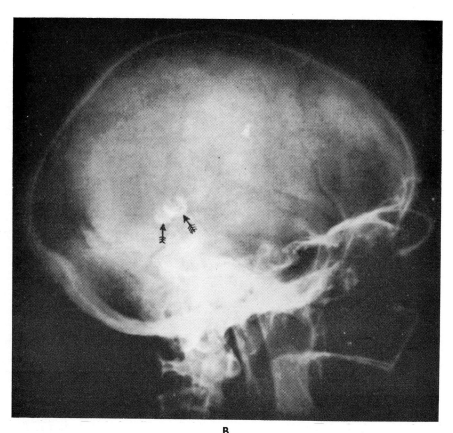

B

FIGURE 6–32 Roentgenogram showing calcification in the glomera of the choroid plexuses. *A*. Towne's position. *B*. Lateral projection.

Apart from *pineal gland* calcification, found in approximately 50 per cent of Caucasian adults and in 10 to 15 per cent of Orientals, intracranial calcification may be found in the following structures: the *glomera of the choroid plexuses* of adults; the *dura* and *falx cerebri;* the *petroclinoid ligaments* posterolateral to the dorsum sellae; the *basal ganglia* (sometimes in association with hyperparathyroidism); and the *caudate nucleus* of the cerebellum. When calcification occurs in children in the pineal gland, it may be indicative of a pinealoma or teratoma; in a glomus of the choroid plexus, there may be an associated choroid plexus papilloma. The *habenular commissure* may also normally undergo calcification.

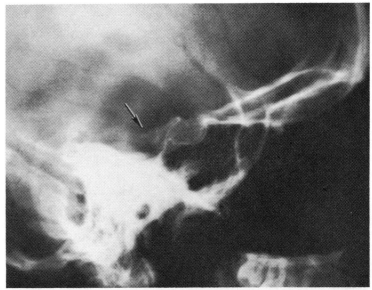

B

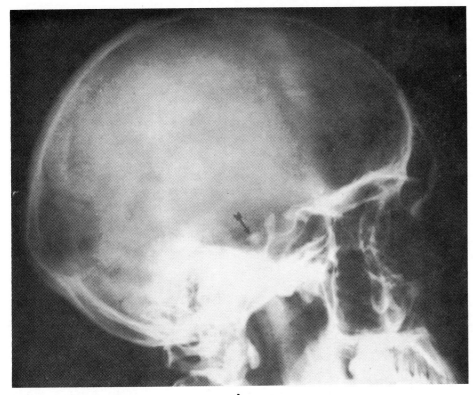

A

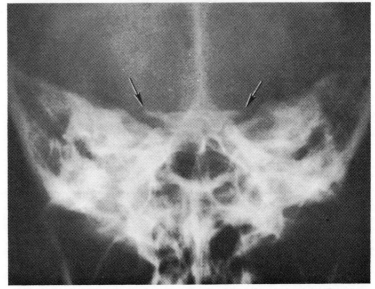

C

FIGURE 6–33 *A*. Radiograph showing calcification in the petroclinoid ligament. *B*. Slightly oblique radiograph showing the configuration of the petroclinoid ligament when the lateral is not true. *C*. Radiograph in Towne's projection showing the petroclinoid ligaments extending between the posterior clinoid processes and dorsum sellae and the petrous ridge (intensified).

ROUTINE RADIOGRAPHIC POSITIONS FOR STUDY OF THE SKULL

Posteroanterior Projection with a 15-Degree Tilt of the Tube Caudally (Caldwell's Projection) (Fig. 6–34)

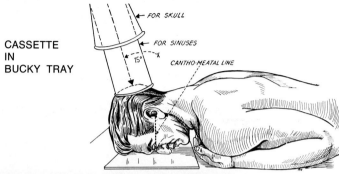

CASSETTE
IN
BUCKY TRAY

FOR SKULL

FOR SINUSES

15°

CANTHO-MEATAL LINE

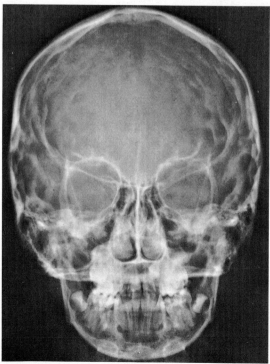

POINTS OF PRACTICAL INTEREST ABOUT FIGURE 6–34

1. The patient's head is adjusted so that the sagittal plane is perfectly perpendicular to the table top and so that the canthomeatal line (outer canthus of the eye to the tragus of the ear or external acoustic meatus) is perpendicular to the plane of the film also. It may be necessary to support the patient's chin on either his fist or a folded towel.

2. The central ray is centered to the glabella and angled toward the feet approximately 15 degrees with respect to the canthomeatal line.

3. It will be noted that in this view the petrous ridges are projected near the inferior margins of the orbits, and hence a clearer concept of the orbits is obtained than would be possible without the 15 degree angulation. Also the lesser and greater wings of the sphenoid bone are projected in the orbits. In the straight posteroanterior projection of the skull these are obscured by the petrous ridges, which are for the most part projected into the orbits.

4. If the frontal bone in itself is the point of major interest, a straight postero-anterior projection of the frontal bone is obtained without angulation of the tube.

5. The outer rims of the orbit are symmetrical and equidistant from the inner table of the vault of the skull.

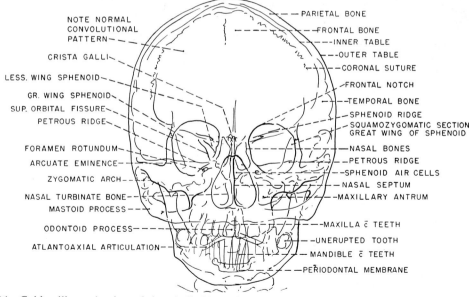

NOTE NORMAL CONVOLUTIONAL PATTERN

CRISTA GALLI

LESS. WING SPHENOID

GR. WING SPHENOID
SUP. ORBITAL FISSURE
PETROUS RIDGE

FORAMEN ROTUNDUM
ARCUATE EMINENCE
ZYGOMATIC ARCH

NASAL TURBINATE BONE
MASTOID PROCESS

ODONTOID PROCESS
ATLANTOAXIAL ARTICULATION

PARIETAL BONE
FRONTAL BONE
INNER TABLE
OUTER TABLE
CORONAL SUTURE
FRONTAL NOTCH
TEMPORAL BONE
SPHENOID RIDGE
SQUAMOZYGOMATIC SECTION GREAT WING OF SPHENOID
NASAL BONES
PETROUS RIDGE
SPHENOID AIR CELLS
NASAL SEPTUM
MAXILLARY ANTRUM
MAXILLA c̄ TEETH
UNERUPTED TOOTH
MANDIBLE c̄ TEETH
PERIODONTAL MEMBRANE

FIGURE 6–34 Caldwell's projection of the skull: Note that patient is positioned so that the canthomeatal line is perpendicular to the film. (The original Caldwell projection for sinuses was 23 degrees with respect to the glabellomeatal line, which is the same as 15 degrees with respect to the canthomeatal line, but more variable and hence a less accurate designation.)

Straight Posteroanterior Projection of the Skull (Fig. 6–34)

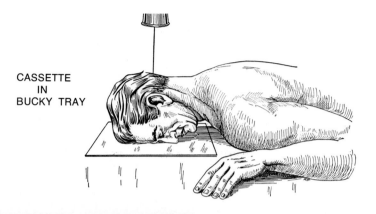

CASSETTE
IN
BUCKY TRAY

POINTS OF PRACTICAL INTEREST ABOUT FIGURE 6–35

1. It will be noted that this view differs from the Caldwell position in that the central ray of the x-ray tube is perpendicular to the film and coincides with the canthomeatal line. It will be noted that the petrous ridges are projected into the orbits, completely obscuring the orbital contents. The sphenoid ridges are projected over the petrous ridges and likewise are considerably obscured.

2. The posterior instead of the anterior cells of the ethmoidal sinuses are shown, and the dorsum sellae is seen as a curved line extending between the orbits just above the ethmoids.

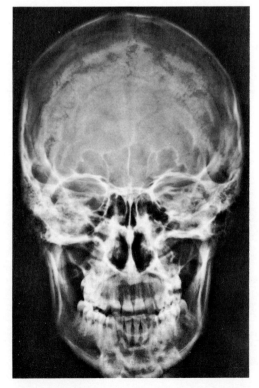

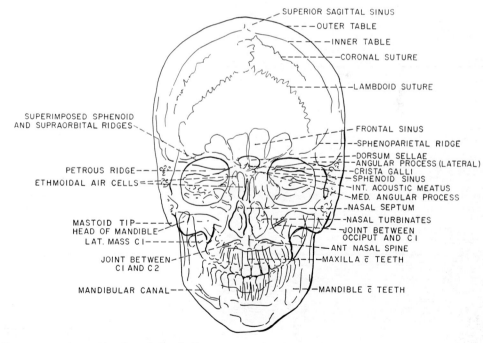

FIGURE 6–35   Posteroanterior projection of the skull.

Anteroposterior Projection with a 30-Degree Tilt of the Tube Caudally (Towne's Position) (Fig. 6–36).

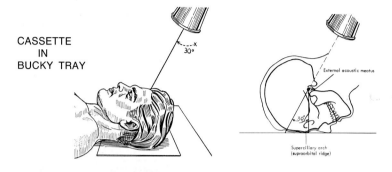

CASSETTE
IN
BUCKY TRAY

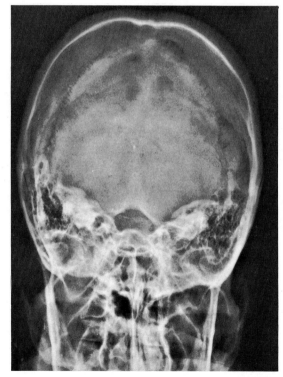

POINTS OF PRACTICAL INTEREST ABOUT FIGURE 6–36

1. The sagittal plane of the patient is placed perpendicular to the table top and along the midline of the table.

2. The head is adjusted so that the canthomeatal line is approximately perpendicular to the table top. This will require that the chin be somewhat depressed upon the neck.

3. The central ray is adjusted at an angle of 30 degrees toward the feet so that it enters the forehead ordinarily at the hairline, and leaves the posterior portion of the cranium in the region of the external occipital protuberance.

4. For better projection of the dorsum sellae into the foramen magnum a somewhat greater angle than 30 degrees may be employed (up to 45 degrees).

5. A view of similar value may be obtained with the patient prone and the tube angled 30 degrees toward the head rather than toward the feet. In the latter instance the central ray enters the head in the region of the external occipital protuberance and leaves the forehead approximately 4 cm. above the superciliary arches. This is called the *reverse Towne's projection*, nuchofrontal projection or Haas position.

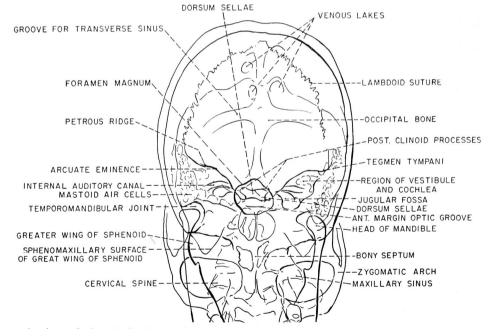

FIGURE 6–36 Towne's projection of the skull (also called Grashey's position).

Both Lateral Projections of the Skull (Fig. 6–37), First with One Side Close to the Film, and Then with the Other Side. (Fig. 6–37)

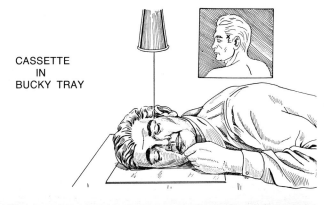

CASSETTE
IN
BUCKY TRAY

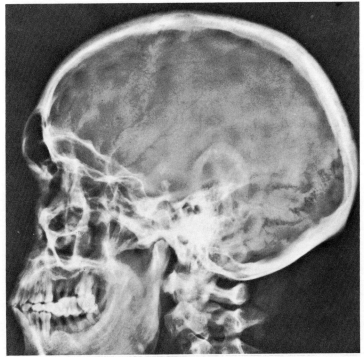

FIGURE 6–37 Lateral projection of skull.

POINTS OF PRACTICAL INTEREST ABOUT FIGURE 6–37

1. The position of the head is adjusted so that its sagittal plane is parallel with the table top and with the film. Its coronal plane is centered to the longitudinal axis of the table. The film is placed transversely in the Potter-Bucky diaphragm beneath the skull.

2. A support is placed under the chin; usually the clenched fist of the patient is adequate in this regard.

3. The central ray passes through a point one inch above the midpoint of the line joining the outer canthus of the eye with the tragus of the ear (cantho-meatal line). This will ordinarily fall immediately over the sella turcica.

4. To evaluate a good lateral projection, the two halves of the mandible should be almost perfectly superimposed over one another and the two orbital roofs should be imposed. If the two rami of the mandible are obliquely projected at fair distances from each other, the projection of the skull is too oblique and should be repeated.

5. It is to be noted that a rather oblique and distorted view of the upper cervical spine is obtained in this lateral view of the skull. This view must not be used routinely for examination of this segment of cervical spine.

6. A "perfect" position for the lateral skull film may be obtained more easily by placing the patient supine and directing the beam horizontally. The cassette in a Bucky tray is then vertical.

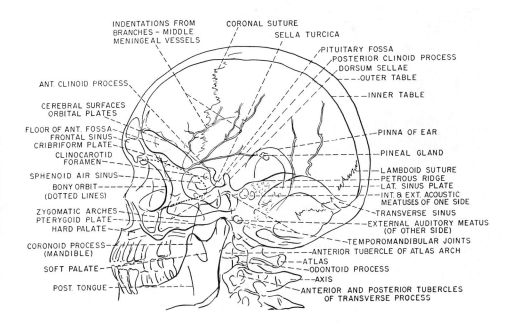

The Axial Projection of the Skull

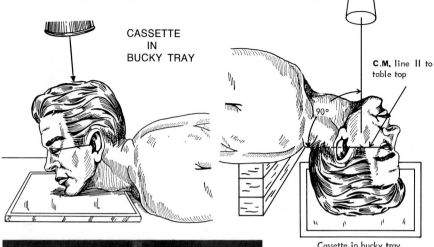

CASSETTE
IN
BUCKY TRAY

C.M. line II to
table top

90°

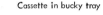

Cassette in bucky tray

POINTS OF PRACTICAL INTEREST ABOUT FIGURE 6–38

1. The head should be rested on the fully extended chin. The more nearly perpendicular the line of the face is to the film, the more satisfactory will be this projection.

2. If possible, the canthomeatal line should be parallel with the table top and film.

3. The central ray should pass through the sagittal plane of the skull perpendicular to the canthomeatal line at its midpoint. It may be necessary to angle the central ray caudally to maintain this relationship if the patient is unable to extend the chin sufficiently.

4. This view is particularly valuable for visualization of the facial bones in tangential projection. It is used along with the frontal view of the facial bones in every instance.

5. This view is also of value for visualization of the posterior ethmoid and sphenoid cells.

6. The "submentovertical position" may be used as an alternate position. The shoulders are elevated, with the head fully extended as shown. The canthomeatal line is parallel to the table top, and the film is in the Bucky tray.

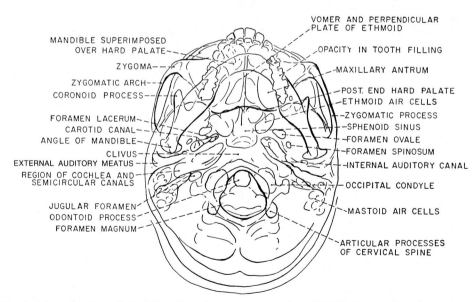

VOMER AND PERPENDICULAR
PLATE OF ETHMOID
MANDIBLE SUPERIMPOSED
OVER HARD PALATE
OPACITY IN TOOTH FILLING
ZYGOMA
MAXILLARY ANTRUM
ZYGOMATIC ARCH
CORONOID PROCESS
POST. END HARD PALATE
ETHMOID AIR CELLS
ZYGOMATIC PROCESS
FORAMEN LACERUM
CAROTID CANAL
SPHENOID SINUS
ANGLE OF MANDIBLE
FORAMEN OVALE
FORAMEN SPINOSUM
CLIVUS
INTERNAL AUDITORY CANAL
EXTERNAL AUDITORY MEATUS
REGION OF COCHLEA AND
SEMICIRCULAR CANALS
OCCIPITAL CONDYLE
JUGULAR FORAMEN
MASTOID AIR CELLS
ODONTOID PROCESS
FORAMEN MAGNUM
ARTICULAR PROCESSES
OF CERVICAL SPINE

FIGURE 6–38 Axial projection of skull (verticosubmental projection; Schüller's position); and submentovertical axial projection.

Posteroanterior Projection of Face (Water's Projection); Skull, or Paranasal Sinuses with Greatest Emphasis in the Latter Upon Showing More Clearly the Maxillary Antra, the Sphenoid (through the Mouth), and the Frontal Sinuses

POINTS OF PRACTICAL INTEREST ABOUT FIGURE 6–39

1. The difference between the skull and the paranasal sinus view is that an extension cylinder (fully extended) is used for visualization of the paranasal sinuses.

2. It is desirable to make these views in the *upright position,* if at all possible, to show fluid levels.

3. The canthomeatal line forms an angle of 37 degrees with the plane of the film. The central ray enters the vertex and emerges at the anterior nasal spine.

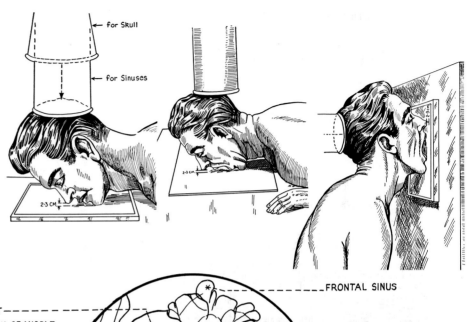

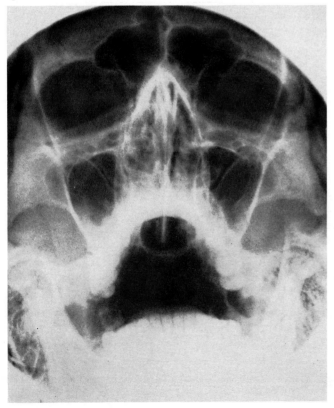

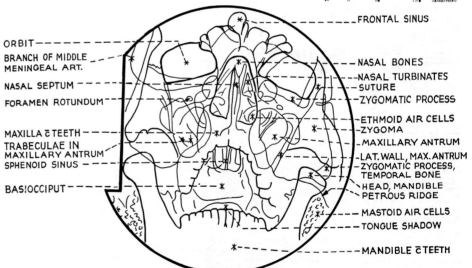

FIGURE 6–39 Water's projection for the paranasal sinuses and skull. Drawings show positioning of patient with mouth closed, with mouth open, and for films taken with patient erect; radiograph and tracing show mouth open. The projection through the open mouth to show the sphenoid sinuses is also called the Pirie transoral projection. Paranasal sinus projections may be obtained with "table top" technique, however, for optimum skull technique, where such close coning is not employed, the cassette should be placed in a Bucky tray and the Bucky technique should be employed.

Alternate Submentovertical Projection of the Skull and Facial Bones (Axial Projection) (Fig. 6–40)

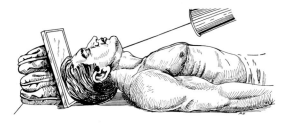

ROUTINE STUDY OF THE ZYGOMATIC ARCHES

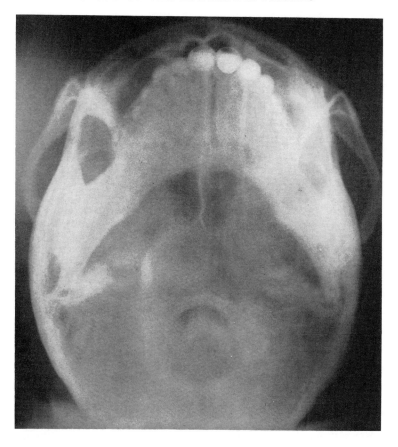

POINTS OF PRACTICAL INTEREST ABOUT FIGURE 6–40

1. The film and the patient's head are placed so that the infraorbital line is parallel with the surface of the film.

2. The central ray is directed perpendicular to the midpoint of the infraorbital line in the sagittal plane of the patient's skull.

3. A similar projection may be obtained in the sitting posture with the patient's head leaned backward against a firm support; or in the supine position by placing a pillow under the upper back. Wherever possible a grid cassette or Potter-Bucky diaphragm should be employed.

4. In this projection a clearer concept of the anterior ethmoidal cells is obtained and ordinarily the facial bones and mandible are projected over one another.

5. This projection is also of value for visualization of the zygomatic arches, since they are thrown into bold relief. However, a lighter exposure technique must be employed for this purpose.

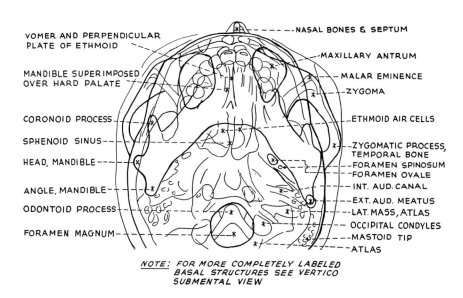

FIGURE 6–40 Axial projection of face (submentovertical projection). Using a slightly "lighter" exposure technique, this projection is utilized for visualization of the zygomatic arches.

POINTS OF PRACTICAL INTEREST ABOUT FIGURE 6–41

1. The sagittal plane of the head is adjusted so that it is perfectly parallel with the film and the table top.

2. The cassette may be placed directly under the head without utilizing the Potter-Bucky diaphragm provided that the extended cone is likewise placed directly in contact with the opposite side of the head.

3. Center to the region of the sella turcica over a point 2.5 cm. anterior to and 2 cm. above the external acoustic meatus. Alternately one may center at a point about 2 cm. above the midpoint of the canthomeatal line.

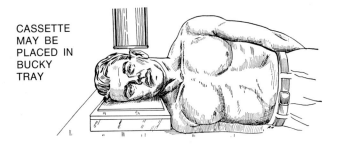

CASSETTE MAY BE PLACED IN BUCKY TRAY

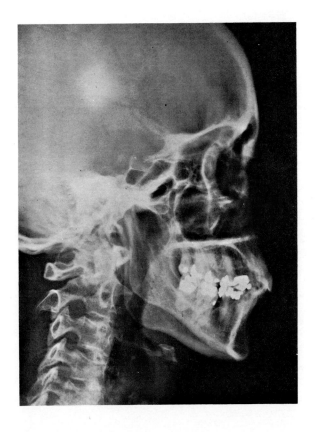

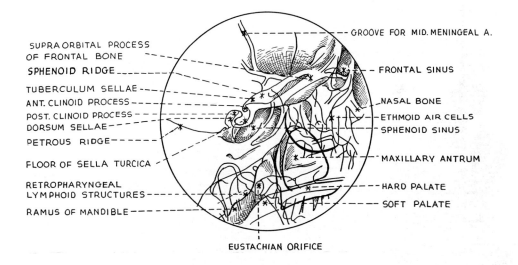

SUPRA ORBITAL PROCESS OF FRONTAL BONE
SPHENOID RIDGE
TUBERCULUM SELLAE
ANT. CLINOID PROCESS
POST. CLINOID PROCESS
DORSUM SELLAE
PETROUS RIDGE
FLOOR OF SELLA TURCICA
RETROPHARYNGEAL LYMPHOID STRUCTURES
RAMUS OF MANDIBLE

GROOVE FOR MID. MENINGEAL A.
FRONTAL SINUS
NASAL BONE
ETHMOID AIR CELLS
SPHENOID SINUS
MAXILLARY ANTRUM
HARD PALATE
SOFT PALATE

EUSTACHIAN ORIFICE

FIGURE 6–41 Lateral projection of face.

Posteroanterior Projections of the Mandible

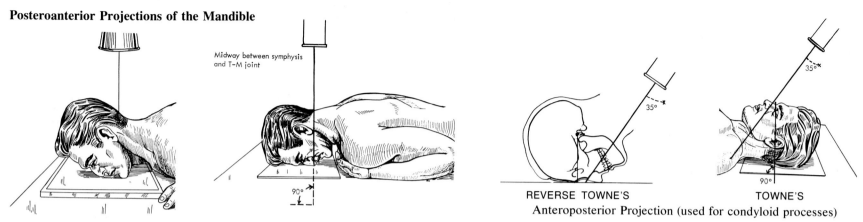

Midway between symphysis and T-M joint

90°

REVERSE TOWNE'S

TOWNE'S

Anteroposterior Projection (used for condyloid processes)

POINTS OF PRACTICAL INTEREST ABOUT FIGURE 6-42

1. The central ray is directed midway between the mandible symphysis and the temporomandibular joint.
2. The Bucky tray is used for placement of the film in each of these views.

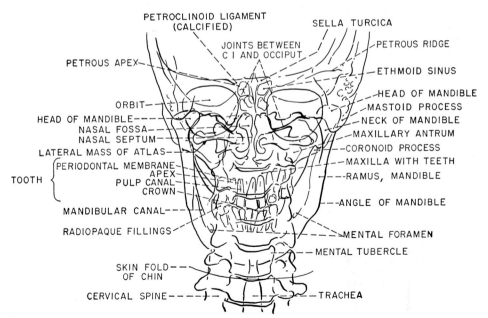

PETROCLINOID LIGAMENT (CALCIFIED)
SELLA TURCICA
JOINTS BETWEEN C I AND OCCIPUT
PETROUS RIDGE
PETROUS APEX
ETHMOID SINUS
HEAD OF MANDIBLE
ORBIT
MASTOID PROCESS
HEAD OF MANDIBLE
NECK OF MANDIBLE
NASAL FOSSA
MAXILLARY ANTRUM
NASAL SEPTUM
CORONOID PROCESS
LATERAL MASS OF ATLAS
MAXILLA WITH TEETH
PERIODONTAL MEMBRANE
TOOTH { APEX
RAMUS, MANDIBLE
PULP CANAL
CROWN
ANGLE OF MANDIBLE
MANDIBULAR CANAL
RADIOPAQUE FILLINGS
MENTAL FORAMEN
MENTAL TUBERCLE
SKIN FOLD OF CHIN
CERVICAL SPINE
TRACHEA

FIGURE 6-42 Posteroanterior projections of mandible.

Oblique Projection of Each Side of the Mandible

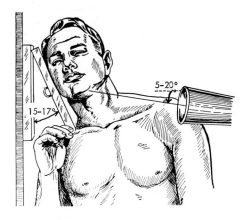

1. The film is placed against the patient's cheek at an angle of approximately 15 degrees from the vertical.

2. The broad surface of the mandibular body is placed parallel to the plane of the film.

3. To avoid distortion a long target-to-film distance may be employed.

4. For better detail of the ramus of the mandible, the central ray may be directed inward, centering over the ramus, which may be brought into a position more directly parallel with the plane of the film.

5. If more information is desired regarding the body of the mandible near the symphysis, the head is rotated so that this area is nearer the film.

6. It is ordinarily easier to obtain an erect position of the injured mandible than the recumbent, although the recumbent view may be obtained in somewhat similar fashion.

7. The central ray is directed to the midpoint of the film at a point midway between the angle and the symphysis of the jaw.

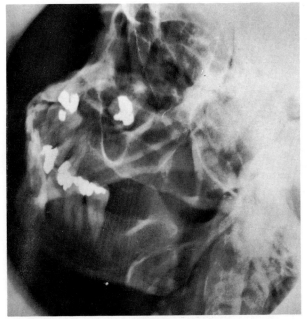

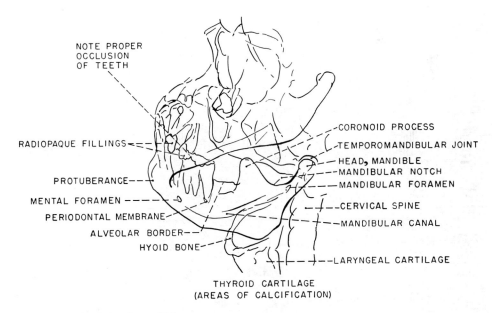

FIGURE 6–43 Oblique projection of mandible.

Special Projection of the Temporomandibular Articulation (Fig. 6–44)

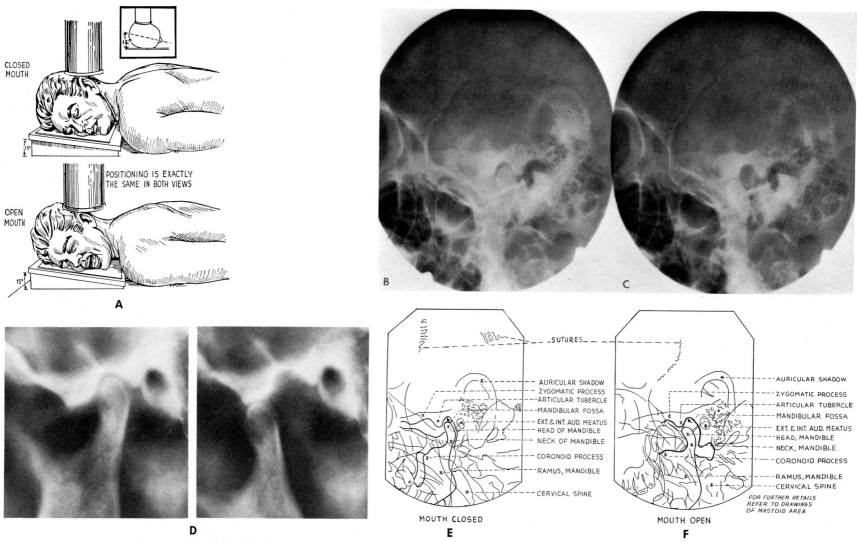

FIGURE 6–44 Projections of temporomandibular joint with the mouth open and closed. *A*, Position of patient with mouth open, with mouth closed. *B* and *C*. Radiographs so obtained (*B*, mouth closed; *C*, mouth open). *D*. Tomographs of temporomandibular joint (*D'*, mouth closed; *D"*, mouth open). *E* and *F*. Tracings of *B* and *C*, respectively. For the body section radiograph, the patient is positioned for a true lateral skull view. The cuts are taken through the joint closest to the film, first with the mouth open and then with the mouth closed, as shown above.

Intraoral Projection of the Body of the Mandible (Fig. 6–45)

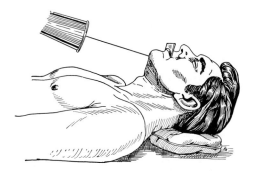

This is obtained by placing an occlusal film in the mouth as far back as possible, and directing the central ray through the submental region.

Panoramic and Pantomographic Views of the Mandible

Panoramic views of the mandible may be obtained by several methods. In one technique the centered electron beam hits a pyramid-shaped anticathode, which has been introduced as a focus into the oral cavity. The rays are reflected outward from the oral cavity and pharynx, striking the film which has been placed on the outside of the mandible. A plain panoramic view of the mandibular arch is obtained with this technique.

There are at least three other panoramic x-ray units available, all having the following features in common: (1) the x-ray source rotates around the patient's head, and (2) the x-ray film is held in a cassette with intensifying screens which also rotates around the patient's head.

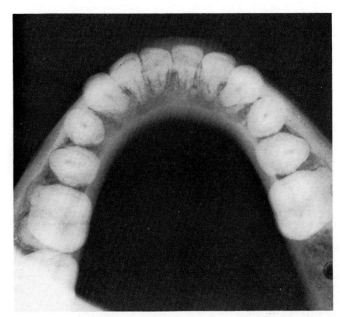

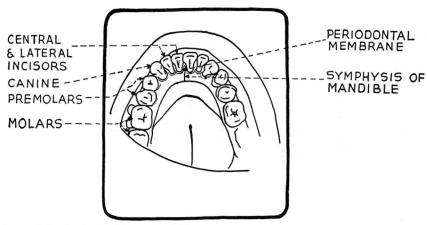

CENTRAL & LATERAL INCISORS

CANINE

PREMOLARS

MOLARS

PERIODONTAL MEMBRANE

SYMPHYSIS OF MANDIBLE

FIGURE 6–45 Intraoral projection of mandible obtained with occlusal film.

Pantomography of the Mandible

Apart from radiography of the mandible and maxilla, this technique can also be applied in sialography and in clinical pantomography of the jaws (Soila and Paatero; Pappas and Wallace). There is an inherent enlargement factor in these units because of the short distance between the x-ray tube-target and the film, and the great distance between the film and the object being radiographed.

These units are capable of recording curved sections of the body, an advantage which is especially useful in radiography of the dental arch. Actually, in the dental arch three arcs are usually filmed: (a) the left buccal segment, (b) an anterior segment, and (c) a right buccal segment. Centers of rotation of the two sides of the mandible are located behind the third mandibular molar tooth on the side opposite that being radiographed. The anterior segment has a center of rotation just behind the incisors at about the level of the mandibular bicuspids.

The cassette is made of a flexible plastic material with intensifying screens wrapped around a curved metal film holder. Films are ordinarily 6 by 12 inches in size. Grids are usually not employed.

If the system is very slightly eccentric to the mandible, either one of the parotid glands may be brought into focus by rotating the head so that the midsaggittal plane is 20 to 25 degrees from the vertical center line.

Pantomography (Soila and Paatero)* has been developed to obtain body section radiographs of curved surfaces. Again, the jaws are especially suitable targets for this technique, but it has been used in other areas of the body as well. As described earlier, the method employs a fixed source of radiation while the object and film are rotated on holders having equal radii and moving at equal speeds through a peripheral frictional arrangement.

For concentric pantomography, which is best suited to structures like the jaw, the object is placed concentrically on the holder. In eccentric pantomography, the object is placed eccentrically on the holder. Stereoscopic films may be produced by shifting the tube horizontally or vertically.

*References may be obtained in Meschan, I.: An Atlas of Anatomy Basic to Radiology. Philadelphia, W. B. Saunders Co., 1975.

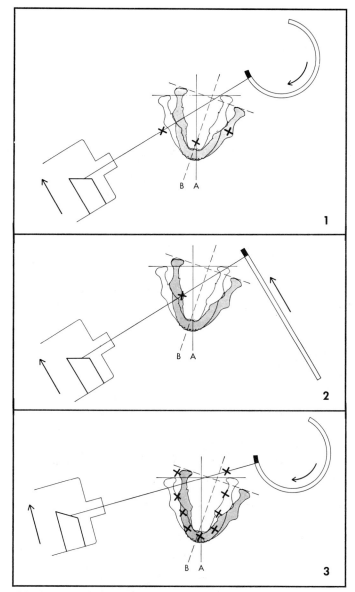

FIGURE 6–46 Schematic drawings of three panoramic x-ray units. The *X's* in drawings 1 and 2 indicate the centers of rotation for the x-ray source. These shift as the x-ray source moves around the face. The *X's* in drawing 3 indicate the path that the x-ray source follows as it moves around the face. (From Pappas, G. C., and Wallace, W. R.: Dent. Radiogr. Photogr. *43*(2):27, 1970.)

Panoramic View of the Mandible

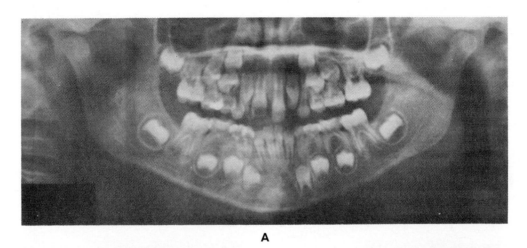

A

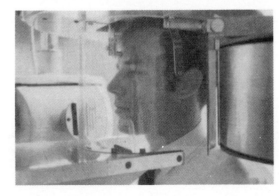
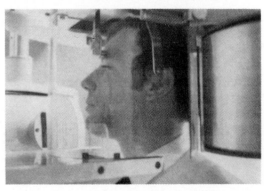

B

FIGURE 6–47 *A*. Routine panoramic radiograph. *B*. Position of the patient's head when the x-ray unit in Figure 6–46 is used for panoramic radiography. *Left*, Conventional position. *Right*, Modified position. (From Pappas, G. C., and Wallace, W. R.: Dent. Radiogr. and Photogr., *43*(2):27, 1970.)

Intraoral Views of the Teeth

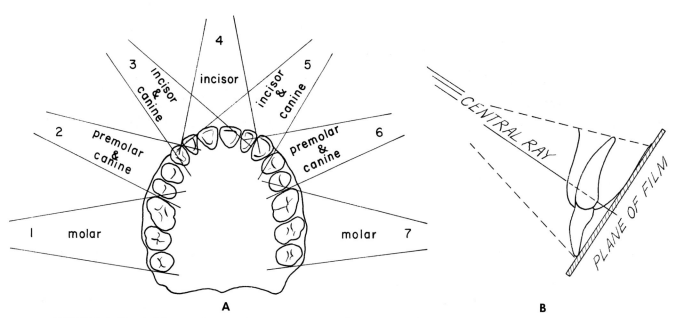

A   **B**

FIGURE 6-48 *A.* The usual seven intraoral dental films obtained for each dental arch. *B.* The angulation of the central ray with respect to the tooth and film. ("Bite-wing films" for demonstration of crown cavities are not illustrated. Refer to dental x-ray technique manuals.)

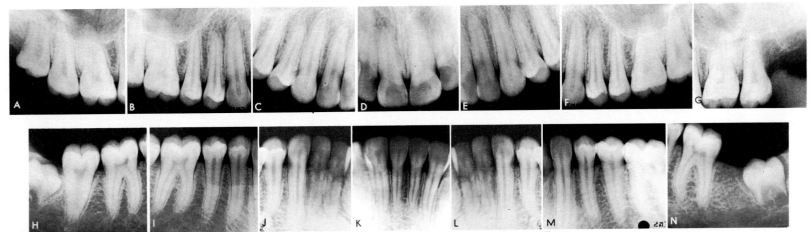

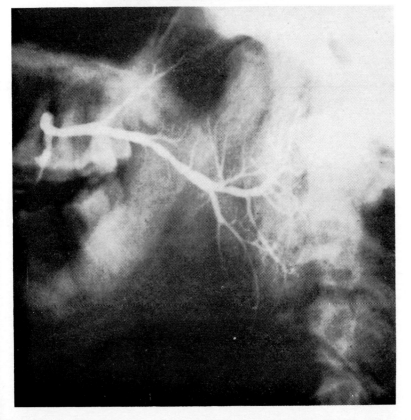

FIGURE 6–49 Representative intraoral dental films: *A*. Right upper molar area. *B*. right upper bicuspid area. *C*. right upper cuspid area. *D*. upper incisor area. *E*. left upper cuspid area. *F*. left upper bicuspid area. *G*. left upper molar area. *H*. right lower molar area. *I*. right lower bicuspid area. *J*. right lower cuspid area. *K*. lower incisor area. *L*. left lower cuspid area. *M*. left lower bicuspid area. *N*. left lower molar area.

Notes About Use of Occlusal Films Around the Mouth

These are frequently used for detection of calculi in salivary glands and ducts, and in conjunction with oblique and lateral films of the face in "sialograms"—radiographs of the salivary ducts and glands following the injection of Sinografin® into the appropriate duct.

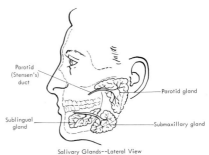

Parotid (Stensen's) duct

Parotid gland

Sublingual gland

Submaxillary gland

Salivary Glands--Lateral View

FIGURE 6–50 Normal sialogram of the parotid gland (supplied by Dr. L. B. Morettin, Galveston, Texas).

FIGURE 6–51 Lateral view of nasolacrimal system. (*a*) lacrimal puncta. (*b*) canaliculi. (*c*) lacrimal sac. (*d*) lacrimal duct. Contrast medium, 1 to 2 cc. warmed Beck's bismuth and oil paste. (From Pendergrass, E. P., et al.: The Head and Neck in Roentgen Diagnosis, 2nd ed. Springfield, Ill., Charles C Thomas, Publisher, 1956. Courtesy of Charles C Thomas, Publisher.)

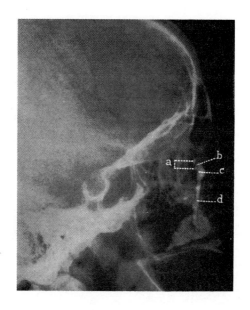

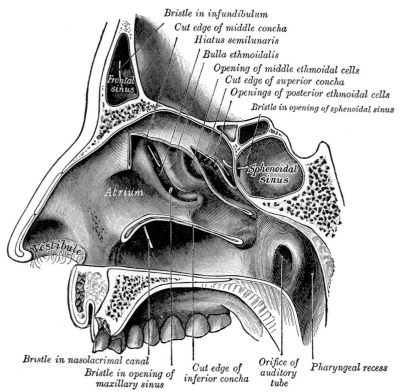

FIGURE 6–52 Lateral wall of nasal cavity to demonstrate apertures leading into it. (From Gray, H. *in* Goss, C. M. (ed.): Gray's Anatomy of the Human Body. Philadelphia, Lea & Febiger, 1973.)

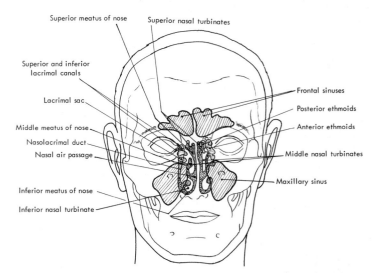

FIGURE 6–53 Frontal diagram of face showing position of nasal air passages and related frontal and maxillary paranasal sinuses.

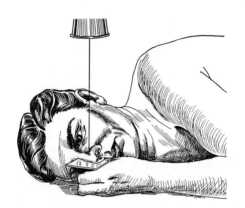

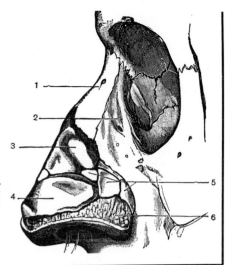

FIGURE 6–54 Diagram to illustrate bones and cartilages of external nose. (*1*) Nasal bone. (*2*) Frontal processes of maxilla. (*3*) Lateral cartilage. (*4*) Greater alar cartilage. (*5*) Lesser alar cartilage. (*6*) Fatty tissue of ala nasi. (From West, C. M., *in* Cunningham, D. J.: Textbook of Anatomy. London, Oxford University Press.)

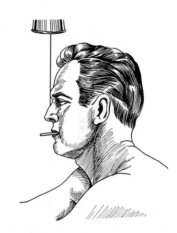

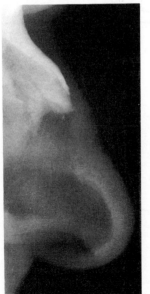

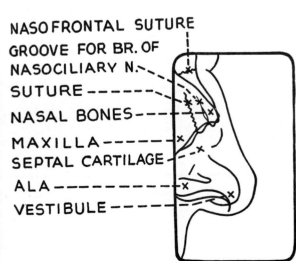

NASOFRONTAL SUTURE
GROOVE FOR BR. OF NASOCILIARY N.
SUTURE
NASAL BONES
MAXILLA
SEPTAL CARTILAGE
ALA
VESTIBULE

FIGURE 6–55 Lateral view of nasal bone.

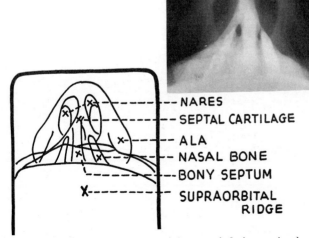

NARES
SEPTAL CARTILAGE
ALA
NASAL BONE
BONY SEPTUM
SUPRAORBITAL RIDGE

FIGURE 6–56 Tangential superoinferior projection of nasal bones.

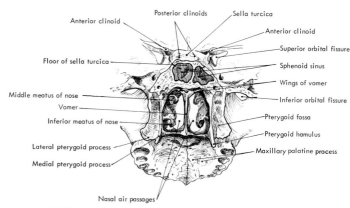

Anterior clinoid

Posterior clinoids

Sella turcica

Anterior clinoid

Superior orbital fissure

Floor of sella turcica

Sphenoid sinus

Wings of vomer

Middle meatus of nose

Inferior orbital fissure

Vomer

Inferior meatus of nose

Pterygoid fossa

Pterygoid hamulus

Lateral pterygoid process

Maxillary palatine process

Medial pterygoid process

Nasal air passages

FIGURE 6–57 Coronal section through nasopharynx viewed from posterior aspect and showing osseous posterior nasal apertures.

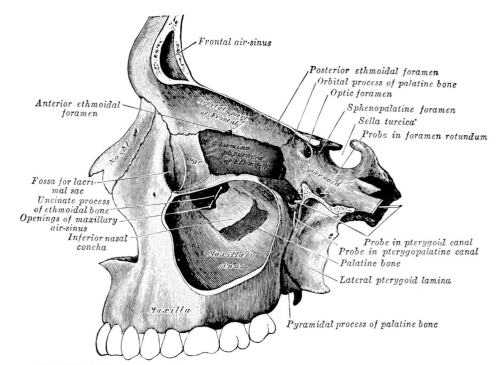

Frontal air-sinus

Posterior ethmoidal foramen

Orbital process of palatine bone

Optic foramen

Sphenopalatine foramen

Sella turcica

Probe in foramen rotundum

Anterior ethmoidal foramen

Nasal

Orbital part of Frontal

Lamina papyracea of ethmoid

Lac

Sphenoid

Fossa for lacri- mal sac

Uncinate process of ethmoidal bone

Openings of maxillary air-sinus

Inferior nasal concha

Maxillary sinus

Probe in pterygoid canal

Probe in pterygopalatine canal

Palatine bone

Lateral pterygoid lamina

Maxilla

Pyramidal process of palatine bone

FIGURE 6–58 Left maxillary sinus opened from lateral side. (From Gray, H. *in* Goss, C. M. (ed.): Gray's Anatomy of the Human Body. Philadelphia, Lea & Febiger.)

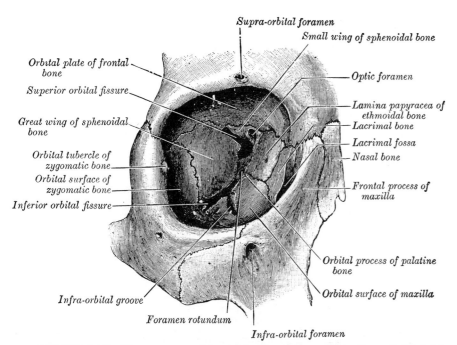

FIGURE 6–59 The anatomy of the orbit. (From Gray, H. in Goss, C. M. (ed.): Gray's Anatomy of the Human Body. Philadelphia, Lea & Febiger.)

Labels for Figure 6–59:
- Supra-orbital foramen
- Small wing of sphenoidal bone
- Orbital plate of frontal bone
- Optic foramen
- Superior orbital fissure
- Lamina papyracea of ethmoidal bone
- Lacrimal bone
- Great wing of sphenoidal bone
- Lacrimal fossa
- Orbital tubercle of zygomatic bone
- Nasal bone
- Orbital surface of zygomatic bone
- Frontal process of maxilla
- Inferior orbital fissure
- Orbital process of palatine bone
- Infra-orbital groove
- Orbital surface of maxilla
- Foramen rotundum
- Infra-orbital foramen

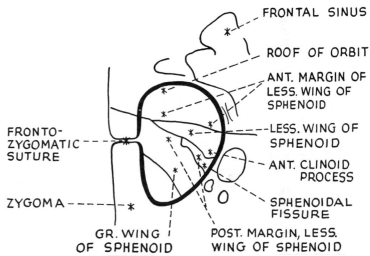

FIGURE 6–60 Tracing of orbital projection obtained by Caldwell's position.

Labels for Figure 6–60:
- FRONTAL SINUS
- ROOF OF ORBIT
- ANT. MARGIN OF LESS. WING OF SPHENOID
- FRONTO-ZYGOMATIC SUTURE
- LESS. WING OF SPHENOID
- ANT. CLINOID PROCESS
- ZYGOMA
- SPHENOIDAL FISSURE
- GR. WING OF SPHENOID
- POST. MARGIN, LESS. WING OF SPHENOID

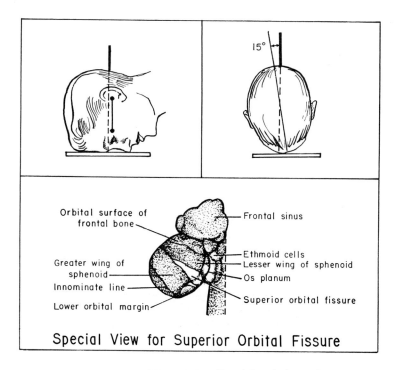

Special View for Superior Orbital Fissure

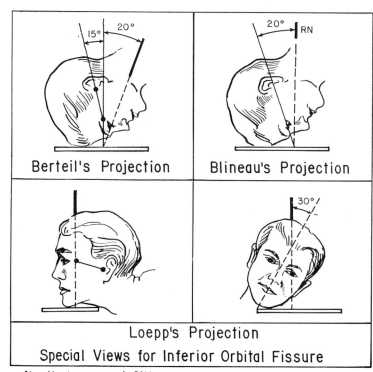

Berteil's Projection

Blineau's Projection

Loepp's Projection

Special Views for Inferior Orbital Fissure

after Hartmann and Gilles

FIGURE 6–61   Special techniques for examination of the orbit, apart from the usual views of the facial bones previously demonstrated.

Comments on the Radiologic Examination of the Orbits

1. The closed-mouth Water's projection (Fig. 6–39) may be used.

2. With the lateral projection of the face (Fig. 6–37), the central ray should be centered at the outer canthus.

3. The posteroanterior projection of the face or skull (Fig. 6–34) — Caldwell's projection should also be employed.

4. Oblique: The head is rotated 20 degrees from the midline of the skull, and the glabellomeatal line is perpendicular to the film. The tube is angled 35 degrees caudad, with the central ray exiting at the nasion. Both sides are studied in this manner.

5. When a "blow-out" fracture is suspected, body-section radiographs are obtained additionally in the posteroanterior and lateral projections. *Additionally,* the posteroanterior projection is repeated, with the tube angled 30 degrees instead of the 12 to 15 degrees of the typical Caldwell's view.

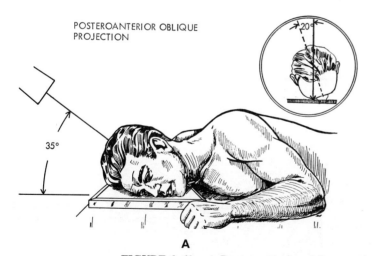

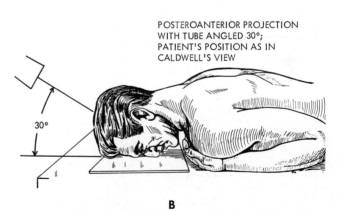

FIGURE 6–62 *A*. Posteroanterior oblique projection of the orbit. *B*. Posteroanterior projection of the skull with the tube angled 30 degrees caudad. The patient's position is the same as that in Caldwell's view, but the primary purpose of this view is for radiologic examination of the orbits.

Parieto-orbital Projection

1. The head is rested on the zygoma, nose, and chin.
2. The acanthomeatal line is perpendicular to the film plane.
3. The head and central ray are rotated as shown.

POINTS OF PRACTICAL INTEREST ABOUT FIGURE 6–63

Alternate Projection:

1. The position of the patient in this projection is identical to that of Stenver's projection of the petrous ridges. The central ray of the x-ray beam, however, is directed 12 degrees *toward the feet,* if the angulated beam is employed, instead of 12 degrees *toward the head* (Stenver's projection).

2. When one studies optic foramina, the two sides are compared with one another; hence, equivalent projections of the two sides must be obtained.

3. The ethmoid air cells are also clearly delineated here to best advantage.

4. In the Rhese position, the patient's head is angled 50 degrees, and the central ray is not angled.

5. The plane of the acanthomeatal line is perpendicular to the film.

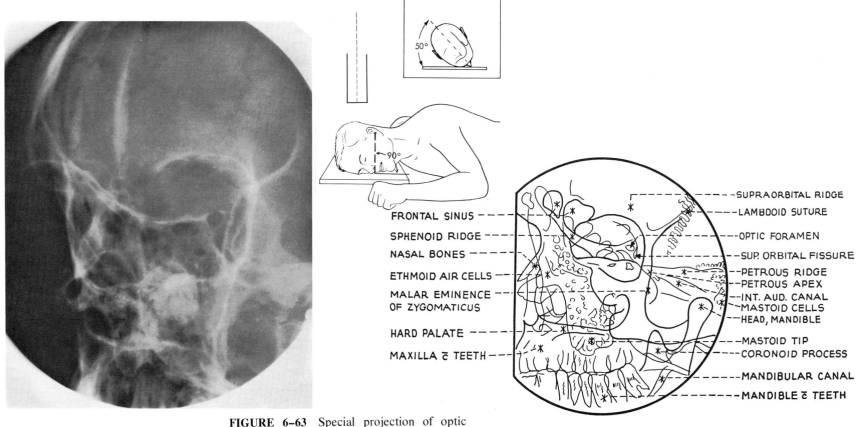

FRONTAL SINUS
SPHENOID RIDGE
NASAL BONES
ETHMOID AIR CELLS
MALAR EMINENCE OF ZYGOMATICUS
HARD PALATE
MAXILLA c̄ TEETH

SUPRAORBITAL RIDGE
LAMBDOID SUTURE
OPTIC FORAMEN
SUP. ORBITAL FISSURE
PETROUS RIDGE
PETROUS APEX
INT. AUD. CANAL
MASTOID CELLS
HEAD, MANDIBLE
MASTOID TIP
CORONOID PROCESS
MANDIBULAR CANAL
MANDIBLE c̄ TEETH

FIGURE 6–63 Special projection of optic foramina.

METHODS FOR DEMONSTRATION OF THE JUGULAR FORAMEN (Figs. 6–64 and 6–65). There are several possible techniques for visualization of the jugular foramen.

(a) A modified Water's projection may be used, in which the mouth is open as wide as possible and the canthomeatal line and roentgenographic table form an angle of 37 degrees (35 to 37 degrees). The x-ray beam is directed perpendicularly to the table in the posteroanterior (or anteroposterior) projection at the level of the external auditory meatus. A cone is employed to include both the jugular foramina for best detail (Kim and Capp).*

(b) A modified Law's position may be used for demonstration of the jugular foramen. The left side of the face is against the roentgenographic table when the left jugular foramen is examined (and vice versa for the right jugular foramen). The face is tilted to the side toward the table to make a 5 degree angle between the sagittal suture line and the table. The chin is tilted toward the table to make a 15 degree angle between the nasal axis line and the table. The x-ray tube is tilted 15 degrees caudad, and the central beam is directed to the external auditory meatus of the ear to be examined (Kim and Capp).*

(c) Transoral projection, open mouth.
(1) Patient is supine with one pillow elevating his ipsilateral shoulder.
(2) The x-ray beam is perpendicular to the table and midline over the patient.
(3) Patient's mouth is opened wide with a cork or other non-opaque object.

(4) With the patient's nose and chin in the midline, extend or flex his head as necessary to align the central beam through the infratragal notch of the ear and the gap between the upper and lower molars as palpated through the cheek.
(5) Exposure factors are slightly less than those used for the base of the skull (Strickler).

(d) Oblique open mouth projection. Follow steps (1) through (4) as for the transoral projection of Strickler. Keeping the patient's chin and nose in a straight line parallel to the midplane, roll the patient's head 10 degrees or less to one side. This maneuver centers the x-ray beam over the jugular foramen and along the jugular canal on the side away from which the face is turned. Repeat, turning the face to the opposite side for the other jugular foramen.

(e) In this projection the patient is supine with pillows elevating his shoulders. The x-ray beam is perpendicular to the table and midline over the patient. With the patient's mouth closed and his nose and chin in the midline, raise the patient's chin until the central ray is aligned through (a) the infratragal notch of the ear, and (b) the point 2 cm. caudad to the lower edge of the chin as viewed from the lateral position. Edentulous patients are positioned the same way.

Roentgenograms and tracings of them are shown for each of these positions.

If POLYTOMOGRAPHY is available, this technique offers the optimum method for demonstration of the jugular foramen—even for separation of the *pars nervosa* from the *pars vasculare*.

(The demonstration of the jugular foramen with opaque media is shown in Figure 6–81.)

---

*References may be obtained in Meschan, I.: An Atlas of Anatomy Basic to Radiology. Philadelphia, W. B. Saunders Co., 1975.

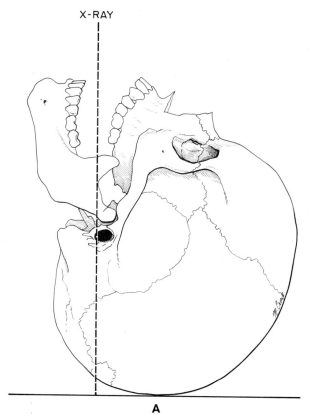

X-RAY

A

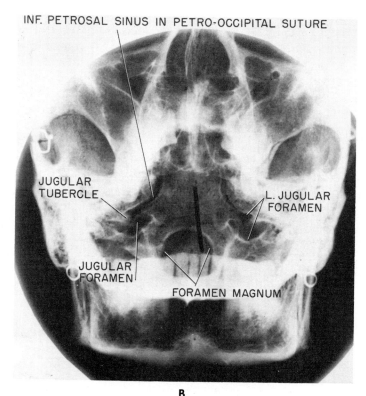

INF. PETROSAL SINUS IN PETRO-OCCIPITAL SUTURE

JUGULAR
TUBERCLE

L. JUGULAR
FORAMEN

JUGULAR
FORAMEN

FORAMEN MAGNUM

B

FIGURE 6–64 *A*. Transoral projection. The x-ray beam perpendicular to the film passes between the molars and through the plane of the jugular foramina, which lies just caudad to the external auditory meatus at the infratragal notch. *B*. Transoral view of both jugular foramina in a dry skull. (From Strickler, J. M.: Am. J. Roentgenol., *97*:601–606, 1966.)

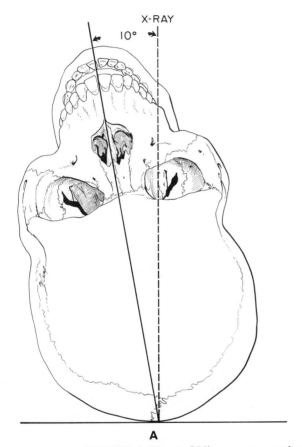

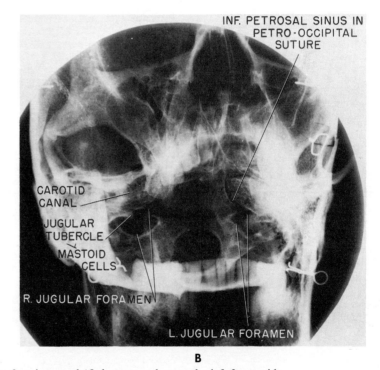

A

B

FIGURE 6–65 *A*. Oblique open-mouth projection. When the face is turned 10 degrees or less to the left from midline, the x-ray beams remains perpendicular to the film and becomes centered through the right jugular foramen. *B*. Oblique open-mouth view of right jugular foramen in a dry skull. The walls of the carotid canal are clear and sharp in this "down the hatch" view. (From Strickler, J. M.: Am. J. Roentgenol., *97:*601–606, 1966.)

Blood Supply of the Orbit

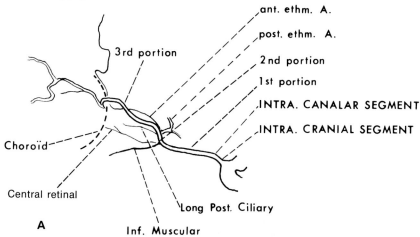

- ant. ethm. A.
- post. ethm. A.
- 2nd portion
- 1st portion
- INTRA. CANALAR SEGMENT
- INTRA. CRANIAL SEGMENT

3rd portion

Choroïd

Central retinal

Long Post. Ciliary

Inf. Muscular

A

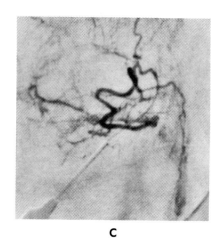

C

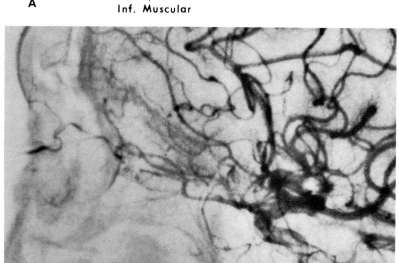

B

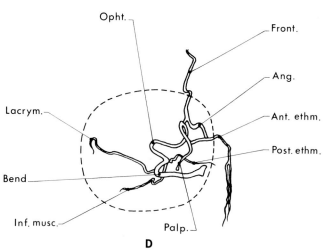

Opht.

Front.

Ang.

Lacrym.

Ant. ethm.

Post. ethm.

Bend

Inf. musc.

Palp.

D

FIGURE 6–66 *A* and *B*. Lateral view of the normal ophthalmic artery. Internal carotid angiography. *C* and *D*. Ophthalmic artery arteriography by catheterization of the exposed angular artery; infra-optic variety; the semicircle is concave medially. There is good visibility of the ethmoidal arteries. Note the opacification of the mucosa of the medial nasal wall by the anterior ethmoidal artery; and the opacification of the lacrimal artery, the inferior muscular artery, and the medial palpebral artery. No supraorbital artery is demonstrated.

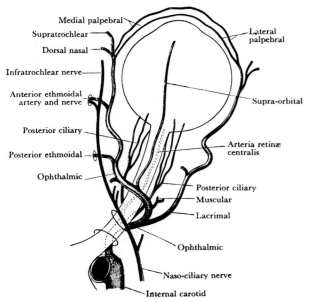

FIGURE 6-67 Diagram of the ophthalmic artery and its branches. (From Cunningham's Manual of Practical Anatomy, 12th ed. Vol. 3. London, Oxford University Press, 1959.)

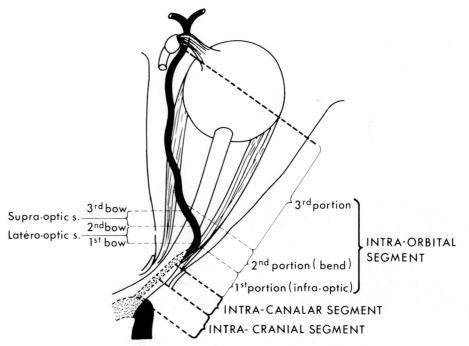

FIGURE 6-68 The different segments of the ophthalmic artery. (From Vignard, J., Clay, C., and Aubin, M. L.: Radiol. Clin. North Am., *10* (1):39–61. 1972.)

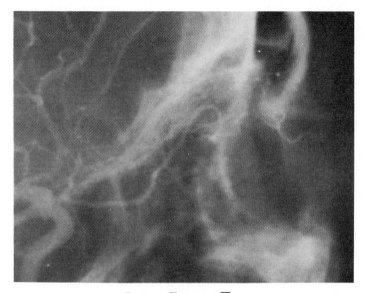

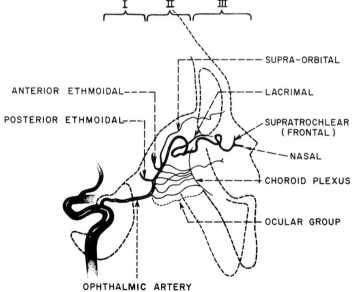

I   II   III

ANTERIOR ETHMOIDAL

POSTERIOR ETHMOIDAL

SUPRA-ORBITAL

LACRIMAL

SUPRATROCHLEAR (FRONTAL)

NASAL

CHOROID PLEXUS

OCULAR GROUP

OPHTHALMIC ARTERY

FIGURE 6–69   Lateral arteriogram and schematic drawing showing normal ophthalmic arterial complex. (Roman numerals indicate division into zones.) (From Wheeler, E. C., and Baker, H. I.: Radiology, *83*:26, 1964.)

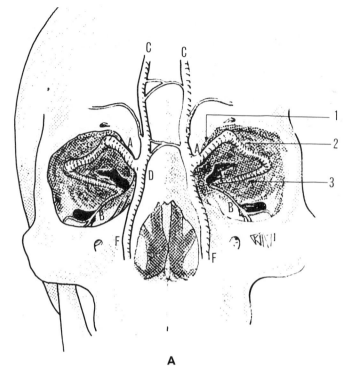

A

Figure 6–70   *See legend on opposite page.*

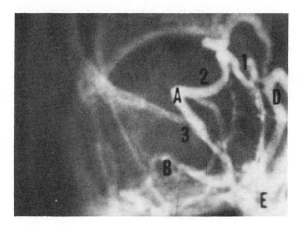
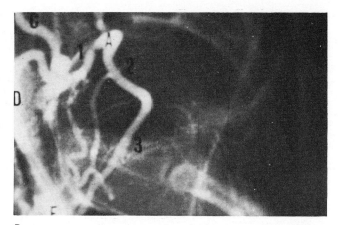

B

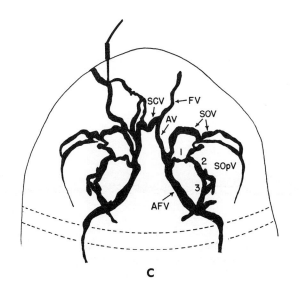

C

FIGURE 6–70 *A*. Schematic drawing of normal orbital veins. *B*. Composite of two cases (right and left) taken in the angled anteroposterior direction. Normal studies. (A) Superior ophthalmic veins divided into three portions (*1, 2, 3*). (B) inferior ophthalmic veins (inconstantly visualized). (C) frontal veins, (D) angular veins. (E) cavernous sinus, (F) facial veins. (From Russell, D. B., and Miller, J. D. R.: Radiology, *103*:267, 1972.) *C*. A tracing of the orbital venogram in Water's projection. (FV) Frontal vein, (AV) angular vein, (SCV) superficial connecting vein, (SOV) supraorbital vein, (SOpV) superior ophthalmic vein. (AFV) anterior facial vein, (1) first segment, (2) second segment, (3) third segment.

Frontal, angular, superficial connecting, and supraorbital veins in order of decreasing choice of venous puncture. (From Lee, K. F., and Lin, S. R.: Am. J. Roentgenol., *112*:341, 1971.)

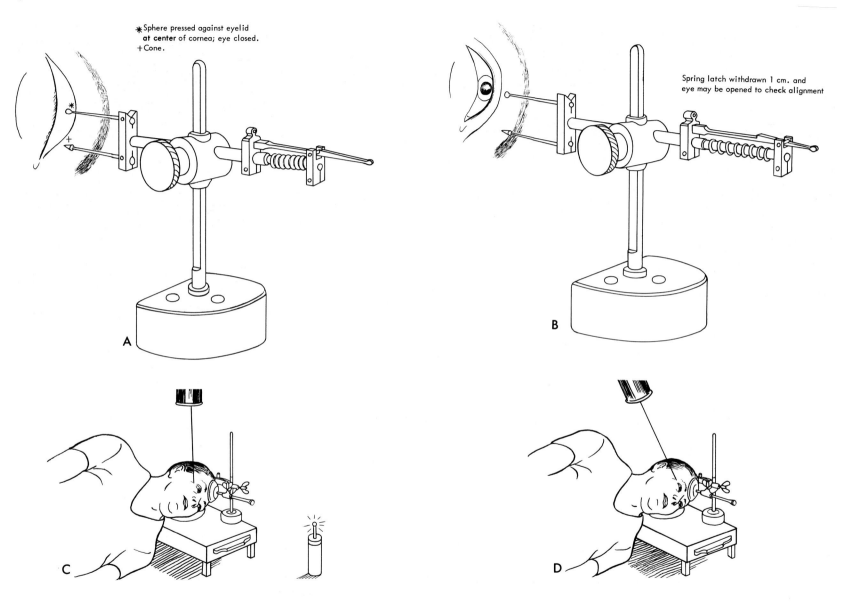

*Sphere pressed against eyelid
at center of cornea; eye closed.
+Cone.

Spring latch withdrawn 1 cm. and
eye may be opened to check alignment

Figure 6–71 *See legend on opposite page.*

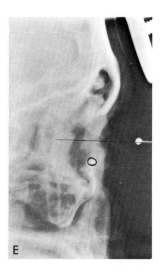
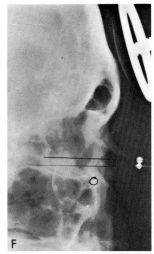
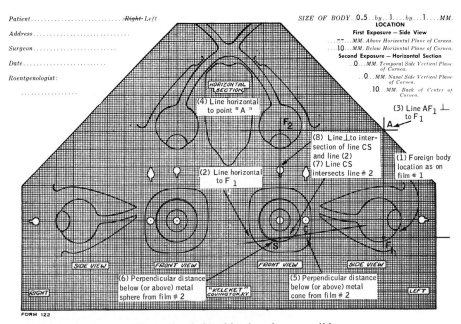

FIGURE 6–71 Sweet method for localization of foreign bodies in the eye. The patient's head is placed upon a slide tunnel so constructed that one-half of an 8 by 10 inch cassette is protected while the other half is being exposed. *A.* The indicator ball of the localizer apparatus is adjusted to the center of the eye with the eyelid closed. The cone-shaped metal tip lies directly below the ball. *B.* Upon release of the trigger, both the cone and ball rebound a carefully calibrated distance of 10 millimeters. *C.* The first exposure is made with the central ray of the x-ray beam perpendicular to the plane of the film and parallel to the patient's eyes, passing through both corneas and superimposing the shadows of the indicator ball and cone and their supporting stems. During exposure, the patient is asked to fix his gaze on a small light source or mark on the wall, eyes open, looking straight forward. *D.* For the second exposure the x-ray tube is shifted 4 to 5 inches toward the patient's feet and tilted so that the central ray passes through the ball of the localizer, making an angle of some 10 to 15 degrees with the vertical; the cassette tray is moved to its second position. The films obtained are shown in *E* and *F.*

The method of transferring data from the films to the localizer chart: (1) From straight lateral film #1 the foreign body is indicated in its exact relationship to the superimposed metal ball and cone (F1); (2) a line is drawn horizontally with respect to F1; (3) a line is drawn perpendicularly from F1 to derive point A; (4) a horizontal line is drawn through A across the horizontal plane depiction; (5) from film #2 the perpendicular distance below (or above) the metal cone is measured and plotted (point C); (6) from film #2 the perpendicular distance below (or above) the metal sphere is measured and plotted (point S); (7) line CS is drawn (note here that CS intersects horizontal line #2); (8) a line is drawn perpendicular to intersection of line CS and line #2.

Point F1 indicates position of foreign body behind the center of the cornea and below the horizontal plane. Point F2 indicates the position of the foreign body medial or lateral to the center of the cornea, and thus all three dimensions are noted.

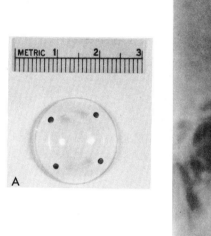

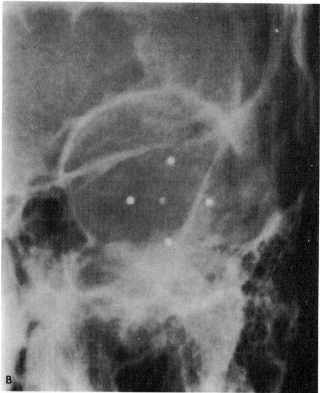

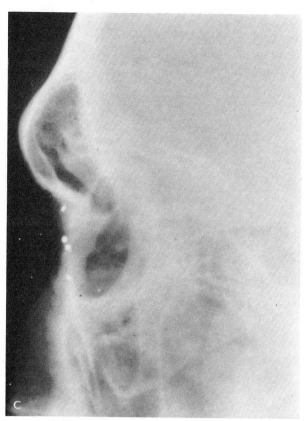

FIGURE 6–72 Foreign body localization in the eye with the aid of the Thorpe plastic lens. The conjunctiva is anesthetized by the physician, and the lens placed into proper position over the cornea of the eye. Straight posteroanterior and lateral projections of the eye are then obtained. *A.* Photograph of the lens. *B.* Posteroanterior radiograph of the eye with the lens in place over the cornea. *C.* Lateral projection. The position of the foreign body is noted and measured with respect to the lead markers on the lens. This is a modification of the Pfeiffer-Comberg method. (The plastic lens was obtained from the House of Vision, Inc., Chicago, Illinois—Catalogue No. XP 3611.)

THE TEMPORAL BONE

The temporal bone is usually divided into three portions: (a) the squamous portion, (b) the tympanic portion, and (c) the petrous portion (Fig. 6–10). These are practical subdivisions in the adult bone, but do not represent separate portions developmentally.

The *squamous portion* is largely a bony plate that helps form the calvaria laterally. It also contributes to the mastoid process posterior to the external acoustic meatus.

The *tympanic portion* contributes to the wall of the tympanic cavity and develops in conjunction with the external acoustic meatus; ultimately it constitutes most of the bony wall of this external acoustic passage.

Of the three portions of the temporal bone, the most important is the *petrous portion,* containing the vestibulocochlear organ. Participating in both the lateral wall and the floor of the skull, the petrous element develops originally as an otic capsule. Intracranially, this capsule contains the internal acoustic opening that transmits the facial and vestibulocochlear nerves; on its tympanic surface, it presents the oval and round windows (fenestra vestibuli and fenestra cochleae). The development of the styloid process is closely related to that of the petrous part.

The *mastoid portion* is formed from both the squamous and petrous portions, and this junction is indicated by the petrosquamous suture, which is somewhat variable in appearance and must not be misconstrued as a fracture.

The mastoid process itself is perforated by numerous foramina—the largest being the mastoid foramen, which transmits the mastoid branch of the occipital artery and a vein to the transverse sinus. The sigmoid groove for the transverse sinus is found on the inner aspect of the mastoid process.

The interior of the mastoid process contains numerous air cells opening into a common chamber—the mastoid or tympanic antrum (Fig. 6–11). The latter communicates with the upper part of the tympanic cavity or epitympanic recess. There are three groups of cells in the mastoid portion: the anteroposterior, the middle, and the apical. These have been further subdivided according to position into: (1) eustachian, (2) zygomatic, (3) cells along the floor of the middle fossa, (4) sublabyrinthine, (5) squamous, (6) lateral sinus, (7) marginal, (8) retrofacial, and (9) mastoid tip.

The degree of pneumatization is very variable.

Middle Ear. The middle ear contains: (1) the tympanic cavity, (2) a tympanic antrum or mastoid antrum that is continuous with the air spaces in the mastoid portion of the temporal bone, and (3) an auditory tube located mostly within the temporal bone that communicates with the nasal part of the pharynx. It also contains the three ear bones that transmit vibrational effects from the tympanic membrane to the inner ear. These structures are shut off from the external ear by the tympanic membrane and from the chambers that form the internal ear by the structures occupying the cochlear and vestibular windows.

The *tympanic cavity* (Fig. 6–11) may be divided into two regions: a lower region at the level of the tympanic membrane (the tympanic cavity proper), and an upper region known as the *epitympanic recess.* The latter is about half the size of the former. The posterior end of the epitympanic recess communicates with the tympanic antrum via the *aditus ad antrum.* Bounding the tympanic cavity are many vital structures such as the internal jugular vein, the carotid artery, and other structures within the middle and inner ear. Overlying the epitympanic recess is the rooflike *tegmen tympani,* and medially to it are the *semicircular canals and prominence of the facial canal.* Laterally is the *scutum,* which forms a point of attachment for the tympanic membrane; inferiorly is the *fossa for the incus.* The boundary line between the tympanic cavity proper and the epitympanic recess is the prominence of the facial canal medially and the fossa of the incus inferiorly.

ROUTINE STUDY OF THE PETROUS RIDGES AND MASTOID PROCESSES

Lateral Projection of the Mastoid Process (Law's Position) (Fig. 6–73)

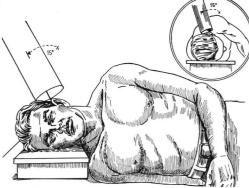

POINTS OF PRACTICAL INTEREST ABOUT FIGURE 6–73

1. There are actually two different ways of obtaining this projection—both acceptable. The alternative to the one shown is by placing a 15 degree angle board under the patient's head and utilizing a central ray that is perpendicular to the table top and centered to the mastoid process which is closest to the film. Thus, instead of angling the tube as shown here, the patient's head is angled an equivalent amount instead.

2. The routine recommended for study of this projection is as follows:

   (a) Note the degree of pneumatization, and whether the cells are diploic, small, mixed or large.

   (b) Note the relative radiolucency of the cells, and the integrity of their walls.

   (c) Trace the integrity of the lateral sinus plate.

   (d) Locate and state the size of the emissary vein.

   (e) Study the auditory meatuses for erosion or enlargement.

   (f) Note the integrity of the temporomandibular joint.

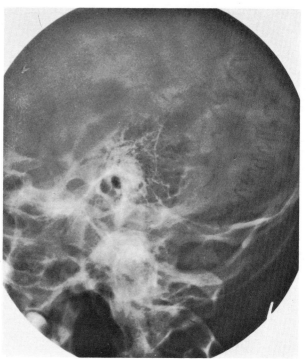

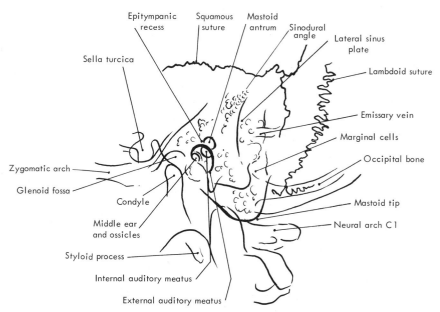

FIGURE 6–73 Lateral projection of mastoid process (Law's position).

Tangential Projection of the Mastoid Tips (Fig. 6–74)

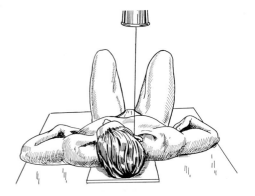

POINTS OF PRACTICAL INTEREST ABOUT FIGURE 6–74

1. The auricles of the ears should be folded forward to avoid the projection of the pinna over the mastoid structures.

2. The smallest possible cone should be employed at a fairly close target-to-film distance (25 to 30 inches). The head is rotated 45 degrees away from the side being radiographed, and the tube is angled 15 degrees caudally, centering over the midpoint of the canthomeatal line.

3. In this projection the mastoid process is projected away from the rest of the calvaria, and the mastoid cells in the tip of the process are shown to best advantage. A rather light exposure technique must be employed to gain this projection. This same projection, however, may also be used to visualize the petrous portion of the temporal bone if a somewhat heavier exposure technique is employed.

4. Comparison films between the two mastoids are always obtained.

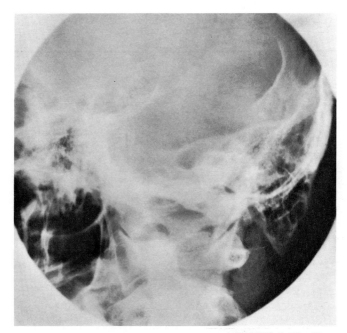

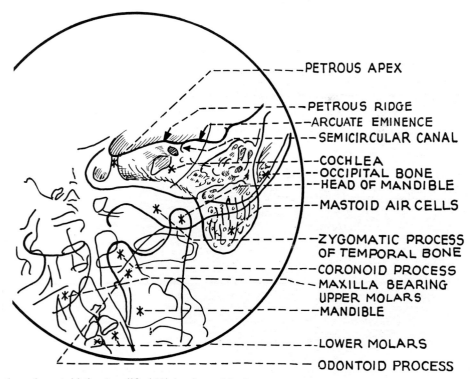

PETROUS APEX

PETROUS RIDGE
ARCUATE EMINENCE
SEMICIRCULAR CANAL

COCHLEA
OCCIPITAL BONE
HEAD OF MANDIBLE

MASTOID AIR CELLS

ZYGOMATIC PROCESS
OF TEMPORAL BONE
CORONOID PROCESS
MAXILLA BEARING
UPPER MOLARS
MANDIBLE

LOWER MOLARS
ODONTOID PROCESS

FIGURE 6–74 Tangential projection of mastoid tips (modified Hickey's position).

Posteroanterior Projection of the Petrous Ridge with the Ridge Placed Parallel to the Film (Stenver's Position) (Fig. 6–75)

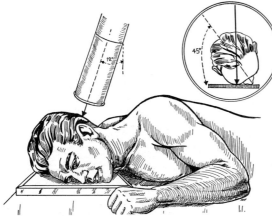

POINTS OF PRACTICAL INTEREST ABOUT FIGURE 6–75

1. Position the patient's head so that the tip of the nose, the point of the chin, and the outer canthus of the eye are all in contact with the plane of the film. This will place the head at an angle of approximately 45 degrees with respect to the film.

2. Adjust the central ray so that it passes to the midpoint of the film at an angle of 12 degrees.

3. In this position the petrous ridge is parallel with the plane of the film and its longest axis is shown to best advantage.

4. This projection may also be utilized for visualization of the tips of the mastoid cells if a lighter exposure technique is employed. However, when satisfactory exposure factors are utilized to see the innermost aspect of the petrous ridge, the mastoid air cells and the tips of the mastoids will not be seen to good advantage except in an extremely bright light.

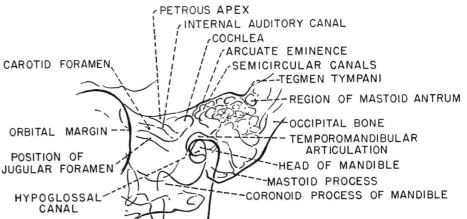

FIGURE 6–75 Posteroanterior projection of the petrous ridge with the ridge parallel to the film (Stenver's position).

Superoinferior Projection of the Petrous Ridges. This is obtained by means of Towne's position already described. This is the anteroposterior projection with a 30 to 35 degree tilt of the tube caudally. As previously indicated, an excellent perspective of both petrous ridges is obtained, along with the projection of the occipital bone, foramen magnum, and dorsum sellae.

Mayer's Position of the Mastoids (Fig. 6–76)

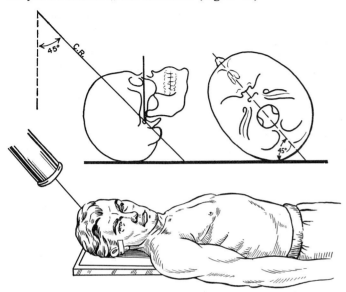

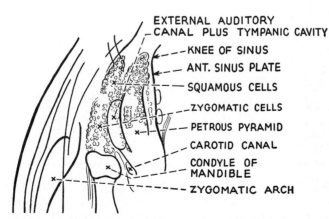

EXTERNAL AUDITORY
CANAL PLUS TYMPANIC CAVITY
— KNEE OF SINUS
— ANT. SINUS PLATE
— SQUAMOUS CELLS
— ZYGOMATIC CELLS
— PETROUS PYRAMID
— CAROTID CANAL
— CONDYLE OF MANDIBLE
— ZYGOMATIC ARCH

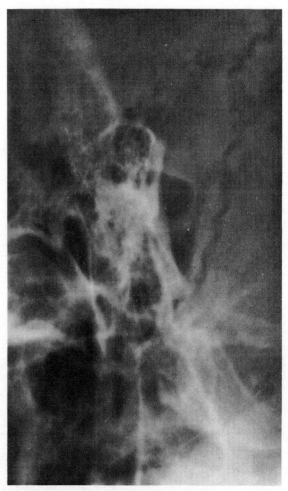

FIGURE 6–76 Mayer's position for examination of petrous ridge and mastoids. Schematic drawings made from a radiograph. This view is especially useful in separation of the anatomic structures of the middle ear as a prerequisite for fenestration operations. It is difficult to duplicate this view from patient to patient; hence, the anatomic depiction is somewhat variable and must be extrapolated from the above diagram.

Runström Projection of the Mastoid Process (Fig. 6–77). This resembles Law's lateral projection, except that the mastoid antrum is separated from the other structures by greater angulation, making this projection especially valuable in the study of the middle ear.

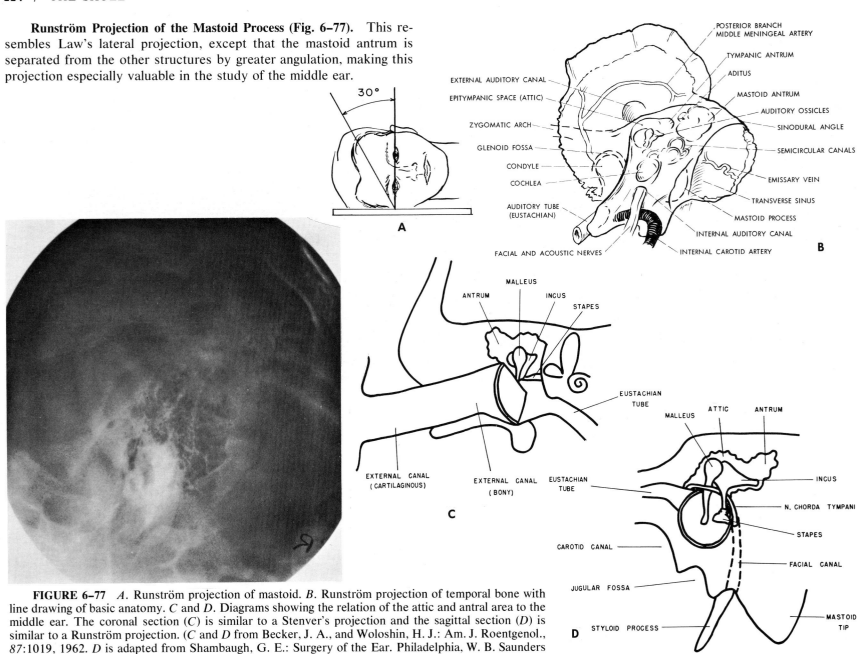

FIGURE 6–77   *A*. Runström projection of mastoid. *B*. Runström projection of temporal bone with line drawing of basic anatomy. *C* and *D*. Diagrams showing the relation of the attic and antral area to the middle ear. The coronal section (*C*) is similar to a Stenver's projection and the sagittal section (*D*) is similar to a Runström projection. (*C* and *D* from Becker, J. A., and Woloshin, H. J.: Am. J. Roentgenol., *87*:1019, 1962. *D* is adapted from Shambaugh, G. E.: Surgery of the Ear. Philadelphia, W. B. Saunders Co., 1959.)

Submentovertical Projection to Demonstrate Tympanic Cavity (After Etter and Cross) (Fig. 6–78)

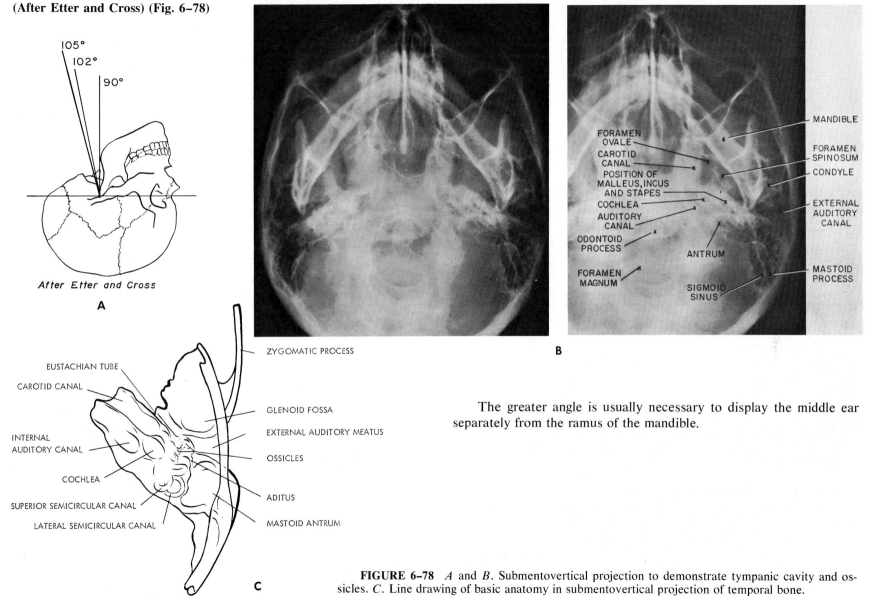

After Etter and Cross

A

ZYGOMATIC PROCESS

B

EUSTACHIAN TUBE

CAROTID CANAL

INTERNAL AUDITORY CANAL

COCHLEA

SUPERIOR SEMICIRCULAR CANAL

LATERAL SEMICIRCULAR CANAL

GLENOID FOSSA

EXTERNAL AUDITORY MEATUS

OSSICLES

ADITUS

MASTOID ANTRUM

FORAMEN OVALE

CAROTID CANAL

POSITION OF MALLEUS, INCUS AND STAPES

COCHLEA

AUDITORY CANAL

ODONTOID PROCESS

FORAMEN MAGNUM

ANTRUM

SIGMOID SINUS

MANDIBLE

FORAMEN SPINOSUM

CONDYLE

EXTERNAL AUDITORY CANAL

MASTOID PROCESS

The greater angle is usually necessary to display the middle ear separately from the ramus of the mandible.

C

FIGURE 6–78 *A* and *B*. Submentovertical projection to demonstrate tympanic cavity and ossicles. *C*. Line drawing of basic anatomy in submentovertical projection of temporal bone.

Laminagraphy of the Ear (Schaefer;* Valvassori).† The examination of the small structures of the internal and middle ear has already been previously described (see Figures 6–13 through 6–16). Laminagraphy—polytomography in particular—has made available to the radiologist immense possibilities in the visualization of minute anatomic details. The Massiot polytome (or its equivalent in other apparatus) allows a separating capacity of thicknesses of 1 mm. and a coefficient of distinctness about five times as great as that which can be obtained with linear tomography (Valvassori).†·‡

Three projections, occasionally a fourth, are used for polytomography of the ear: lateral, frontal, Stenver's, and occasionally, axial.

The frontal and axial views are best for demonstration of the canal in its full length, and the lateral view is best for visualization of the canal in cross section. In Stenver's view, the internal auditory canal is foreshortened. Polytomography is best employed for visualization of the canal and its minute details.

These views demonstrate the longer anterior wall and the shorter posterior wall with its medial concave lip (Fig. 6–78). In a study by Valvassori and Pierce, comparison between the posterior walls of the right and left canals of the same patient showed a variation of up to 1 mm. in 86 per cent of the patients and a variation of 1 to 2 mm. in 13 per cent. The variation between the two sides was 2 to 3 mm. in only 1 per cent of the patients.

The anterior wall of the internal auditory canal was also measured. Its greatest length was 19 mm., the shortest was 6 mm., and the average was 12 mm. Comparison between the internal auditory canals of the same patient showed a variation of up to 1 mm. in 85 per cent of the patients, 1 to 2 mm. in 8 per cent, and 2 to 3 mm. in 7 per cent.

In a study of 100 petrous bones for crista falciformis detail, it was noted that in 85 per cent of the patients the crista appeared as a linear density ranging from 1 to 7 mm. Its thickness appeared to decrease progressively from its lateral origin to its medial end. In 15 per cent of the patients only the origin of the crista was detectable as a definite knob of increased density. *The origin of the crista falciformis was located at, or above, the midpoint of the vertical diameter in all of the patients studied.*

Thus, although the length of the crista falciformis is variable, its position in relation to the height of the canal is consistent. *If the crista falciformis can be identified below the midpoint of the canal, an abnormal situation may be identified.* (The above measurements have been corrected for magnification and represent the true anatomic size.)

Positive Contrast Demonstration of Normal Internal Acoustic Meatus, Meckel's Cave, and Jugular Foramen (Posterior Fossa Cisternomyelography) (Reese and Bull; Baker; Gass; Scanlan)* Method. Nine ml. of iophendylate (Pantopaque) is introduced into the lumbar subarachnoid space as in myelography. The head is maintained in full extension by a small hard pillow. After all of the oil is pooled in the cervical region and appropriate roentgenograms are made, the table is slowly tilted down with the head in extension, while the oil advances onto the clivus to the base of the dorsum sellae. When the oil is over the tip of the clivus and into the middle fossa, it is irretrievable, so that the head must be carefully controlled at this time. By very carefully turning the head while it is in extension, the oil may be moved from the clivus into the cerebellopontine angle cistern. After anteroposterior and lateral roentgenograms of the clivus have been made, the table is returned to the horizontal position and the oil on the clivus returns to the cervical region (Fig. 6–80).

The head and shoulders are then rotated to one side or the other at least 30 degrees while the head is in hyperextension. The table is tilted downward and the contrast medium is observed closely on the fluoroscope as it flows from the cervical region into the cerebellopontine angle cistern. Roentgenograms are then made in the anteroposterior and cross table lateral projections (Fig. 6–81).

*Schaeffer, R. E.: Roentgen anatomy of the temporal bone: tomographic studies. Med. Radiogr. Photogr., 48:2–22, 1972.

†Valvassori, G. E.: Laminagraphy of the ear. Normal roentgenographic anatomy. Am. J. Roentgenol., 89:1155–1167, 1963.

‡Valvassori, G. E., and Buckingham, R. A.: Tomography and cross sections of the ear. Philadelphia, W. B. Saunders Co., 1975.

*Additional references within the text may be obtained in Meschan, I.: An Atlas of Anatomy Basic to Radiology. Philadelphia, W. B. Saunders Co., 1975.

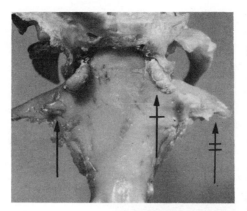
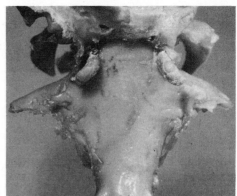

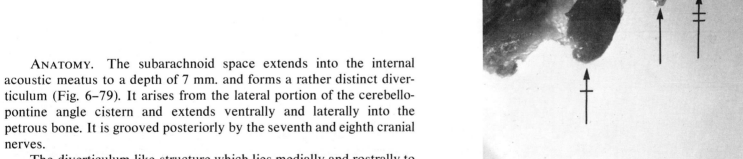

ANATOMY. The subarachnoid space extends into the internal acoustic meatus to a depth of 7 mm. and forms a rather distinct diverticulum (Fig. 6–79). It arises from the lateral portion of the cerebellopontine angle cistern and extends ventrally and laterally into the petrous bone. It is grooved posteriorly by the seventh and eighth cranial nerves.

The diverticulum-like structure which lies medially and rostrally to the internal acoustic meatus is the *Meckel's cave*. At times there is also a smaller diverticulum just caudal to the internal acoustic meatus and in line with it; this is the extension of the arachnoid space into the jugular foramen (Fig. 6–81).

The *roentgenographic appearance* and appropriate diagrams are shown in Figure 6–81.

FIGURE 6–79 Resin-injection casts of the subarachnoid cisterns. *Upper.* Pontine and cerebellopontine angle cisterns seen from below: →, internal auditory canal; ⇸, large Meckel's caves protruding anteriorly: ⇻, cerebellopontine angle cisterns. These pictures are a stereoscopic pair. *Lower.* Oblique crosstable lateral view: ⇻, bulbous Meckel's cave anteriorly; →, internal auditory canal; ⇸, tiny amount of resin in the jugular foramen. (From Reese, D. F., and Bull, J. W. D.: Am. J. Roentgenol., *100*:650–655, 1967.)

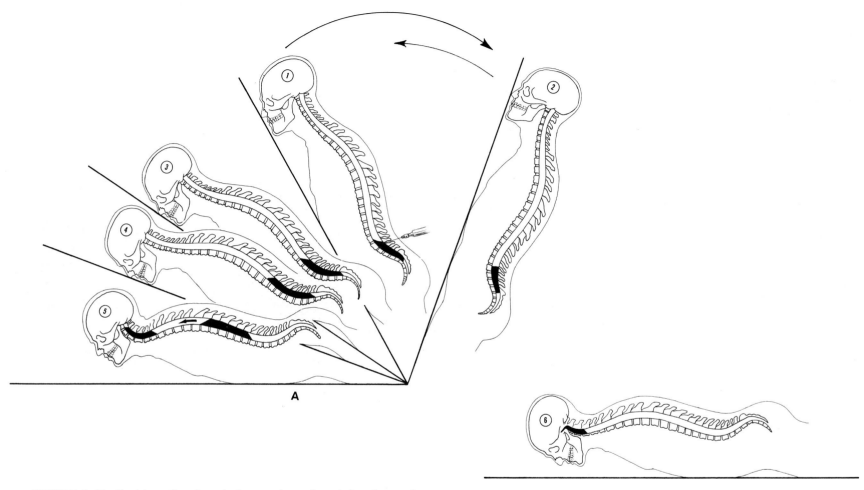

FIGURE 6-80 Position of patient during myelography. *A*. Lumbar and cervical. *B*. For visualization of region of clivus and internal acoustic meatus (see text for description).

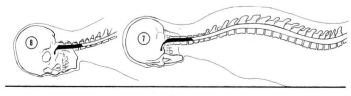

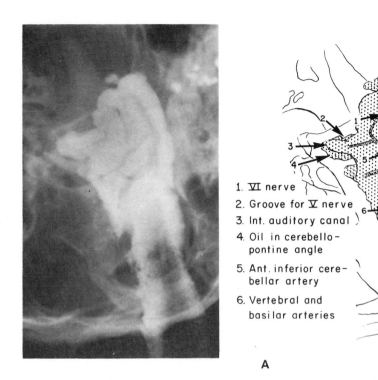

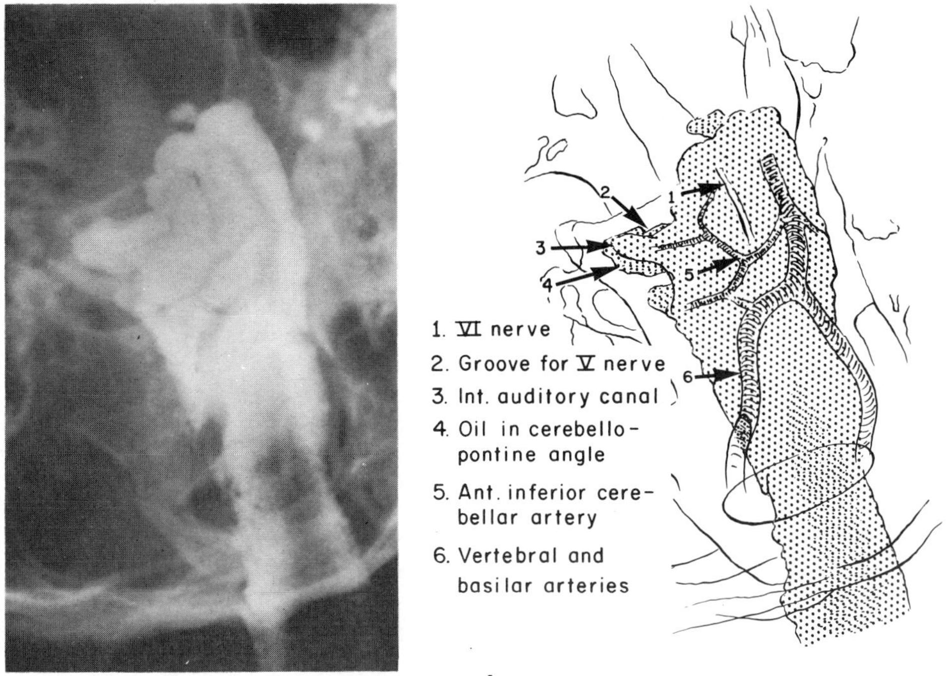

1. VI nerve
2. Groove for V nerve
3. Int. auditory canal
4. Oil in cerebello-
   pontine angle
5. Ant. inferior cere-
   bellar artery
6. Vertebral and
   basilar arteries

A

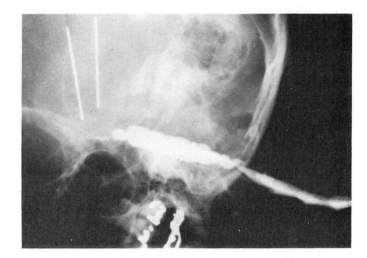

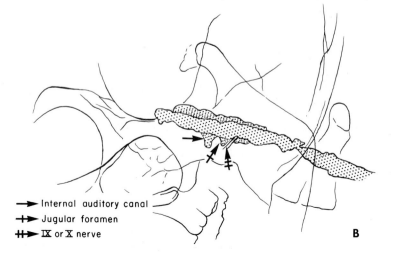

→ Internal auditory canal
↦ Jugular foramen
�* IX or X nerve

B

FIGURE 6–81 *A*. Posteroanterior projection of the pontine and left cerebellopontine angle cisterns, with the head turned to the right 45 degrees. The oil in the
internal auditory canal is somewhat obscured by oil in the overlying cerebellopontine
angle cistern. *B*. Crosstable lateral view, with head in same position as in *A*. The
internal auditory canal and jugular foramen are separated from the oil in the cerebellopontine angle cistern. (From Reese, D. F., and Bull, J. W. D.: Am. J. Roentgenol., *100*:650–655, 1967.)

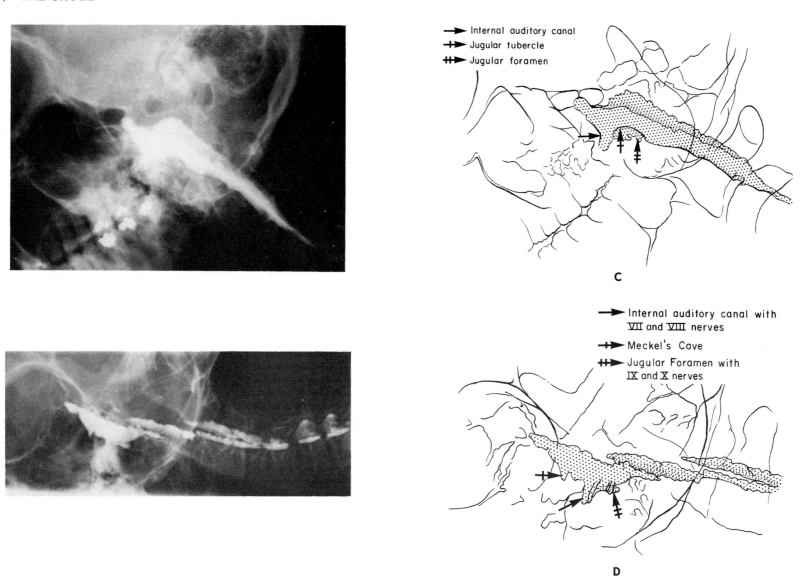

FIGURE 6–81 *Continued.* *C.* Jugular tubercle is faintly seen, with the internal auditory canal directly in front of and below it. *D.* Oil is present in Meckel's cave, internal auditory canal, and jugular foramen. In no case to date have we seen such extensive filling of Meckel's cave as found in the resin-injection cast. (From Reese, D. F., and Bull, J. W. D.: Am. J. Roentgenol., *100*:650–655, 1967.)

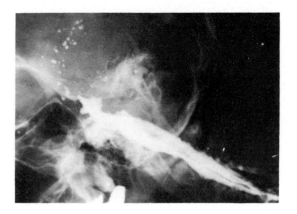

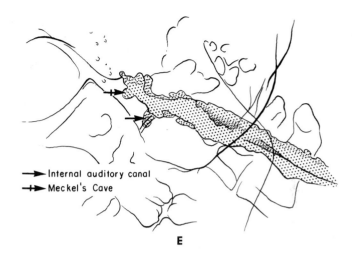

E

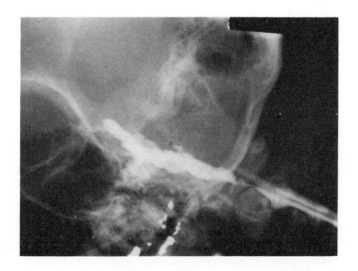

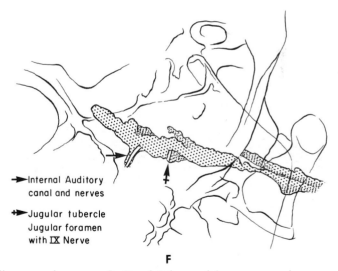

F

FIGURE 6–81 *Continued.* *E.* Meckel's cave and the internal auditory canal are seen. In *D* and *E* the cranial nerves VII and VIII can be seen traversing the posterior portion of the canal. *F.* Jugular foramen and internal auditory canal are filled. The linear shadow in the oil column and the upper cervical part of spinal column is a portion of the dentate ligaments. (From Reese, D. F., and Bull, J. W. D.: Am. J. Roentgenol., *100*:650–655, 1967.)

The Sella Turcica

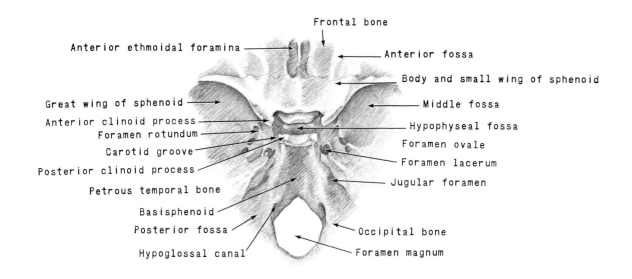

Relations of the Sella Turcica

FIGURE 6-82 En face view of sella turcica.

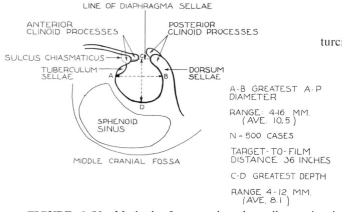

A-B GREATEST A-P DIAMETER

RANGE: 4-16 MM.
(AVE. 10.5)

N = 500 CASES

TARGET-TO-FILM DISTANCE 36 INCHES

C-D GREATEST DEPTH

RANGE 4-12 MM.
(AVE. 8.1)

FIGURE 6-83 Method of measuring the sella turcica in lateral projection.

Hare has proposed that 130 sq. mm. be used as a maximum area for the sella turcica in the lateral projection (Acheson).*

*Acheson, R. M.: Measuring the pituitary fossa from radiographs. Br. J. Radiol., 29:76-80, 1956.

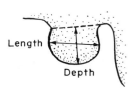
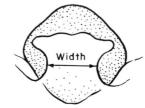

$$V = \frac{1}{2}(L \times D \times W)$$

Minimum	Mean (173 adults)	Maximum
240 mm.^{3}	594 mm.^{3}	1092 mm.^{3}

Accuracy

Prediction of sella size	83 %
Prediction of pituitary size	87 %

FIGURE 6-84 The volume of the sella turcica as determined by DiChiro and Nelson.

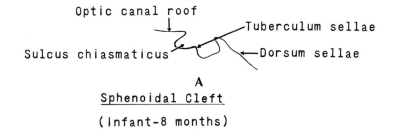

Optic canal roof

Tuberculum sellae

Sulcus chiasmaticus

Dorsum sellae

A

Sphenoidal Cleft

(Infant-8 months)

Floor of anterior fossa

Sella turcica

Intersphenoid synchondrosis

Spheno-occipital synchondrosis

Floor of middle fossa

B

FIGURE 6-86 *A*. Infantile sella turcica. (From Kier, Am. J. Roentgenol., *102*:747, 1968.) *B*. Sellar and parasellar synchondroses. (From Shopfner, C. E., et al.: Am. J. Roentgenol., *104*:186, 1968.)

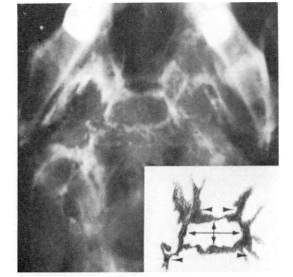

FIGURE 6-85 Normal cavernous sinogram obtained before hypophysectomy for carcinoma of the breast. Submentovertex projection with the catheter in the inferior petrosal sinus (lower arrowheads, insert). Contrast material is noted to outline the cavernous sinus (long double arrow), the intercavernous bridges (short double arrow), and the ophthalmic veins (upper arrowheads). (From Jacobs, J. B., and Grivas, N. E.: Am. J. Roentgenol., *107*:589, 1969.)

AXIAL TOMOGRAPHY OF THE BASE OF THE SKULL (FOR COMPUTED AXIAL TOMOGRAPHY OF THE BRAIN, SEE SECTION UNDER "BRAIN")

Common Legend for Figure 6–87 *A–G**

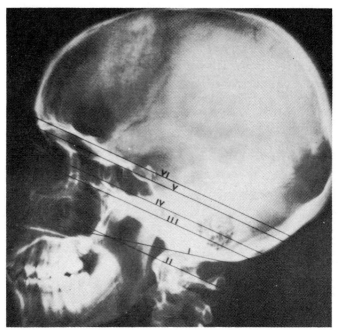

FIGURE 6–87 *A* to *G*, The common legend for parts A–G is given to the right.* *A*, Lateral view, indicating the levels of the base of the skull at which the cadaver heads were sectioned.

Figure continued on opposite page.

1. Anterior arch atlas 92%
2. Anterior clinoid process 34%
3. Anterior condyloid canal
4. Anterior margin middle cranial fossa 87%
5. Anterior wall maxillary antrum
6. Clivus 74%
7. Condyloid fossa
8. Condyloid process of the mandible
9. Cribriform plate
10. Crista galli 88%
11. Dorsum sellae
12. Ethmoid sinus 94%
13. Eustachian tube 10%
14. Exocranial opening, internal carotid artery canal
15. External auditory canal 92%
16. Foramen lacerum 40%
17. Foramen magnum 4%
18. Foramen of Vesalius
19. Foramen ovale 51%
20. Foramen rotundum 10%
21. Foramen spinosum 86%
22. Foramen transversarium 34%
23. Fossa of Rosenmüller 55%
24. Frontal sinus 72%
25. Glenoid fossa 90%
26. Greater palatine foramen 26%
27. Horizontal semicircular canal 37%
28. Inferior orbital fissure 13%
29. Infraorbital nerve canal 5%
30. Internal auditory canal 62%
31. Internal carotid artery
32. Internal carotid artery canal 60%
33. Internal carotid artery groove
34. Jugular foramen 1%
35. Lamina papyracea 92%
36. Lateral pterygoid plate 98%
37. Lateral wall of orbit 87%
38. Mandibular head 91%
39. Mastoid 83%
40. Maxillary antrum 90%
41. Medial pterygoid plate 95%
42. Medial wall maxillary antrum
43. Nasopharynx 46%
44. Occipital condyle 59%
45. Odontoid process
46. Optic foramen
47. Oropharynx
48. Posterior arch C1
49. Posterior clinoid process 5%
50. Posterior condyloid canal 1%
51. Posterior process C2
52. Posterior wall maxillary antrum
53. Pterygopalatine fossa
54. Sella floor
55. Sella side wall 10%
56. Sella turcica
57. Sphenoid sinus 92%
58. Sphenoid sinus septum 94%
59. Superior orbital fissure 10%
60. Styloid process
61. Torus tubarius 51%
62. Tuberculum sellae 56%
63. Turbinate 95%
64. Vidian canal 3%

*The percentages listed after many of the items indicate how often these items were interpreted as normal on review of 50 unselected base views.

(*A*, *B*, and *G*, From Binet, E. F.: *Seminars in Roentgenol.* 9:137, 1974. Used by permission of Grune & Stratton, Inc. Parts *C* to *F* reprinted from Med. Radiogr. Photogr. Courtesy of Radiography Markets Division, Eastman Kodak Company.)

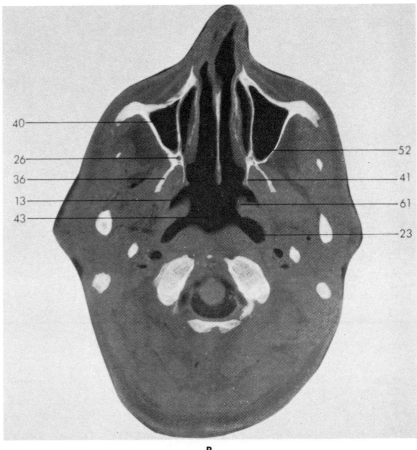

B

(The structures listed below appear in *B*.)

40. Maxillary antrum
26. Greater palatine foramen
36. Lateral pterygoid plate
13. Eustachian tube
43. Nasopharynx

52. Posterior wall maxillary antrum
41. Medial pterygoid plate
61. Torus tubarius
23. Fossa of Rosenmüller

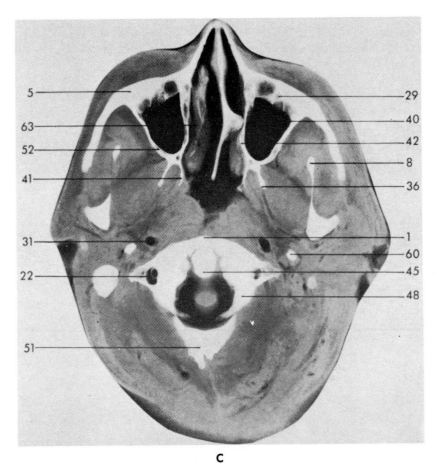

C

(The structures listed below appear in *C*.)

5. Anterior wall maxillary antrum
63. Turbinate
52. Posterior wall maxillary antrum
31. Internal carotid artery
22. Foramen transversarium
51. Posterior process C2

29. Infraorbital nerve canal
40. Maxillary antrum
42. Medial wall maxillary antrum
8. Condyloid process of the mandible
1. Anterior arch atlas
60. Styloid process
45. Odontoid process
48. Posterior arch C1

Figure continued on following page.

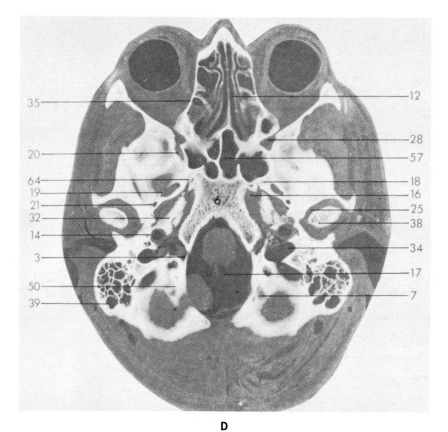

D

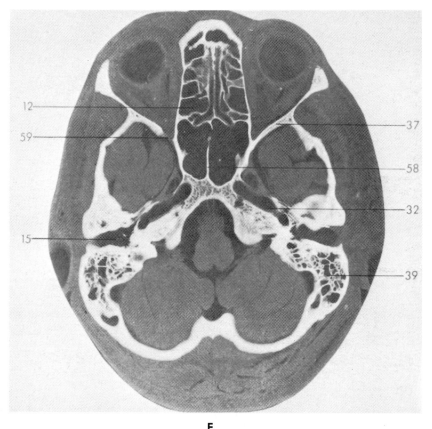

E

FIGURE 6–87 *Continued.* *D.* Clivus (Level III). *E.* Superior orbital fissure (Level IV).

(The structures listed below appear in *D*.)

35. Lamina papyracea	12. Ethmoid sinus
20. Foramen rotundum	28. Inferior orbital fissure
64. Vidian canal	57. Sphenoid sinus
19. Foramen ovale	18. Foramen of Vesalius
21. Foramen spinosum	16. Foramen lacerum
32. Internal carotid artery canal	25. Glenoid fossa
14. Exocranial opening, internal carotid artery canal	38. Mandibular head
	34. Jugular foramen
3. Anterior condyloid canal	17. Foramen magnum
50. Posterior condyloid canal	7. Condyloid fossa
39. Mastoid	

(The structures listed below appear in *E*.)

12. Ethmoid sinus	37. Lateral wall of orbit
59. Superior orbital fissure	58. Sphenoid sinus septum
15. External auditory canal	32. Internal carotid artery canal
	39. Mastoid

Figure continued on opposite page.

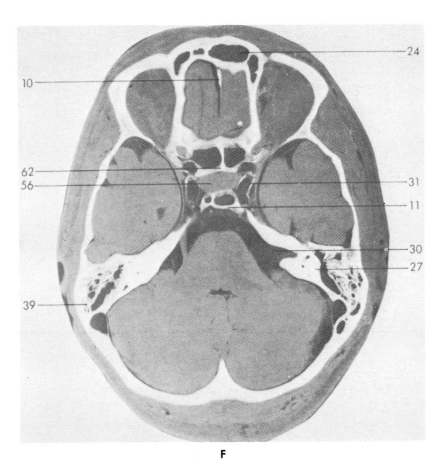

F

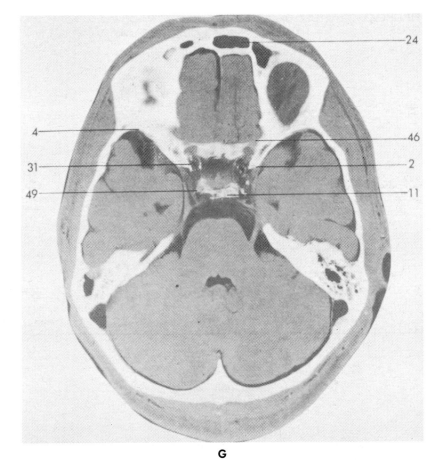

G

FIGURE 6–87 *Continued.* *F.* Internal auditory canal (Level V). *G.* Anterior clinoid process (Level VI).

(The structures listed below appear in *F*.)

10. Crista galli	24. Frontal sinus
62. Tuberculum sellae	31. Internal carotid artery
56. Sella turcica	11. Dorsum sellae
39. Mastoid	30. Internal auditory canal
	27. Horizontal semicircular canal

(The structures listed below appear in *G*.)

4. Anterior margin middle cranial fossa	24. Frontal sinus
31. Internal carotid artery	46. Optic foramen
49. Posterior clinoid process	2. Anterior clinoid process
	11. Dorsum sellae

GENERAL METHOD OF STUDY OF SKULL RADIOGRAPHS

This system of viewing may be applied to all other views of the skull shown radiographically and diagrammatically.

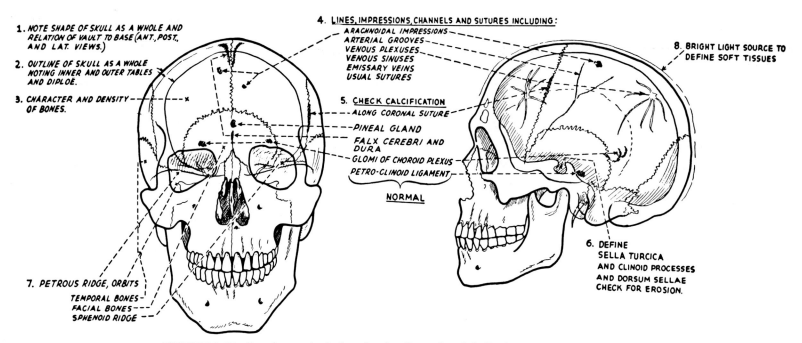

1. *NOTE SHAPE OF SKULL AS A WHOLE AND RELATION OF VAULT TO BASE (ANT., POST. AND LAT. VIEWS.)*

2. *OUTLINE OF SKULL AS A WHOLE NOTING INNER AND OUTER TABLES AND DIPLOË.*

3. *CHARACTER AND DENSITY OF BONES.*

4. *LINES, IMPRESSIONS, CHANNELS AND SUTURES INCLUDING:*
   - *ARACHNOIDAL IMPRESSIONS*
   - *ARTERIAL GROOVES*
   - *VENOUS PLEXUSES*
   - *VENOUS SINUSES*
   - *EMISSARY VEINS*
   - *USUAL SUTURES*

5. *CHECK CALCIFICATION*
   - *ALONG CORONAL SUTURE*
   - *PINEAL GLAND*
   - *FALX CEREBRI AND DURA*
   - *GLOMI OF CHOROID PLEXUS*
   - *PETRO-CLINOID LIGAMENT*

NORMAL

6. *DEFINE SELLA TURCICA AND CLINOID PROCESSES AND DORSUM SELLAE CHECK FOR EROSION.*

7. *PETROUS RIDGE, ORBITS*
   - *TEMPORAL BONES*
   - *FACIAL BONES*
   - *SPHENOID RIDGE*

8. *BRIGHT LIGHT SOURCE TO DEFINE SOFT TISSUES*

FIGURE 6–88   Routine method of study of radiographs of skull—frontal and lateral views. This system of viewing may be applied to all other views of the skull shown radiographically diagrammatically.

7

THE BRAIN

with anatomical sketches by
GEORGE LYNCH

Professor of Medical
Illustration
Bowman Gray School of
Wake Forest University,
Winston-Salem,
North Carolina

GROSS ANATOMY OF THE BRAIN AND MENINGES AS RELATED TO RADIOLOGY

The Meninges

The brain is completely enveloped by three fibrous coverings called meninges, consisting of the following structures: (1) a *pia mater*, a membrane that is closely applied to the surface of the brain with no structures intervening; (2) an *arachnoid membrane*, separated from the pia mater by the *subarachnoid space;* and (3) a *dura mater*, separated from the arachnoid by a potential space, the *subdural space*, and con-

sisting of two layers; an *endosteal layer* closely adherent to the calvaria, and an inner *meningeal layer,* on its inner aspect.

The two layers of the dura contain large blood sinuses: the *dural venous sinuses* and the *venous lacunae* ("lakes") in certain places.

The thin layer of cells lining the central canal of the spinal cord and the ventricles of the brain is called the *ependymal layer.*

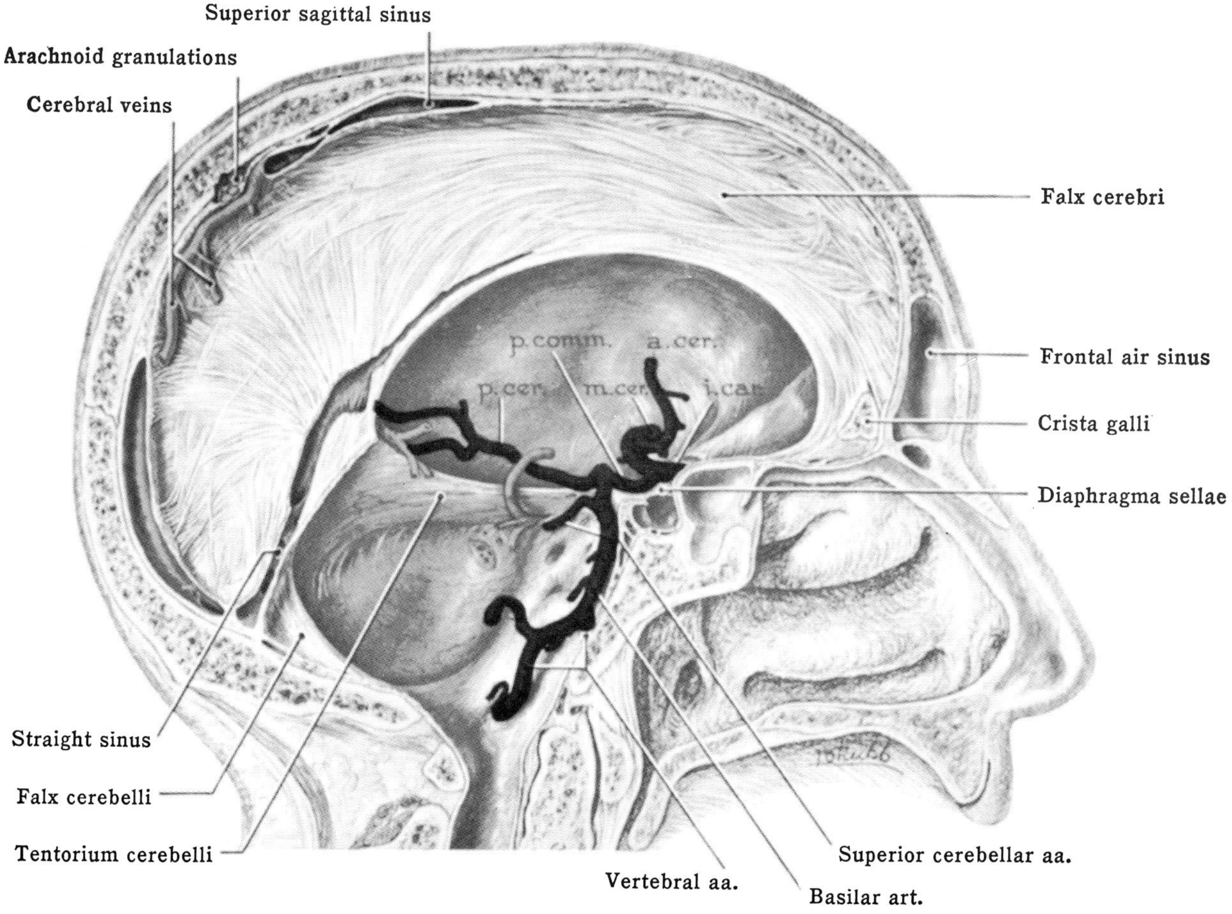

FIGURE 7–1A Folds of the dura mater. There are two vertical sickle-shaped folds—the falx cerebri and the falx cerebelli—and there are two rooflike folds—the tentorium cerebelli and the diaphragma sellae. (Reproduced by permission from J. C. B. Grant: An Atlas of Anatomy, 5th ed. Copyright © 1962, The Williams and Wilkins Company.)

Those aspects of the meninges which are most important to the radiologist are:

1. The reflections or reduplications of the meningeal layer of the dura that form two vertical rigid membranes and two horizontal membranes.
2. The dural venous sinuses.
3. The venous lakes or lacunae into which arachnoidal granulations project.
4. The cerebral spinal fluid cisterns.
5. The meningeal vessels.

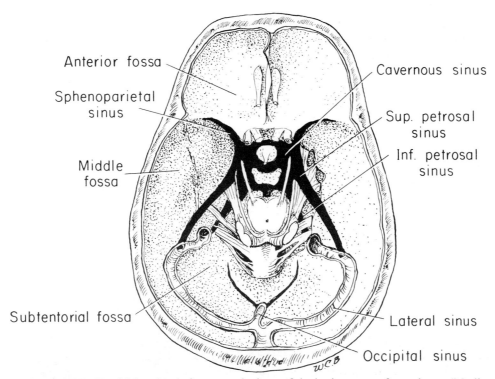

FIGURE 7–1B Major dural sinuses at the base of the brain as seen from above. (Modified from Bailey, P.: Intracranial Tumors. Springfield, Ill., Charles C Thomas, Publisher, 1933. Courtesy of Charles C Thomas, Publisher.)

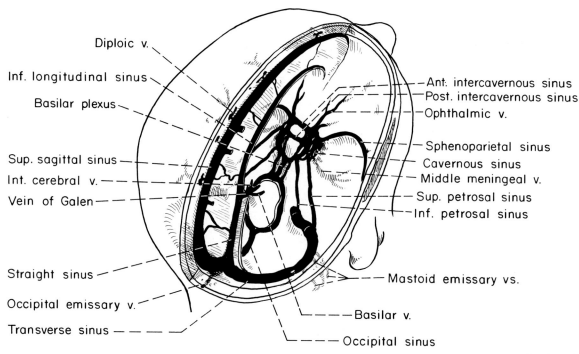

Diploic v.

Inf. longitudinal sinus

Basilar plexus

Sup. sagittal sinus

Int. cerebral v.

Vein of Galen

Straight sinus

Occipital emissary v.

Transverse sinus

Ant. intercavernous sinus
Post. intercavernous sinus
Ophthalmic v.

Sphenoparietal sinus
Cavernous sinus
Middle meningeal v.
Sup. petrosal sinus
Inf. petrosal sinus

Mastoid emissary vs.

Basilar v.

Occipital sinus

FIGURE 7–2 Dural venous sinuses as related to the dura.

FIGURE 7–3 Relations of meninges to brain, cord, and cerebrospinal fluid (based on Rasmussen, Principal Nervous Pathways). (From Pansky, B., and House, E. L.: Review of Gross Anatomy, 2nd ed. New York, Macmillan Co. 1969.)

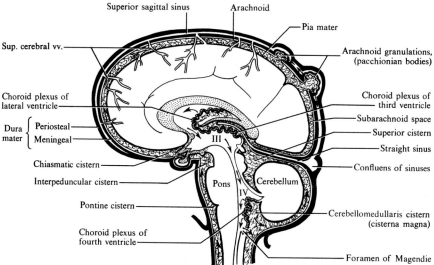

Superior sagittal sinus   Arachnoid

Sup. cerebral vv.

Choroid plexus of
lateral ventricle

Dura { Periosteal
mater { Meningeal

Chiasmatic cistern

Interpeduncular cistern

Pontine cistern

Choroid plexus of
fourth ventricle

Pia mater

Arachnoid granulations,
(pacchionian bodies)

Choroid plexus of
third ventricle

Subarachnoid space

Superior cistern

Straight sinus

Confluens of sinuses

Cerebellomedullaris cistern
(cisterna magna)

Foramen of Magendie

Pons   Cerebellum

III

IV

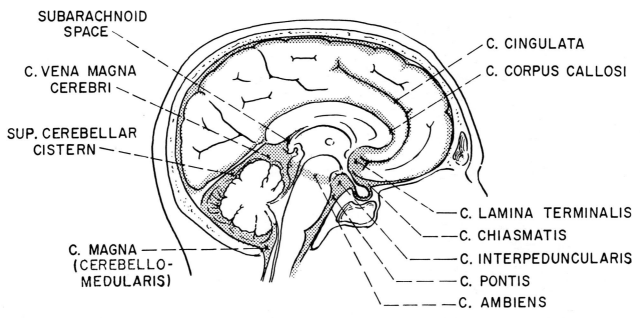

SUBARACHNOID SPACE

C. VENA MAGNA CEREBRI

SUP. CEREBELLAR CISTERN

C. MAGNA (CEREBELLO-MEDULARIS)

C. CINGULATA

C. CORPUS CALLOSI

C. LAMINA TERMINALIS

C. CHIASMATIS

C. INTERPEDUNCULARIS

C. PONTIS

C. AMBIENS

FIGURE 7–4 Diagram illustrating subarachnoid cisterns. (Not shown: C. fossae lateralis cerebri and C. laminae terminalis.)

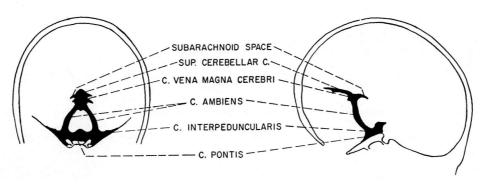

SUBARACHNOID SPACE

SUP. CEREBELLAR C.

C. VENA MAGNA CEREBRI

C. AMBIENS

C. INTERPEDUNCULARIS

C. PONTIS

FIGURE 7–5 Cisterna ambiens in Towne's and lateral projections. (Modified from Robertson, E. G.: Pneumoencephalography. Springfield, Ill., Charles C Thomas, Publisher, Courtesy of Charles C Thomas, Publisher.)

Subdivisions of the Brain

The brain is divided into five principal parts (Fig. 7-6): (1) the cerebrum, composed of two cerebral hemispheres, lying above a plane drawn between the internal occipital protuberance, the petrous ridges, and the floor of the anterior cranial fossa; (2) the cerebellum, composed of two hemispheres and a small central portion called the vermis, lying in the posterior fossa; (3) the midbrain, which lies between the cerebral hemispheres above and the hindbrain below; (4) the pons, lying beneath the fourth ventricle between the cerebral peduncles above and the medulla oblongata below; and (5) the medulla oblongata, which lies immediately above the spinal cord above the level of the foramen magnum.

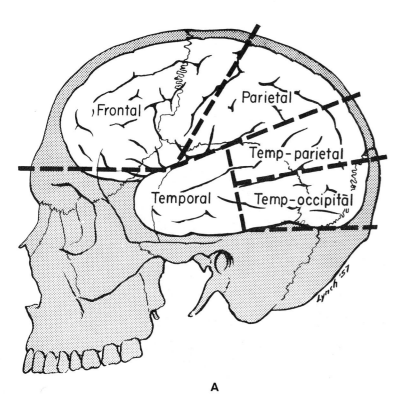

FIGURE 7-6 *A.* Diagram showing the position of various subdivisions of the brain as considered clinically and radiologically (supratentorial).

A

Figure continued on opposite page.

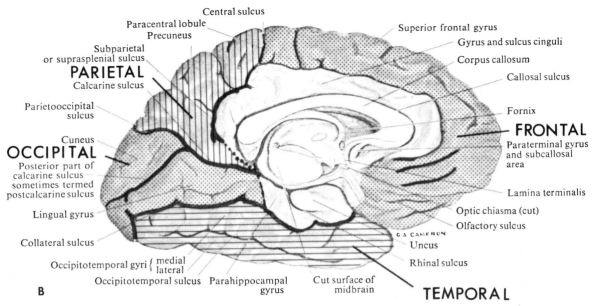

Central sulcus
Paracentral lobule
Precuneus
Subparietal
or suprasplenial sulcus
PARIETAL
Calcarine sulcus
Parietooccipital
sulcus
Cuneus
OCCIPITAL
Posterior part of
calcarine sulcus
sometimes termed
postcalcarine sulcus
Lingual gyrus
Collateral sulcus
Occipitotemporal gyri { medial / lateral
Occipitotemporal sulcus Parahippocampal
gyrus

Superior frontal gyrus
Gyrus and sulcus cinguli
Corpus callosum
Callosal sulcus
Fornix
FRONTAL
Paraterminal gyrus
and subcallosal
area
Lamina terminalis
Optic chiasma (cut)
Olfactory sulcus
Uncus
Rhinal sulcus
Cut surface of
midbrain
TEMPORAL

B

FIGURE 7–6 *Continued. B.* Lobes, gyri, and sulci as seen from the sagittal and somewhat inferior aspect of the brain.

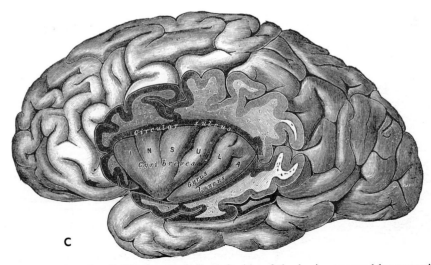

C

FIGURE 7–6 *Continued. C.* The insula of the left side of the brain, exposed by removing the opercula. (From Goss, C. M. (ed.): Gray's Anatomy of the Human Body, 29th ed. Philadelphia, Lea & Febiger, 1973.)

Ventricular System

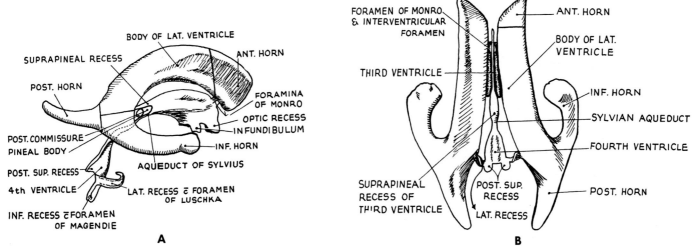

FIGURE 7–7 Ventricular system of the brain. *A*. Lateral view. *B*. Superior view.

The ventricles of the brain are a series of communicating cavities, lined by ependymal epithelium and containing cerebrospinal fluid, which communicate with the subarachnoid space surrounding the brain and the spinal cord and with the central canal of the cord (Figs. 7–7 and 7–8).

The lateral ventricles, one in each cerebral hemisphere, communicate with one another and with the third ventricle via the interventricular foramina. Each consists of a body and three horns—the frontal, the occipital and the temporal.

The third ventricle is a midline slitlike cavity, 2 to 8 mm. wide and about 3 cm. long. Anteriorly, there is an extension from its floor toward the sella turcica (infundibulum, optic recess, and hypothalamic extension). Posteriorly, there is a narrow midline channel extending from the floor that connects the third with the fourth ventricle and is called the cerebral aqueduct (aqueduct of Sylvius). This is an arched structure with a radius of 3.5 to 3.8 cm. with respect to the dorsum sellae, measuring about 1.5 cm. in length and about 2 to 3 mm. in diameter.

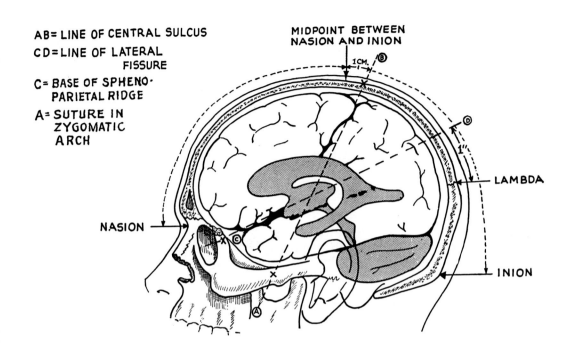

AB = LINE OF CENTRAL SULCUS

CD = LINE OF LATERAL FISSURE

C = BASE OF SPHENO- PARIETAL RIDGE

A = SUTURE IN ZYGOMATIC ARCH

MIDPOINT BETWEEN NASION AND INION

1 CM.

LAMBDA

NASION

INION

FIGURE 7–8 Diagram of the brain: relationship of the central sulcus and lateral fissure to the ventricles and skull.

FIGURE 7–9 Scheme of roof of fourth ventricle. The arrow is in the foramen of Magendie. (From Lewis, W. H. (ed.): Gray's Anatomy of the Human Body, 24th ed. Philadelphia, Lea & Febiger, 1942.)

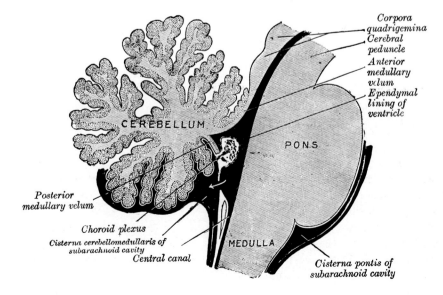

Corpora quadrigemina
Cerebral peduncle
Anterior medullary velum
Ependymal lining of ventricle

CEREBELLUM

PONS

Posterior medullary velum

Choroid plexus

Cisterna cerebellomedullaris of subarachnoid cavity

Central canal

MEDULLA

Cisterna pontis of subarachnoid cavity

The fourth ventricle is a midline cavity, diamond-shaped in frontal projection and triangular in lateral cross section. It communicates anteroinferiorly with the central canal of the medulla oblongata. There are outpouchings laterally (lateral recesses or foramina of Luschka) which communicate with the cisterna magna. Anterior to the choroid plexus of the fourth ventricle, there is a midline foramen (foramen of Magendie) which connects this ventricle with the cisterna cerebellomedullaris. The average measurements of the fourth ventricle are: superoinferiorly, 4 cm.; and from the apex in the roof (fastigium) to the floor, 1.6 cm.

The Subarachnoid Cisterns

The important cisterns are illustrated in Figures 7–4 and 7–5. These appear as lakelike structures on pneumoencephalograms and are helpful in detecting space-occupying lesions.

The fissures and sulci can also on occasion be identified and offer clues to disease processes. When excessively wide, they point toward atrophy. When displaced from a normal relationship, a space-occupying lesion may be suspected.

Cerebrospinal Fluid

It is probable that the cerebrospinal fluid is produced in the three following regions (Fig. 7–10): the *choroid plexuses* (1) of the ventricles, which produce most of the fluid; the *ependyma* of the central canal of the spinal cord (7), lending a small current of fluid which tends to go cephalad; and the *perivascular linings* of the blood vessels that enter and leave the brain in close proximity with the subarachnoid spaces.

The intraventricular fluid flows down the ventricles (2 to 5) to the fourth ventricle (6), and thereafter flows out of the fourth ventricle through the foramina of Magendie and Luschka into the subarachnoid space (8 to 13). There is probably no other communication between the intraventricular fluid and the subarachnoid fluid.

The fluid then distributes itself in the subarachnoid space underlying and covering the brain (8 to 13), and is ultimately absorbed by diffusion through the arachnoid villi (or granulations) into the great dural sinuses (14). There is also a small amount of absorption through the perineural lymphatics.

It is probable that the fluid in the subdural space is produced locally by its own mesothelial cells, but the exact relationship of this fluid to the cerebrospinal fluid is not known.

VENTRICULOGRAPHY

If increased intracranial pressure is present, herniation of brain substance through the foramen magnum (and death) may occur at the time lumbar puncture is performed and cerebrospinal fluid is removed. To prevent this, when air studies of the ventricles are necessary, cerebral puncture is accomplished through the parietal lobes, and cerebrospinal fluid is removed and replaced by air. The same series of films is obtained. The subarachnoid space outside the ventricular system is ordinarily not well demonstrated by this technique.

On occasion, for better visualization of the cerebral aqueduct, 1 to 2 ml. of Pantopaque may be injected into the lateral ventricle. When the patient's head is moved appropriately, the oil, which is heavier than cerebrospinal fluid, will move downward by gravity toward the cerebral aqueduct and fourth ventricle, and films may be taken to demonstrate the adjoining anatomy.

This method of positive contrast ventriculography is utilized particularly when other techniques have failed to reveal sufficient detail for an accurate diagnosis. (New opaque agents are used overseas and experimentally in the U.S.A. but at this writing they have not received F.D.A. approval.)

COMPUTED AXIAL TOMOGRAPHY (CAT OR C/T)

Although this technique is noninvasive and would ordinarily precede pneumography of the brain, it will be described in this text after the pneumography section to allow for a clearer understanding of the anatomy that may be visualized with this newer technique.

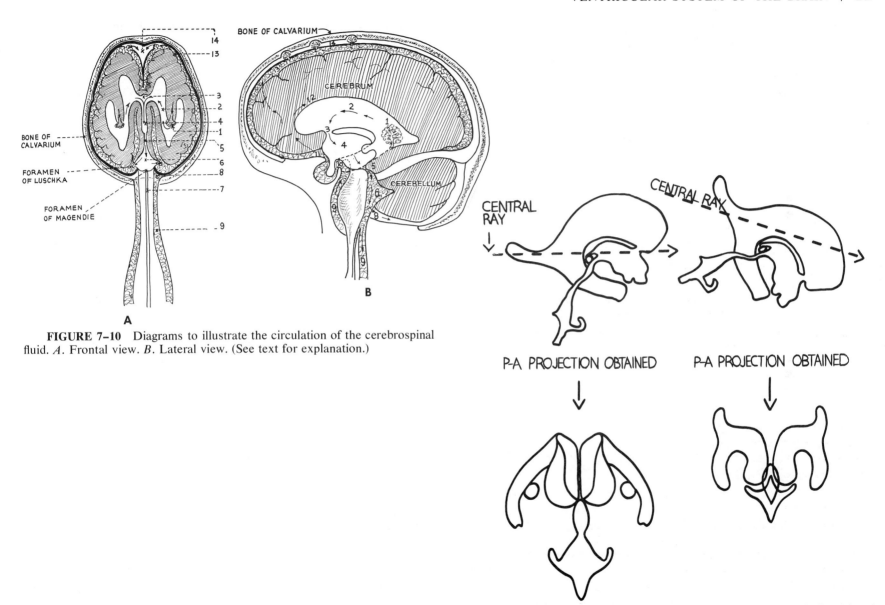

FIGURE 7–10 Diagrams to illustrate the circulation of the cerebrospinal fluid. *A.* Frontal view. *B.* Lateral view. (See text for explanation.)

FIGURE 7–11 Radiographic appearance of ventricles in frontal and lateral perspectives, with appropriate tilted or angle views.

RADIOGRAPHIC STUDY OF THE BRAIN

The radiographic methods of investigating the brain include: plain film studies (for physiologic or abnormal areas of calcification or radiolucency, i.e., lipomas of the corpus callosum); special studies with radioisotopes (outside the scope of the present text); computerized axial tomography; and pneumoencephalography, ventriculography, and cerebral angiography. Pneumoencephalography involves the injection into the subarachnoid space in the spinal region of a gaseous contrast medium that replaces the cerebrospinal fluid so that the ventricles of the brain and the subarachnoid space surrounding it may be visualized. In ventriculography, the contrast medium (usually gaseous) is injected directly into the ventricles of the brain through burr holes in the calvarium or through the space afforded by sutures of the skull. Cerebral angiograms are produced by injecting a contrast medium (opaque and of a type readily excreted by the urinary tract) directly into the arterial system supplying the brain, and immediately thereafter obtaining films during the arterial, capillary, and venous phases in at least two perpendicular projections. Ideally, these are obtained simultaneously and rapidly, as will be described, so that the arterial and venous anatomy can be studied as accurately as possible.

Computerized axial tomography, being noninvasive, should follow plain film studies; it will be described separately.

PNEUMOENCEPHALOGRAMS AND VENTRICULOGRAMS

Some Technical Aspects

Our emphasis in this text is on the elementary aspects studied from the viewpoint of the radiographer and the interested medical trainee.

Greater detail may be obtained from texts devoted exclusively to this subject (Taveras and Wood).*

The gas most frequently employed is air filtered through sterile cotton, although many others have also been used.

The pneumoencephalographic examination is begun with the patient in a sitting position, and the air is introduced by lumbar puncture. The first fraction of 5 to 8 ml. is injected without withdrawal of a significant amount of cerebrospinal fluid, and the air is trapped in the posterior fossa by carefully flexing the head (90 degrees as shown in Figure 7–12). Ideally, at this juncture, fluoroscopy with the aid of image amplification and closed circuit television will indicate whether the position is optimum. Films are obtained in posteroanterior and lateral perspectives. As the degree of flexion of the head is carefully diminished (Fig. 7–12), air may be seen to rise above the tentorium cerebelli into the third and lateral ventricles. The intermittent injection of small amounts of air (following withdrawal of similar amounts of cerebrospinal fluid) will often permit radiographic visualization of important anatomic detail otherwise obscured by superimposed gas shadows.

If the head is immobilized and the patient is strapped in a suitable "tumbling" chair, and if the passage of the air is monitored by closed circuit television, the best positions of the head for optimum filling of the ventricles and subarachnoid space surrounding the brain can be achieved with maximum efficiency. If much cerebrospinal fluid must be drained off, approximately 80 ml. of air may be utilized in the course of the study.

In some instances, for reasons usually difficult to explain, the air will enter the subdural rather than the subarachnoid space. Since this has little diagnostic value, the needle should be repositioned.

---

*Taveras, J. M., and Wood, E. H.: Diagnostic Neuroradiology. Baltimore, Williams & Wilkins, 1964.

Descriptive Terms for Positions and Projections

Anteroposterior (A-P): Beam traverses head from front to back, parallel to Reid's base line (infraorbital-meatal line).

Posteroanterior (P-A): Beam traverses from back to front.

Half axial: May be either P-A, or A-P. Beam is at an angle with respect to Reid's base line, usually between 12 and 35 degrees, although, in the initial pneumoencephalographic films, this may be as much as 90 degrees.

Axial: The beam traverses the skull from base to vertex or vice versa, usually perpendicular to Reid's base line.

Decubitus: The central x-ray beam is in the horizontal plane, and the patient is lying down, *prone* if facing downward, and *supine* if on his back and facing upward.

Brow up, Brow down: Face up or face down respectively.

Lateral: Side projection, named by the side closest to the film.

Oblique: The sagittal axis of the body is turned at an angle to the film; projection is named by the side closest to the film. The angle is usually 45 degrees unless otherwise specified.

The positions are illustrated in the ensuing pages. In every instance, unless the projection is oblique, *the central x-ray beam must be absolutely perpendicular to the sagittal or coronal plane of the head and the film.* A minimum of two views, perpendicular to one another, is usually obtained in each position of the head, as the air shifts from one area to another. These views are illustrated with respect to the position of both the head and the central ray so that radiograph and related anatomy can be properly understood.

Anyone who would attempt radiography of this area must have some basic understanding of the anatomy of the brain. The anatomic sketches included herein are minimal in this respect, although admittedly radiographers probably need fewer reference points of anatomy than do physicians.

Usual Sequence of Head Positions and Projections Obtained

1. Patient sitting, head half axial at 90 degrees, 65 degrees or 45 degrees; posteroanterior and lateral projections (Fig. 7–12).

2. Patient sitting, head erect; anteroposterior and lateral projections (Fig. 7–13).

3. Patient sitting, head erect; Towne's projections, 15 to 35 degrees, as in Figure 7–16, but erect.

4. Patient prone, brow down; posteroanterior and lateral projections (Fig. 7–14) (half-axial projection may also be obtained).

5. Patient supine, brow up; anteroposterior and lateral projections, (Fig. 7–15), and half axial projection if desired, in Towne's projection (Fig. 7–16).

6. Patient prone again, but head turned first to one side and then the other; in each of these two positions, posteroanterior and lateral projections are obtained, the posteroanterior projections utilizing a horizontal beam (Fig. 7–17).

7. Body-section radiographs and tomograms are utilized whenever a clearer view of a given anatomic part is desired. Tomography is a technique whereby the patient's head is slowly rotated on its vertical axis during a lateral exposure, especially of the midline structures such as the cerebral aqueduct or fourth ventricle. This is virtually routine with us as an adjunct to step 1. Subtraction techniques are also added, as required.

The projections and positions usually employed by this author are as follows:

Patient Sitting, Head Half-axial at 90 Degrees, 65 Degrees, 45 Degrees; Anteroposterior and Lateral Projections (Fig. 7–12).

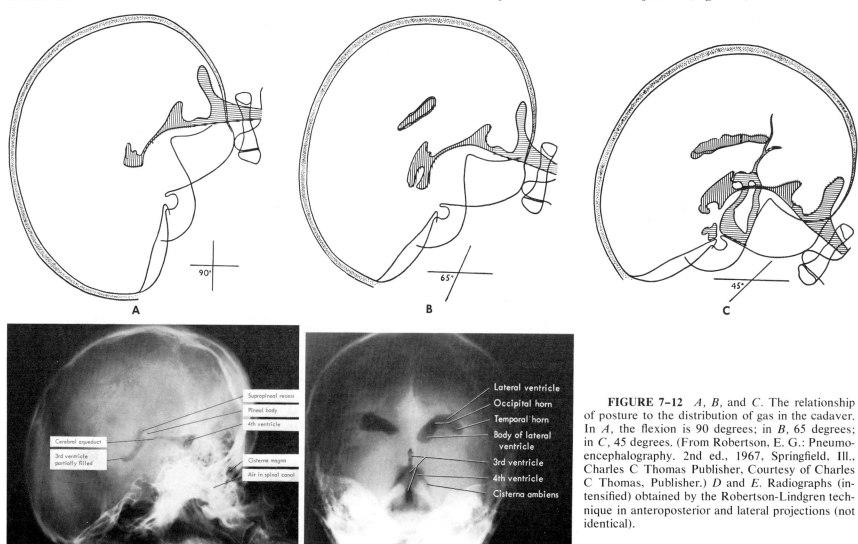

FIGURE 7–12 *A*, *B*, and *C*. The relationship of posture to the distribution of gas in the cadaver. In *A*, the flexion is 90 degrees; in *B*, 65 degrees; in *C*, 45 degrees. (From Robertson, E. G.: Pneumoencephalography. 2nd ed., 1967, Springfield, Ill., Charles C Thomas Publisher, Courtesy of Charles C Thomas, Publisher.) *D* and *E*. Radiographs (intensified) obtained by the Robertson-Lindgren technique in anteroposterior and lateral projections (not identical).

Patient Sitting, Head Erect; Lateral and Anteroposterior Projections (Fig. 7–13).

Patient Sitting, Head Erect; Towne's Projection, 15 to 35 Degrees as in Figure 7–16, But With Patient Erect.

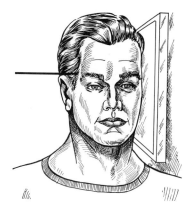

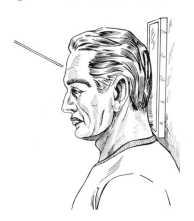

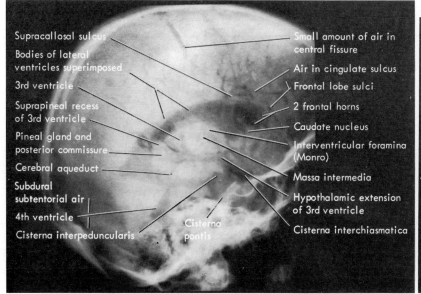

Supracallosal sulcus
Bodies of lateral ventricles superimposed
3rd ventricle
Suprapineal recess of 3rd ventricle
Pineal gland and posterior commissure
Cerebral aqueduct
Subdural subtentorial air
4th ventricle
Cisterna interpeduncularis
Cisterna pontis

Small amount of air in central fissure
Air in cingulate sulcus
Frontal lobe sulci
2 frontal horns
Caudate nucleus
Interventricular foramina (Monro)
Massa intermedia
Hypothalamic extension of 3rd ventricle
Cisterna interchiasmatica

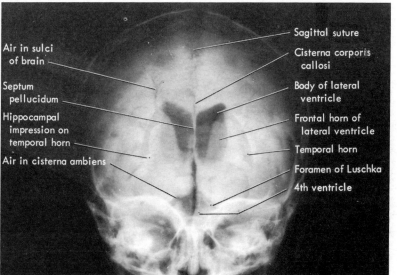

Air in sulci of brain
Septum pellucidum
Hippocampal impression on temporal horn
Air in cisterna ambiens

Sagittal suture
Cisterna corporis callosi
Body of lateral ventricle
Frontal horn of lateral ventricle
Temporal horn
Foramen of Luschka
4th ventricle

FIGURE 7–13 Positioning for and radiographs (intensified) obtained during pneumoencephalography with patient erect and beam horizontal, anteroposterior and lateral projections.

**Patient Prone, Brow Down; Posteroanterior and Lateral Projections
(Fig. 7–14). (Half-axial Views May Also Be Obtained.)**

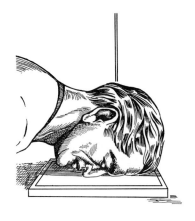

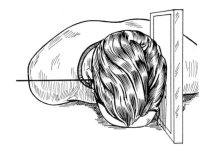

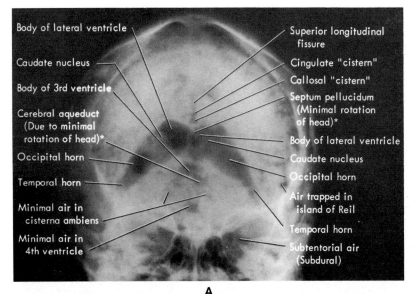

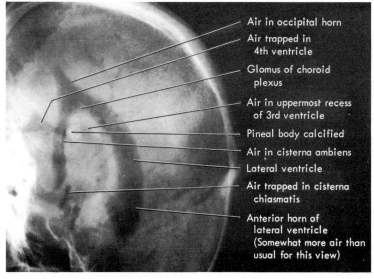

A

B

FIGURE 7–14 Positioning for and radiographs (intensified) obtained during pneumoencephalography with patient prone, brow down. *A.* Vertical beam. *B.* Horizontal beam. *Note that minimal rotation of head as indicated by relationship of mastoid processes with condyloid processes (mandible) may distort the septum pellucidum and third ventricle, as well as make the lateral ventricles appear slightly asymmetrical.

Patient Supine, Brow Up; Anteroposterior and Lateral Projections (Fig. 7–15).

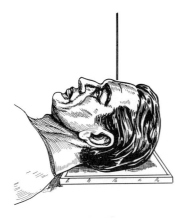

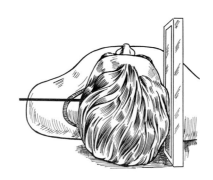

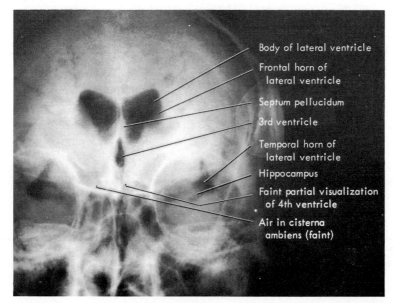

Body of lateral ventricle

Frontal horn of lateral ventricle

Septum pellucidum

3rd ventricle

Temporal horn of lateral ventricle

Hippocampus

Faint partial visualization of 4th ventricle

Air in cisterna ambiens (faint)

A

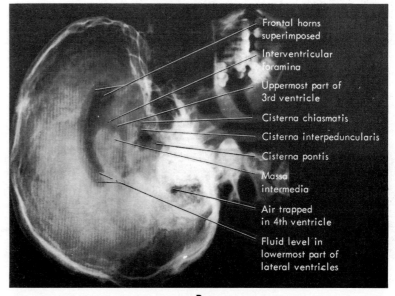

Frontal horns superimposed

Interventricular foramina

Uppermost part of 3rd ventricle

Cisterna chiasmatis

Cisterna interpeduncularis

Cisterna pontis

Massa intermedia

Air trapped in 4th ventricle

Fluid level in lowermost part of lateral ventricles

B

FIGURE 7–15 Positioning for and radiographs (intensified) obtained during pneumoencephalography with patient recumbent, supine, *A*. Vertical beam. A-P: *B*. Horizontal beam, lateral (both laterals may be taken).

Half-axial Projections May Be Obtained in Towne's Projection (Fig. 7–16).

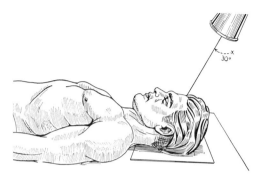

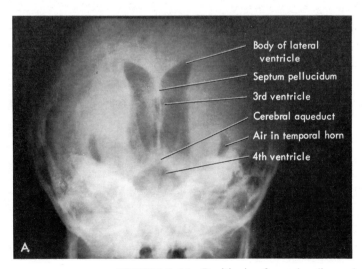

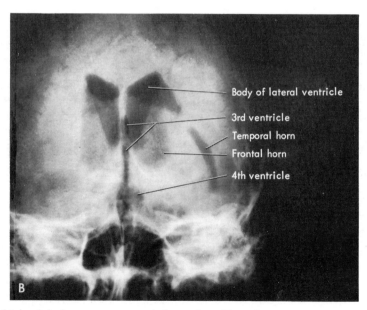

FIGURE 7–16 Positioning for and radiographs (intensified) obtained during pneumoencephalography with patient supine in Towne's projection. *A*, 30-degree angulation of central ray caudad. *B*, 15-degree angulation of central ray caudad.

Patient Prone, Head Turned First to One Side and Then the Other.

In each of these two positions, anteroposterior and lateral projections are obtained, utilizing a horizontal beam (Fig. 7–17). Views employing a vertical beam, reverse Towne's projection, may also be obtained at this time (Fig. 7–18).

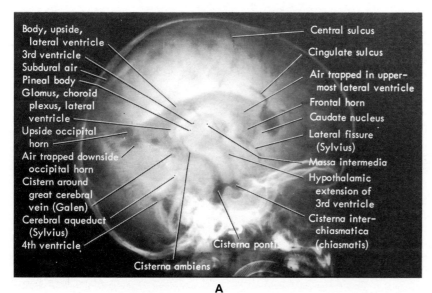

Body, upside, lateral ventricle
3rd ventricle
Subdural air
Pineal body
Glomus, choroid plexus, lateral ventricle
Upside occipital horn
Air trapped downside occipital horn
Cistern around great cerebral vein (Galen)
Cerebral aqueduct (Sylvius)
4th ventricle
Cisterna ambiens
Cisterna pontis
Central sulcus
Cingulate sulcus
Air trapped in uppermost lateral ventricle
Frontal horn
Caudate nucleus
Lateral fissure (Sylvius)
Massa intermedia
Hypothalamic extension of 3rd ventricle
Cisterna interchiasmatica (chiasmatis)

A

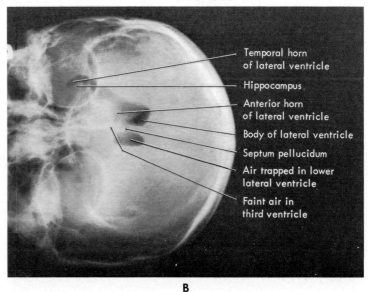

Temporal horn of lateral ventricle
Hippocampus
Anterior horn of lateral ventricle
Body of lateral ventricle
Septum pellucidum
Air trapped in lower lateral ventricle
Faint air in third ventricle

B

FIGURE 7–17 Positioning for and radiographs (intensified) obtained during pneumoencephalography with patient lying down, right side of head uppermost. *A*. Vertical beam. *B*. Horizontal beam. A similar set of two films is obtained with the left side of the head uppermost.

Projections Employing a Vertical Beam, Reverse Towne's Projection, May Also Be Obtained.

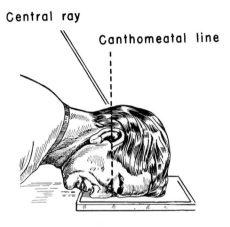

Central ray

Canthomeatal line

POINTS OF PRACTICAL INTEREST ABOUT FIGURE 7–18

1. Since the air rises to the uppermost portions of the ventricular system, this projection has its chief application in visualization of the occipital horns, the posterior portions of the lateral ventricles, the posterior part of the third ventricle, and the fourth ventricle.

2. The true Towne position, with the patient supine and the central ray angled 35 degrees toward the feet, is most applicable to visualization of the temporal horns and the anterior sectors of the lateral ventricles.

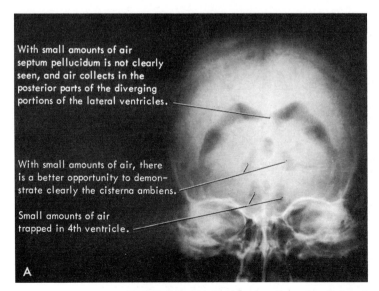

With small amounts of air septum pellucidum is not clearly seen, and air collects in the posterior parts of the diverging portions of the lateral ventricles.

With small amounts of air, there is a better opportunity to demonstrate clearly the cisterna ambiens.

Small amounts of air trapped in 4th ventricle.

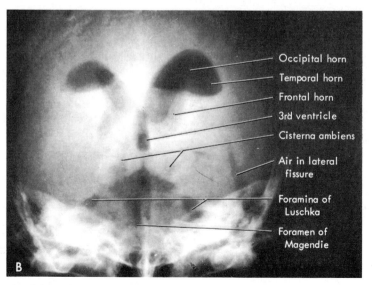

Occipital horn
Temporal horn
Frontal horn
3rd ventricle
Cisterna ambiens
Air in lateral fissure
Foramina of Luschka
Foramen of Magendie

FIGURE 7–18 Positioning for and radiographs (intensified) obtained during pneumoencephalography with patient prone, reverse Towne's projection. *A.* Central ray angled 12 degrees to canthomeatal line. *B.* Central ray angled 25 degrees to canthomeatal line. (Foramina of Luschka label probable, not certain.)

A Basovertical Projection with the Patient Prone, Positioned as Shown in Figure 7–19, May Also be Obtained.

Body section radiographs and tomograms are utilized whenever a clear view of a given anatomic part is desired. Autotomography is a technique whereby the patient's head is slowly rotated on its vertical axis during a lateral exposure, especially when a view of the midline structures such as the cerebral aqueduct and fourth ventricle is desired. For structures other than those in the midline, special tomographic devices are necessary.

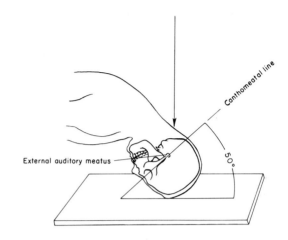

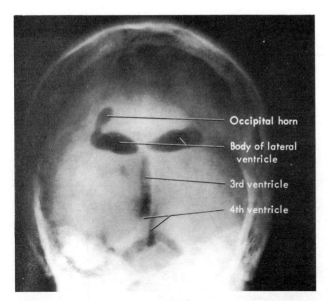

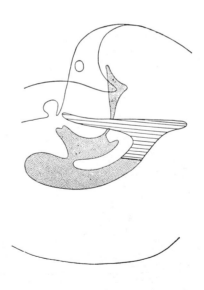

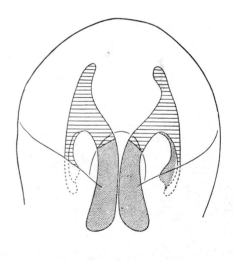

FIGURE 7–19 Positioning for radiograph (intensified) and tracings of basovertical projection; patient prone, beam vertical. A horizontal beam lateral view (diagram, center) is also obtained with the patient in this position. (Tracings from Robertson, E. G.: Pneumoencephalography. Springfield, Ill., Charles C Thomas, Publisher, 1967. Courtesy of Charles C Thomas, Publisher.)

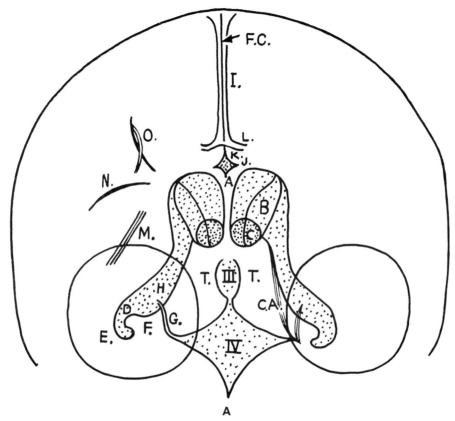

FIGURE 7–20   Diagram illustrating the various anatomic parts seen in pneumoencephalography. *A*. Anteroposterior projection. (A) Corpus callosum. (B) caudate nucleus, (C) choroid plexus, (D) temporal horns, (E) eminentia collateralis, (F) fornix, (G) lateral recess of fourth ventricle, (H) foramen of Luschka, (I) longitudinal fissure, (J) callosal sulcus, (K) cisterna corpus callosi, (L) cingulate sulcus, (M) air in depths of Sylvian fissure, (N) superior frontal sulcus, (O) interparietal sulcus, (T–T) thalamus, (CA) cisterna ambiens, (FC) falx cerebri.

FIGURE 7–20 *Continued.* *B.* Lateral projection. (A) Lamina terminalis, (B) cerebellar folia, (C) posterior cerebral artery, (D) basilar artery, (E) optic chiasm, (F) anterior communicating artery, (G) colliculi, (H) cerebral peduncles (mammillary bodies), (I) tuber cinereum, (J) superior medullary velum, (K) oculomotor nerve, (L) cingulate sulcus, (M) cingulate gyrus, (N) cisterna ambiens, (P) pulvinar, (CN) caudate nucleus, (FO) fornix, (AC) anterior commissure, (MC) middle commissure, (PC) posterior commissure, (CA) calcar avis, (PI) pineal, (R) infundibulum, (CS) callosal sulcus-cisterna corpus callosi, (PX) parieto-occipital sulcus, (CF) calcarine fissure, (SP) subparietal sulcus, (PO) parolfactory sulcus, (Cen. S.) central sulcus (Rolando), (CT) cerebellar tonsil, (TC) tentorium cerebelli, (Z) air outlining cerebellum, (GCP) glomus of the choroid plexus.

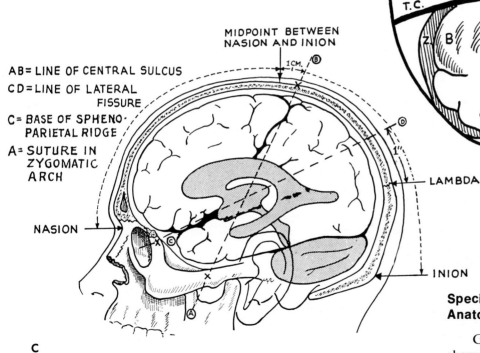

FIGURE 7–20 *Continued.* *C.* Medial sagittal section of the brain. Relationship of the central sulcus and lateral fissure to the ventricles and skull.

Special Demonstrations of Pneumoencephalographic Anatomy

Gross demonstrations of pneumoencephalographic anatomy are shown in the following illustrations (Figs. 7–21 to 7–27), but in these several demonstrations, finer detail of brain anatomy can be achieved by polytomography, as indicated in other portions of this chapter.

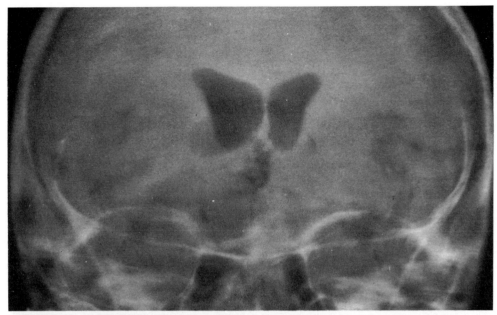

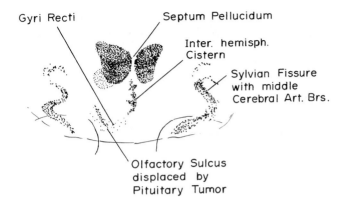

Gyri Recti Septum Pellucidum

Inter. hemisph. Cistern

Sylvian Fissure with middle Cerebral Art. Brs.

Olfactory Sulcus displaced by Pituitary Tumor

FIGURE 7–21 Labeled pneumoencephalographic details in a normal person, posteroanterior projection.

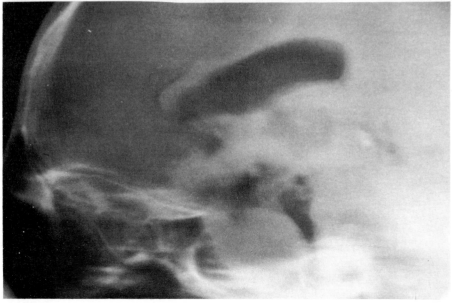

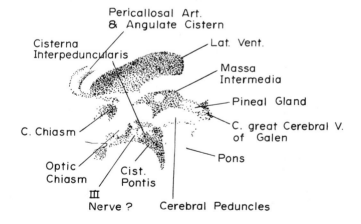

Pericallosal Art. & Angulate Cistern

Cisterna Interpeduncularis Lat. Vent.

Massa Intermedia

Pineal Gland

C. Chiasm

C. great Cerebral V. of Galen

Optic Chiasm Cist. Pontis Pons

III Nerve ? Cerebral Peduncles

FIGURE 7–22 Labeled pneumoencephalographic details in a normal person, lateral projection.

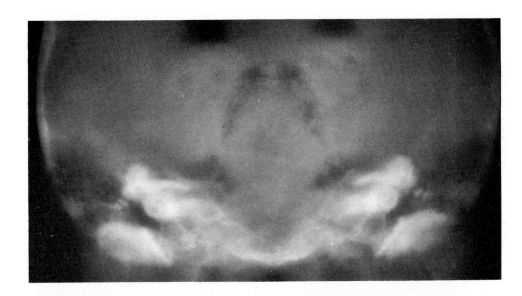

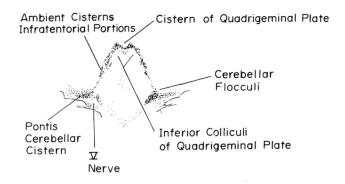

FIGURE 7–23 Labeled pneumoencephalographic details in a normal person, reverse Towne's projection, patient erect.

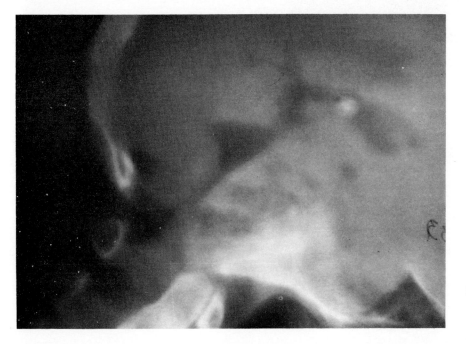

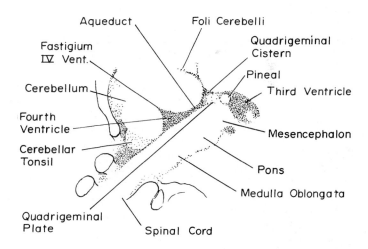

FIGURE 7–24 Labeled pneumoencephalographic details in a normal person, lateral projection, with head flexed slightly in lateral projection.

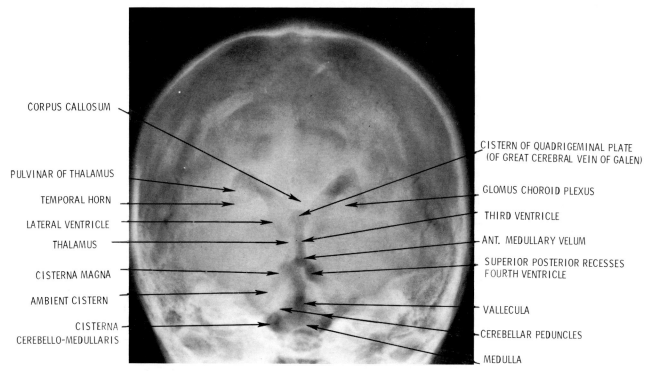

CORPUS CALLOSUM

PULVINAR OF THALAMUS

TEMPORAL HORN

LATERAL VENTRICLE

THALAMUS

CISTERNA MAGNA

AMBIENT CISTERN

CISTERNA
CEREBELLO-MEDULLARIS

CISTERN OF QUADRIGEMINAL PLATE
(OF GREAT CEREBRAL VEIN OF GALEN)

GLOMUS CHOROID PLEXUS

THIRD VENTRICLE

ANT. MEDULLARY VELUM

SUPERIOR POSTERIOR RECESSES
FOURTH VENTRICLE

VALLECULA

CEREBELLAR PEDUNCLES

MEDULLA

FIGURE 7–25 Labeled posteroanterior pneumoencephalogram in reverse
Towne's projection, patient erect.

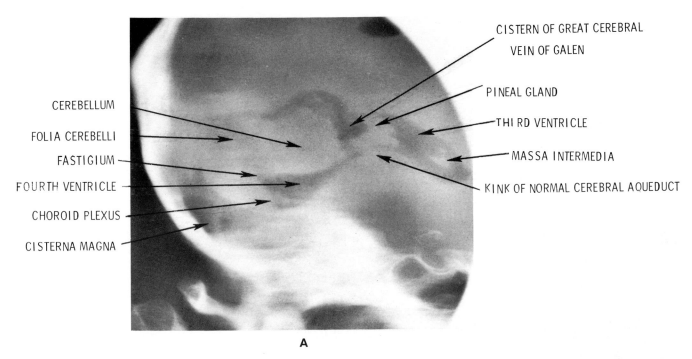

CISTERN OF GREAT CEREBRAL
VEIN OF GALEN

CEREBELLUM

FOLIA CEREBELLI

FASTIGIUM

FOURTH VENTRICLE

CHOROID PLEXUS

CISTERNA MAGNA

PINEAL GLAND

THIRD VENTRICLE

MASSA INTERMEDIA

KINK OF NORMAL CEREBRAL AQUEDUCT

A

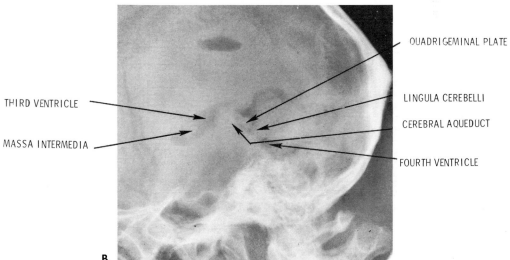

QUADRIGEMINAL PLATE

THIRD VENTRICLE

MASSA INTERMEDIA

LINGULA CEREBELLI

CEREBRAL AQUEDUCT

FOURTH VENTRICLE

B

FIGURE 7–26 *A*. Pneumoencephalogram of posterior fossa obtained after autotomography, showing improved detail. *B*. Pneumoencephalogram in a patient who is erect with head slightly flexed, demonstrating special structures in the third ventricle and fourth ventricle as well as the structures between.

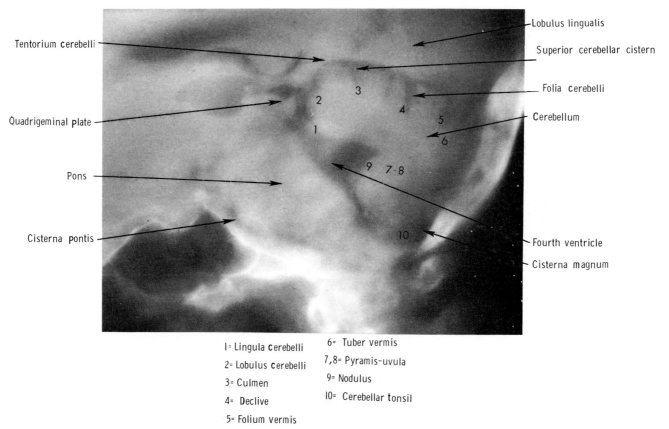

Tentorium cerebelli

Quadrigeminal plate

Pons

Cisterna pontis

Lobulus lingualis

Superior cerebellar cistern

Folia cerebelli

Cerebellum

Fourth ventricle

Cisterna magnum

I= Lingula cerebelli
2= Lobulus cerebelli
3= Culmen
4= Declive
5= Folium vermis

6= Tuber vermis
7,8= Pyramis-uvula
9= Nodulus
IO= Cerebellar tonsil

FIGURE 7–27 Tomographic view of the posterior fossa with particular emphasis on the detail associated with the cerebellum. Apart from those areas labeled directly there are the following: (1) lingula cerebelli, (2) lobulus cerebelli, (3) culmen, (4) declive, (5) folium vermis, (6) tuber vermis, (7, 8) pyramis and uvula, (9) nodulus, (10) cerebellar tonsil.

ANATOMY BASIC TO CEREBRAL ANGIOGRAPHY

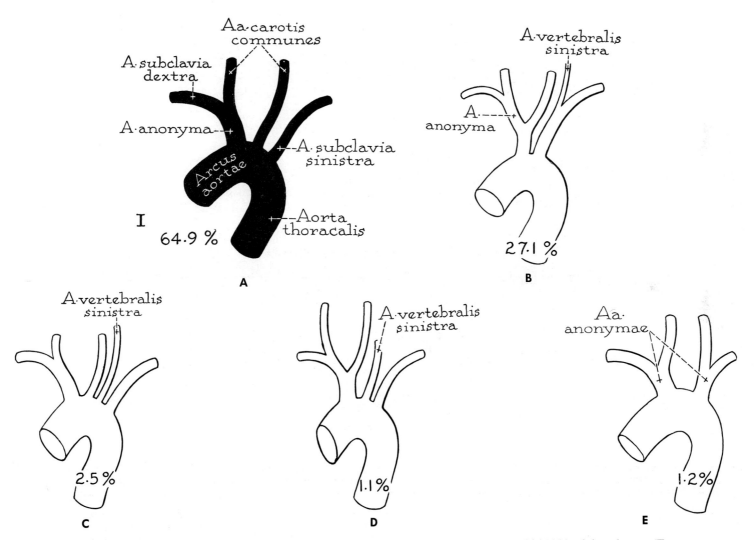

FIGURE 7–28 The most frequent types of branching of the aortic arch encountered in 1000 adult cadavers. (From Anson, B. J.: An Atlas of Human Anatomy, 2nd ed. Philadelphia, W. B. Saunders Co., 1963.) (*Sinistra* is "left"; *dextra* is "right"; *A, anonyma* is the truncus brachiocephalicus.)

CEREBRAL ANGIOGRAPHY

Comment on Examination Technique

Basically, this method of examination involves the direct or indirect introduction of a suitable contrast agent into the major blood vessels of the brain. This may be accomplished by needle puncture of the carotid arteries or the vertebral artery, by threading a catheter *via* the brachial or femoral artery to an appropriate position for injection, or by the retrograde injection of the contrast agent into the brachial or subclavian artery directly.

If the injection is made directly into the carotid or vertebral artery, usually 6 to 8 ml. will suffice if injected rapidly; if it is made into the arch of the aorta or more peripherally, a greater volume, such as 30 to 40 ml., may be necessary.

Serial exposures are routinely made in anteroposterior half axial (Fig. 7–57) and lateral projections (horizontal beam), simultaneously, at two per second for three seconds, and one per second for four seconds. The half axial angulation is 15 to 20 degrees for carotid angiography and 30 degrees for vertebral. Occasionally, 30 degree oblique or basilar projections are also obtained.

If the injection is made below the bifurcation of the common carotid artery, a visualization of the external carotid artery is also obtained, although its circulation is a few seconds slower than the internal carotid. (This technique is especially helpful in meningiomas.) If it is made into the subclavian artery, the vertebral artery of that side is visualized simultaneously, along with its flow pattern with respect to the basilar artery and its major ramifications.

The ideal frontal perspective in most instances is one in which the supraorbital ridge is directly superimposed over the petrous ridge. The condyloid processes of the mandible must be absolutely symmetrical with respect to the mastoid processes. In the lateral projections, there must be a perfect superimposition of the rami of the mandible and the temporomandibular joints.

It will be noted that if emphasis on the vertebral circulation is required, the horizontal x-ray beam is centered 3 cm. below the external auditory meatus for the lateral views. In carotid angiography, the horizontal beam is centered 3 cm. above and 1 cm. anterior to the meatus (Fig. 7–57).

The exposures are begun near the end of the injection period. Injections may be repeated with somewhat different timing after the initial films are seen. In general, the arterial phase occurs within the first two seconds; the capillary phase, two seconds thereafter; and the venous phase in the final two to three seconds. These sequences may have to be varied depending upon individual requirements.

Anatomy

External Carotid Artery (Fig. 7–33). Radiologically, the important branches for identification are: (1) the occipital; (2) the superficial temporal; and (3) the internal maxillary, which in turn gives rise to the middle meningeal and small orbital branches that communicate with the ophthalmic branch of the internal carotid.

Internal Carotid Artery (Fig. 7–34). The important parts and branches for radiologic identification are: (1) the carotid sinus and (2) the ophthalmic; (3) the posterior communicating (joining the posterior cerebral); (4) the anterior choroidal; and (5) and (6), terminally, the anterior and middle cerebral arteries.

The important branches of the anterior cerebral for identification on both frontal and lateral perspectives are: (1) the frontopolar; (2) the pericallosal; and (3) the callosomarginal. The anterior communicating is usually too small to identify.

The important branches of the middle cerebral for identification are: (1) the lenticulostriate arterial twigs; (2) the ascending frontoparietal; (3) the posterior parietal; (4) the angular; and (5) the posterior temporal.

A few of the important relationships of these main branches are indicated in Figures 7–29 to 7–63.

Vertebral Artery. The vertebral arteries ordinarily arise from the subclavian on either side (Fig. 7–29). They enter the foramen transversarium on each side at the level of the sixth cervical vertebra and ascend in the foramen transversarium of each successive cervical vertebra to the C 2 level, where each artery swings laterally for about 1 cm. It then traverses the foramen transversarium of C 1 and enters the cranial cavity at the lateral border of the foramen magnum. Its important branches, apart from small muscular branches in the neck, are the following: (1) the posterior meningeal, (2) the anterior and posterior spinal and (3) the posterior inferior cerebellar. This latter branch is of great importance, since it lies, in its first part, close to the medial part of the cerebellar tonsil, and more distally, close to the floor of the fourth ventricle and its choroid plexus. If it can be identified 5 mm. or more below the level of the foramen magnum, it is virtually certain that there is a downward herniation of the cerebellar tonsil through the foramen magnum. Near the upper medulla, the two vertebral arteries merge medially to form the basilar artery.

Basilar Artery. This artery runs between the clivus and the pons, in the cisterna pontis (Fig. 7–42). In the interpeduncular cistern, it divides into the two posterior cerebral arteries. The main branches to be identified are: (1) the pontine twigs and (2) the internal auditory, (3) the anterior inferior cerebellar and (4) the superior cerebellar arteries. The last-mentioned encircles the brain stem in the cisterna ambiens, but unlike the posterior cerebral, it finally ramifies beneath the tentorium cerebelli over the upper part of the cerebellum.

Unfortunately for our diagnostic accuracy, the appearance of the basilar artery varies considerably, as it wanders from one side to the other of the brain stem.

Posterior Cerebral Artery (Fig. 7–43). Beyond the posterior communicating artery, it is important to identify the following branches: (1) the thalamostriate; (2) the posterior choroidal, three on each side; (3) the anterior and posterior temporal; (4) the posterior occipital; and (5) the calcarine arteries, terminally ramifying over the temporal and occipital lobes. The posterior cerebral follows the midbrain in the cisterna ambiens, near the edge, but above the tentorial notch. Herniation downward may be detected with protrusion of the brain stem through this notch.

Circle of Willis (Fig. 7–32). This anastomotic arterial circle consists of: (1) the two anterior cerebrals connected by the anterior communicating and (2) the internal carotids connected with the posterior cerebrals by the two posterior communicating arteries. The basilar artery forms the common linkage posteriorly.

Deep Cerebral Veins (Figs. 7–53 to 7–56). The important deep veins to identify are: (1) the septal; (2) the anterior caudate or terminal; (3) the striothalamic; (4) the internal cerebral, which courses medially along the roof of the third ventricle to fuse posteriorly to form (5) the great cerebral vein of Galen, the midline vein that courses slightly upward and posteriorly to empty into the straight venous sinus; and (6) the basal vein of Rosenthal, which winds its way around the midbrain near the brain stem to empty into the great cerebral vein of Galen.

The Venous Sinuses (Figs. 7–1 and 7–2). As previously indicated, the venous sinuses are contained within the dura mater. Those that are important to identify are: (1) the superior longitudinal sinus, (2) the inferior longitudinal sinus, (3) the straight sinus, (4) the lateral sinus, (5) the superior petrosal sinus, (6) the inferior petrosal sinus, (7) the sphenoparietal sinus, and (8) the cavernous sinus.

The Superficial Cerebral Veins (Figs. 7–54 and 7–62). These drain into the dural venous sinuses and consist of the following main groups: (1) the anastomotic veins of Trolard, superiorly; (2) the anastomotic vein of Labbé, inferiorly; (3) the middle cerebral vein in the lateral (Sylvian) fissure, emptying into the sphenoparietal and cavernous sinuses, and (4) the superior cerebral veins, which are superficial and empty into the superior longitudinal sinus.

The Venous Angle. It will be noted that this represents the confluent point of the striothalamic vein, and the septal vein, and the origin of the internal cerebral vein (Fig. 7–53). Anatomically, the angle is usually situated at the interventricular foramen on each side of the midline. These veins are of considerable importance, since they serve to delineate much of the body and anterior horn of the lateral ventricle and the roof of the third ventricle. The basal vein of Rosenthal, which together with the internal cerebral vein empties into the great cerebral vein of Galen, winds its way around the midbrain in close approximation to the posterior cerebral artery.

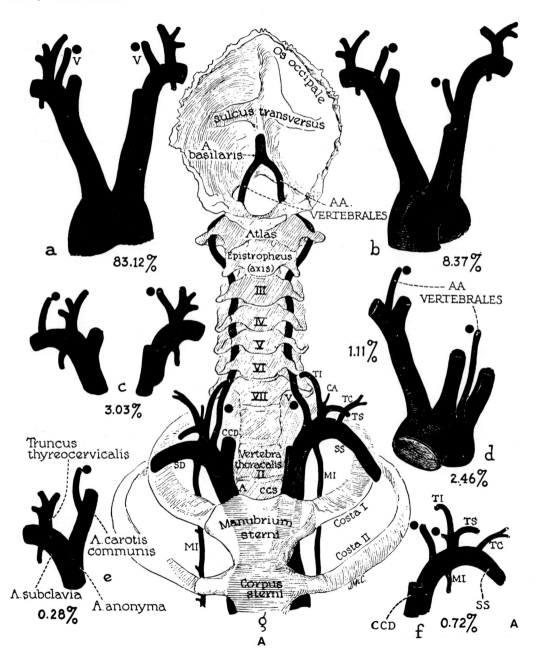

FIGURE 7–29 *A.* Variations in the origin of the vertebral artery, (From Anson, B. J.: Atlas of Human Anatomy, 2nd ed. Philadelphia, W. B. Saunders Co., 1963.) (A. anonyma is truncus brachiocephalicus.)

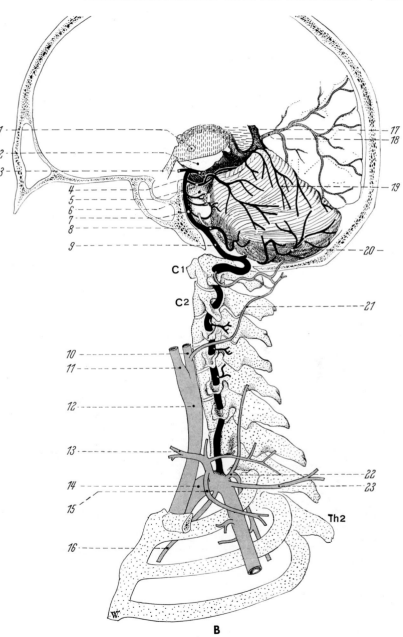

FIGURE 7–29 *Continued. B.* Extracranial and intracranial course of the vertebral artery and its branches. Vascular supply of the posterior portion of the circle of Willis. (From Krayenbühl, H. A., and Yasargil, M. G.: Zerebrale Angiographie, 2nd ed. Stuttgart, G. Thieme Verlag, 1965.)

(1) Massa intermedia
(2) Cerebral peduncle
(3) Posterior communicating artery
(4) Posterior cerebral artery
(5) Superior cerebellar artery
(6) Pons
(7) Basilar artery
(8) Anterior inferior cerebellar artery
(9) Left vertebral artery
(10) External carotid artery
(11) Internal carotid artery
(12) Common carotid artery

(13) Thyreocervical arteries
(14) Subclavian artery
(15) Suprascapular artery
(16) Internal mammillary artery
(17) Splenium
(18) Right posterior cerebral artery
(19) Superior cerebellar artery
(20) Posterior inferior cerebellar artery
(21) Occipital artery
(22) Costocervical artery
(23) Transverse artery of the neck

B

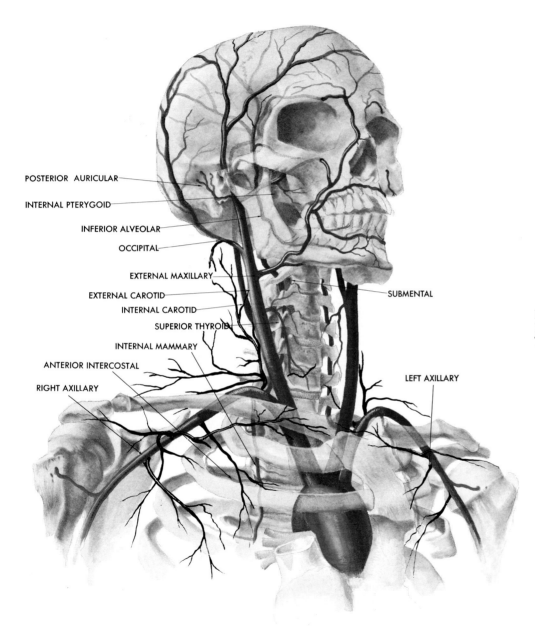

POSTERIOR AURICULAR

INTERNAL PTERYGOID

INFERIOR ALVEOLAR

OCCIPITAL

EXTERNAL MAXILLARY

EXTERNAL CAROTID

INTERNAL CAROTID

SUPERIOR THYROID

INTERNAL MAMMARY

ANTERIOR INTERCOSTAL

RIGHT AXILLARY

SUBMENTAL

LEFT AXILLARY

FIGURE 7–30 Deep circulation of the head and neck. (From Bierman, H. C.: Selective Arterial Catheterization. Springfield, Ill., Charles C Thomas, Publisher, 1969. Courtesy of Charles C Thomas, Publisher.)

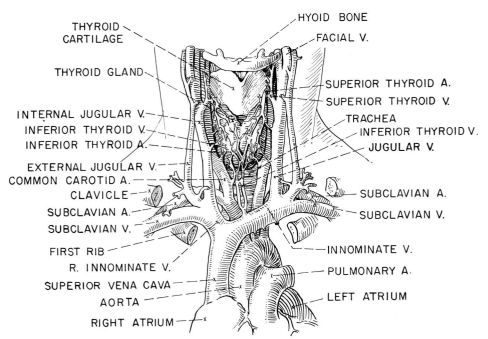

FIGURE 7–31 Diagram of major circulation in the neck. (Innominate V. is truncus brachiocephalicus vein.)

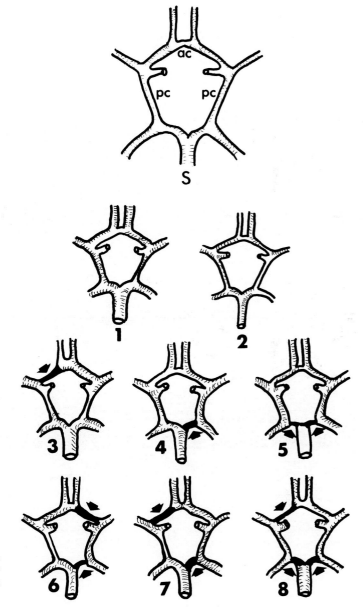

FIGURE 7–32 Variations of the circle of Willis (after Riggs). (S) standard relationships, (ac) anterior communicating artery, (pc) posterior communicating artery. The blackened segments represent agenesis or absence. Hypoplastic segments are shown narrower in caliber than the others.

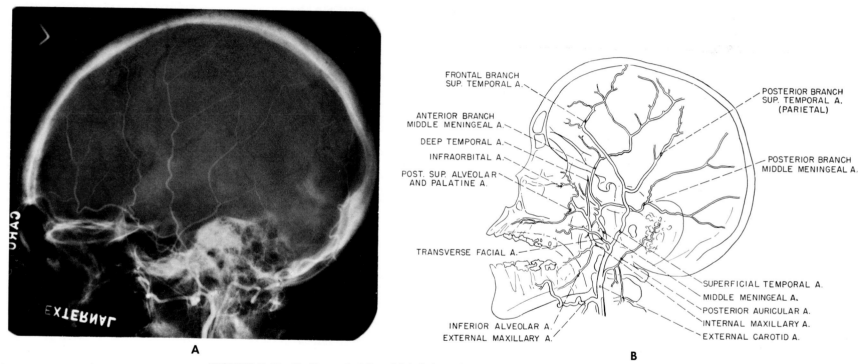

FIGURE 7-33 Radiograph *(A)* and labeled tracing *(B)* of external carotid arteriogram.

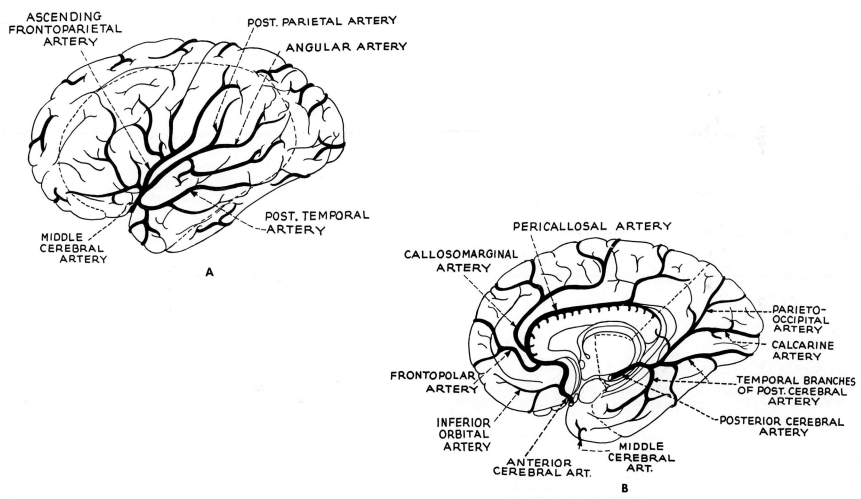

FIGURE 7–34 Chief divisions of the internal carotid artery. *A*. Lateral aspect. *B*. Median sagittal aspect.

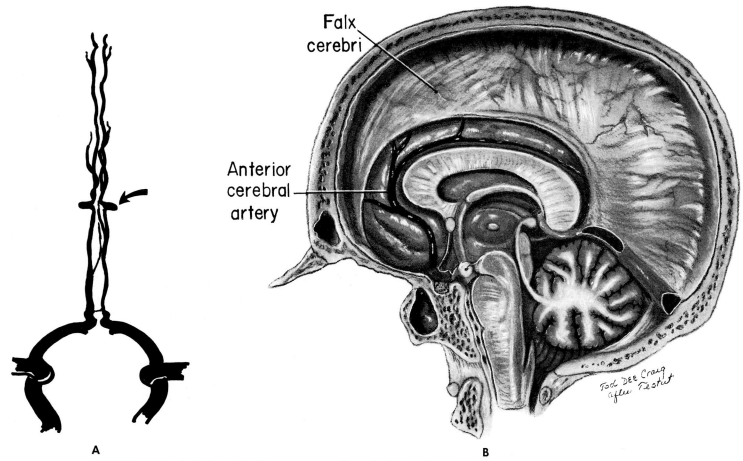

Falx
cerebri

Anterior
cerebral
artery

A   B

FIGURE 7–35 *A.* "Moustache" appearance of terminal branches of the pericallosal in the lateral longitudinal sulcus of the corpus callosum. *B.* Diagram of longitudinal section of skull and brain. The falx is much thinner on its anterior aspect and becomes thicker as it goes posteriorly to join the tentorium. The anterior cerebral artery gives off branches which, as they extend peripherally, go beyond the edge of the falx. Therefore, when these arteries are displaced, they must return to the midline as they reach the falx edge. (From Taveras, J. M., and Wood, E. H.: Diagnostic Neuroradiology. Baltimore, The Williams & Wilkins Co., 1964.)

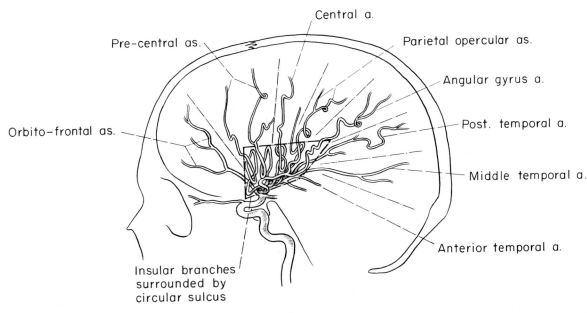

Central a.

Pre-central as.

Parietal opercular as.

Angular gyrus a.

Orbito-frontal as.

Post. temporal a.

Middle temporal a.

Anterior temporal a.

Insular branches
surrounded by
circular sulcus

A

FIGURE 7–36 *A*. Position of the insular portion of the middle cerebral artery in the Sylvian triangle. *A*. Lateral diagram. *B*. Sulci and gyri of the insula. The opercula has been removed to show the surface of the insula surrounded by the circular sulcus. (1,2,3) Short gyri on frontal part of insula; (4,5) long gyrus partly divided. (From Cunningham's Manual of Practical Anatomy, 12th ed. Vol. 3. London, Oxford University Press, 1958.)

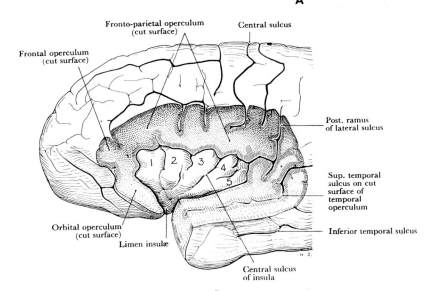

Fronto-parietal operculum
(cut surface)

Central sulcus

Frontal operculum
(cut surface)

Post. ramus
of lateral sulcus

Sup. temporal
sulcus on cut
surface of
temporal
operculum

Orbital operculum
(cut surface)

Inferior temporal sulcus

Limen insulæ

Central sulcus
of insula

B

SPHENO-PARIETAL GROOVE
WHERE IT PROJECTS OVER
BODY OF SPHENOID BONE

1"

LAMBDA

MIDDLE CEREBRAL ARTERY
SHOULD NOT BE OFF THIS
LINE BY MORE THAN 6 MM.
IN ADULTS (SLIGHTLY MORE IN CHILDREN)

FIGURE 7–37 Author's technique for illustrating the correct anatomic position of the axis of the middle cerebral artery group of vessels on the basis of bony landmarks of the skull, provided the lateral projection is a perfect one. As noted, the line is drawn from the sphenoparietal groove where it projects over the body of the sphenoid bone to a point 1 inch above lambda. Although this line is somewhat different from that proposed by Taveras and Wood, it has generally been found that the middle cerebral artery should not vary from this line by more than 6 mm. in adults and slightly more in children.

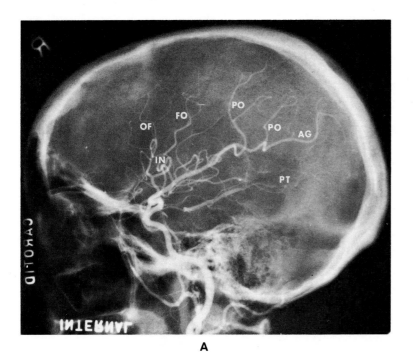

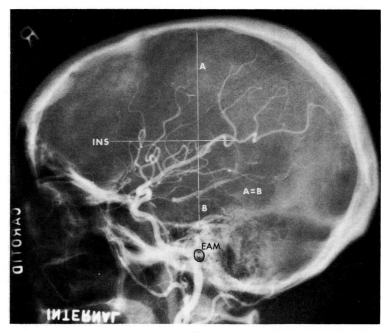

A

B

FIGURE 7–38 *A.* Visualization of the middle cerebral artery and its major branches without interference from the anterior cerebral artery. (OF) Orbitofrontal artery, (FO) frontal opercular arteries (precentral artery), (PO) parietal opercular arteries (central artery). (PO) (without the C) is another parietal opercular artery, (AG) the angular gyrus artery, (PT) posterior temporal artery.

B. Diagram for evaluation of the position of the middle cerebral artery in the lateral view (modified from Vlahovitch et al., 1964). (INS) alignment of insular branches. Line AB is drawn perpendicular to this line from the external auditory meatus (EAM). Line A is equal in length to line B, suggesting correct position of the insular branches, and line A divides the frontal branches from the parietal branches.

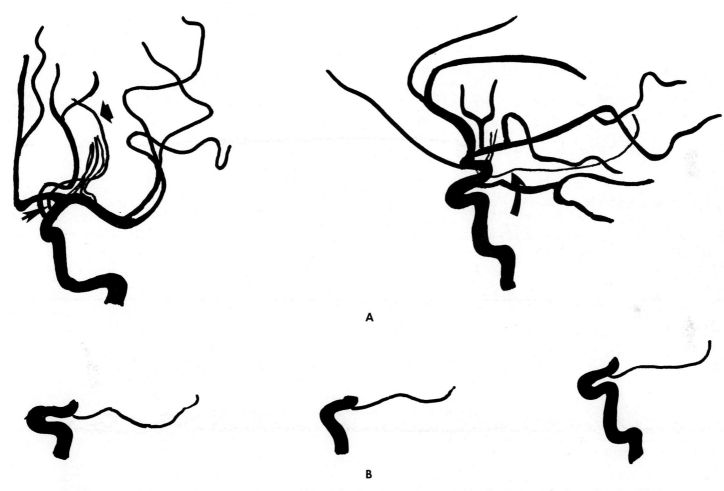

A

B

FIGURE 7–39 *A*. Line drawings of the main ramifications of the internal carotid artery in frontal and lateral perspective, with particular reference to the anterior choroidal artery (arrow). The origin of the anterior choroidal artery can vary as described in the text. *B*. Variations in the appearance of the anterior choroidal artery in the lateral projection. The details of termination of the anterior choroidal artery will be shown more specifically in relation to the branches of the posterior choroidal artery in a later section.

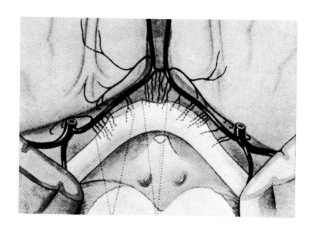

A

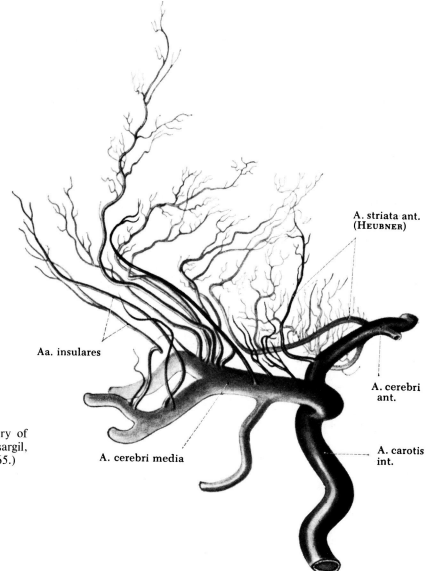

A. striata ant.
(Heubner)

Aa. insulares

A. cerebri
ant.

A. cerebri media

A. carotis
int.

B

FIGURE 7–40 *A* and *B*. Perforating branches and recurrent artery of Heubner (anterior cerebral branch). (From Krayenbühl, H. A., and Yasargil, M. G.: Zerebrale Angiographie, 2nd ed. Stuttgart, G. Thieme Verlag, 1965.)

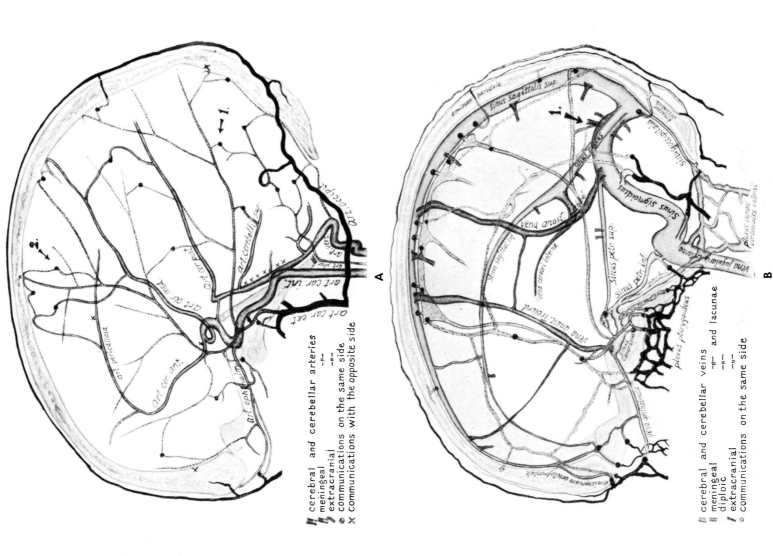

A

cerebral and cerebellar arteries
-"-   meningeal
-"-   extracranial
• communications on the same side
✕ communications with the opposite side

B

cerebral and cerebellar veins
-"-   meningeal
-"-   diploic
/   extracranial
○ communications on the same side

FIGURE 7–41 *A.* Diagram of the arteries supplying the cranium, with special reference to their communications, indicated by arrows. The arterial system of the auditory apparatus has been omitted from the diagram. *B.* Diagram of the veins and dural sinuses of the cranium and their communications. The venous system of the auditory apparatus has been omitted from the diagram. (From Lindblom, K.: Acta Radiol. (Stockholm), Suppl. 30, 1936.)

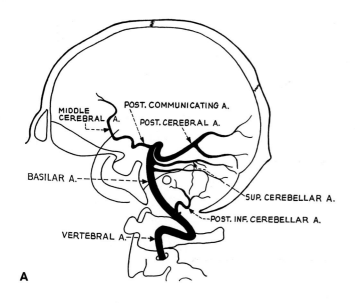

A

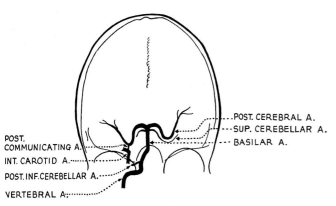

B

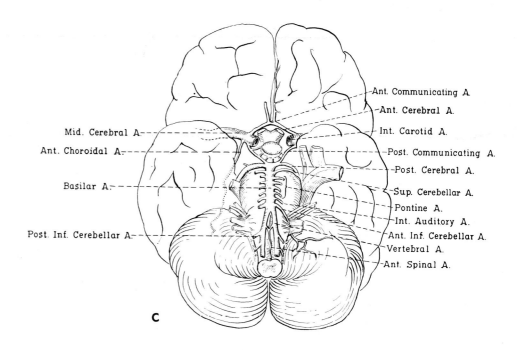

C

FIGURE 7–42 *A.* Diagram of vertebral angiogram, lateral projection. *B.* Towne's projection. *C.* Anatomy of the vertebral artery and branches in relation to the base of the brain.

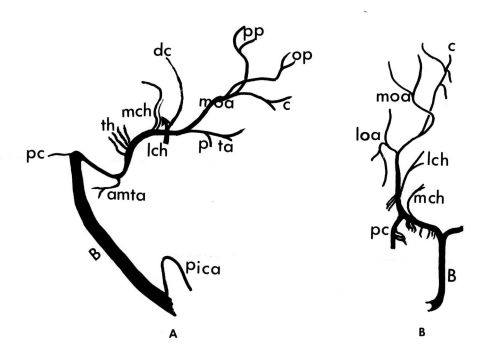

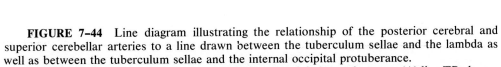

FIGURE 7-43 Line diagrams of the posterior cerebral arteries in Towne's anteroposterior (*A*) and lateral (*B*) projections.

(amta) anterior and middle temporal arteries, (B) basilar arteries, (c) calcarine artery, (dc) dorsal callosal artery, (lch) lateral posterior choroidal artery, (loa) lateral occipital artery. (mch) median posterior choroidal artery, (moa) medial occipital artery, (op) occipitoparietal artery, (pc) posterior communicating artery, (pica) posterior inferior cerebellar artery, (pp) posterior parietal artery, (pta) posterior temporal artery, (ta) temporal artery, (th) thalamic artery.

FIGURE 7-44 Line diagram illustrating the relationship of the posterior cerebral and superior cerebellar arteries to a line drawn between the tuberculum sellae and the lambda as well as between the tuberculum sellae and the internal occipital protuberance.

(T) tuberculum sellae, (L) lambda, (Iop) internal occipital protuberance, (A) line TB, drawn 60° from line T−IOP, crosses at A, the medial branch of the posterior choroidal artery in this projection; (B) crossing of the lateral branch of the posterior choroidal artery. (Modified from Pachtman, H., Hilal, F. K., and Wood, E. H.: Radiology, *112*:343–352, 1974.)

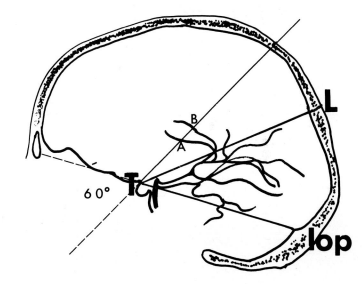

$$\frac{TA}{T\text{-}Iop} \times 100 = 46.1\% \pm 0.56$$

$$\frac{TB}{T\text{-}Iop} \times 100 = 53.4\% \pm 0.58$$

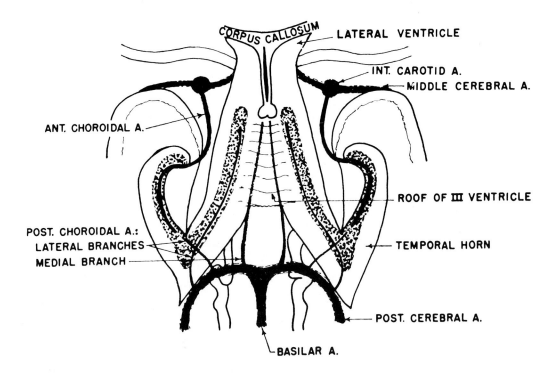

FIGURE 7–45 Diagram of the blood supply of the choroid plexus of the lateral ventricle. The ventricles are exposed from above. (From Lemay, M. J., and Jackson, D. M.: Am. J. Roentgenol., *92*:776–785, 1964.)

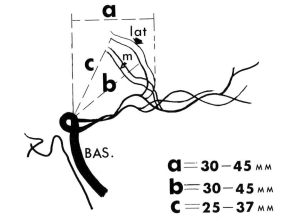

$$a = 30-45 \text{ MM}$$
$$b = 30-45 \text{ MM}$$
$$c = 25-37 \text{ MM}$$

FIGURE 7–46 *A.* Method of measurement of the medial and lateral branches of the posterior choroidal arteries. Three distances are measured from the bifurcation between the basilar artery and the posterior cerebral artery to the lateral posterior choroid artery forming the largest curve.

(a) the distance to the tangent to the posterior part of the posterior choroid artery as measured along a line parallel to the longitudinal direction of the posterior cerebral artery, (b) the greatest distance to the posterior choroid artery (lateral branch), (c) the distance to the anterior upper part of the posterior choroid artery (lateral branch). (lat) lateral branch, (m) medial branch, (BAS) basilar artery. (After Lofgren, F. O.: Acta Radiol., *50*:108–124, 1958.)

B. Diagrams of anterior (ac), lateral (lat), and medial (m) choroidal arteries. The posterior communicating artery (pc) is also shown for orientation. (Modified from Galloway, J. R., and Greitz, T.: Acta Radiol., *53*:353–366, 1960.)

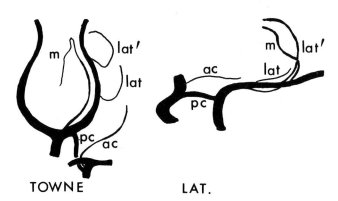

TOWNE   LAT.

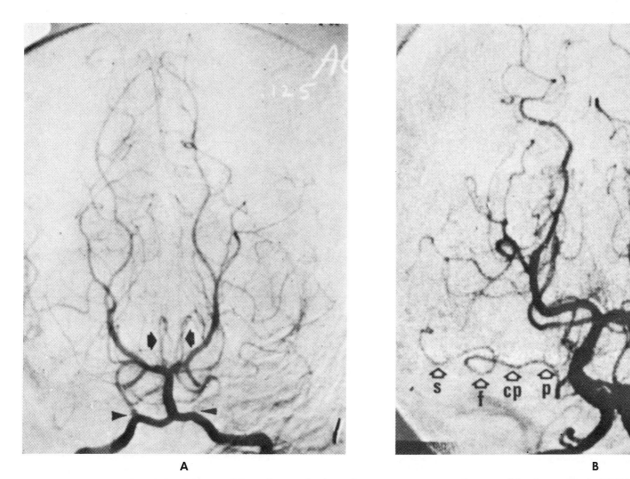

A   **B**

FIGURE 7–47 *A*. Normal vertebral angiogram, anteroposterior arterial phase. Both PICA's are opacified (lower arrows). The posterior medullary segments (upper arrows) delineate the lateral walls of the vallecula. *B*. Normal vertebral angiogram, anteroposterior arterial phase. The posterior cerebral, superior cerebellar and right anterior inferior cerebellar (arrows) arteries are well demonstrated. (p) Pontine segment, (cp) cerebellopontine angle segment, (f) floccular segment, (s) semilunar segment. Subtraction films. (From George, A. E.: Radiol. Clin. North Am., *12*:371–399, August, 1974.)

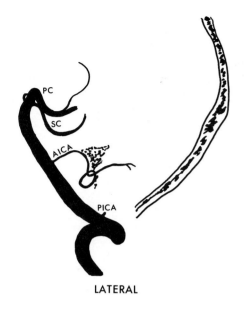

LATERAL

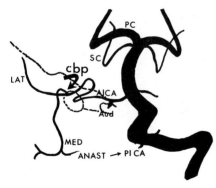

TOWNE'S

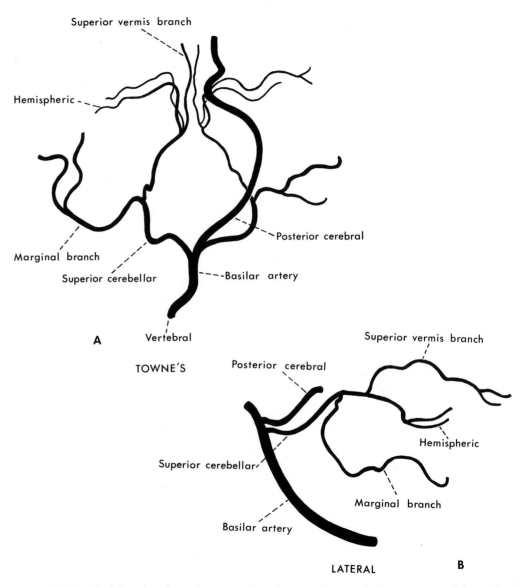

FIGURE 7–48 Anterior inferior cerebellar artery (AICA). The lateral and Towne's projections are shown diagrammatically. (PC) posterior cerebral artery, (SC) superior cerebellar artery. (Aud) auditory branch, (cbp) cerebellopontine angle. The artery varies and anastomoses with the other two cerebellar arteries.

FIGURE 7–49 Line drawings demonstrating the superior cerebellar artery and its major branches. (Modified from Mani, R. L., Newton, T. H., and Glickman, M. G.: Radiology, *91*:1102–1108, 1968.)

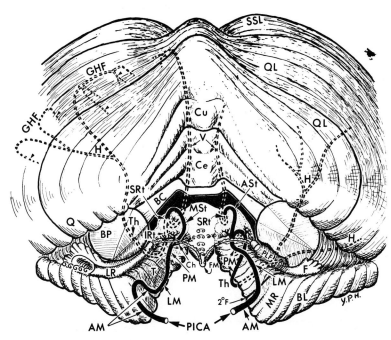

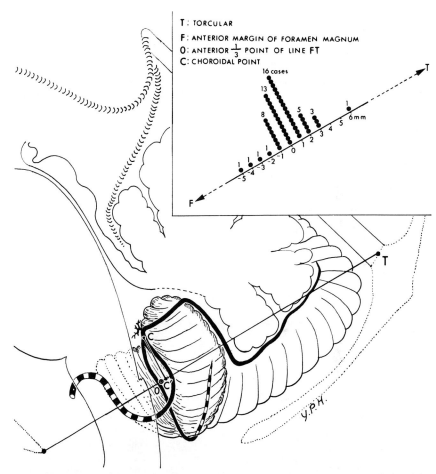

FIGURE 7–50 Diagrams showing the anatomic relationships of the posterior inferior cerebellar artery (PICA).

Covered portions of the arteries are shown in dashed fashion. The portions covered by the posterior medullary velum are, however, shown with solid lines. Labeled structures are the anterior medullary segment (AM), apical supratonsillar segment (ASt), brachium conjunctivum (BC), biventral lobule (BL), brachium pontis (BP), central lobule (Ce), choroidal branches (Ch), culmen (cu), declive (Dc), flocculus (F), fastigium (Fa), foramen of Luschka (FL), foramen of Magendie (FM), great horizontal fissure (GHF), hemispheric segment (H), inferior colliculus (I), inferior retrotonsillar segment (IRt), lateral medullary segment (LM), lateral recess (LR), medullary ridge (MR) of the biventral lobule, medial supratonsillar segment (MSt), pyramid (P), posterior inferior cerebellar artery (PICA), posterolateral fissure (PLF), posterior medullary segment (PM), quadrangular lip (Q), quadrangular lobule (QL), superior colliculus (S), suprapyramidal branch (Sp), superior retrotonsillar segment (SRt), superior semilunar lobule (SSL), cerebellar tonsil (T), tonsillohemispheric branch (Th), tuber (Tu), and vermian segment (V). The location of the copula pyramidis is indicated by an asterisk (*). The secondary fissure (2°F), third and fourth ventricles ($_3$V, $_4$V) are also labeled. (From Huang, Y. P., and Wolf, B. S.: Am. J. Roentgenol., *107*:543–564, 1969.)

FIGURE 7–51 Normal measurements of the "choroidal point" (C) of the posterior inferior cerebellar artery in relation to other anatomic landmarks. The choroidal point is chosen as the point at which the posterior medullary segment joins the supratonsillar segment. Geometrically, the slope of the curve begins to decrease at this point or there may be an acute angulation. FT is a line drawn from the anterior margin of the foramen magnum to the torcula.

C′ = the foot of a perpendicular dropped from C to FT. The insert shows the relation of C′ to the anterior one-third point (0) of FT in 50 presumably normal adult cases. In 90 per cent of cases, C′ was located from 1 mm. anterior to 3 mm. posterior to the anterior one-third point. (From Huang, Y. P., and Wolf, B. S.: Am. J. Roentgenol., *107*:543–564, 1969.)

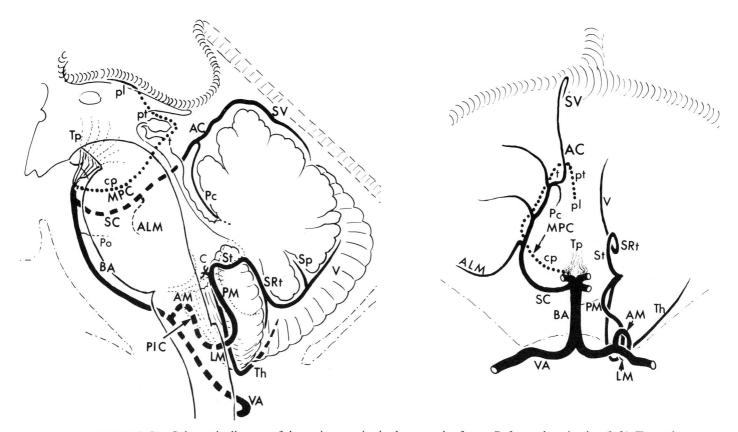

FIGURE 7–52 Schematic diagram of the major arteries in the posterior fossa. *D.* Lateral projection (left). Towne's projection (right). (AC) Anterior culminate segment. (ALM) anterior lateral marginal branch, (AM) anterior medullary segment, (BA) basilar artery, (C) choroidal arteries, (cp) circumpeduncular segment, (LM) lateral medullary segment, (MPC) medial posterior choroidal artery, (No) nodular branch, (Pc) precentral cerebellar artery, (PIC) posterior inferior cerebellar artery, (pl) plexal segment, (PM) posterior medullary segment, (Po) pontine artery, (pt) pretectal segment, (SC) superior cerebellar artery, (Sp) suprapyramidal branch of the posterior inferior cerebellar artery. (SRt) superior retro-tonsillar segment of the posterior inferior cerebellar artery, (St) supratonsillar segment of the posterior inferior cerebellar artery, (SV) vermian segment, (Th) tonsillohemispheric branch, (Tp) thalamoperforate arteries, (V) vermian segment, (VA) vertebral artery, (t) tectal segment. (From Huang, Y. P., and Wolf, B. S.: Neuroradiology, *1*:4, 1970.)

FIGURE 7–53 *A.* Diagrammatic representation of the deep cerebral veins.

The two thalamostriate veins are seen to join the septal vein to form the internal cerebral vein on each side. The internal cerebral veins are contained within the velum interpositum and join posteriorly to form the vein of Galen. The choroid plexus was removed on the right side to show the choroid vein. The thalamostriate vein is drawn to the temporal horn. This is seen sometimes but is by no means a constant feature. Variation in the configuration of the veins is, of course, the rule.

(1) Septal vein, (2) anterior horn at the junction with the body of the lateral ventricle. (3) thalamostriate vein, (4) internal cerebral veins, (5) the two leaves of the velum interpositum, (6) vein of Galen, (7) occipital horn, (8) tentorium, (9) quadrigeminal tubercles, (10) choroid plexus, (11) initial segment of the thalamostriate vein or terminal vein, (12) choroidal vein, (13) temporal horn, (14) frontal horn of the lateral ventricle. See also Part B.

Medial to the thalamostriate vein is the thalamus and anterolaterally is the caudate nucleus.

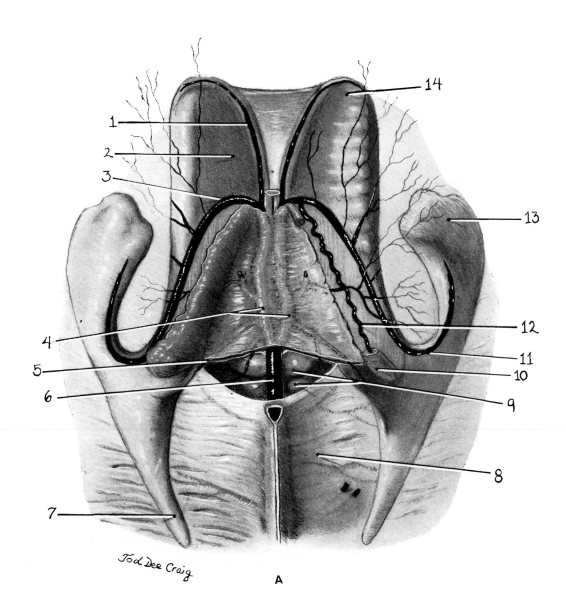

Tod Dee Craig

A

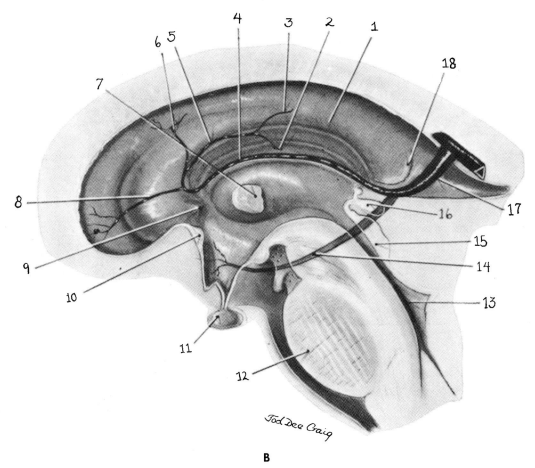

B

FIGURE 7–53 *Continued.* *B.* Diagrammatic representation of the deep cerebral veins and their relation to the adjacent brain structures in lateral projection.

(1) Lateral ventricle, (2) terminal branch of thalamostriate vein, (3) posterior caudate veins, (4) internal cerebral vein, (5) thalamostriate vein, (6) anterior caudate vein, (7) mass intermedia, (8) septal vein, (9) foramen of Monro, (10) anterior commissure, (11) hypophysis, (12) pons, (13) fourth ventricle, (14) basilar vein passing schematically behind the midbrain, (15) quadrigeminal plate, (16) pineal, (17) vein of Galen, (18) splenium of corpus callosum. (*A* and *B* from Taveras, J. M., and Wood, E. H.: Diagnostic Neuroradiology. Baltimore, The Williams & Wilkins Co., 1964.)

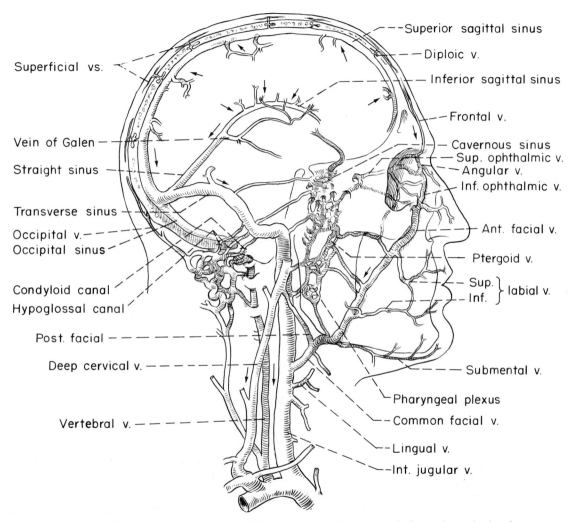

FIGURE 7-54 Diagram showing the flow pattern of the venous drainage from the head.

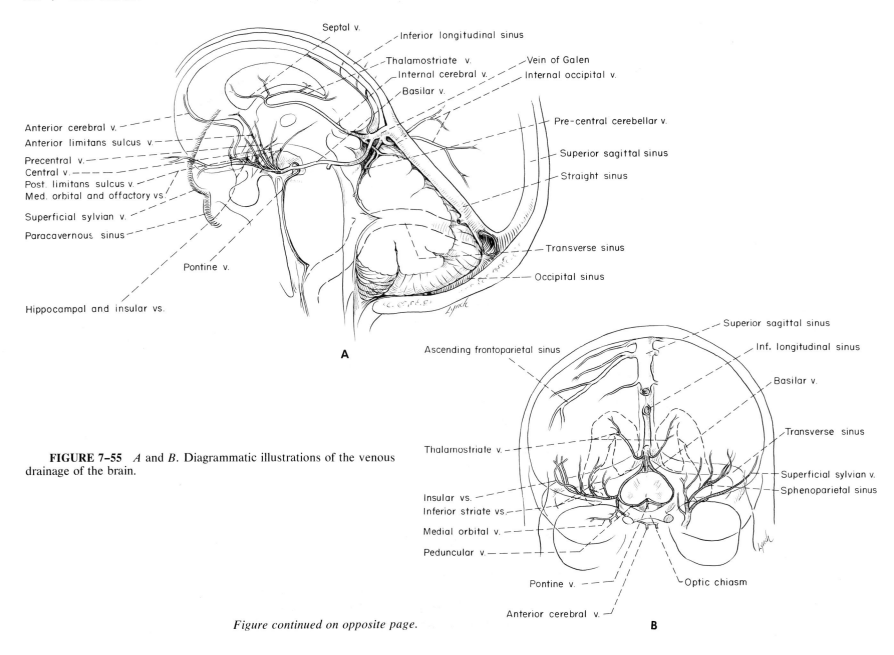

Septal v.

Inferior longitudinal sinus

Thalamostriate v.

Internal cerebral v.

Vein of Galen

Internal occipital v.

Basilar v.

Anterior cerebral v.

Anterior limitans sulcus v.

Precentral v.

Central v.

Post. limitans sulcus v.

Med. orbital and offactory vs.

Superficial sylvian v.

Paracavernous sinus

Pontine v.

Hippocampal and insular vs.

Pre-central cerebellar v.

Superior sagittal sinus

Straight sinus

Transverse sinus

Occipital sinus

A

Superior sagittal sinus

Inf. longitudinal sinus

Ascending frontoparietal sinus

Basilar v.

Transverse sinus

Thalamostriate v.

Superficial sylvian v.

Sphenoparietal sinus

Insular vs.

Inferior striate vs.

Medial orbital v.

Peduncular v.

Pontine v.

Optic chiasm

Anterior cerebral v.

B

FIGURE 7–55 *A* and *B*. Diagrammatic illustrations of the venous drainage of the brain.

Figure continued on opposite page.

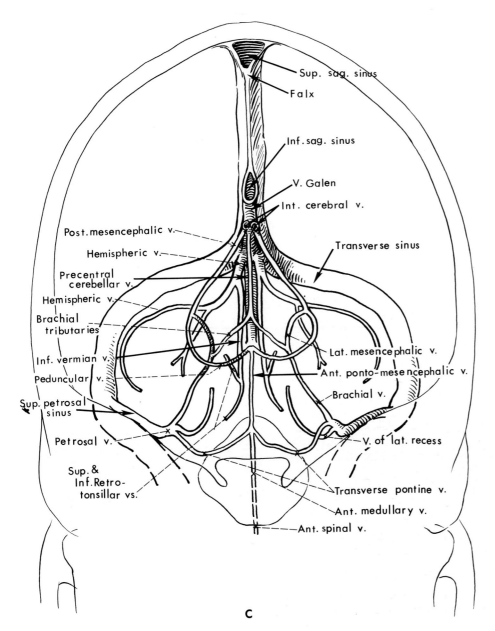

C

FIGURE 7–55 *Continued.* *C.* Diagrammatic illustration of the venous drainage of the brain. Posterior fossa in Towne's projection (Modified from Wolf, B. S., and Huang, Y. P.: Am. J. Roentgenol., *90:* 472–489, 1963.)

Figure continued on following page.

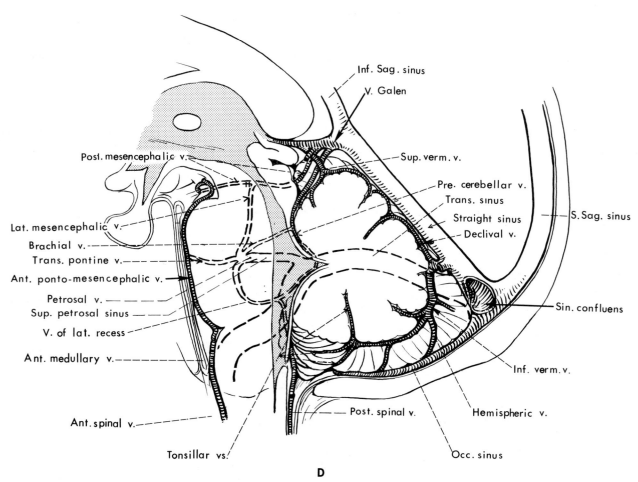

Inf. Sag. sinus

V. Galen

Post. mesencephalic v.

Sup. verm. v.

Pre. cerebellar v.

Trans. sinus

Straight sinus

S. Sag. sinus

Lat. mesencephalic v.

Brachial v.

Trans. pontine v.

Declival v.

Ant. ponto-mesencephalic v.

Petrosal v.

Sup. petrosal sinus

V. of lat. recess

Sin. confluens

Ant. medullary v.

Inf. verm. v.

Ant. spinal v.

Post. spinal v.

Hemispheric v.

Tonsillar vs.

Occ. sinus

D

FIGURE 7–55 *Continued.* *D.* Diagram of the venous drainage of the posterior fossa in lateral projection.

FIGURE 7–56 Schematic. Lateral venous phase, normal vertebral angiogram. *1.* (APM) Anterior pontomesencephalic vein, (AM) anterior medullary vein, (AS) anterior spinal vein, (PMV) posterior mesencephalic vein, (LM) lateral mesencephalic vein, (PC) precentral cerebellar vein, (SV) superior vermian vein, (IV) inferior vermian vein.

2. The petrosal vein (P) and its tributaries have been added to the basic venous diagram. (VLR) Vein of the lateral recess, (IH) inferior hemispheric vein, (SH) superior hemispheric vein. A brachial tributary of the petrosal vein joins the brachial tributary of the precentral cerebellar vein (arrows).

3. The relationship of the precentral cerebellar vein to Twining's line. (T) Tuberculum, (To) torcula, (X) point of perpendicular intersection. (TX) = XTo ± 5 per cent.

4. The relationship of the copular point (CP) to the F-T line. (F) Anterior lip of the foramen magnum, (T) torcula, (X) point of perpendicular intersection, (M) midpoint of the F-T line. (MX) = approximately 4 mm. (*E1–4* from George, A. E.: Radiol. Clin. North Am., *12:*371–399, 1974.)

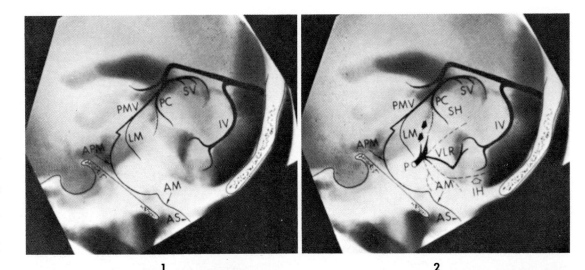

1

2

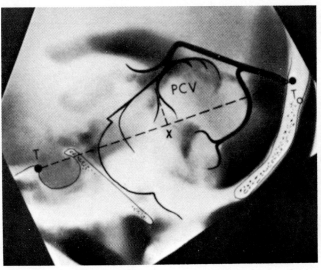

3

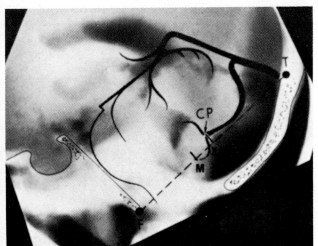

4

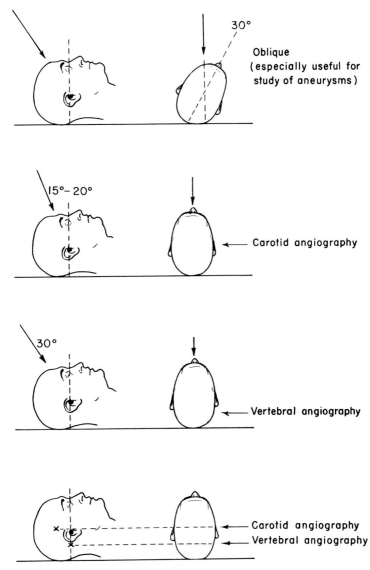

30°

Oblique
(especially useful for
study of aneurysms)

15°–20°

Carotid angiography

30°

Vertebral angiography

Carotid angiography
Vertebral angiography

FIGURE 7–57 Positioning for carotid and vertebral angiography. The axial view may also be used on occasion to demonstrate the basilar artery and its branches.

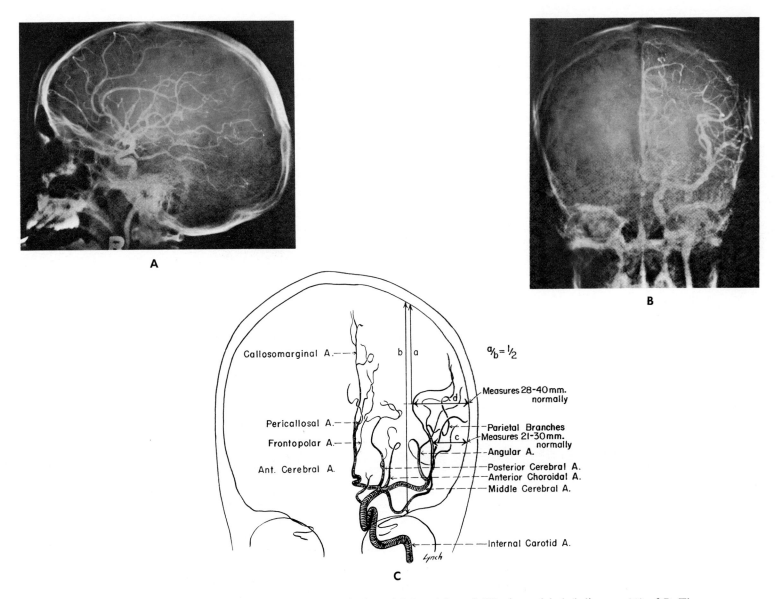

FIGURE 7–58 Internal carotid arteriograms in lateral (*A*) and frontal (*B*) views; labeled diagram (*C*) of B. The labeled diagram shows the various relationships, especially of the parts of the middle cerebral artery in frontal views.

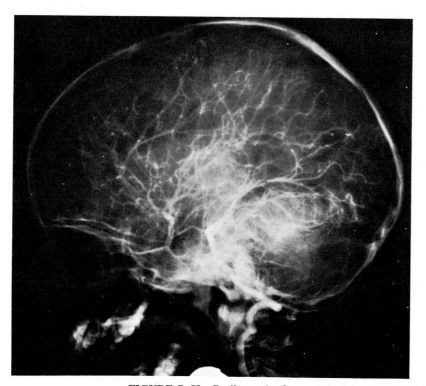 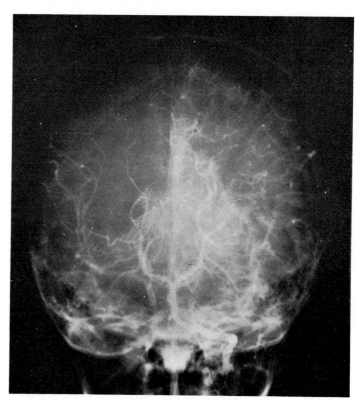

FIGURE 7–59   Radiographs for vertebral-basilar arterial studies. *A*, Lateral projection. *B*. Towne's anteroposterior projection.

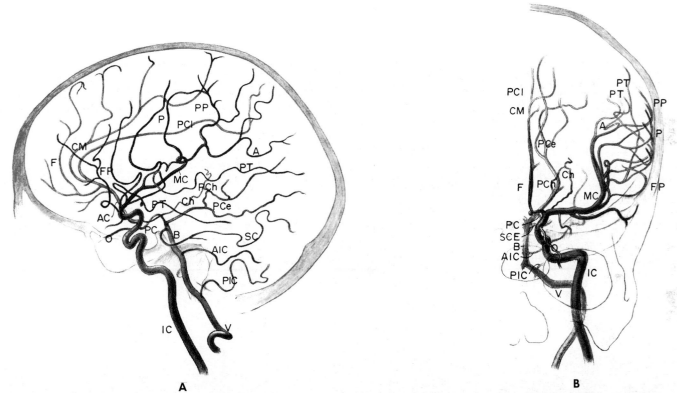

A

B

FIGURE 7–60 Internal carotid and basilar arteriograms. *A*. Diagram of lateral view. *B*. Diagram of anteroposterior view. (A) angular, (AC) anterior cerebral, (AIC) anterior inferior cerebellar, (B) basilar, (Ch) choroidal, (CM) calloso-marginal, (F) frontopolar, (FP) frontoparietal, (IC) internal carotid, (MC) middle cerebral, (O) ophthalmic, (P) parietal, (PC) posterior communicating, (PCe) posterior cerebral, (PCh) posterior choroidal, (PCl) pericollosal, (PIC) posterior inferior cerebellar, (PP) posterior parietal, (PT) posterior temporal, (SC) superior cerebellar, (SCE) superior cerebellar, (V) vertebral.

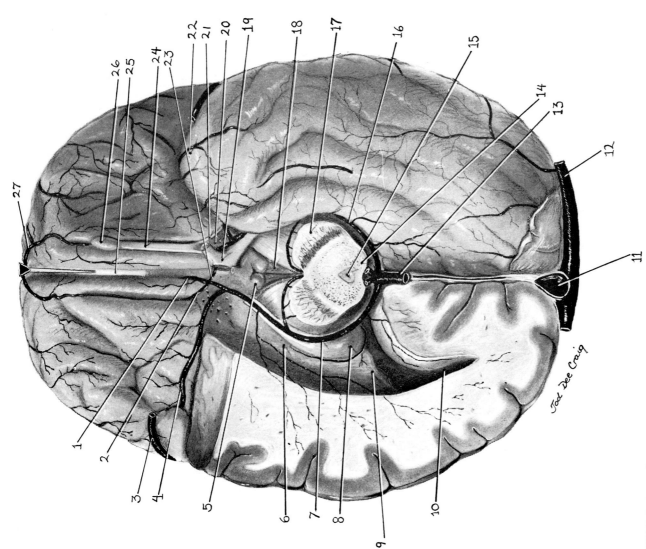

FIGURE 7–61 Diagram depicting the basal vein, its origins and relations with the midbrain. The tip of the temporal lobe on the right side has been removed and a horizontal cross section of the temporal and occipital lobes has been done to open the temporal horn, occipital horn, and atrium of the ventricle. (1) Anterior cerebral vein, (2) olfactory vein, (3) superficial middle cerebral vein, (4) deep middle cerebral vein, (5) mammillary body, (6) temporal horn of the lateral ventricle, (7) basilar vein, (8) hippocampus major, (9) collateral eminence, (10) posterior horn of the lateral ventricle, (11) superior sagittal sinus joining (12) transverse sinus, (13) vein of Galen, (14) quadrigeminal plate, (15) aqueduct of Sylvius, (16) basilar vein, (17) cerebral peduncle, (18) posterior perforated substance, (19) optic chiasm, (20) anterior perforated substance, (21) lateral olfactory striae, (22) anterior tip of the temporal lobe, (23) anterior communicating vein, (24) olfactory tract, (25) longitudinal (interhemispheric) fissure, (26) olfactory bulb, (27) superficial cerebral veins. (From Taveras, J. M. and Wood, E. H.: Diagnostic Neuroradiology. Baltimore, The Williams & Wilkins Co., 1964.)

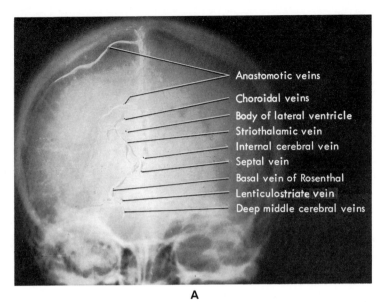

Anastomotic veins
Choroidal veins
Body of lateral ventricle
Striothalamic vein
Internal cerebral vein
Septal vein
Basal vein of Rosenthal
Lenticulostriate vein
Deep middle cerebral veins

A

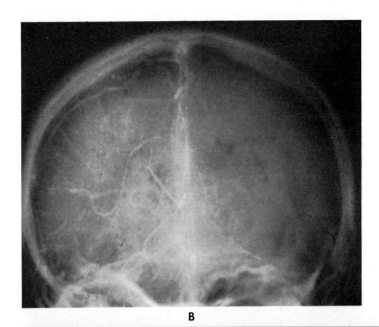

B

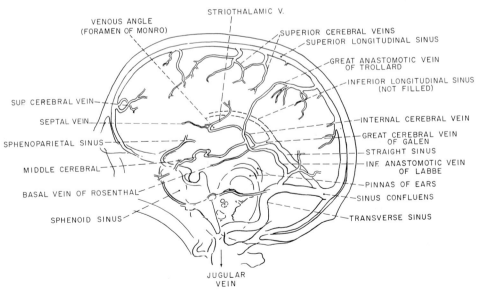

VENOUS ANGLE
(FORAMEN OF MONRO)

STRIOTHALAMIC V.

SUPERIOR CEREBRAL VEINS
SUPERIOR LONGITUDINAL SINUS

GREAT ANASTOMOTIC VEIN
OF TROLLARD

INFERIOR LONGITUDINAL SINUS
(NOT FILLED)

SUP. CEREBRAL VEIN
SEPTAL VEIN
SPHENOPARIETAL SINUS
MIDDLE CEREBRAL
BASAL VEIN OF ROSENTHAL
SPHENOID SINUS

INTERNAL CEREBRAL VEIN
GREAT CEREBRAL VEIN
OF GALEN
STRAIGHT SINUS
INF. ANASTOMOTIC VEIN
OF LABBE
PINNAS OF EARS
SINUS CONFLUENS
TRANSVERSE SINUS

JUGULAR
VEIN

C

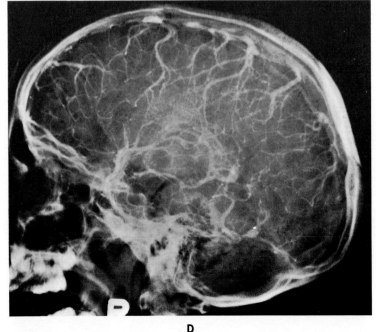

D

FIGURE 7-62 Internal carotid venograms in anteroposterior (*A* and *B*) and lateral (*D*) projections. *A*. Labeled radiograph of anteroposterior venogram. *C*. Labeled diagram of lateral view.

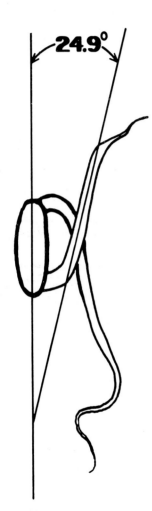

24.9°

TABLE 7–1. Normal Angles Between the Internal Cerebral
Vein and Striothalamic Vein*

	Half-Axial	Anteroposterior
Mean	24.9 degrees	18.2 degrees
Range	17.3–32.0 degrees	13.5–2.0 degrees
Standard deviation	4.06 degrees	2.45 degrees

Note: The angle varies significantly with projection.
   *From Richardson, H. D., and Bednarz, W. W.: The depiction of ventricular size by the striothalamic vein in the anteroposterior phlebogram. Radiology, *81*:604–609, 1963.

   (For other techniques of measurement of the venous angle, and distortions of the septal veins with projection, see Meschan, I.: An Atlas of Anatomy Basic to Radiology. Philadelphia, W. B. Saunders Co., 1975.)

FIGURE 7–63 Diagram showing the method of measurement of the angle between the striothalamic and internal cerebral vein. A vertical line is drawn through the internal cerebral vein perpendicular to the base of the skull. Another line is drawn along the relatively straight laterally inclined segment of the striothalamic vein to intersect the vertical line. The intervening angle is measured.
   Normal angles are shown in the table (the angle varies significantly with the projection). (From Richardson, H. D., and Bednarz, W. W.: Radiology, *81*:604–609, 1963.)

ANGIOGRAPHIC DIAGNOSIS OF POSTERIOR FOSSA MASS LESIONS (FIG. 7–56)*†

The precentral cerebellar vein and the pontomesencephalic vein, as well as the choroidal branch of the posterior inferior cerebellar artery, are extremely important indicators.

Having established from the lateral view the posterior fossa compartment in which a mass is present, one then turns to the anteroposterior view to determine, if possible, the side on which the mass is located. *The most important indicator for this purpose is the vermis branch of each posterior inferior cerebellar artery (PICA). This vessel is normally at or within about 2 millimeters of the midline and normally courses ipsilaterally,* never contralaterally, to the side of its origin. Lateral or cerebellar hemisphere mass lesions displace it contralaterally. If a lesion, however, is situated in the inferior portion of the cerebellar hemisphere, it may not affect the vermian branches of PICA but only the distal PICA in the region of the choroidal loop, just proximal to the origin of the vermian artery. Therefore, one must carefully evaluate the entire course of the PICA to ascertain this factor. It must be added that if a lesion is bilateral it may not have an effect on the vermian

artery, and other indicators such as herniation of important arterial or venous components toward the spinal canal are important. Actually, if the angiogram indicates hydrocephalus from a posterior fossa mass lesion and the PICA loops and vermis artery branches are well seen in normal positions, a midline mass may be suspected; such a mass may give direct evidence of its presence by spreading the choroidal loop of the PICA.

The anterior inferior cerebellar artery (AICA) passes, as has been previously shown, through the ipsilateral cerebellopontine angle cistern, looping near the porus of the internal auditory canal and then coursing around the anterior surface of the cerebellum. Its displacement in the region of the internal acoustic canal is of great importance in indicating a local mass.

If the posterior cerebral and superior cerebral arteries are widely separated and have lost their normal undulations as they course around the brain stem, enlargement of the brain stem is suggested.

The superior vermian veins, unfortunately, are apparently not displaced significantly from their essentially midline position even with large masses in the posterior fossa.

The petrosal vein, which is between the cerebellum and the superior petrosal sinus, may perhaps be useful in a negative fashion. If it is not seen in the presence of good filling of the ipsilateral PICA, a mass in the angle cistern is suggested. The reverse should also be true. The clinical usefulness, however, of this latter sign is not fully established.

---

*Davis, D. O., and Roberson, G. H.: Angiographic diagnosis of posterior fossa mass lesions. Semin. Roentgenol., 6:89–102, 1971.

†George, A. E.: A systematic approach to the interpretation of posterior fossa angiography. Radiol. Clin. North Am., *12*:371–400, 1974.

GENERAL COMMENTS REGARDING CEREBRAL ARTERIOGRAPHY AND VENOGRAPHY

Wolf and Huang have addressed themselves generally to the diagnostic value of cerebral veins in mass lesions of the brain. From their extensive experience they have drawn the following conclusions:

1. Displacements of superficial cortical veins are of some significance in relation to such processes as subdural hematomas or epidural mass lesions. However, premature visualization of a cortical vein may be the most important evidence of a vascular intracerebral mass lesion. In contrast to the superficial veins the subependymal veins within the walls of a lateral ventricle often show marked displacement and deformity and are therefore of great value in diagnosis.

2. The usefulness of the deep veins is of course particularly evident in cases of displacement and deformity of the internal cerebral vein. The internal cerebral vein adjoins the midline in the roof of the third ventricle and its displacement is an indicator of a mass lesion.

3. Displacement of the striothalamic veins toward the periphery of the skull is also significant because it points toward a dilated lateral ventricular system that may be indicative of either unilateral or bilateral obstructive hydrocephalus.

4. Displacement of the basal vein of Rosenthal inferiorly is a common feature of downward tentorial herniation. Apparently such herniation underneath the falx can sometimes be recognized even in the absence of contralateral displacement of the anterior cerebral artery.

5. Abnormalities of the frontal lobe may be recognized by posterior displacement of the inferior striate and uncal veins.

6. As pointed out by Davis and Roberson, the precentral cerebellar vein is of special significance since it is located in the cleft between the upper portion of the cerebellum and the brain stem.

7. Displacements of the petrosal vein or the great anterior cerebellar vein have been demonstrated with masses in the cerebellopontine angles — specifically, acoustic neuromas.

One can hardly leave this subject of cerebral angiography without emphasizing its importance in the evaluation of patients with cerebrovascular disease generally.* Abnormalities of blood vessels are outside the scope of this text, but arteriosclerotic cerebrovascular disease is indeed one of the leading causes of death in the United States and is probably more frequently the underlying cause of neurologic deficit than all other disease processes combined. It is therefore important to identify not only the position of the vessels but also their size, degree of filling, contour alterations, and abnormalities of the intima. The blood supply of the brain by way of both carotid arteries and the vertebral arteries forms a communicating network of potential collateral channels in the neck, the face, the scalp, the base of the brain, and over the cerebral surface, as we have already emphasized.

---

*Chase, N. E., and Kricheff, I. I.: Cerebral angiography in the evaluation of patients with cerebrovascular disease. Radiol. Clin. North Am., *4*:131–144, 1966.

COMPUTED TOMOGRAPHY OF THE BRAIN AND ORBIT

In 1972, Godfrey Hounsfield, electronic engineer and physicist, and Dr. James Ambrose, neuroradiologist (both of England), reported the first computed transverse axial x-ray scanning technique of the head. In essence, the machine they developed consisted of an x-ray device that produces a slitlike beam or thin sheet of x-rays, which passes through the head. The x-ray tube produces this beam at 1-degree intervals, eventually moving through 180 degrees. By careful collimation, this "sheet of x-rays" can delimit a slice of tissue from 0.4 to 1.3 cm. in width. At each degree pause, the "remnant radiation" emitted is detected by phosphorescent crystals, and the number of photons so recorded is transmitted to a computer. The volume of tissue traversed in the 180-degree arc is theoretically divided into thousands of small units (*volume elements,* or *"voxels"*). The absorption of x-ray photons in each of these voxels is related to the average tissue structure, or its average absorption coefficient. Tissues are now classified in relation to this absorption in so-called Hounsfield units, in an effort to relate the absorption coefficients of the voxels to water. The ultimate reconstruction of the image is made from the total photons absorbed by each voxel in the computer to a gray scale read-out device (*direct display console,* or *DDC*), by an appropriate algorithm and use of the computer language. Tissues with only minimally differing absorption coefficients may thereby be differentiated.

Water absorption is used as the basis for comparison with all other absorption values (Fig. 7–64). Photographs of a computed tomographic unit are shown in Figure 7–65 *A* and *B*. A diagrammatic representation of the scanning process is shown in Figure 7–66.

The scanning process may be started from any angle, moving 1 degree at a time, but it is usually begun with the x-ray tube in its lowermost position, with the patient "brow-up." The patient must be motionless, with anesthesia required where the patient cannot cooperate to this extent.

With more recent models of CT units, fan beams from one or more x-ray tubes are recorded on 600 or more stationary gaseous or crystalline detectors, thereby speeding up the scan time to one or two seconds.

If "contrast enhancement" is required to demonstrate blood vessels and selective absorption across the "blood-brain barrier," 150 to 300 ml. of 25 per cent meglumine diatrizoate is injected by drip or rapidly, and the entire scanning sequence is repeated.

There should be full cognizance that some patients may have undesirable reactions to the contrast agent and may require immediate treatment, as described in the section on the urinary tract (the agents used are identical).

A "window width" on the control panel adjusts the range of absorption coefficients and, in turn, varies the range of contrast in the image. The "window level" control sets the center of the window width to any desired point on the scale of x-ray absorption coefficients.

In the usual settings, cerebrospinal fluid appears black; bone appears white; and the brain appears various shades of gray. With appropriate use of the controls, it is possible to measure the absorption coefficient of any given portion of the image to assist in interpretation.

For greater detail, the student is referred to the text on this subject by New and Scott[*] and to information provided by the manufacturer of the unit being utilized.

The brief "atlas of anatomy" included in this chapter and ensuing chapters, where this method has application, is for introductory purposes only. See Chapter 16 for a list of references on CT scanning and for more complete discussion.

---

[*]New, P. F. J., and Scott, W. R.: Computerized Tomography of the Brain and Orbit (EMI Scanning). Baltimore, Williams & Wilkins Co., 1975.

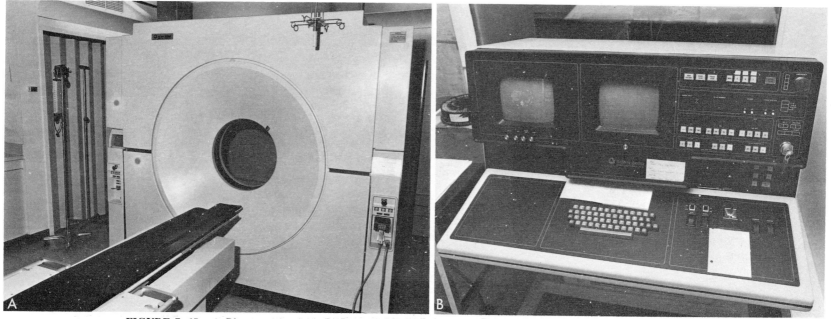

HOUNSFIELD UNITS

-1000 -100 -75 -50 -25 0 25 50 75 100 1000

WATER
BONE
SPLEEN
PANCREAS
GRAY MATTER
WHITE MATTER
BLOOD
LIVER
KIDNEY
FAT
AIR
IODINE 2.4 mg/ml, 3 SD value*
CaCl2 40 mg/ml, 3 SD value*
NORMAL SALINE, 2 SD value*

*Zatz 1977

FIGURE 7-64 Classification of tissue density in computed tomography. By algorithmic conversion of the absorption of photons in volume elements (voxels), the computer can reconstruct images that display differences of density far smaller than those shown by conventional radiography, but there is some sacrifice in resolution, or definition, of the "picture" obtained, depending upon the size of the voxel. (*Modified from Zatz, L. M.: "The EMI scanner: Collimator design, polychromatic artifacts, and selective material imaging." In Ter-Pogossian, M. (ed.) Workshop on Reconstruction Tomography in Diagnostic Radiology and Nuclear Medicine (Proceedings). Baltimore, University Park Press, 1977.)

FIGURE 7-65 *A.* Photograph of gantry into which the patient's body part is placed. The patient lies on the cot. *B.* Photograph of console of tomographic unit, showing display tubes and selector buttons.

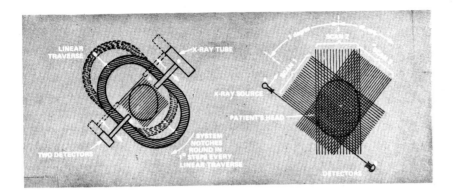

FIGURE 7–66 Diagrammatic representation of scanning sequence, which comprises a series of 180 parallel traverses of the accurately aligned x-ray beam and two photon detectors, with 1 degree rotation of the gantry after each linear sweep. Each block of tissue in each of the two simultaneously scanned sections (slices) will have been scanned 180 times at the completion of a scan sequence, and the photon transmission measurements obtained are averaged for each small tissue block. The readings are digitized and fed to the computer, which solves 28,800 simultaneous equations for each slice to derive absorption (attenuation) values in each block. (From New, P. F. J., and Scott, W. R.: Computerized Tomography of the Brain and Orbit (EMI Scanning). Baltimore, Md., The Williams & Wilkins Co., 1975.)

FIGURE 7–67 Orientation for usual tomographic slices obtained and those illustrated in this chapter (25–30 degrees to RBL).

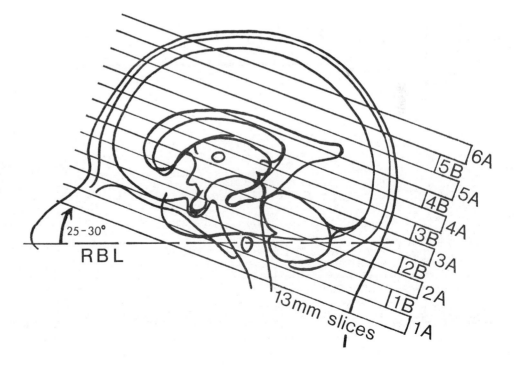

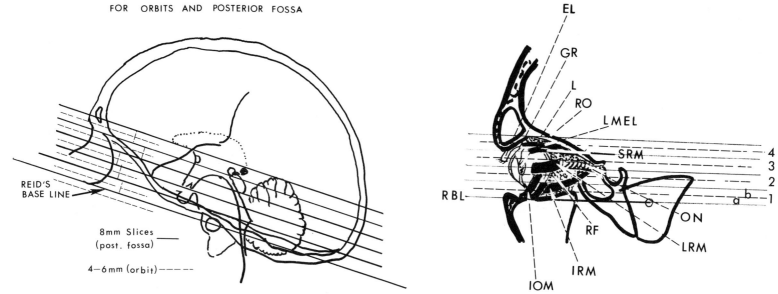

FOR ORBITS AND POSTERIOR FOSSA

REID'S BASE LINE

8mm Slices (post. fossa)

4—6mm (orbit)

EL
GR
L
RO
LMEL
SRM
RBL
RF
ON
LRM
IRM
IOM

4
3
2
a b 1

FIGURE 7-68 *A.* Orientation for orbital and posterior fossa tomographic slices. Occasionally posterior fossa slices are taken at narrower intervals as well, but since a lesser number of photons is collected in each of the "voxels," the images so obtained are coarser. The window width and level usually require different settings for the orbit, as compared with posterior fossa brain settings (see manufacturer's manual for details).

B. Close-up diagram of the orbit and its contents, showing the anatomic structures in their usual relationship to the "tomographic cuts" obtained. (EL) eyelid, (GR) global rim, (L) lens of eye, (RO) roof of orbit, (LMEL) levator muscle of upper eyelid, (SRM) superior rectus muscle, (ON) optic nerve, (LRM) lateral rectus muscle, (RF) retrobulbar fat, (IRM) inferior rectus muscle, (IOM) inferior oblique muscle, (RBL) infraorbital meatal line (Reid's base line).

1, 2, 3, 4 represent the cuts shown; and "a" and "b" are subdivisions within these cuts. A total of eight cuts, approximately 5 mm. apart, is obtained usually.

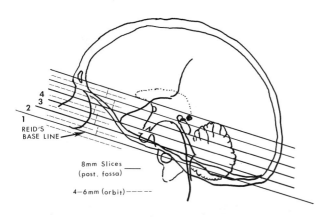

FOR ORBITS AND POSTERIOR FOSSA

4
3
2
1

REID'S
BASE LINE

8mm Slices
(post. fossa)

4–6mm (orbit) ––––––

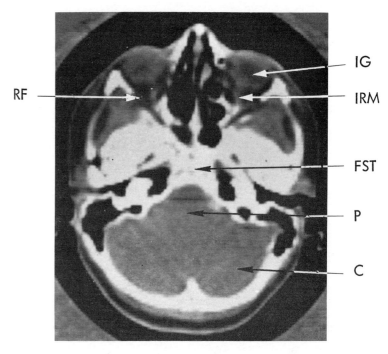

RF

IG

IRM

FST

P

C

RF = RETRO-ORBITAL FAT
IG = INF. GLOBE
IRM = INF. RECTUS MUSCLE
FST = FLOOR, SELLA TURCICA
P = PONS
C = CEREBELLUM

FIGURE 7–70 Orbital section 21B (EMI settings: 5/200).

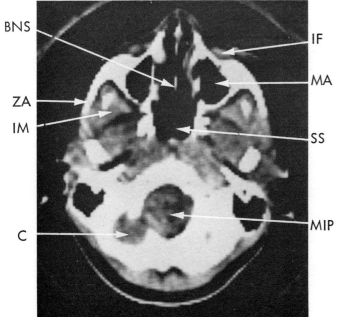

BNS

IF

ZA

MA

IM

SS

C

MIP

FIGURE 7–69 Orbital section 21A (EMI settings: 18/75).

BNS = BONE NASAL SEPTUM
ZA = ZYGOMATIC ARCH
IM = INFRATEMPORAL MUSCLES
C = CEREBELLUM
IF = INFRAORBITAL FAT
MA = MAXILLARY ANTRUM
SS = SPHENOID SINUS
MIP = MEDULLA AND/OR INFERIOR PONS

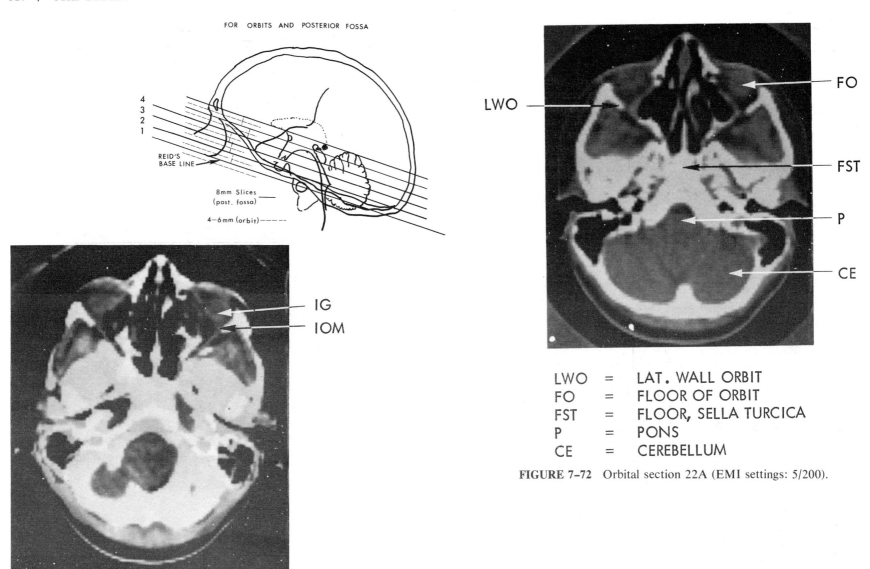

FOR ORBITS AND POSTERIOR FOSSA

REID'S
BASE LINE

8mm Slices
(post. fossa)

4—6mm (orbit)

LWO

FO

FST

P

CE

LWO	=	LAT. WALL ORBIT
FO	=	FLOOR OF ORBIT
FST	=	FLOOR, SELLA TURCICA
P	=	PONS
CE	=	CEREBELLUM

FIGURE 7–72 Orbital section 22A (EMI settings: 5/200).

IG
IOM

| IG | = | INF. GLOBE |
| IOM | = | INF. OBLIQUE MUSCLE |

FIGURE 7–71 Repeat orbital section 21B on another patient for special visualization of inferior oblique muscle (EMI settings: 5/200). (Second cut.)

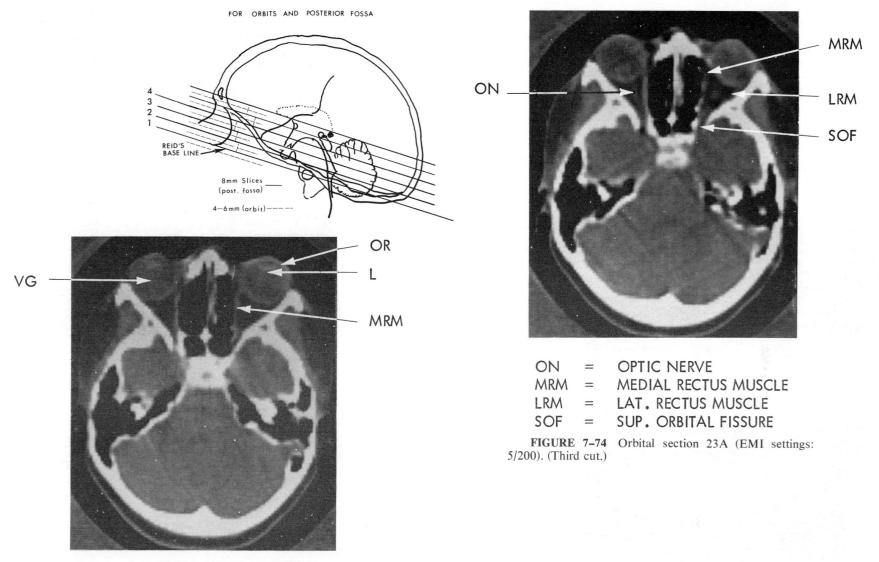

FOR ORBITS AND POSTERIOR FOSSA

4
3
2
1

REID'S
BASE LINE

8mm Slices
(post. fossa)

4–6mm (orbit)

ON = OPTIC NERVE
MRM = MEDIAL RECTUS MUSCLE
LRM = LAT. RECTUS MUSCLE
SOF = SUP. ORBITAL FISSURE

FIGURE 7–74 Orbital section 23A (EMI settings: 5/200). (Third cut.)

VG = VITREOUS OF GLOBE
OR = OCULAR RIM
L = LENS
MRM = MEDIAL RECTUS MUSCLE

FIGURE 7–73 Orbital section 22B (EMI settings: 5/200).

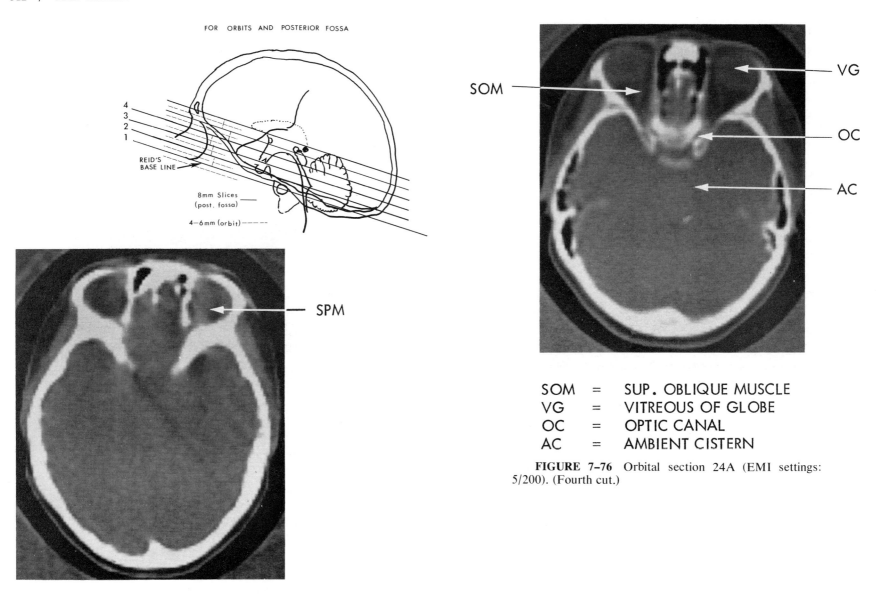

FOR ORBITS AND POSTERIOR FOSSA

REID'S BASE LINE

8mm Slices (post. fossa)

4—6mm (orbit)

SOM

VG

OC

AC

SPM

SOM = SUP. OBLIQUE MUSCLE
VG = VITREOUS OF GLOBE
OC = OPTIC CANAL
AC = AMBIENT CISTERN

FIGURE 7–76 Orbital section 24A (EMI settings: 5/200). (Fourth cut.)

SPM = SUPERIOR PALPEBRAL MUSCLE

FIGURE 7-75 Orbital section 23B (EMI settings: 5/200).

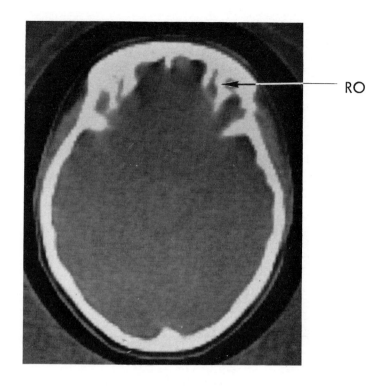

RO = ROOF OF ORBIT

FIGURE 7–77   Orbital section 24B (EMI settings: 5/200).

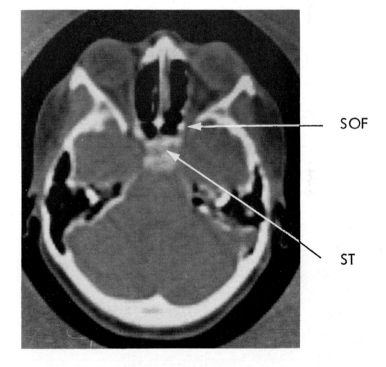

SOF = SUP. ORBITAL FISSURE
ST = SELLA TURCICA

FIGURE 7–78   Orbital section 23A for superior orbital fissure (EMI settings: 0/400).

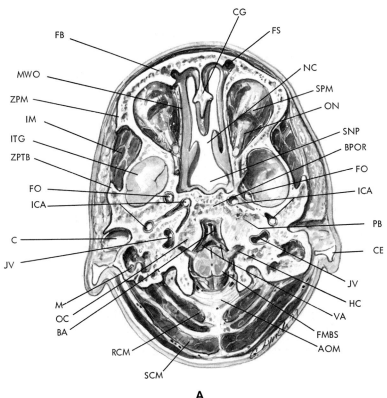

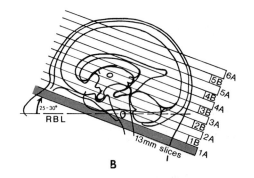

B

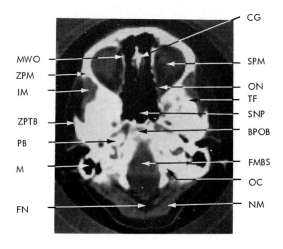

A

FIGURE 7–79 *A*. Anatomic sketch equivalent to section 1A of brain scan. *B*. Miniature of Figure 7–67 for orientation. *C*. Labeled scan at this level. (FB) frontal bone, (MWO) medial wall of orbit, (ZPM) zygomatic process of maxilla, (IM) infratemporal muscles (mastication), (ITG) inferior temporal gyrus, (ZPTB) zygomatic process of temporal bone, (FO) foramen ovale, (ICA) internal carotid artery, (C) condyloid process, (JV) jugular vein, (M) mastoid, (OC) occipital condyle, (BA) basilar artery, (RCM) rectus capitis muscle, (SCM) semispinalis capitis muscle, (AOM) atlanto-occipital membrane, (FMBS) foramen magnus with brain stem, (VA) vertebral arteries, (HC) hypoglossal canal, (JV) jugular vein, (CE) cerebellum, (PB) petrous bone, (ICA) internal carotid artery, (FO) foramen ovale, (BPOR) basilar part of occipital bone, (SNP) superior nasopharynx, (ON) optic nerve, (SPM) superior palpebral muscle, (NC) nasal cavity, (FS) frontal sinus, (CG) crista galli.

MWO	=	MEDIAL WALL, ORBIT	FB	=	FRONTAL BONE
ZPM	=	ZYGOMATIC PROCESS MAXILLA	ITG	=	INF. TEMPORAL GYRUS
IM	=	INFRATEMPORAL MUSCLES (MASTICATION)	C	=	CONDYLOID PROCESS
ZPTB	=	ZYGOMATIC PROCESS, TEMPORAL BONE	BA	=	BASILAR ARTERY
PB	=	PETROUS BONE	RCM	=	RECTUS CAPITIS MUSCLE
M	=	MASTOID	SCM	=	SEMISPINALIS CAPITIS MUSCLE
FN	=	FASCIA OF NECK	FS	=	FRONTAL SINUS
SPM	=	SUP. PALPEBRAL MUSCLE	NC	=	NASAL CAVITY
ON	=	OPTIC NERVE	FO	=	FORAMEN OVALE
SNP	=	SUPERIOR NASOPHARYNX	ICA	=	INT. CAROTID ARTERY
BPOB	=	BASILAR PART. OCCIPITAL BONE	CE	=	CARTILAGE OF EAR
FMBS	=	FORAMEN MAGNUM WITH BRAIN STEM	JV	=	JUGULAR VEIN
OC	=	OCCIPITAL CONDYLE	HC	=	HYPOGLOSSAL CANAL
NM	=	NECK MUSCLES	VA	=	VERTEBRAL ARTERIES
CG	=	**CRISTA GALLI**	AOM	=	ATLANTO-OCCIPITAL MEMBRANE

C

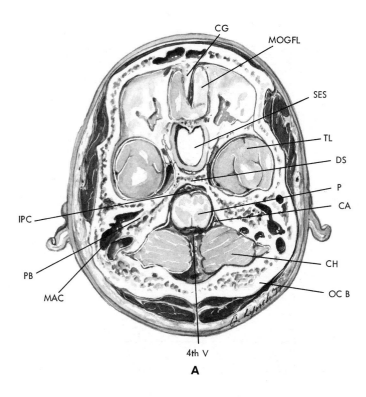

A

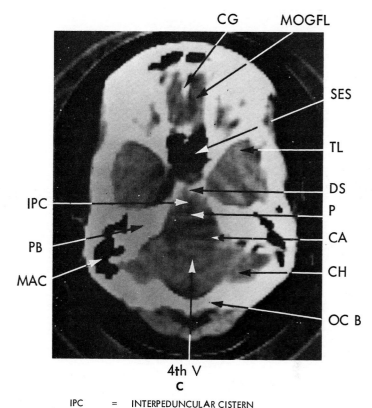

C

IPC	=	INTERPEDUNCULAR CISTERN
PB	=	PETROUS BONE
MAC	=	MASTOID AIR CELLS
CG	=	CRISTA GALLI
MOGFL	=	MED. ORBITAL GYRUS-FRONTAL LOBE
SES	=	SPHENOID AND ETHMOID SINUSES
TL	=	TEMPORAL LOBE
DS	=	DORSUM SELLAE
P	=	PONS
CA	=	CISTERNA AMBIENS
CH	=	CEREBELLAR HEMISPHERE
OC B	=	OCCIPITAL BONE
4th V	=	4th VENTRICLE

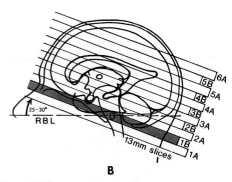

B

FIGURE 7–80   *A*, Diagram of brain section and skull at 1B level. *B*, Miniature of Figure 7–67 for orientation. *C*, Labeled computed tomograph at this level.

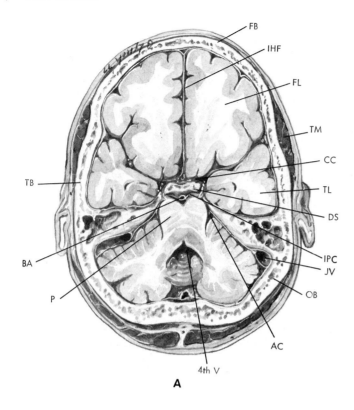

A

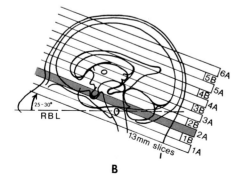

B

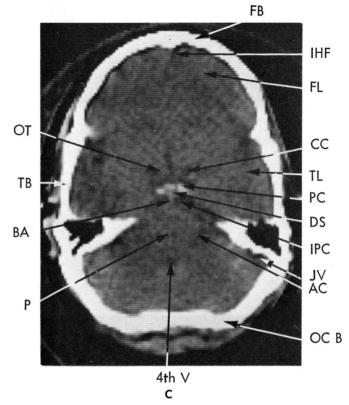

C

OT	=	OPTIC TRACT
TB	=	TEMPORAL BONE
BA	=	BASILAR ARTERY
P	=	PONS
FB	=	FRONTAL BONE
IHF	=	INTERHEMISPHERIC FISSURE
FL	=	FRONTAL LOBE
CC	=	CHIASMATIC CISTERN
TL	=	TEMPORAL LOBE
PC	=	POSTERIOR CLINOIDS
DS	=	DORSUM SELLAE
IPC	=	INTERPEDUNCULAR CISTERN
JV	=	JUGULAR VEIN
AC	=	AMBIENT CISTERN
OC B	=	OCCIPITAL BONE
4th V	=	4th VENTRICLE

FIGURE 7–81 *A.* Diagram of the brain at the 2A level. *B.* Miniature of Figure 7–67 for orientation. *C.* Tomographic scan at the 2A level.

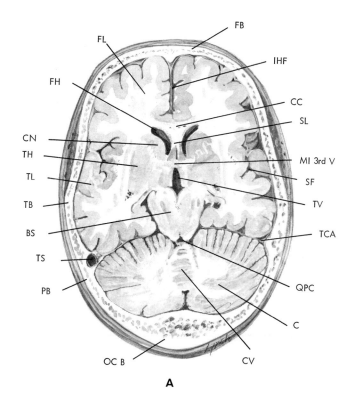

A

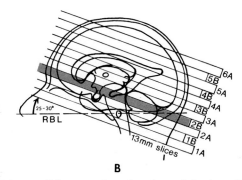

B

FIGURE 7–82 *A.* Diagram of section through brain at 2B level. *B.* Miniature of Figure 7–67 for orientation. *C.* Tomographic scan at the 2B level.

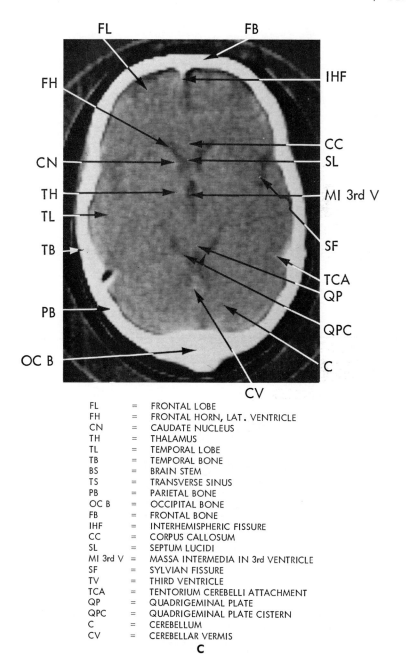

FL	=	FRONTAL LOBE
FH	=	FRONTAL HORN, LAT. VENTRICLE
CN	=	CAUDATE NUCLEUS
TH	=	THALAMUS
TL	=	TEMPORAL LOBE
TB	=	TEMPORAL BONE
BS	=	BRAIN STEM
TS	=	TRANSVERSE SINUS
PB	=	PARIETAL BONE
OC B	=	OCCIPITAL BONE
FB	=	FRONTAL BONE
IHF	=	INTERHEMISPHERIC FISSURE
CC	=	CORPUS CALLOSUM
SL	=	SEPTUM LUCIDI
MI 3rd V	=	MASSA INTERMEDIA IN 3rd VENTRICLE
SF	=	SYLVIAN FISSURE
TV	=	THIRD VENTRICLE
TCA	=	TENTORIUM CEREBELLI ATTACHMENT
QP	=	QUADRIGEMINAL PLATE
QPC	=	QUADRIGEMINAL PLATE CISTERN
C	=	CEREBELLUM
CV	=	CEREBELLAR VERMIS

C

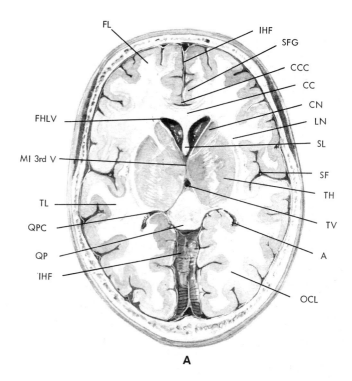

A

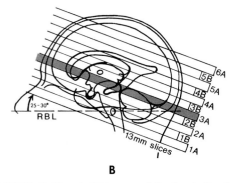

B

FIGURE 7–83 *A*. Diagram of brain at the 3A level. *B*. Miniature of Figure 7–67 for orientation. *C*. Tomographic cut at the 3A level.

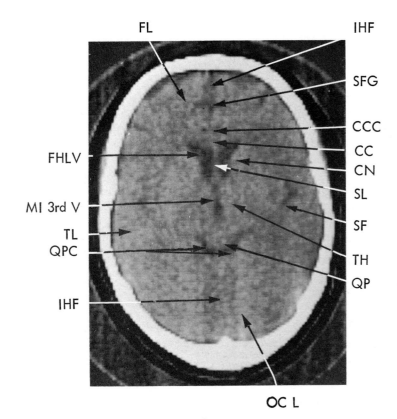

C

FL	=	FRONTAL LOBE
FHLV	=	FRONTAL HORN, LAT. VENTRICLE
MI 3rd V	=	MASSA INTERMEDIA IN 3rd VENTRICLE
TL	=	TEMPORAL LOBE
QPC	=	QUADRIGEMINAL PLATE CISTERN
IHF	=	INTERHEMISPHERIC FISSURE
IHF	=	INTERHEMISPHERIC FISSURE
SFG	=	SUPERIOR FRONTAL GYRUS
CCC	=	CISTERNA CORPUS CALLOSI
CC	=	CORPUS CALLOSUM
CN	=	CAUDATE NUCLEUS
SL	=	SEPTUM LUCIDI
SF	=	SYLVIAN FISSURE
TH	=	THALAMUS
QP	=	QUADRIGEMINAL PLATE
OC L	=	OCCIPITAL LOBE
LN	=	LENTICULAR NUCLEUS
TV	=	THIRD VENTRICLE
A	=	ATRIUM

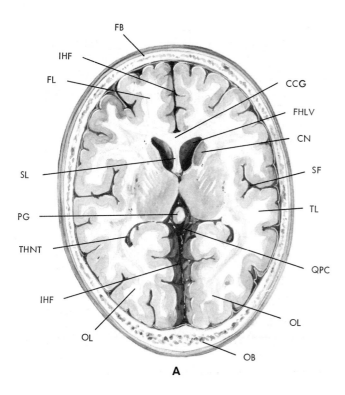

A

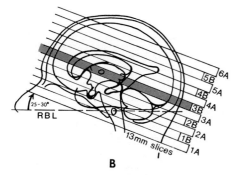

B

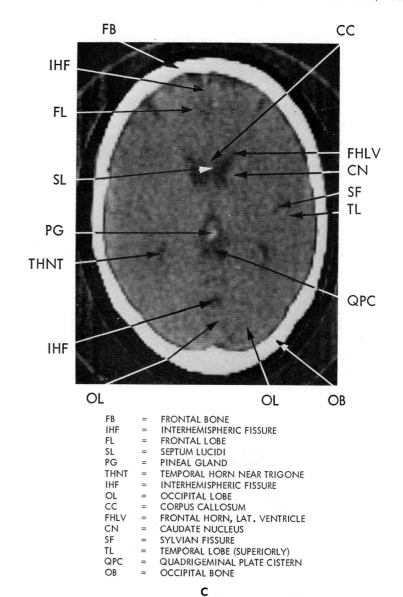

C

FB	=	FRONTAL BONE
IHF	=	INTERHEMISPHERIC FISSURE
FL	=	FRONTAL LOBE
SL	=	SEPTUM LUCIDI
PG	=	PINEAL GLAND
THNT	=	TEMPORAL HORN NEAR TRIGONE
IHF	=	INTERHEMISPHERIC FISSURE
OL	=	OCCIPITAL LOBE
CC	=	CORPUS CALLOSUM
FHLV	=	FRONTAL HORN, LAT. VENTRICLE
CN	=	CAUDATE NUCLEUS
SF	=	SYLVIAN FISSURE
TL	=	TEMPORAL LOBE (SUPERIORLY)
QPC	=	QUADRIGEMINAL PLATE CISTERN
OB	=	OCCIPITAL BONE

FIGURE 7–84 *A*. Diagram of brain at the 3B level. *B*. Miniature of Figure 7–67 for orientation. *C*. Tomographic cut at the 3B level.

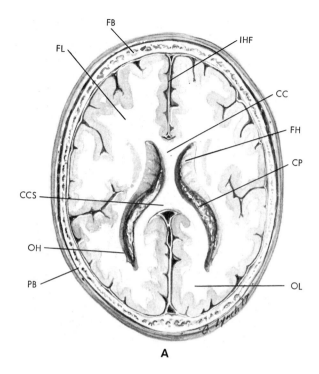

A

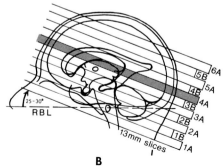

B

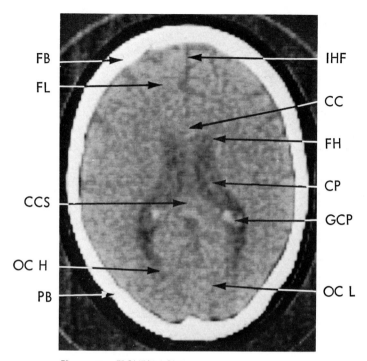

FB = FRONTAL BONE
FL = FRONTAL LOBE
CCS = CORPUS CALLOSUM SPLENIUM
OC H = OCCIPITAL HORN, LAT. VENT.
PB = PARIETAL BONE
IHF = INTERHEMISPHERIC FISSURE
CC = CORPUS CALLOSUM
FH = FRONTAL HORN, LAT. VENT.
CP = CHOROID PLEXUS, LAT. VENT.
GCP = GLOMUS (WITH CALCIUM),
        CHOROID PLEXUS IN TRIGONE, LAT. VENT.
OC L = OCCIPITAL LOBE

C

FIGURE 7–85 *A*. Diagram of brain through at 4A level. *B*. Miniature of Figure 7–67 for orientation. *C*. Tomographic slice at 4A level.

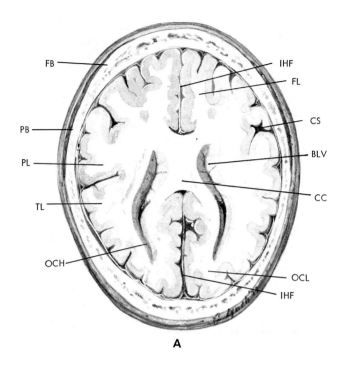

A

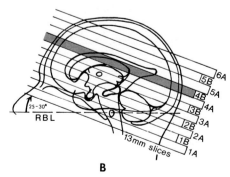

B

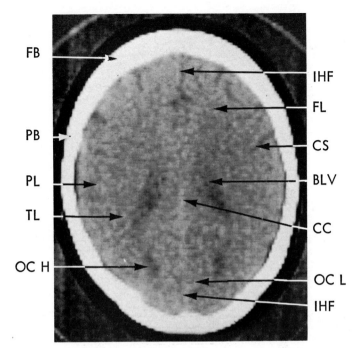

FB	=	FRONTAL BONE
PB	=	PARIETAL BONE
PL	=	PARIETAL LOBE
TL	=	TEMPORAL LOBE
OC H	=	OCCIPITAL HORN, LAT. VENT.
IHF	=	INTERHEMISPHERIC FISSURE
FL	=	FRONTAL LOBE
CS	=	CENTRAL SULCUS
BLV	=	BODY, LAT. VENTRICLE
CC	=	CORPUS CALLOSUM
OC L	=	OCCIPITAL LOBE
IHF	=	INTERHEMISPHERIC FISSURE

C

FIGURE 7–86 *A*. Diagram of brain at the 4 B level. *B*. Miniature of Figure 7–67 for orientation. *C*. Tomographic slice at level 4 B.

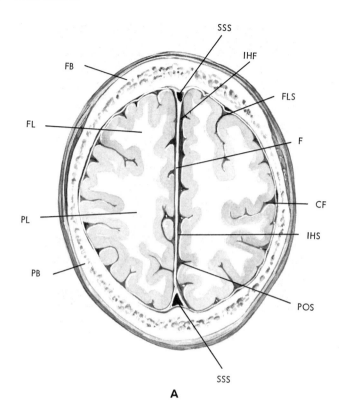

A

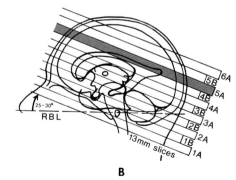

B

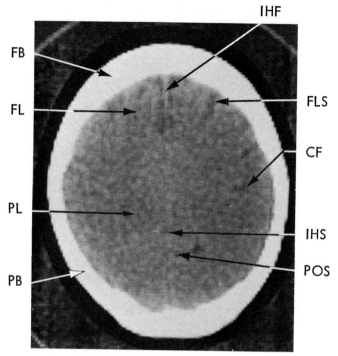

FB	=	FRONTAL BONE
FL	=	FRONTAL LOBE
PL	=	PARIETAL LOBE
PB	=	PARIETAL BONE
IHF	=	INTERHEMISPHERIC FISSURE
FLS	=	FRONTAL LOBE SULCUS
CF	=	CENTRAL FISSURE
IHS	=	INTERHEMISPHERIC SULCUS
POS	=	PARIETO-OCCIPITAL SULCUS
SSS	=	SUPERIOR SAGITTAL SINUS
F	=	FALX
SSS	=	SUPERIOR SAGITTAL SINUS

C

FIGURE 7–87 *A*. Diagram of brain at the 5 A level.
B. Miniature of Figure 7–67 for orientation. *C*. Tomographic slice at the 5 A level.

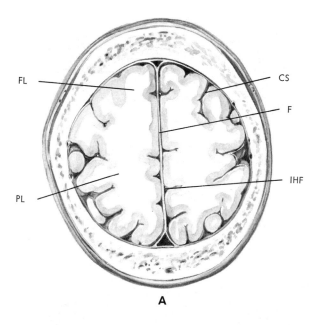

A

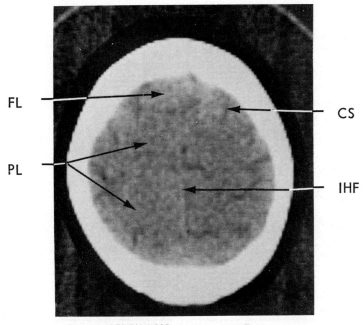

FL = FRONTAL LOBE
PL = PARIETAL LOBE
CS = CENTRAL SULCUS
IHF = INTERHEMISPHERIC (LONGITUDINAL) FISSURE
F = FALX

C

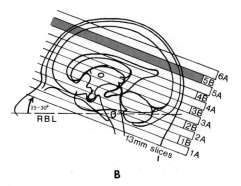

B

FIGURE 7-88 *A*. Diagram of brain at the 5B level. *B*. Miniature of Figure 7-67 for orientation. *C*. Tomographic slice at the 5B level.

ACA   MCA

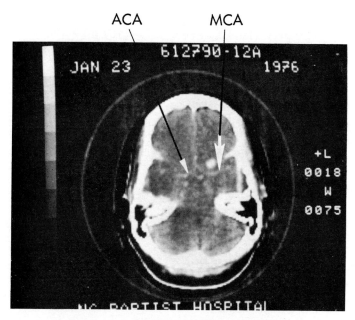

ACA - ANT. CEREBRAL ART.
MCA - MIDDLE CEREBRAL ART.

FIGURE 7–89 Computed tomograph at the 2A level immediately following the infusion of 300 ml. of 25 per cent Reno-M-30-DIP (diatrizoate meglumine) for contrast enhancement of the blood vessels and other structures in the brain. Note the demonstration of the internal carotid artery in cross section as it divides into the anterior cerebral and middle cerebral arteries. The middle cerebral artery in its first portions is clearly shown.

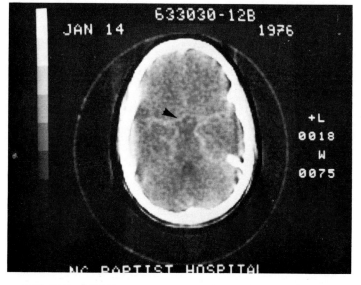

⟶ CIRCLE OF WILLIS WITH CONTRAST AGENT

FIGURE 7–90 Computed tomograph at the 2B level with contrast infusion (enhancement) demonstrating the circle of Willis.

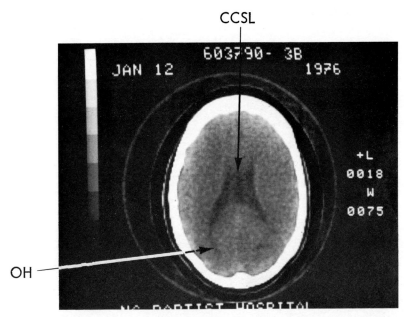

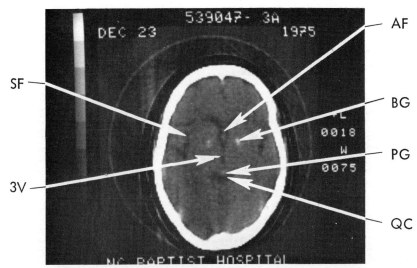

CCSL — CISTERNA CAVUM SEPTUM LUCIDI
OH — OCCIPITAL HORN, LAT. VENTRICLE

FIGURE 7-92 Computed tomograph at the 3B level, 25 to 30 degrees to Reid's base line, showing clearly the cisterna cavum septi pellucidi as well as the occipital horns of the lateral ventricle.

SF — SYLVIAN FISSURE
3V — THIRD VENTRICLE
AF — ANTERIOR FORNIX
BG — CALCIFIED BASAL GANGLIA
PG — PINEAL GLAND
QC — QUADRIGEMINAL CISTERN

FIGURE 7-91 Computed tomograph at the 3A level, showing more clearly some of the structures that have been previously depicted. There is calcium deposit in the basal ganglia, structures much more frequently calcified by computed tomography than on conventional radiography.

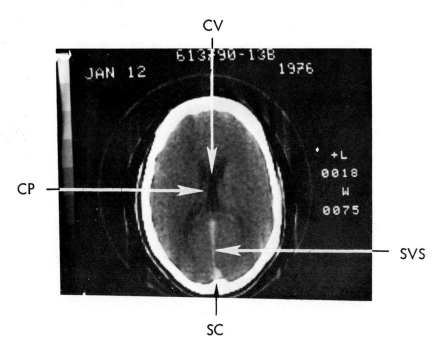

CV — CAVUM VERGI
CP — CHOROID PLEXUS, LAT. VENTRICLE
SC — SINUS CONFLUENS
SVS — STRAIGHT VENOUS SINUS

FIGURE 7–93 Computed tomograph at the 3B level following contrast enhancement with infusion of contrast agent and showing such structures as the cavum vergi, the choroid plexuses of the lateral ventricles, the straight venous sinus, and the sinus confluens.

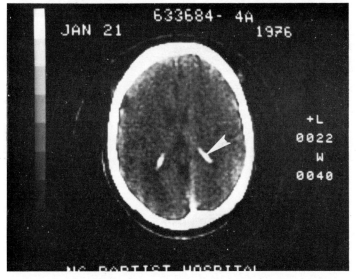

BILAT. CALCIFIED GLOMERA OF CHOROID PLEXUSES

FIGURE 7–94 Computed tomograph at the 4A level, 25 to 30 degrees to Reid's base line. This shows bilateral calcified glomera of the choroid plexuses (arrow).

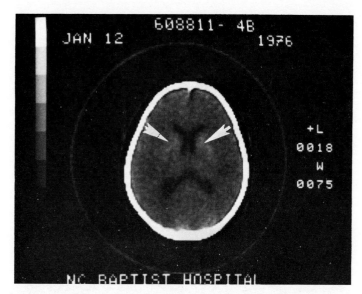

→ FAINTLY CALCIFIED BASAL GANGLIA

FIGURE 7–95 Computed tomograph at the 4B level showing faintly calcified basal ganglia. The anterior and posterior limbs of the internal capsules separate the head of the caudate nucleus, partially calcified, from the putamen, also partially calcified. Even the thalamus can be separated.

8

THE VERTEBRAL COLUMN
AND SPINAL CORD

THE VERTEBRAL COLUMN

The vertebral column is composed of separate articulating segments called vertebrae. These are 33 in number and distributed as follows: 7 cervical, 12 thoracic, 5 lumbar, 5 sacral, and 4 coccygeal (Fig. 8–1).

Occasionally there is an extra vertebra in either the thoracic or lumbar spine, or there may be one less vertebra than normal, particularly in the lumbar spine. In the latter case, there may be an extra vertebra fused with the sacrum or coccyx, either completely or partially.

A vertebra consists of the following parts: (1) the body, (2) the transverse process on each side, (3) the pedicles, (4) the laminae, (5) the superior articular processes, (6) the inferior articular processes, (7) the spinous processes, and (8) the partes interarticulares situated between the two articular processes.

In the cervical spine, the transverse and costal processes fuse to form the "lateral mass," with the foramen transversaria between. In the thoracic spine, the costal process remains separate and participates in the formation of the head and neck of the rib with which it articulates. In the lumbar and sacral spine, the costal and transverse processes are completely fused.

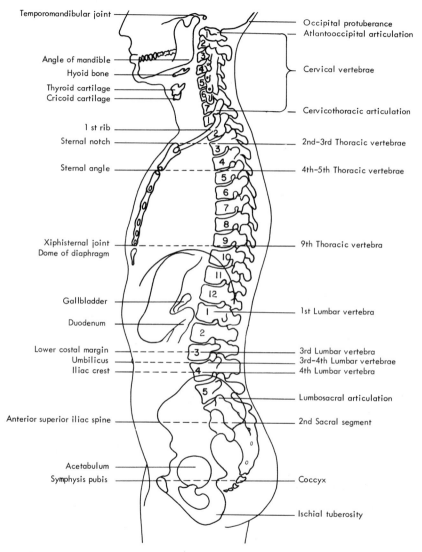

FIGURE 8–1 Lateral view of the spinal column in relation to some anterior structures. (Modified from Clark, K. C.: Positioning in Radiography. London, Ilford Ltd. William Heineman Medical Books, 1964.)

The following joints are identified in the spinal column: (1) amphiarthrodial joints between the vertebral bodies (intervertebral disk); (2) synovial joints (diarthrodial joints) between the articular processes on each side of adjoining vertebrae (also called apophyseal joints); (3) costovertebral joints which represent synovial joints at the junction of ribs and vertebrae; and (4) synovial joints between the posterolateral margins of the lower five cervical vertebral bodies (joints of Luschka) (Fig. 8-2A and B).

The intervertebral disk which lies between each two vertebral bodies (from C2 to S1) is composed of fibrocartilage, with a gelatinous central matrix known as the nucleus pulposus. It is firmly attached to adjoining vertebral bodies.

The thoracic spine has several distinguishing characteristics. The vertebral bodies of the upper eight segments articulate with two ribs on each side, and the lower four articulate only with the one rib with which they are numerically associated. There are also small costal facets on each transverse process of the upper 10 thoracic vertebrae. The two different joints formed are called the costovertebral and costotransverse joints, respectively, with separate synovial cavities and joint capsules in each instance.

The paraspinal line (paravertebral soft tissue shadows, Fig. 8-20), well delineated in frontal radiographs of the thoracic spine, must be differentiated from manifestations of disease. A left paraspinal shadow, delimited by the left pleural reflection, is commonly visualized on films of the thoracic spine. It roughly parallels the left margin of the vertebral column and the aorta, and lies between these two structures.

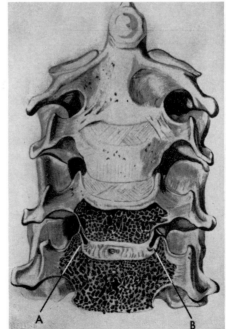
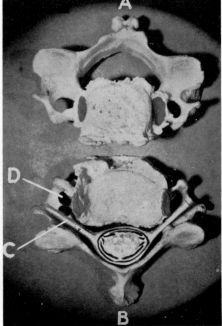

FIGURE 8-2 *A*. Reproduction from Luschka's "Monograph," showing the joints (A and B) between the posterolateral aspects of the sectioned lower cervical vertebral bodies. *B*. Photograph of the fifth (A) and sixth (B) cervical vertebrae showing Luschka joints in relationship to the mixed nerve roots and vertebral foramina. The joints are painted for contrast; the female segment is seen on A and the male part on B. It is apparent that Luschka joints are situated ventromedial to the nerves (C) which emerge through the intervertebral foramina and also medial to the vertebral vessels and sympathetics which pass through the vertebral foramina (D). (From Boreadis, A. G., and Gershon-Cohen, J.: Radiology, *66*, 1956.)

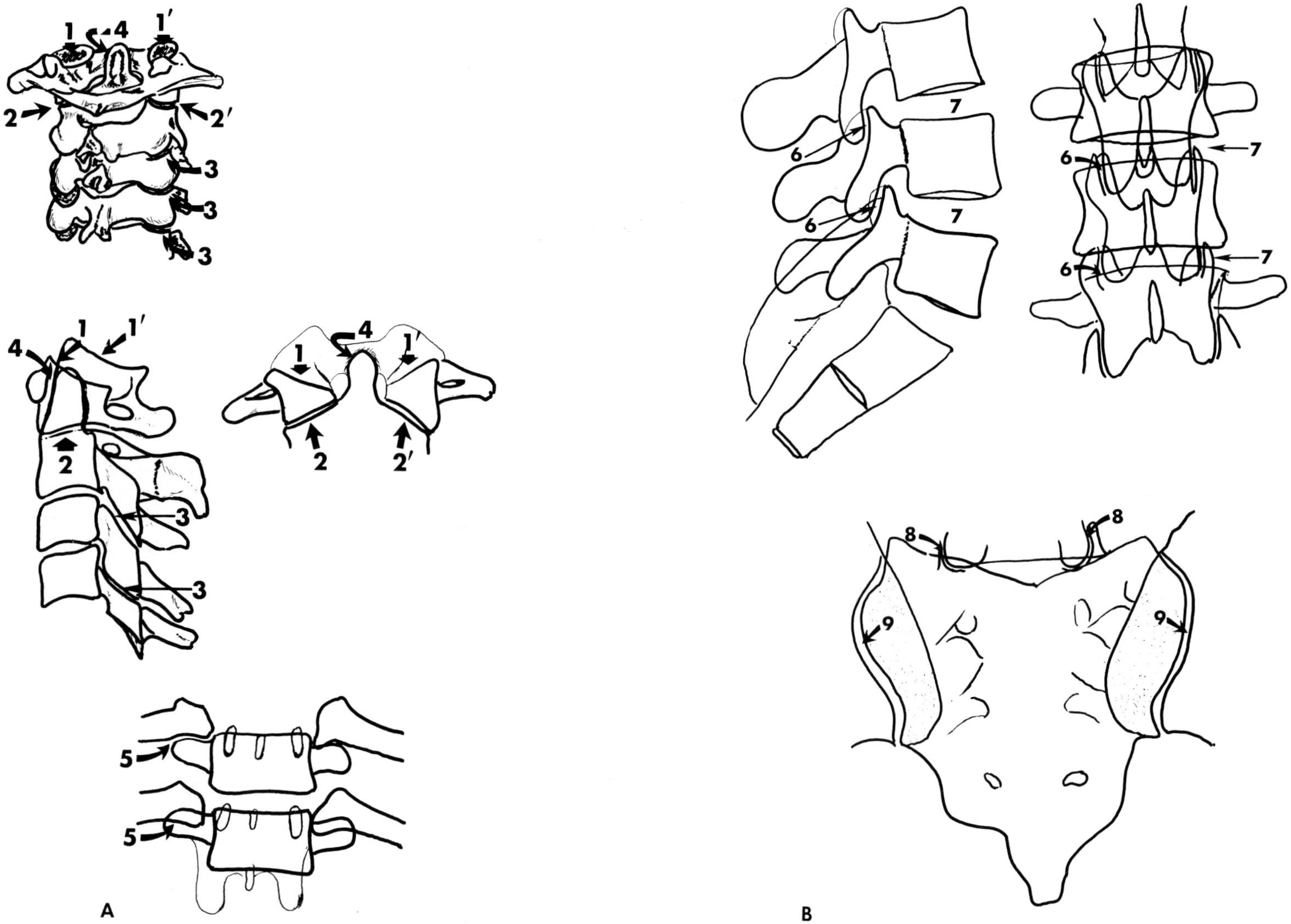

FIGURE 8–3 *A* and *B*. Diagrams of the various joints of the spine. (1) Superior joint surface articulating with occipital condyles, (2) apophyseal joint between the atlas and the axis (C1 and C2), (3) apophyseal joint of the rest of the cervical spine, (4) joint between the anterior tubercle of C1 and the odontoid process of C2, (5) costovertebral joint, (6) apophyseal joints of the lumbar region, (7) intervertebral joint, (8) the synovial joints between L 5 and the superior sacrum, (9) sacroiliac joint.

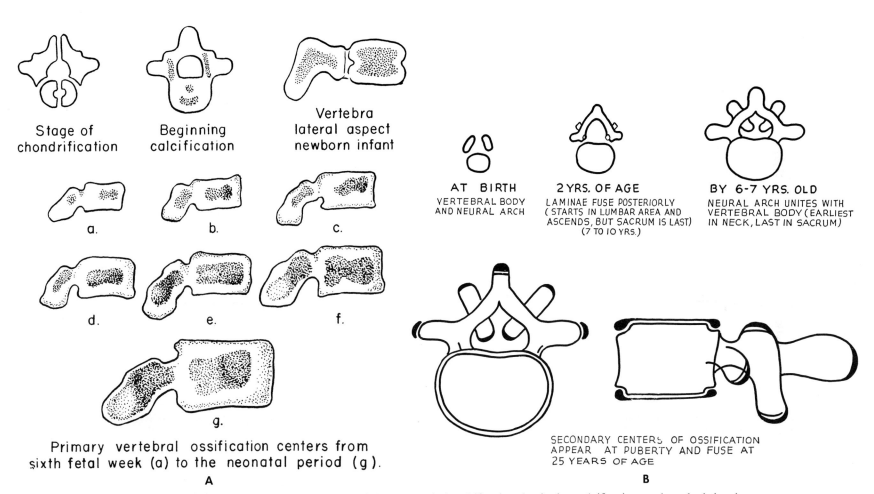

Stage of chondrification

Beginning calcification

Vertebra lateral aspect newborn infant

a.

b.

c.

d.

e.

f.

g.

Primary vertebral ossification centers from sixth fetal week (a) to the neonatal period (g).

A

AT BIRTH
VERTEBRAL BODY AND NEURAL ARCH

2 YRS. OF AGE
LAMINAE FUSE POSTERIORLY (STARTS IN LUMBAR AREA AND ASCENDS, BUT SACRUM IS LAST) (7 TO 10 YRS.)

BY 6-7 YRS. OLD
NEURAL ARCH UNITES WITH VERTEBRAL BODY (EARLIEST IN NECK, LAST IN SACRUM)

SECONDARY CENTERS OF OSSIFICATION APPEAR AT PUBERTY AND FUSE AT 25 YEARS OF AGE

B

FIGURE 8–4 *A.* Further diagrams of the stage of chondrification, beginning calcification, and gradual development of ossification in the vertebral body of the newborn. *B.* Diagrams illustrating time of union of the laminae and the joining of the neural arches with the body. The secondary centers of ossification are also illustrated.

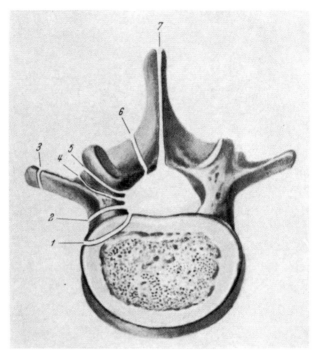

FIGURE 8–5 Diagram illustrating the various areas for defective ossification in the neural arch and pedicles: (1) Retrosomatic hiatus, (2) hiatus in the pedicle, (3) persistent epiphysis of the transverse process, (4 and 5) defects in the pars interarticularis, (6) retroisthmic hiatus, (7) bifid posterior spinous process. (From Köhler, A. and Zimmer, E. A.: Borderlands of the Normal and Early Pathologic in Skeletal Roentgenology. 11th ed. New York, Grune & Stratton, 1968. Used by permission.)

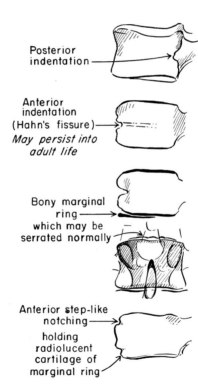

Posterior indentation

Anterior indentation (Hahn's fissure) — *May persist into adult life*

Bony marginal ring — which may be serrated normally

Anterior step-like notching — holding radiolucent cartilage of marginal ring

FIGURE 8–6 The normal appearance of posterior and anterior indentations on vertebral bodies in relation to blood supply and venous drainage. The anterior steplike notching changes the contour in relation to the cartilaginous end plates of the vertebral body.

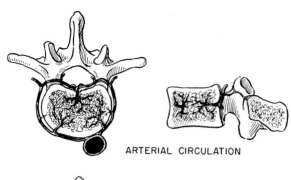

ARTERIAL CIRCULATION

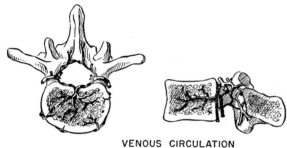

VENOUS CIRCULATION

FIGURE 8–7 Diagrams illustrating the arterial and venous circulation of a vertebral body and its neural arch.

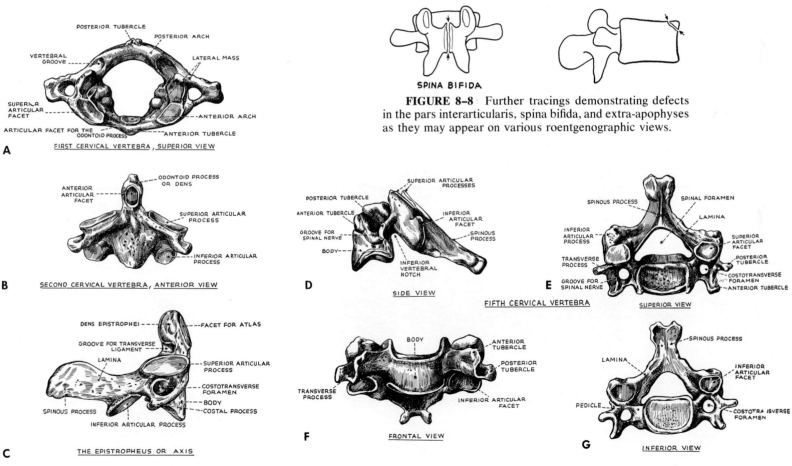

DEFECTS IN OSSIFICATION OF VERTEBRAE

DEFECTS IN PARS INTERARTICULARIS

EXTRA-APOPHYSES

SPINA BIFIDA

FIGURE 8-8 Further tracings demonstrating defects in the pars interarticularis, spina bifida, and extra-apophyses as they may appear on various roentgenographic views.

A
FIRST CERVICAL VERTEBRA, SUPERIOR VIEW

POSTERIOR TUBERCLE
POSTERIOR ARCH
VERTEBRAL GROOVE
LATERAL MASS
SUPERIOR ARTICULAR FACET
ARTICULAR FACET FOR THE ODONTOID PROCESS
ANTERIOR ARCH
ANTERIOR TUBERCLE

B
SECOND CERVICAL VERTEBRA, ANTERIOR VIEW

ODONTOID PROCESS OR DENS
ANTERIOR ARTICULAR FACET
SUPERIOR ARTICULAR PROCESS
INFERIOR ARTICULAR PROCESS

C
THE EPISTROPHEUS OR AXIS

DENS EPISTROPHEI
FACET FOR ATLAS
GROOVE FOR TRANSVERSE LIGAMENT
LAMINA
SUPERIOR ARTICULAR PROCESS
COSTOTRANSVERSE FORAMEN
BODY
COSTAL PROCESS
SPINOUS PROCESS
INFERIOR ARTICULAR PROCESS

D
SIDE VIEW

SUPERIOR ARTICULAR PROCESSES
POSTERIOR TUBERCLE
ANTERIOR TUBERCLE
INFERIOR ARTICULAR FACET
GROOVE FOR SPINAL NERVE
SPINOUS PROCESS
BODY
INFERIOR VERTEBRAL NOTCH

F
FRONTAL VIEW

BODY
ANTERIOR TUBERCLE
POSTERIOR TUBERCLE
TRANSVERSE PROCESS
INFERIOR ARTICULAR FACET

FIFTH CERVICAL VERTEBRA

E
SUPERIOR VIEW

SPINOUS PROCESS
SPINAL FORAMEN
LAMINA
INFERIOR ARTICULAR PROCESS
SUPERIOR ARTICULAR FACET
TRANSVERSE PROCESS
POSTERIOR TUBERCLE
COSTOTRANSVERSE FORAMEN
GROOVE FOR SPINAL NERVE
ANTERIOR TUBERCLE

G
INFERIOR VIEW

SPINOUS PROCESS
LAMINA
INFERIOR ARTICULAR FACET
PEDICLE
COSTOTRANSVERSE FORAMEN

FIGURE 8-9 Distinguishing characteristics of cervical vertebrae.

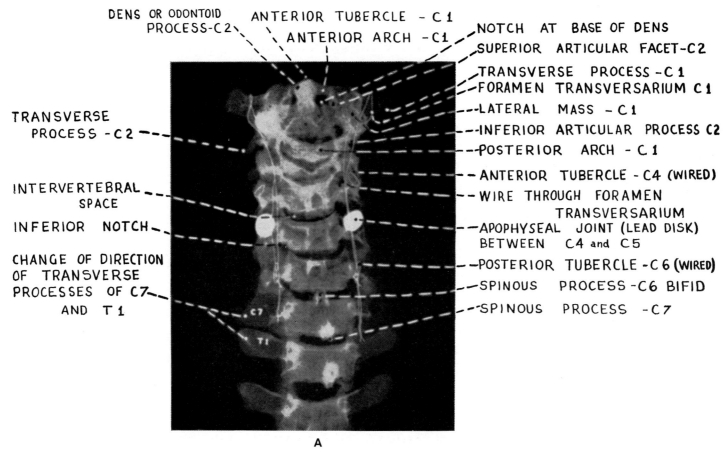

DENS OR ODONTOID PROCESS-C2

ANTERIOR TUBERCLE - C1

ANTERIOR ARCH - C1

NOTCH AT BASE OF DENS

SUPERIOR ARTICULAR FACET-C2

TRANSVERSE PROCESS - C1

FORAMEN TRANSVERSARIUM C1

LATERAL MASS - C1

INFERIOR ARTICULAR PROCESS C2

POSTERIOR ARCH - C1

ANTERIOR TUBERCLE - C4 (WIRED)

WIRE THROUGH FORAMEN TRANSVERSARIUM

APOPHYSEAL JOINT (LEAD DISK) BETWEEN C4 and C5

POSTERIOR TUBERCLE - C6 (WIRED)

SPINOUS PROCESS -C6 BIFID

SPINOUS PROCESS - C7

TRANSVERSE PROCESS - C2

INTERVERTEBRAL SPACE

INFERIOR NOTCH

CHANGE OF DIRECTION OF TRANSVERSE PROCESSES OF C7 AND T1

A

FIGURE 8–10 *A*. Radiograph of a cervical spine specimen with certain anatomic features indicated, anteroposterior projection.

Figure continued on opposite page.

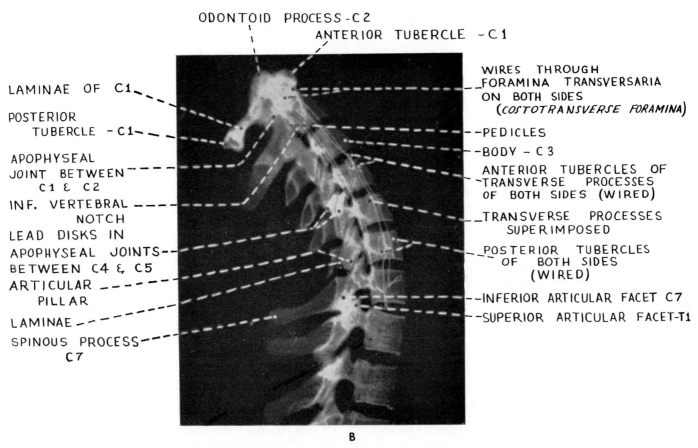

ODONTOID PROCESS-C2
ANTERIOR TUBERCLE - C1

LAMINAE OF C1

POSTERIOR
    TUBERCLE - C1

APOPHYSEAL
JOINT BETWEEN
    C1 & C2

INF. VERTEBRAL
        NOTCH
LEAD DISKS IN
APOPHYSEAL JOINTS
BETWEEN C4 & C5
ARTICULAR
    PILLAR

LAMINAE

SPINOUS PROCESS
        C7

WIRES THROUGH
FORAMINA TRANSVERSARIA
ON BOTH SIDES
(COSTOTRANSVERSE FORAMINA)

PEDICLES

BODY - C3

ANTERIOR TUBERCLES OF
TRANSVERSE PROCESSES
OF BOTH SIDES (WIRED)

TRANSVERSE PROCESSES
    SUPERIMPOSED

POSTERIOR TUBERCLES
    OF BOTH SIDES
        (WIRED)

INFERIOR ARTICULAR FACET C7

SUPERIOR ARTICULAR FACET-T1

B

FIGURE 8–10 *Continued. B.* Radiograph of a cervical spine specimen with certain anatomic features indicated, lateral projection.

Figure continued on following page.

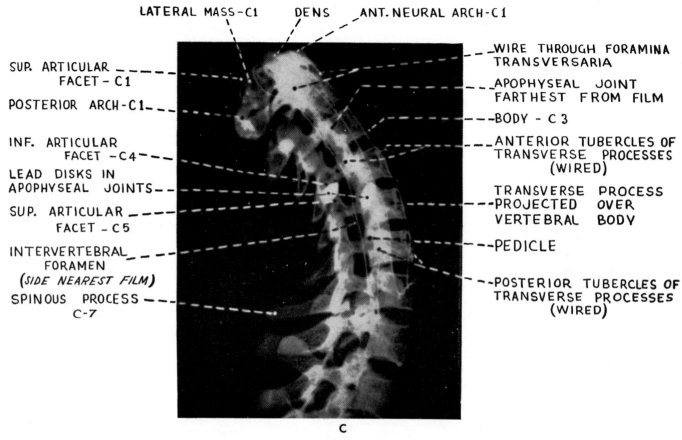

LATERAL MASS-C1   DENS   ANT. NEURAL ARCH-C1

SUP. ARTICULAR
FACET - C1

POSTERIOR ARCH-C1

INF. ARTICULAR
FACET -C4

LEAD DISKS IN
APOPHYSEAL JOINTS

SUP. ARTICULAR
FACET - C5

INTERVERTEBRAL
FORAMEN
(SIDE NEAREST FILM)

SPINOUS PROCESS
C-7

WIRE THROUGH FORAMINA
TRANSVERSARIA

APOPHYSEAL JOINT
FARTHEST FROM FILM

BODY - C3

ANTERIOR TUBERCLES OF
TRANSVERSE PROCESSES
(WIRED)

TRANSVERSE PROCESS
PROJECTED OVER
VERTEBRAL BODY

PEDICLE

POSTERIOR TUBERCLES OF
TRANSVERSE PROCESSES
(WIRED)

C

FIGURE 8–10 *Continued. C.* Radiograph of a cervical spine specimen with certain anatomic features indicated, oblique projection.

INTRODUCTION TO RADIOGRAPHIC STUDIES OF THE VERTEBRAL COLUMN

UNDER NO CONDITION MUST A PATIENT BE MOVED FROM HIS STRETCHER IF A FRACTURE IS SUSPECTED, UNTIL EXPLORATORY FILMS PROVE THAT THERE HAS BEEN NO FRACTURE.

By employing a mobile x-ray unit, survey films are first made with a horizontal beam (for the lateral view) in the anteroposterior and lateral projections without moving the patient from the stretcher.

Anteroposterior Projection of the Cervical Spine

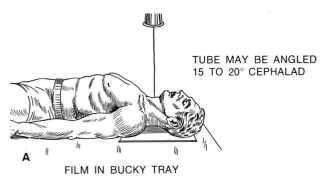

TUBE MAY BE ANGLED
15 TO 20° CEPHALAD

A

FILM IN BUCKY TRAY

POINTS OF PRACTICAL INTEREST ABOUT FIGURE 8–11

1. The sagittal plane of the head is centered to the longitudinal axis of the table and the patient's chin is extended sufficiently so that the lower edge of his anterior teeth is in the same perpendicular line as the tip of the mastoid processes.

2. The head should be immobilized by means of either sandbags or head clamps. These have been omitted in the drawings for the sake of clarity.

3. The central ray passes through the most prominent point of the thyroid cartilage. This ordinarily lies anterior to the fourth cervical segment.

4. Alternately, the central ray may be angled 15 or 20 degrees toward the head, which gives one a somewhat clearer concept of the lower intervertebral spaces and a better view for demonstration of possible cervical ribs.

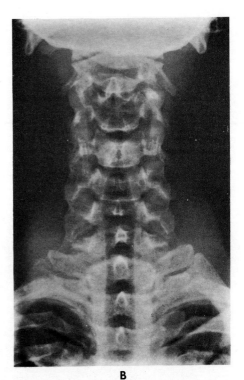

B

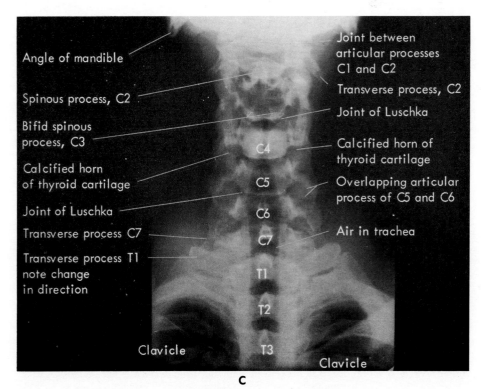

C

FIGURE 8–11 Anteroposterior projection of the cervical spine. *A*, Position of tube and patient. *B*, Radiograph so obtained. *C*. Same radiograph, labeled.

Anteroposterior Projection of the Upper Cervical Spine Through the Open Mouth or with the Mandible in Motion

POINTS OF PRACTICAL INTEREST ABOUT FIGURE 8–12

1. The patient's mouth is opened as widely as possible and it may be kept in this position by a large cork or balsa wood block.

2. A line drawn between the lower margin of the anterior upper teeth and the tip of the mastoid process must be perpendicular to the film.

3. If the patient will softly say "Ah" during the exposure, the tongue will be more closely fixed to the floor of the mouth so that its shadow will not be projected over the atlas and axis.

4. Body-section radiographs of the odontoid process and adjoining joints are frequently very helpful (Fig. 8–13).

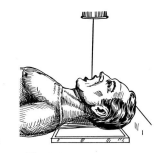

A

FILM IN BUCKY TRAY

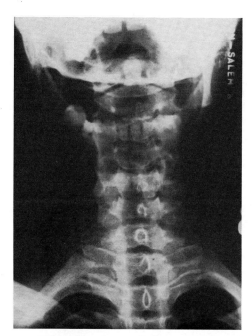

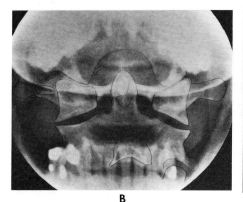

B

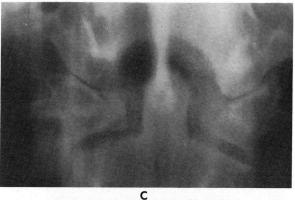

C

FIGURE 8–13 Anteroposterior projection of upper cervical spine with mouth open to show the odontoid process in particular. (Radiograph intensified.) *A*. Position of patient. *B*. View so obtained. *C*. Tomographic projection of the odontoid process so obtained. *D*. Radiograph in *B* with anatomic parts labeled.

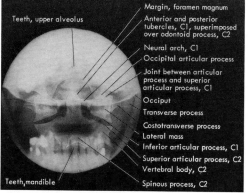

Teeth, upper alveolus

Margin, foramen magnum
Anterior and posterior tubercles, C1, superimposed over odontoid process, C2
Neural arch, C1
Occipital articular process
Joint between articular process and superior articular process, C1
Occiput
Transverse process
Costotransverse process
Lateral mass
Inferior articular process, C1
Superior articular process, C2
Vertebral body, C2
Spinous process, C2

Teeth, mandible

D

FIGURE 8–12 Anteroposterior projection of the cervical spine obtained with a rhythmic motion of the lower jaw during the exposure. The head, of course, is rigidly immobilized to prevent movement of the cervical spine. When a view is obtained in this manner, a concept of the upper two cervical segments may be obtained that otherwise is not possible in this projection, since these segments, invariably, are obscured by the shadow of the mandible (Ottonello method).

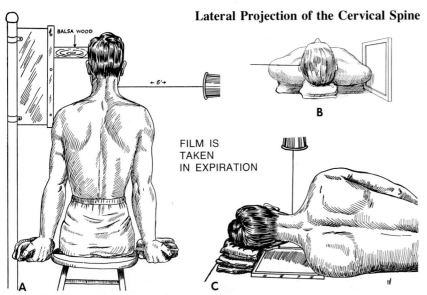

POINTS OF PRACTICAL INTEREST ABOUT FIGURE 8–14

1. The shoulders should be lowered by weights held in the patient's hands, and all *seven* cervical vertebrae must be clearly seen.

2. The hand is supported in a perfectly vertical position, with the sagittal plane perfectly parallel to the cassette.

This places the cervical spine a considerable distance from the film. *Distortion and magnification are very considerable under these circumstances, unless a long film-target distance is employed* (6 feet). Every effort is made to preserve the normal curvature of the cervical spine, but frequently this curvature disappears in the event of muscular spasm. The normal alignment previously described is only slightly disturbed under these circumstances.

In this projection, the lateral mass is projected in part over the vertebral body, particularly in its costal element. The articular processes, however, are shown very clearly.

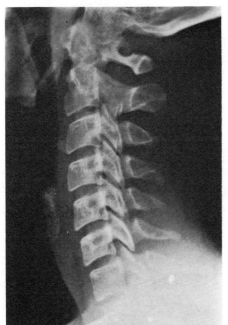

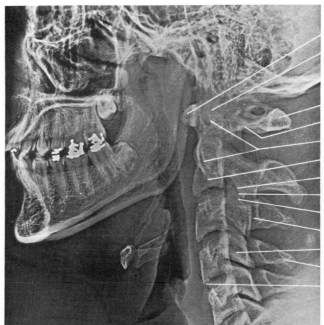

ANTERIOR TUBERCLE, C1
DENS (ODONTOID PROCESS)

POSTERIOR TUBERCLE, C1
POSTERIOR ARCH, C1
TRANSVERSE PROCESSES, C1–C2
BODY, C2
INFERIOR ARTICULAR PROCESS, C3
APOPHYSEAL JOINT
SUPERIOR ARTICULAR PROCESS, C4
LAMINAE, C3
ARTICULAR PILLAR
SPINOUS PROCESS, C4
INTERVERTEBRAL SPACE

FIGURE 8–14 Lateral projection of cervical spine; various methods of obtaining this projection; radiographs so obtained. *A.* Patient erect and a 6 foot film-to-target distance employed. *B.* Patient lying flat and a horizontal beam employed; *C.* Patient lying on his side and a vertical beam employed. *D.* Radiograph so obtained. (Please note that seven segments should be identified.) *E.* Radiograph of *D* with labels of anatomic parts superimposed (xeroradiograph employed for increased clarity).

TABLE 8–1. Normal Sagittal Measurements*

Region Evaluated	Normal Sagittal Measurements for Children 15 Years and Under (120 cases)		Normal Sagittal Measurements for Adults (480 cases)	
	AVERAGE (MM.)	RANGE (MM.)	AVERAGE (MM.)	RANGE (MM.)
Retropharyngeal space	3.5	2–7	3.4	1–7
Retrotracheal space	7.9	5–14	14.0	9–22
Cervical spinal canal:				
At first cervical vertebra	21.9	18–27	21.4	16–30
At second cervical vertebra	20.9	18–25	19.2	16–28
At third cervical vertebra	17.4	14–21	19.1	14–25
At fifth cervical vertebra	16.5	14–21	18.5	14–25
At seventh cervical vertebra	16.0	15–20	17.5	13–24

*From Whiley, M. H., et al.: Radiology, *71*:350, 1958.

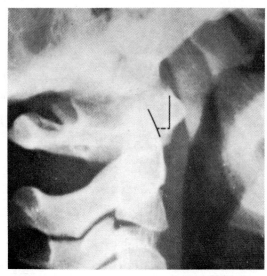

FIGURE 8–15 Upper cervical spine showing the distance measured (broken line) between the posterior inferior portion of the anterior arch of the atlas and the anterior border of the dens. (From Locke, G. R., Gardner, J. I., and Van Epps, E. F.: Am. J. Roentgenol., *97*:135–140, 1966.)

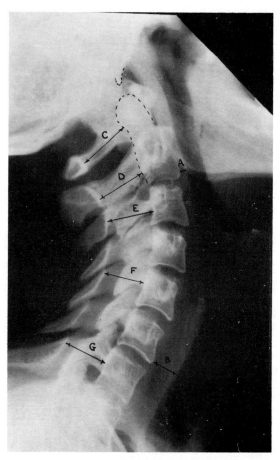

FIGURE 8–16 Normal lateral view of neck indicating regions evaluated. (A) retropharyngeal space, second cervical vertebra; (B) retrotracheal space, sixth cervical vertebra; (C to G) cervical spinal canal; (C) first cervical vertebra; (D) second cervical vertebra; (E) third cervical vertebra; (F) fifth cervical vertebra; (G) seventh cervical vertebra. (From Wholey, M. H., Brewer, A. J., and Baker, H. L., Jr.: Radiology, *71*:350, 1958.)

Oblique Projection of the Cervical Spine

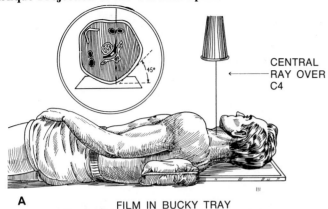

CENTRAL
RAY OVER
C4

A

FILM IN BUCKY TRAY

POINTS OF PRACTICAL INTEREST ABOUT FIGURE 8–17

1. This view may be obtained in either the *erect* or *recumbent* position.

2. The entire body of the patient is rotated, and if he is supine, sandbags are placed beneath the shoulder and the buttocks to support his position at an angle of 45 degrees with the table top. The sagittal axis of the patient's head is perfectly straight with regard to that of the entire body.

3. The central ray is directed over the cervical spine at the level of the fourth cervical segment (at the level of the most prominent portion of the thyroid cartilage).

4. Alternately, an additional angulation of the tube 15 degrees toward the head may be employed, with the patient in the position just described.

5. It is best to employ a focal-film distance of at least 48 inches since the cervical spine is at such a great distance from the film in this projection.

6. Oblique studies of both sides are routinely obtained.

7. The intervertebral foramina that are farthest from the film are the ones that are shown most clearly.

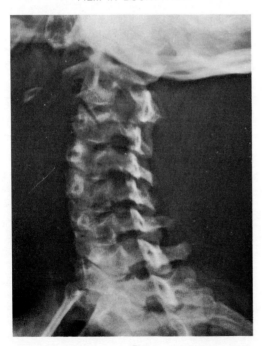

B

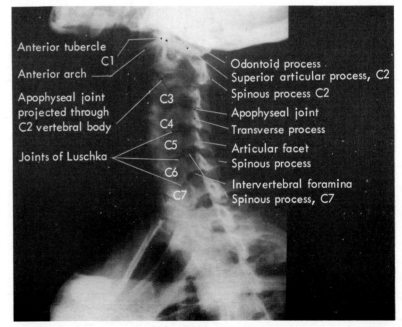

Anterior tubercle
C1
Anterior arch

Apophyseal joint
projected through
C2 vertebral body

C3

C4

C5

Joints of Luschka

C6

C7

Odontoid process
Superior articular process, C2
Spinous process C2
Apophyseal joint
Transverse process
Articular facet
Spinous process
Intervertebral foramina
Spinous process, C7

C

FIGURE 8–17 Oblique projection of cervical spine. *A*. Position of patient and central ray of x-ray tube. *B*. Right anteroposterior oblique projection so obtained. *C*. Radiograph with labels for anatomic parts superimposed.

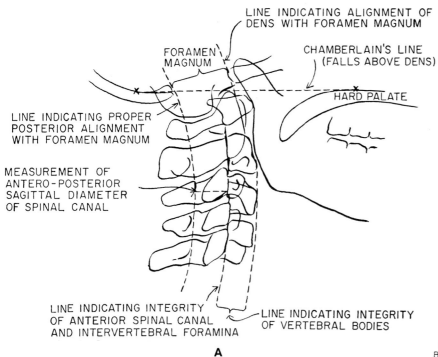

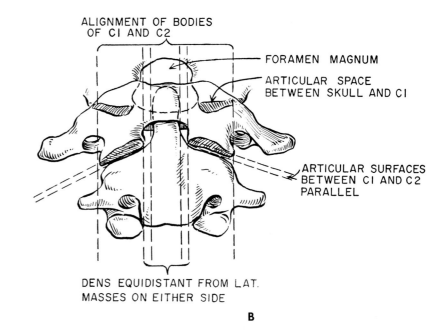

FIGURE 8–18 Alignment of cervical segments with respect to each other and to the skull. *A*. Lateral projection. *B*. Odontoid projection. *C*. Various roentgen criteria for the normal relationship of the odontoid to the mastoid processes and the foramen magnum.

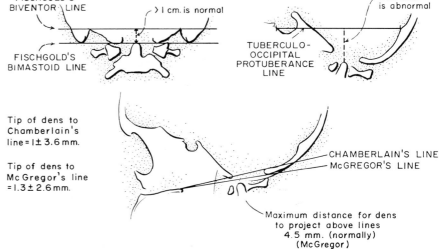

The Thoracic or Dorsal Spine

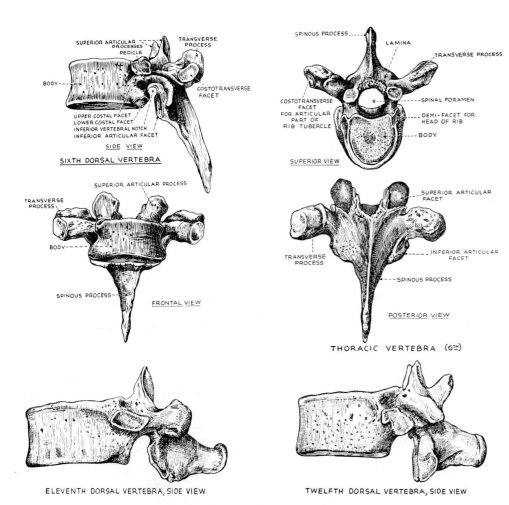

SUPERIOR ARTICULAR
PROCESSES
PEDICLE
TRANSVERSE
PROCESS

BODY

COSTOTRANSVERSE
FACET

UPPER COSTAL FACET
LOWER COSTAL FACET
INFERIOR VERTEBRAL NOTCH
INFERIOR ARTICULAR FACET

SIDE VIEW

SIXTH DORSAL VERTEBRA

SUPERIOR ARTICULAR PROCESS

TRANSVERSE
PROCESS

BODY

SPINOUS PROCESS

FRONTAL VIEW

SPINOUS PROCESS

LAMINA

TRANSVERSE PROCESS

COSTOTRANSVERSE
FACET
FOR ARTICULAR
PART OF
RIB TUBERCLE

SPINAL FORAMEN

DEMI-FACET FOR
HEAD OF RIB

BODY

SUPERIOR VIEW

SUPERIOR ARTICULAR
FACET

TRANSVERSE
PROCESS

INFERIOR ARTICULAR
FACET

SPINOUS PROCESS

POSTERIOR VIEW

THORACIC VERTEBRA (6ᵀᴴ)

ELEVENTH DORSAL VERTEBRA, SIDE VIEW

TWELFTH DORSAL VERTEBRA, SIDE VIEW

FIGURE 8–19 Distinguishing characteristics of dorsal vertebrae.

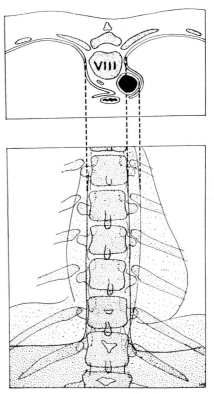

FIGURE 8–20 *Above.* Cross section through the posterior mediastinum at the level of the eighth thoracic vertebra. *Below.* Diagram taken from a roentgenogram depicting the posterior portions of the visceral and parietal pleura as lines along the vertebral column. Dotted lines indicate anatomical substrates of pleural lines and aortic lines in cross section. (From Lachman, E.: Anat. Rec., *83*, 1942.)

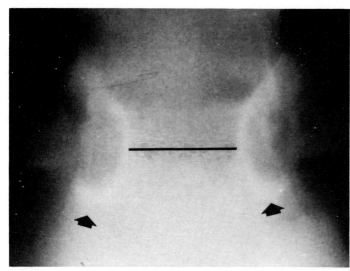

FIGURE 8–21 Radiograph showing the advantage of tomography for the demonstration of pedicles and interpediculate distance.

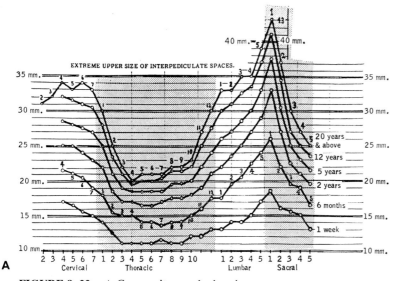

A

FIGURE 8–22 *A.* Composite graph showing extreme upper measurements of interpediculate spaces in various age groups. Variations of 2 mm. or more are considered significant, suggesting a mass lesion of the spinal canal. (From Schwarz, C. S.: Am. J. Roentgenol., 76:476, 1956.) *B.* Chart for determination of interpedicular distances of the spine, adapted from chart in *A.*

Normal Interpediculate Distances in Children and Adults. A concept of the width of the spinal canal may be obtained by measurement of the distances between the inner margins of the pedicle as portrayed on the anteroposterior projections of the spine (Figs. 8–21 and 8–22).

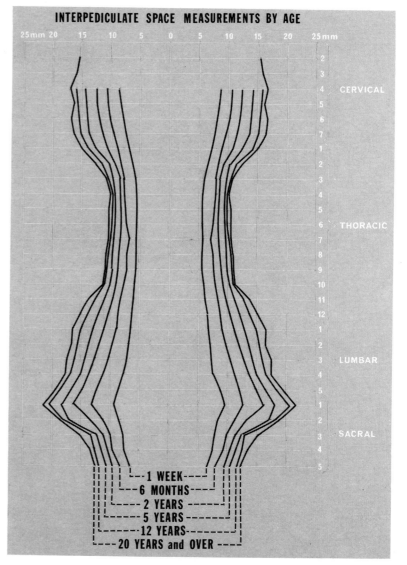

B

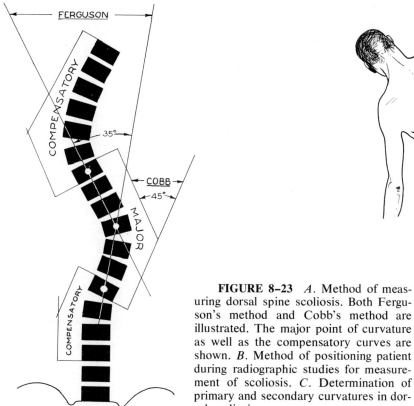

A

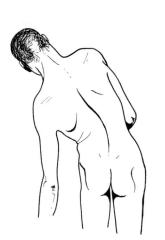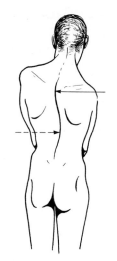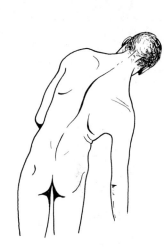

Primary curvature remains relatively constant (——➤).
Secondary curvature tends to correct itself (– – ➤).

B

FIGURE 8–23 *A.* Method of measuring dorsal spine scoliosis. Both Ferguson's method and Cobb's method are illustrated. The major point of curvature as well as the compensatory curves are shown. *B.* Method of positioning patient during radiographic studies for measurement of scoliosis. *C.* Determination of primary and secondary curvatures in dorsal scoliosis.

DETERMINATION OF PRIMARY AND SECONDARY
CURVATURES IN DORSAL SCOLIOSIS

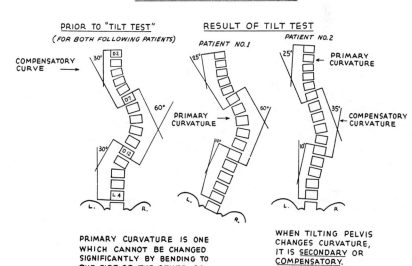

C

STUDIES FOR ABNORMALITIES IN SPINAL CURVATURE

Definition of Terms

Scoliosis: Rotation or torsion of several vertebrae in their longitudinal axis.

Lordosis: Increased concavity of the spine on its posterior aspect.

Kyphosis: Angulation of the spine on its posterior aspect.

Gibbus: Posterior angulation of the spine with no significant disturbance in the line of weight bearing.

ROUTINE RADIOGRAPHIC POSITIONS AND RADIOGRAPHIC ANATOMY OF THE THORACIC SPINE

Anteroposterior Projection of the Thoracic Spine (Fig. 8–24). A film is centered directly under the midpoint between the superior border of the manubrium and the xiphoid process of the sternum. The patient is instructed to suspend respiration and hold his breath during the exposure. A vertical beam is employed.

This position may also be made with the patient and the Bucky erect through the use of a horizontal beam.

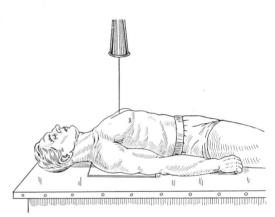

FILM IN BUCKY TRAY

A

FIGURE 8–24 Anteroposterior projection of the thoracic spine. *A.* Positioning of patient, with respect to central ray. *B*, Radiograph so obtained. *C.* Radiograph with anatomic parts intensified and labeled.

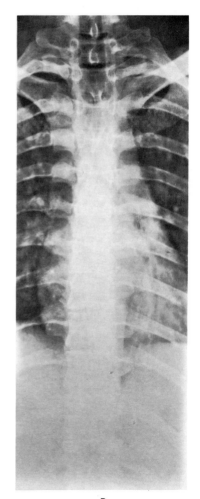

B

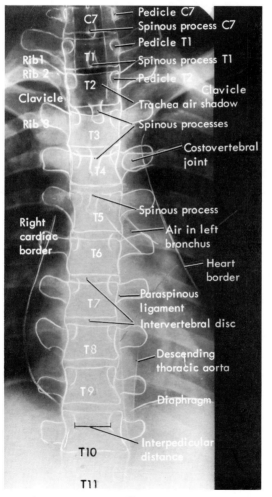

C

Lateral View of the Thoracic Spine (Fig. 8–25). The lateral projection gives an excellent perspective of the vertebral bodies and spinal canal. The various processes and synovial joints are obscured to a great extent by the overlapping laminae, spinous processes, and ribs, as are the upper two thoracic segments.

The gas shadows of the lung structures overlie the vertebral bodies of the thoracic spine and frequently make the interpretation of minimal trabecular abnormality virtually impossible. In cases of doubt, body section radiographs are of considerable help. The patient may breathe during the exposure, blurring the lung markings; the diaphragmatic motion improves the appearance of the lower thoracic segments also.

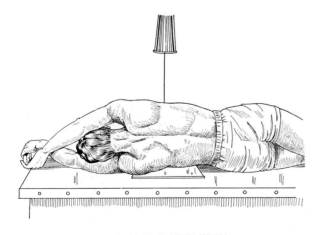

A LINE MAY BE DRAWN BETWEEN THE FIRST AND TWELFTH VERTEBRAE. THE TUBE IS CENTERED OVER THE MIDPOINT OF THIS LINE.

FILM IN BUCKY TRAY

A

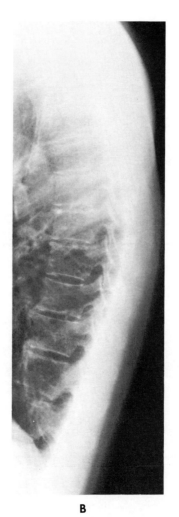

B

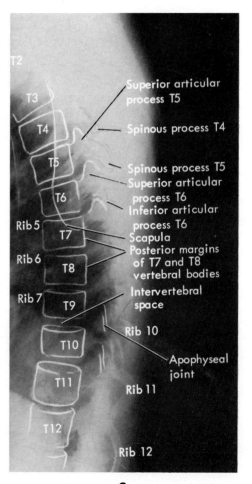

T2

T3

T4

T5

T6

Rib 5

Rib 6

Rib 7

T7

T8

T9

T10

T11

T12

Superior articular process T5

Spinous process T4

Spinous process T5
Superior articular process T6
Inferior articular process T6
Scapula
Posterior margins of T7 and T8 vertebral bodies

Intervertebral space

Rib 10

Apophyseal joint

Rib 11

Rib 12

C

FIGURE 8–25 Lateral projection of the thoracic spine. *A.* Positioning of patient with respect to central ray. *B.* Radiographic view so obtained. *C.* Radiograph with anatomic parts intensified and labeled.

Lateral (Slightly Oblique) Projection of the Upper Two Thoracic Segments

POINTS OF PRACTICAL INTEREST ABOUT FIGURE 8–26

1. The patient's midaxillary plane is placed against the midline of the film. The shoulder that is farthest from the film is depressed as much as possible with a heavy weight in the hand, whereas that which is closest to the film is rotated forward by placing the hand on the head and flexing the elbow. There may be a very slight rotation of the patient's body, 5 to 10 degrees as shown.

2. The patient's axilla closest to the film is centered on the film, and the central ray is directed perpendicular to the film at this central point.

3. The central ray is perpendicular to the film if the remote shoulder can be depressed adequately, but an angle of 15 degrees toward the feet may be employed when the shoulder cannot be well depressed.

4. A view of the uppermost two thoracic segments is not obtained on a routine lateral thoracic spine film, and when these two segments must be visualized some special means such as this must be employed.

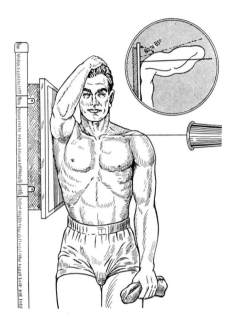

USUALLY PHYSICAL EXPOSURE
FACTORS UTILIZED IN LUMBAR
RADIOGRAPHY ARE EMPLOYED.

GREATER OBLIQUITY TO EVEN
45 DEGREES MAY BE USED IN THE
SUPINE POSITION, CENTERING
OVER THE TOP OF THE MANUBRIUM
IF THIS VIEW IS NOT SUCCESSFUL.

A

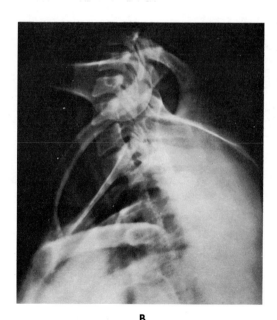

B

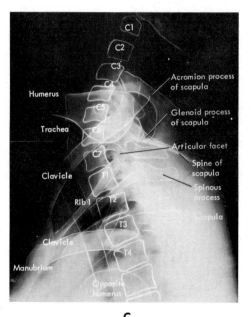

C

FIGURE 8–26 Lateral (slightly oblique) view of upper two thoracic segments. (Twining position). *A*. Position of patient with respect to central ray. *B*. Radiograph so obtained. *C*. Radiograph with anatomic parts intensified and labeled.

Lumbar and Sacral Vertebrae

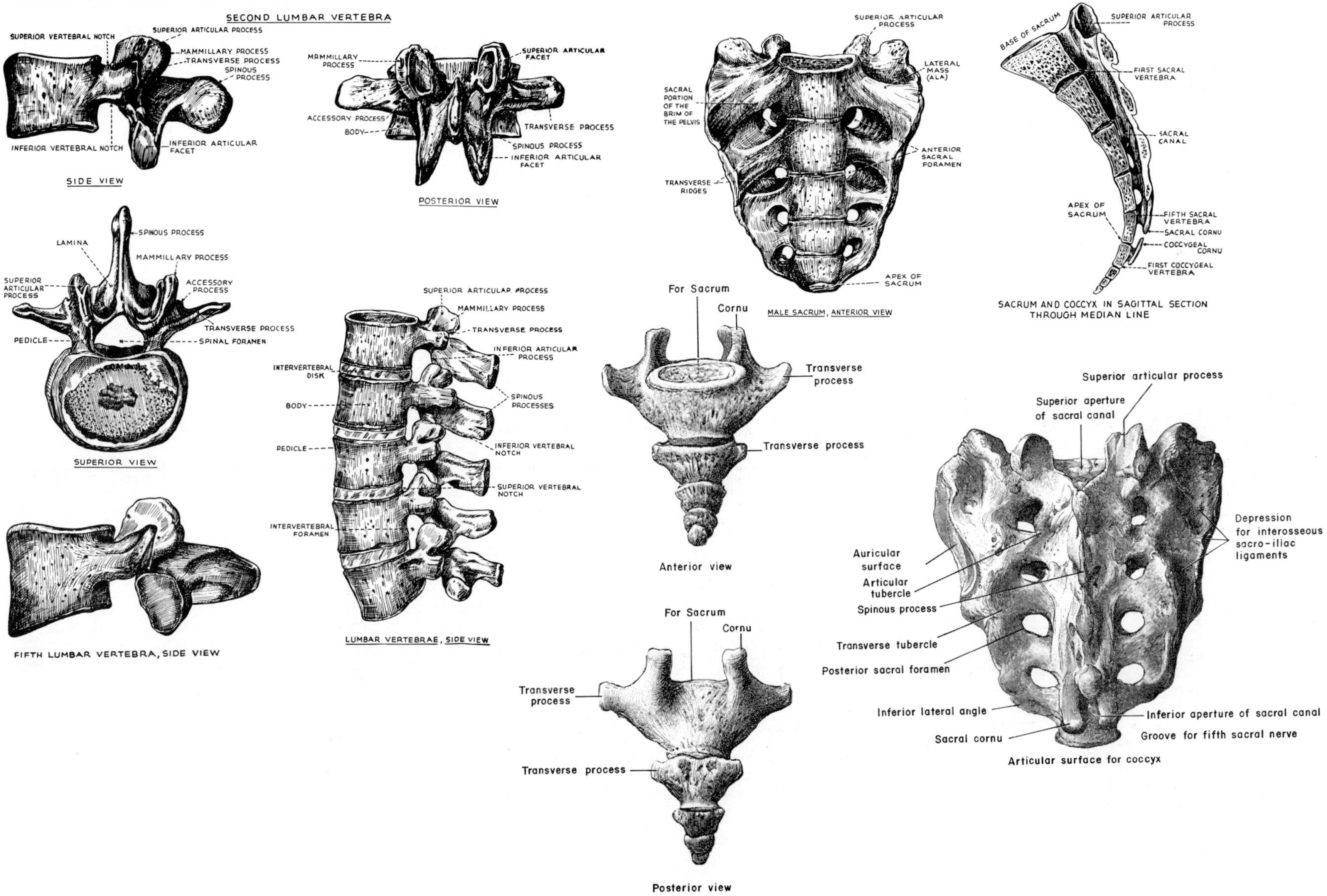

SECOND LUMBAR VERTEBRA

SUPERIOR VERTEBRAL NOTCH
SUPERIOR ARTICULAR PROCESS
MAMMILLARY PROCESS
TRANSVERSE PROCESS
SPINOUS PROCESS
INFERIOR VERTEBRAL NOTCH
INFERIOR ARTICULAR FACET

SIDE VIEW

MAMMILLARY PROCESS
SUPERIOR ARTICULAR FACET
ACCESSORY PROCESS
BODY
TRANSVERSE PROCESS
SPINOUS PROCESS
INFERIOR ARTICULAR FACET

POSTERIOR VIEW

LAMINA
SPINOUS PROCESS
MAMMILLARY PROCESS
ACCESSORY PROCESS
SUPERIOR ARTICULAR PROCESS
TRANSVERSE PROCESS
PEDICLE
SPINAL FORAMEN

SUPERIOR VIEW

FIFTH LUMBAR VERTEBRA, SIDE VIEW

SUPERIOR ARTICULAR PROCESS
MAMMILLARY PROCESS
TRANSVERSE PROCESS
INFERIOR ARTICULAR PROCESS
INTERVERTEBRAL DISK
BODY
SPINOUS PROCESSES
PEDICLE
INFERIOR VERTEBRAL NOTCH
SUPERIOR VERTEBRAL NOTCH
INTERVERTEBRAL FORAMEN

LUMBAR VERTEBRAE, SIDE VIEW

SUPERIOR ARTICULAR PROCESS
SACRAL PORTION OF THE BRIM OF THE PELVIS
LATERAL MASS (ALA)
TRANSVERSE RIDGES
ANTERIOR SACRAL FORAMEN
APEX OF SACRUM

MALE SACRUM, ANTERIOR VIEW

For Sacrum
Cornu
Transverse process
Transverse process

Anterior view

For Sacrum
Cornu
Transverse process
Transverse process

Posterior view

BASE OF SACRUM
SUPERIOR ARTICULAR PROCESS
FIRST SACRAL VERTEBRA
SACRAL CANAL
APEX OF SACRUM
FIFTH SACRAL VERTEBRA
SACRAL CORNU
COCCYGEAL CORNU
FIRST COCCYGEAL VERTEBRA

SACRUM AND COCCYX IN SAGITTAL SECTION THROUGH MEDIAN LINE

Superior articular process
Superior aperture of sacral canal
Depression for interosseous sacro-iliac ligaments
Auricular surface
Articular tubercle
Spinous process
Transverse tubercle
Posterior sacral foramen
Inferior lateral angle
Sacral cornu
Inferior aperture of sacral canal
Groove for fifth sacral nerve
Articular surface for coccyx

FIGURE 8–27 Various views of lumbar, sacral, and coccygeal vertebrae.

Films for Demonstration of Instability or Subluxation

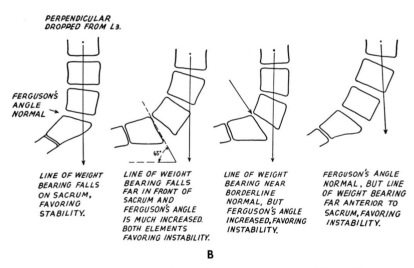

FIGURE 8-28 Analysis of two factors in lumbosacral instability. (Modified from Ferguson, A. B.: Roentgen Diagnosis of Extremities and Spine. New York, Paul B. Hoeber, Inc., 1949.)

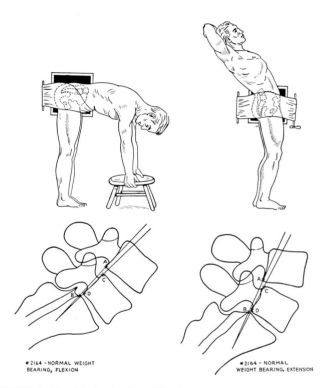

FIGURE 8-29 Method of positioning patient for measuring stability at the lumbo-sacral angle. The technique includes obtaining films that show weight-bearing in flexion and extension as well as measuring the alignment of the fifth lumbar vertebra with respect to the fourth lumbar vertebra and the sacrum.

RELATIONSHIP OF CERVICAL VERTEBRAL BODIES IN
FLEXION, NEUTRAL, AND EXTENSION POSITIONS

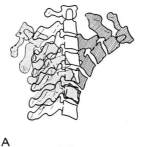

A

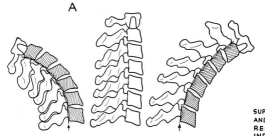

—NOTE STEPLIKE RELATIONSHIP OF POSTERIOR MARGINS
OF VERTEBRAL BODIES IN NORMAL ALIGNMENT.

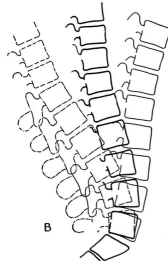

B

SUPERIMPOSED TRACINGS OF LUMBAR SPINE IN FLEXION
AND EXTENSION AS WELL AS NEUTRAL POSITION.
RELATIVE MOVEMENTS OF L3, L4, AND L5 GIVE SOME
INDICATION OF PRESENCE OR ABSENCE OF DISC
ABNORMALITIES, SINCE A RELATIVE IMMOBILITY
IS NOTED UNDER THESE CIRCUMSTANCES.

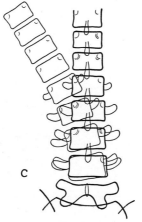

C

RELATIVE MOVEMENT OF L3, L4, and L5
MAY ASSIST IN LOCALIZING INTRASPINAL
DISEASE. NORMAL RELATIONSHIPS ARE
SHOWN ABOVE. IMMOBILITY MAY ASSIST
IN LOCALIZING DISEASE.

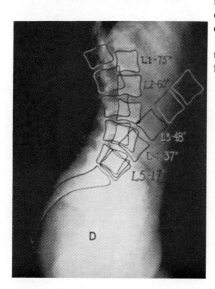

D

Sites of Subluxation or Dislocation in the Spine

Subluxation or dislocation occurs most frequently at the following sites: (1) the first two cervical segments; (2) the levels of C4, C5, C6, and C7; and (3) the lower lumbar region in relation to a phenomenon known as spondylolisthesis.

Spondylolisthesis refers to the slipping forward of a vertebral body with respect to the adjoining body, usually because of defective ossification, and hence inadequate bony support, at the pars interarticularis.

FIGURE 8–30 *A* to *C.* Flexion and extension studies of the cervical and lumbar spine. *D.* A lateral view of the lumbar spine with tracing superimposed on the lumbar spine in flexion, neutral position, and extension. A method is devised for determining the total change of angulation of each vertebral body. If these angles were plotted, a smooth curve would be obtained. Any change in the smoothness of this curve may be significant in localizing altered mobility from any cause.

ROUTINE RADIOGRAPHIC POSITIONS AND RADIOGRAPHIC ANATOMY OF THE LUMBAR SPINE

Anteroposterior Projection of the Lumbosacral Spine

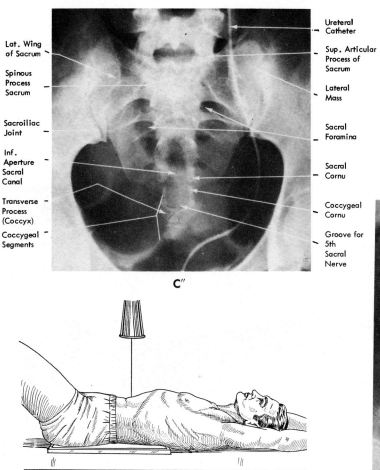

Ureteral Catheter

Lat. Wing of Sacrum

Sup. Articular Process of Sacrum

Spinous Process Sacrum

Lateral Mass

Sacroiliac Joint

Sacral Foramina

Inf. Aperture Sacral Canal

Sacral Cornu

Transverse Process (Coccyx)

Coccygeal Cornu

Coccygeal Segments

Groove for 5th Sacral Nerve

C''

A

POINTS OF PRACTICAL INTEREST ABOUT FIGURE 8–31

1. The lumbar curvature will impose a degree of distortion and magnification on those lumbar vertebrae which are farthest from the film. To diminish this effect, the knees are flexed as shown in Figure 8–31, which straightens the lumbar spine to some extent.

2. The student should acquire sufficient knowledge of anatomy to visualize the entire vertebral segment from the frontal and lateral perspectives. This can best be accomplished by studying the labeled radiographs with vertebrae in hand.

3. In some instances, erect films are required to detect the effect of standing and weight-bearing.

4. The arms are extended as shown.

5. The pelvis is adjusted so that there is no rotation.

6. A compression band may be placed across the abdomen to insure immobilization and diminish the anteroposterior thickness (with less secondary radiation).

7. The film is in the Bucky tray, centered to a point half-way between the crests of the ilium.

8. The film is made during expiration.

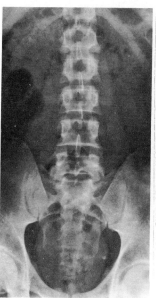

B

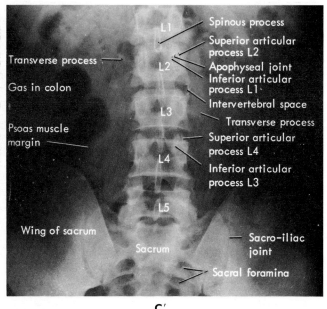

L1

Spinous process

Superior articular process L2

Transverse process

Apophyseal joint

Gas in colon

L2

Inferior articular process L1

Intervertebral space

L3

Transverse process

Psoas muscle margin

Superior articular process L4

L4

Inferior articular process L3

L5

Wing of sacrum

Sacro-iliac joint

Sacrum

Sacral foramina

C'

FIGURE 8–31 Anteroposterior projection of lumbosacral spine. *A*. Positioning of patient with respect to central ray. *B*. Radiograph so obtained. *C'* and *C''*, Radiographs with anatomic parts labeled.

Lateral Projection of the Lumbosacral Spine

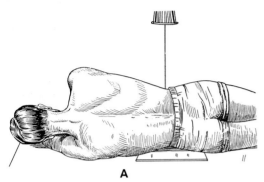

A

FILM IN BUCKY TRAY

FIGURE 8–32 Lateral projection of the lumbosacral spine. *A.* Positioning of the patient with respect to central ray. *B.* Radiographic view so obtained. *C.* Radiograph with anatomic parts labeled.

POINTS OF PRACTICAL INTEREST ABOUT FIGURE 8–32

1. The hips and knees are flexed to a comfortable position, and balsa wood blocks are placed in the depression above the iliac crest so that the thoracic spine, lumbar spine, and sacrum are parallel with the table top. A Potter-Bucky diaphragm is always employed.

2. Usually, a separate exposure is required for the fifth lumbar, sacrum and coccyx, since more penetrating x-rays are required. A suitable wedge filter may be employed to combine the two on a single exposure.

3. The patient's arms are brought forward; the uppermost arm grasps the table for support. A pillow may be placed between the knees to assist in the proper alignment of the spine to the horizontal plane. If the spine is not parallel to the table top, the tube or table may be tilted appropriately. The patient holds breath in expiration.

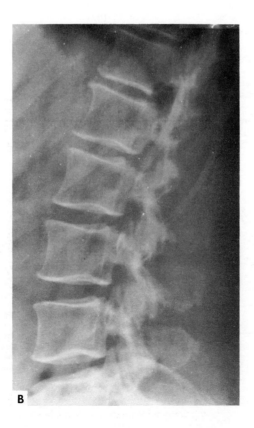

B

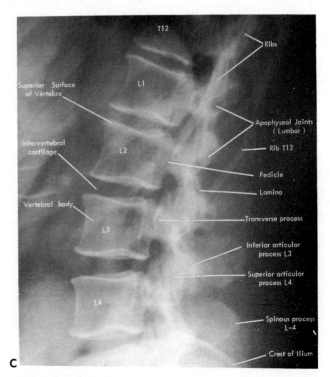

C

Lateral Projection of the 5th Lumbar Vertebra, Sacrum and Coccyx

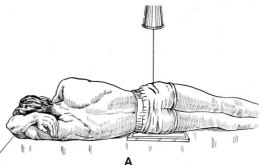

A

CASSETTE IN BUCKY TRAY

POINTS OF PRACTICAL INTEREST ABOUT FIGURE 8–33

1. To help immobilize the patient, his hips and knees are flexed to a comfortable position.

2. The coronal plane passing 3 inches posterior to the midaxillary line is adjusted to the longitudinal axis of the table.

3. It is usually desirable to place folded sheets or balsa wood blocks in the depression above the iliac crest to maintain the lower thoracic spine in a perfectly parallel relationship with the table top.

4. Although the film here is demonstrated immediately beneath the patient, a Potter-Bucky diaphragm is always employed.

5. If it is the coccyx that is the major interest, a somewhat lighter exposure technique must be employed and less detail with regard to the sacrum will then be obtained.

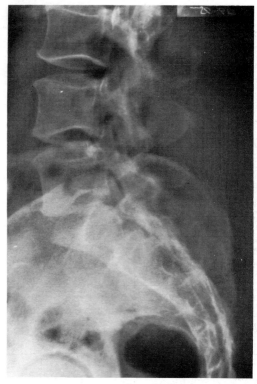

B

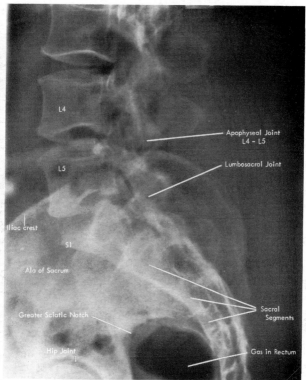

C

FIGURE 8–33 Special lateral projection of fifth lumbar vertebra, sacrum, and coccyx. *A.* Positioning of patient with respect to central ray. *B.* Radiographic view so obtained. *C.* Radiograph with anatomic parts labeled. *D.* Lateral projection of sacrum and coccyx.

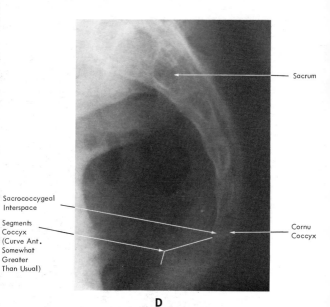

D

Oblique Projection of the Lumbosacral Spine

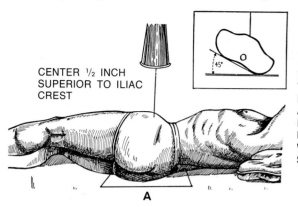

CENTER ½ INCH SUPERIOR TO ILIAC CREST

ANTERIOR SUPERIOR ILIAC SPINES MUST BE IN SAME TRANSVERSE PLANE. ANKLES AND KNEES ARE SUPPORTED WITH SANDBAGS.

A

CASSETTE IN BUCKY TRAY

POINTS OF PRACTICAL INTEREST ABOUT FIGURE 8-34

1. The patient's body is placed obliquely with respect to the table top at an angle of 25 to 45 degrees. The coronal plane passing through the spinous processes is centered to the midline of the table.

2. If the lower lumbar apophyseal joints are of greatest interest, the central ray passes through the level of the raised iliac crest. If the upper lumbar apophyseal joints are desired, the central ray passes through a point about 1 inch above the raised iliac crest.

3. The apophyseal joints closest to the film will be shown to best advantage, but occasionally it will require several attempts with varying degrees of angulation to obtain a clear view of all the apophyseal joints. This may be necessary since the plane of the joint varies somewhat as one descends the lumbar spine.

4. The sacroiliac joint that is farthest from the film will be opened up to best advantage. An angle of approximately 25 degrees is usually most satisfactory for the sacroiliac joint depiction.

FIGURE 8-34 Oblique projection of lumbosacral spine. *A.* Positioning of patient with respect to central ray. *B.* Radiographic view so obtained. *C.* Radiograph with anatomic parts labeled.

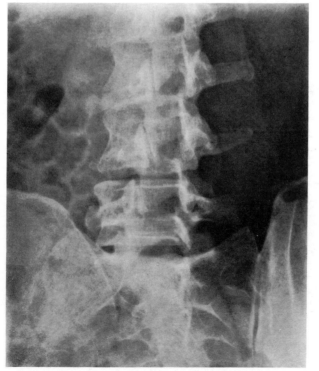

B

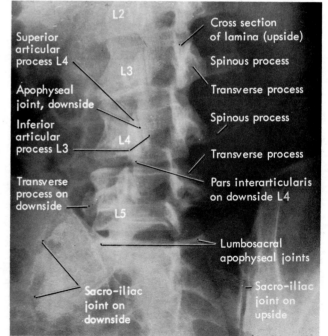

C

Structure of the Intervertebral Disk (Fig. 8–35)

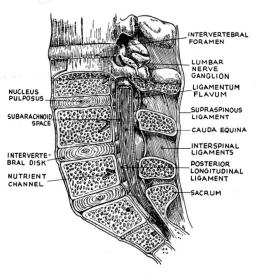

FIGURE 8–35 Structure of intervertebral disk and its relationship to the subarachnoid space and adjoining ligamentous structures.

There is an intervertebral disk between each vertebral body between the second cervical and first sacral segments. Its development has already been described. This structure is described here in considerable detail, as it may cause compression of the spinal cord when degenerated and posteriorly herniated.

The annulus fibrosus forms the major portion of the disk and is composed of lamellated fibrocartilage intimately attached to the epiphyseal bony ring of the adjacent vertebral bodies. Its periphery is reinforced by the longitudinal ligaments.

The nucleus pulposus is the residuum of the notochord and is composed of gelatinous matrix interspersed with fibers from the inner zone of the annulus fibrosus, with which it blends. Its apparent function is to distribute the pressure evenly over the vertebral bodies.

There is a cartilaginous plate cemented to the adjoining surface of the vertebral body, which fuses with the epiphyseal ring of the body. There are vacuolated spaces in this calcified cartilage through which nutrition diffuses for maintenance of the intervertebral disk.

There are numerous places of congenital weakness in the intervertebral disks and cartilaginous end plates which are residua of small vascular channels that have disintegrated and become filled by cartilage as the individual grows and develops. These weaknesses in both the cartilaginous end plates and the disks permit the nucleus pulposus to protrude in one direction or another. When this protrusion occurs into the adjoining vertebral bodies centrally, the phenomenon is referred to as a "Schmorl's node." When, however, the protrusion is posterior or lateral, a compression of a nerve structure may result. Thus, simple Schmorl's nodes of a central type are relatively frequent and asymptomatic. However, protrusion elsewhere may be of definite pathologic significance, producing clinical symptoms and signs.

Other abnormalities in the configuration and dimensions of the intervertebral disk are related to the underlying bone. Thus, for example, when osteoporotic bone is compressed the central portion of the intervertebral disk is in turn depressed; this produces the so-called "fish vertebra," an ellipsoid expansion of the intervertebral disk. In many cases of sickle cell disease or thalassemia, a cuplike defect is produced.

THE VERTEBRAL CANAL AND SPINAL SUBARACHNOID SPACE

Radiographic Anatomy. The vertebral canal tends to be triangular in shape, relatively large in the cervical and lumbar areas, and small and ovoid in the thoracic area. It is bounded by the following structures: (1) Anteriorly lie the posterior longitudinal ligament, the posterior portions of the vertebral bodies, and the posterior margins of the intervertebral disks. (2) Laterally are situated the pedicles of the vertebral bodies, the intervertebral foramina, and the articulating facets. (3) Posteriorly lie the laminae, the ligamenta flava, and the spinous processes. The vertebral canal contains the following structures (Fig. 8–36): (*a*) Centrally, the spinal cord and its meninges are longitudinally placed. (*b*) The spinal nerves and vessels traverse the intervertebral foramina. (*c*) Between the inner margins of the vertebral canal and the meninges is the epidural space. This contains considerable fat, venous plexuses, and nerves (supplying the meninges, intervertebral disks, and ligaments). The fat is most abundant in the thoracic region. There is a small recurrent nerve from the spinal nerves adjoining the division of the latter into anterior and posterior rami that supplies the structures within the vertebral canal.

All of these structures are important in that their aberrations may cause encroachment on the vertebral canal; the site of involvement may be easily determined, but the exact nature of anatomic and pathologic processes may remain obscure.

It will be recalled that the spinal cord lies loosely within its meninges and extends from the foramen magnum to the lower border of the first lumbar vertebra. It has two bulbous enlargements innervating the upper and lower extremities respectively, and below the lower enlargement, it narrows to a cone-shaped structure, the conus medullaris, from which a slender filament, the filum terminale, extends downward to the first segment of the coccyx.

As in the case of the brain, the dura is normally closely applied to the arachnoid, with only a potential subdural space between them. The dura ends in a cone-shaped cul-de-sac, usually in the vicinity of the first or second sacral segment, occasionally somewhat higher. The space between the arachnoid and pia mater investing the cord, the subarachnoid space, is bathed in spinal fluid and is in direct communication with the ventricles of the brain and its surrounding spaces.

The spinal nerves arise at considerably higher levels than their corresponding intervertebral foramina. The cauda equina is formed by the spinal nerves extending below the termination of the spinal cord at L1 level, and these nerves lie free in the subarachnoid space with one exception: just as they leave the vertebral canal they are invested for a short distance by the meningeal covering of the cord, called the nerve sheath. There is a small pouch on the inferior aspect of the nerve sheath near the point of exit called the axillary pouch or subarachnoid pouch (Fig. 8–36 *A*). In the lumbar region, the nerve sheath curves under the vertebral pedicle to reach its exit, and thus has a relatively long extradural but intravertebral course compared with other regions of the spine. The point of exit is below the inferior margin of the intervertebral disk, a fact that is of considerable importance when an aberration of the disk exists because it allows pressure upon the nerve in this vulnerable location.

Pockets of the subarachnoid and dural membranes appear to extend through the intervertebral foramina, accompanying the anterior and posterior roofs of the foramina. The arachnoid membrane thus participates in the formation of a posterior ligament. This ligament, coupled with the ligamentum denticulum, serves to keep the cord in the midline and to prevent its undue rotation. The ligamentum denticulum divides the spinal subarachnoid space into anterior and posterior compartments, but these interconnect considerably. The various nerve roots, both anterior and posterior, cross through the spinal subarachnoid space, receiving a prolongation of the arachnoidal membrane down to a level below the intervertebral foramina.

The posterior part of the spinal subarachnoid space in both the cervical and dorsal regions is subdivided into lateral parts by means of a posterior septum of the arachnoidal membrane. This septum may not be complete and may indeed be very thin and hardly detectable (Fig. 8–36 *B*).

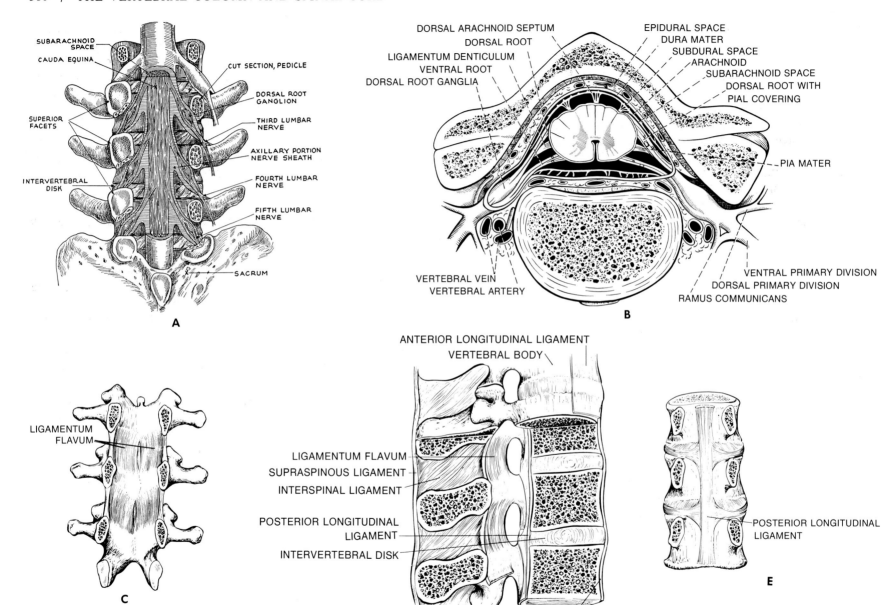

A

SUBARACHNOID SPACE
CAUDA EQUINA
SUPERIOR FACETS
INTERVERTEBRAL DISK

CUT SECTION, PEDICLE
DORSAL ROOT GANGLION
THIRD LUMBAR NERVE
AXILLARY PORTION NERVE SHEATH
FOURTH LUMBAR NERVE
FIFTH LUMBAR NERVE
SACRUM

B

DORSAL ARACHNOID SEPTUM
DORSAL ROOT
LIGAMENTUM DENTICULUM
VENTRAL ROOT
DORSAL ROOT GANGLIA

EPIDURAL SPACE
DURA MATER
SUBDURAL SPACE
ARACHNOID
SUBARACHNOID SPACE
DORSAL ROOT WITH PIAL COVERING
PIA MATER

VERTEBRAL VEIN
VERTEBRAL ARTERY

VENTRAL PRIMARY DIVISION
DORSAL PRIMARY DIVISION
RAMUS COMMUNICANS

C

LIGAMENTUM FLAVUM

D

ANTERIOR LONGITUDINAL LIGAMENT
VERTEBRAL BODY

LIGAMENTUM FLAVUM
SUPRASPINOUS LIGAMENT
INTERSPINAL LIGAMENT
POSTERIOR LONGITUDINAL LIGAMENT
INTERVERTEBRAL DISK

ANTERIOR LONGITUDINAL LIGAMENT

E

POSTERIOR LONGITUDINAL LIGAMENT

See legend on opposite page.

General Features of the Spinal Cord

The spinal cord is approximately 45 cm. long (on the average) in the adult male, and 43 cm. in the adult female. Until the third month of intrauterine life it occupies the entire length of the vertebral canal. However, since the spinal canal grows faster than the spinal cord, the cord terminates at various levels, ranging from the middle of the body of T12 to the superior border of the body of L3; usually, however, it ends somewhere between the inferior border of the body of L1 and the superior border of the body of L2. At birth the lower end of the cord is at the level of the body of L3.

In certain abnormal states, the lower end of the spinal cord remains tethered to the lowest portion of the spinal canal, giving rise to the so-called "tethered cord syndrome."

The spinal cord remains suspended within the spinal canal by lateral ligaments called *ligamenta denticulata*. There is also a cushion of adipose tissue between the dura and spinal cord that contains a considerable venous plexus.

The cord contains an ellipsoid expansion, or bulge, in its contour in the lower half of the cervical spine to accommodate the brachial plexus, and in the region of the lumbosacral to accommodate the lumbosacral plexus. These bulges correspond with the nerve supply of the upper and lower extremities. The greatest dimension of the cord is opposite C5, where it measures 12 to 14 mm. In the lumbar region the cord is enlarged from T10 to T12, with the greatest dimension at T12, where it measures approximately 11 to 13 mm. The cord tapers to its conus medullaris below this level.

The *filum terminalus* is about 6 inches long from the lowest portion of the spinal cord to approximately the level of L2. Generally, it adheres to the posterior aspect of the coccyx. There are two parts to the filum terminalus, internal and external. The internal part is a simple fibrous thread strengthened by dura mater, and the external part is composed largely of pia mater. The latter encloses the terminal part of the central spinal canal in its superior half.

As implied before, the nerves are largest when they form the trunks of the upper and lower limbs and smallest in the coccyx. The thoracic nerves, except for the first, are slender. The cervical nerve roots diminish in size from bottom to top.

Method of Study of the Spinal Subarachnoid Space

Contrast Myelography. The contents of the vertebral canal are studied radiographically by introducing contrast media into either the subarachnoid space or the epidural space (usually the former). The two major methods of study involve the use of either negative or positive contrast media in the subarachnoid space. Dandy (1919) first advocated the use of air, and Sicard and Forestier (1922, 1926) introduced the use of iodized oil (Lipiodol, iodized poppy-seed oil). Various other media have been used. Aqueous media like Thorotrast have been used,

FIGURE 8–36 *A*. Relationship of spinal nerve roots to axillary pouches of the subarachnoid space. *B*. Diagram of the cross section of the spinal cord, showing its meningeal coverings and the manner of exits of the spinal nerves. (After Rauber in Buchana's Functional Anatomy.) *C*. Diagram showing the relationship of the ligamentum flavum adherent to the laminae of adjacent vertebra. *D*. Diagram of ligaments of the spine; anatomical parts are labeled. *E*. The posterior longitudinal ligament is shown in relationship to the spine. (*B–E* modified from Vakili, H.: The Spinal Cord. New York, Intercontinental Medical Book Corp., 1967.)

but they are irritating, and the removal of Thorotrast is very tedious. It has an inherent radioactivity and cannot be left in the vertebral canal; its use in the United States is now forbidden by the Food and Drug Administration. Skiodan is another aqueous contrast medium, but it is irritating and does not produce as satisfactory contrast as do the iodized oils. Experiments with other water-soluble media are being performed with some success. At this writing, the Food and Drug Administration has not approved these for general use.

The best results have been obtained with the oil-type media. Among these, Pantopaque (ethyl-iodophenylundecylenate, discovered in 1944) has been found most satisfactory. It is absorbed at the rate of about 1 cc. per year if left in the vertebral canal, and it may be slightly less irritating than Lipiodol. Ordinarily it is removed following the examination.

TECHNIQUE. With the patient in the prone position, 6 to 15 ml. of the iodized oil is introduced at the level of the third or fourth lumbar interspace (Fig. 8–37 A). It is desirable if possible to avoid the interspace in which the pathologic condition is suspected, since the introduction of the needle at this level may introduce a small area of hemorrhage that may complicate the interpretation of the findings. The needle is usually left in place to facilitate removal of the contrast medium after completion of the examination, unless it is desired to examine the thoracic subarachnoid space particularly.

First the patient is almost erect, so that the caudal sac may be studied in posterior, anterior, oblique, and lateral decubitus projections. The patient is then slowly moved into a horizontal position (Fig. 8–37 B), with each interspace studied fully. The horizontal beam study is particularly valuable, because it may outline a posteriorly herniated disk with the patient prone, whereas other techniques may not show this as clearly (Fig. 8–38 D). Then, with the patient still prone, the table is tilted under fluoroscopic control until the medium reaches the thoracic spine. At this point, the oil column may break up, but by tilting the table and at the same time hyperextending the patient's head, the oil medium, being heavier than spinal fluid, will be trapped in the cervical region. Once the main bulk of the medium is in this region, the table may be turned back to horizontal level. By carefully flexing the patient's head and tilting the table head downward at the same time, the entire cervical subarachnoid space can be visualized to the level of the foramen magnum. Again, posteroanterior and lateral decubitus films are obtained (Fig. 8–38 E and F).

If it is desirable to delineate the internal acoustic meatus and clivus, the following procedure should be carefully carried out. After the oil medium is on the clivus but not in the cranial cavity itself, the patient's head is carefully rotated with the chin toward the right, and then lowered just enough to trap a droplet of oil in the internal acoustic meatus. When this has been done, appropriate films are immediately obtained and the oil is once again returned to its position on the clivus (Fig. 8–39 A). In the same way, the head is then rotated to the opposite side and a similar film and fluoroscopic study of the opposite meatus is obtained. It is best to place an opaque object such as a lead number in each external auditory meatus to facilitate orientation during fluoroscopy. It is imperative during this procedure that there be close cooperation between the fluoroscopist and the person holding the patient's head. Moreover, image amplification and closed circuit television fluoroscopy are useful if best results are to be achieved. Usually all of the Pantopaque can be recovered through the lumbar needle by appropriately tilting the table and the patient.

If a special examination of the thoracic subarachnoid space is desired, the needle may be removed, the patient turned to the supine position, and the Pantopaque collected in the concavity of the thoracic spine. Usually larger volumes of the Pantopaque are necessary for a satisfactory examination of this region.

The width of the myelographic shadow varies considerably in accordance with the width of the vertebral canal. *If the width of the column is less than 16 mm., it is considered that the examination will not accurately reflect anatomic changes in the vertebral canal.*

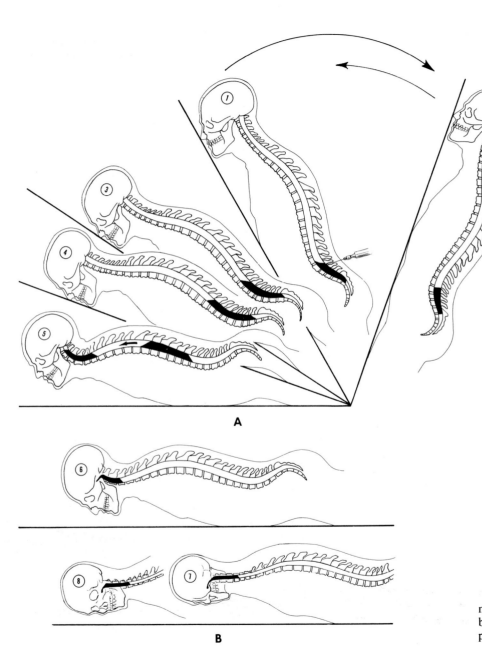

A

B

FIGURE 8–37 Position of patient during myelography. *A.* Position for lumbar and cervical segments. *B.* Position for visualization of region of clivus and internal acoustic meati (see text for description of movements).

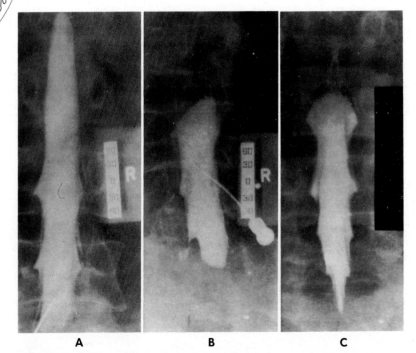

A   **B**   **C**

FIGURE 8–38 Sample radiographs of lumbar cervical and thoracic myelograms. *A,* Lumbar myelogram. *B.* Oblique view of lower lumbar and beginning entry to caudal sac. *C.* Lower lumbar and caudal sac, antero-posterior view.

Legend continued on following page.

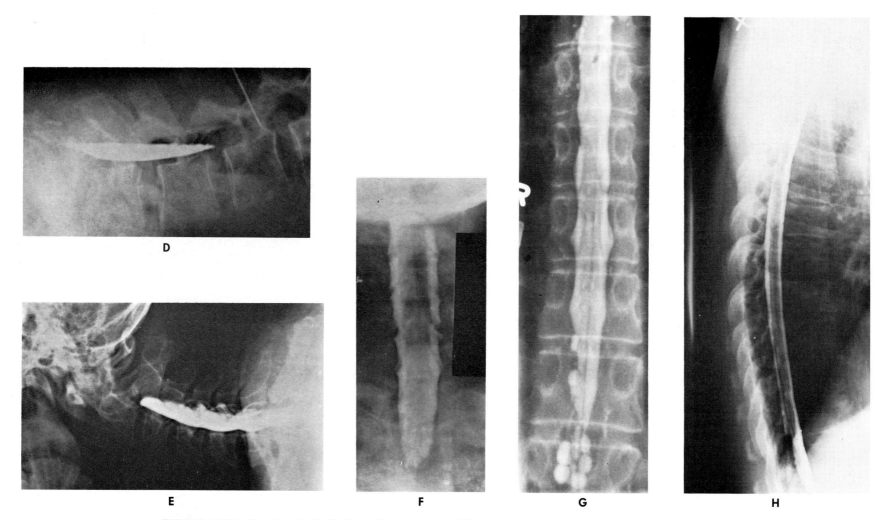

FIGURE 8–38 *Continued. D.* Horizontal beam study of lower lumbar and lumbosacral junction. *E.* Horizontal beam study of cervical segments, see third to seventh cervical segments. *F.* Anteroposterior cervical myelogram; see third to seventh cervical segments. *G* and *H.* Normal anteroposterior and horizontal beam lateral views of the thoracic myelograms.

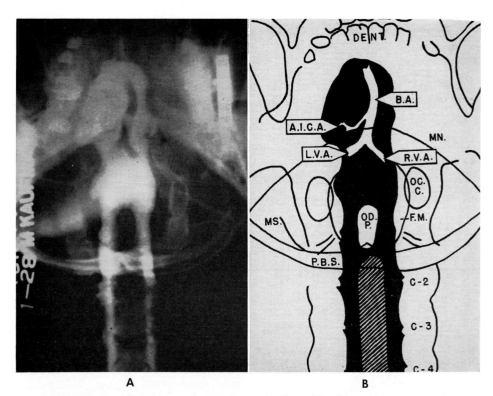

A

B

FIGURE 8–39 Normal anteroposterior projection of the foramen magnum and clivus myelogram. (From Malis, L. I.: Radiology, *70*:196–221, 1958.) *A*. Radiograph. *B*. Diagrammatic tracing of radiograph with anatomic parts labeled. (A.I.C.A.) anterior inferior cerebellar artery, (L.V.A.) left verterbral artery, (R.V.A.) right verterbral artery, (B.A.) basilar artery, (MS.) mastoids, (F.M.) foramen magnum, (O.D.P.) odontoid process; (P.B.S.) posterior base of skull.

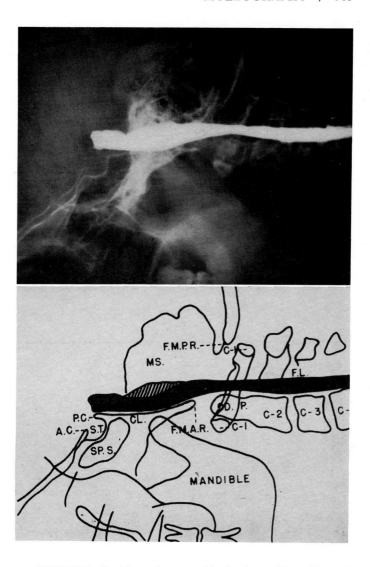

FIGURE 8–40 Normal cross-table (horizontal beam) lateral view of cervical myelogram with Pantopaque on the clivus, in same position as in Figure 8–39. (F.M.P.R.) foramen magnum posterior rim, (MS.) mastoids, (P.C.) posterior clinoids, (A.C.) anterior clinoids, (S.T.) sella turcica, (SP.S.) sphenoid sinus, (CL) clivus, (F.M.A.R.) foramen magnum, anterior rim, (OD.P.) odontoid process, (F.L.) fluid level of Pantopaque. The cervical segments are labeled by number. (From Malis, L. I.: Radiology, *70*:196–221, 1958.)

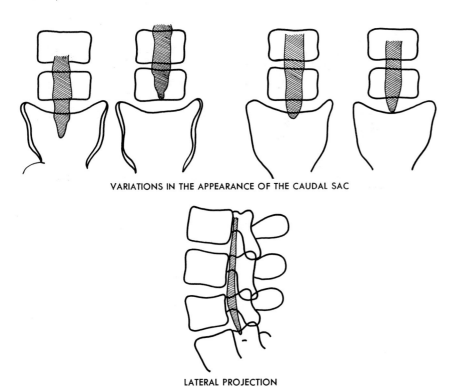

VARIATIONS IN THE APPEARANCE OF THE CAUDAL SAC

LATERAL PROJECTION

FIGURE 8–41 Variations in appearance of the terminal theca with the patient in the erect position.

According to Gates* (1976), with the head of the table elevated 60 degrees from the horizontal, thereby insuring the filling of the distal subarachnoid space, and by angling the overhead tube 15 degrees cranially and directing the central ray at the lumbosacral junction, a 45-degree

relationship between the plane of the table and the radiographic beam is produced. A cross-table horizontal beam study with the film perpendicular to the table top may also be produced at this time. The resulting radiographs have allowed for improved assessment of nerve root detail in the region of the fifth lumbar vertebra and below.

Air Contrast Studies of the Spinal Subarachnoid Space. Air in the spinal subarachnoid space for diagnosis and localization of spinal cord lesions has been utilized since 1925 (Dandy). The method of Girout has probably achieved the widest use, with some modifications (Girout; Lindgren; Murtagh et al.; Wende and Beer).* The procedure is performed as follows: the patient is placed in a sitting position with the cervical spine anteflexed so that the cervical spinal cord is at the highest level of the cerebrospinal fluid pathway (Fig. 8–43). This position is maintained by a head rest under the forehead of the patient. A lumbar puncture is performed in a routine manner, but no fluid is withdrawn. Next, 20 cubic cm. of air is slowly injected and an upright roentgenogram is taken in the lateral projection. Additional air is then injected in 20 cubic cm. increments until the upper cervical spinal cord is completely visualized. An average volume of 40 cc. of air is used for cervical air myelography, but volumes of 80 cc. or more are occasionally required. High kilovoltage technique and tomography are essential for best results. Murtagh et al. tilted the patient in different positions for visualization of different parts of the spinal cord.

The Blood Supply of the Spinal Cord

The main blood supply of the spinal cord is formed by: (1) the *anterior spinal artery,* beginning at the junction of the corresponding branches of the vertebral arteries; (2) the *posterior spinal arteries,* which are continuations of the posterior spinal branches of the vertebral arteries; and (3) extensive *segmental anastomoses between the anterior*

---

*Gates, G. F.: 45-degree central ray angulation for improved lumbosacral myelography. Radiol. Technol., *47*:301–305, 1976.

*The additional references may be obtained in Meschan, I.: An Atlas of Anatomy Basic to Radiology. Philadelphia, W. B. Saunders Co., 1975.

and posterior spinal arteries through their pial branches as described earlier. The anterior spinal artery extends the length of the spinal cord in the anterior longitudinal fissure, and the posterior spinal arteries run the length of the cord in the posterolateral sulci. There are additional *radicular arteries,* as described.

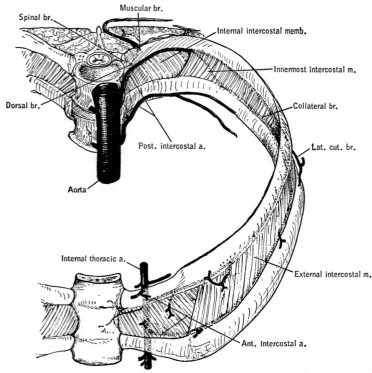

FIGURE 8–42 Diagram showing the plan of branching of the anterior and posterior intercostal arteries. (From Anson, B. J. (ed.): Morris's Human Anatomy, 12th ed. Copyright © 1966 by McGraw-Hill, Inc. Used by permission of McGraw-Hill Book Company.)

The major supplying vessel of the dorsal and lumbar cord is the *artery of Adamkiewicz* (also called the arterioradicularis magna [ARM]). In 75 per cent of cases it arises on the left between the ninth and the twelfth thoracic nerve roots. An intercostal artery in this area branches into the artery of the dorsal lumbar enlargement, which in turn divides into two rami, one supplying the posterior spinal artery and the other the artery of Adamkiewicz, with an anterior destination.

The ARM has a characteristic hairpin-like appearance and a slender ascending branch that joins the thoracic portion of the anterior spinal artery (Fig. 8–45). It has a somewhat larger descending branch that anastomoses with the posterior spinal arteries and the lumbosacral radicular arteries to form the vascular terminal conus. During arteriography, subtraction techniques are often necessary to demonstrate these delicate and sinuous arteries.

It should be emphasized that the ARM represents the major segmental arterial supply to the lower dorsal and lumbar segments of the spinal cord. The relationship of spinal cord complications following aortography and aortic surgery to injury of the ARM is well recognized. The ARM arises as the largest anterior radicular branch from one of the lower intercostal or upper lumbar (T8 to L4) segmental arteries. Unusual origins from as high as T5 or as low as L5 have been reported. In over 60 per cent of cases it is left-sided and passes through the intervertebral foramen with a corresponding anterior nerve root. It turns cranially and ascends along the lateral and anterior surface of the cord to the anterior median sulcus, where it bifurcates into a small ascending and a large descending branch. These branches become the anterior spinal artery at this cord level, usually anastomosing with a very small descending branch in the midthoracic area. As it turns into the anterior spinal region to become the anterior spinal artery of the lower cord and conus, the hairpin configuration is very noticeable.

The *vertebral veins* (Fig. 8–46) are derived from the substance of the spinal cord and terminate in a plexus in the pia mater, in which six longitudinal channels have been described. The vertebral veins, which terminate in the cranium, are also known as *Batson's plexus.*

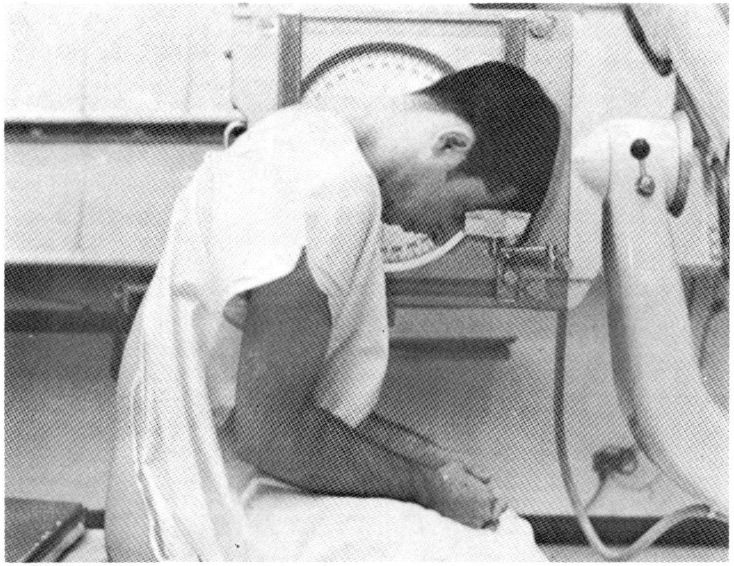

A

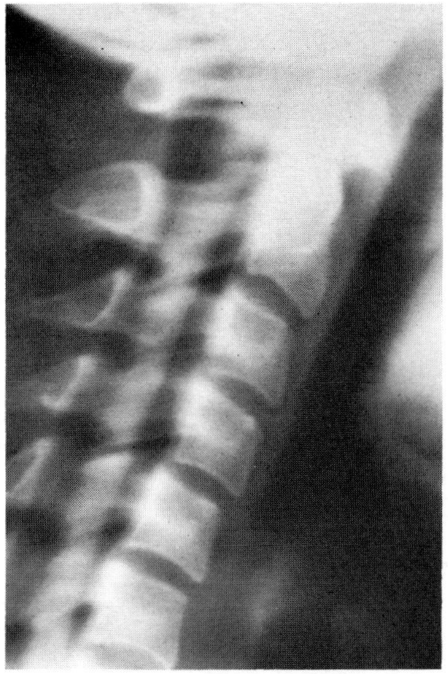

B

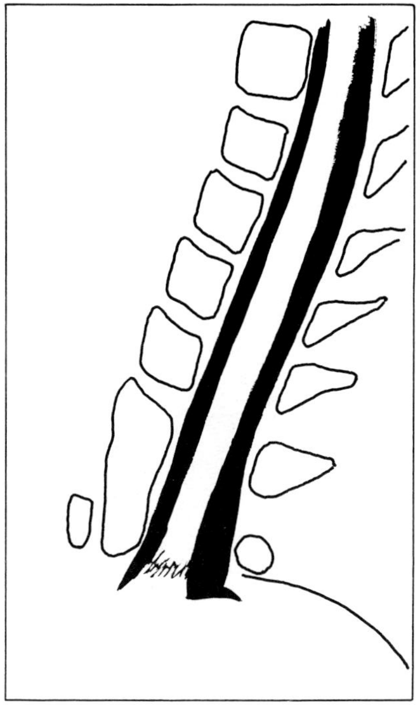

C

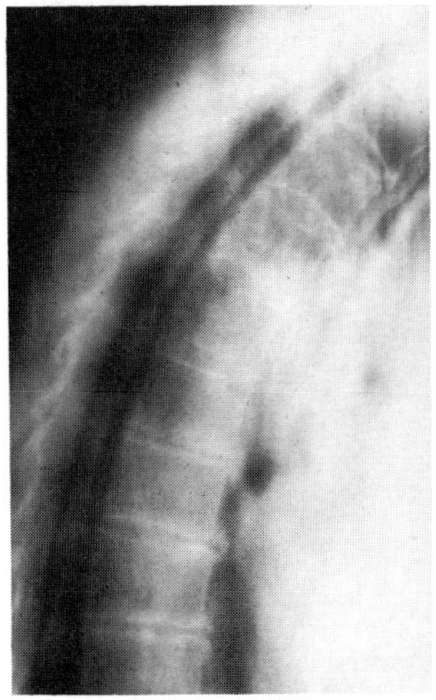

D

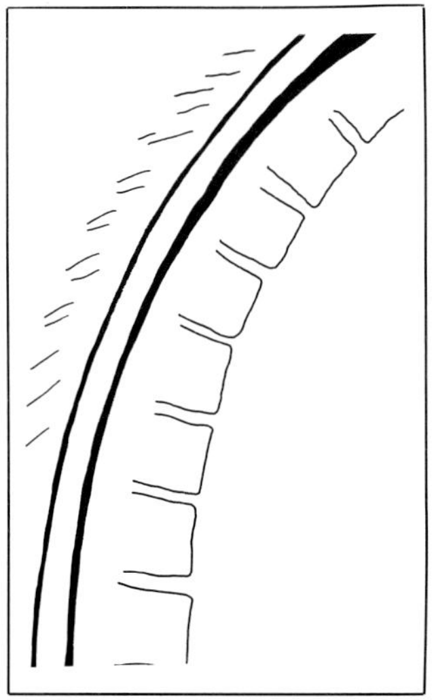

E

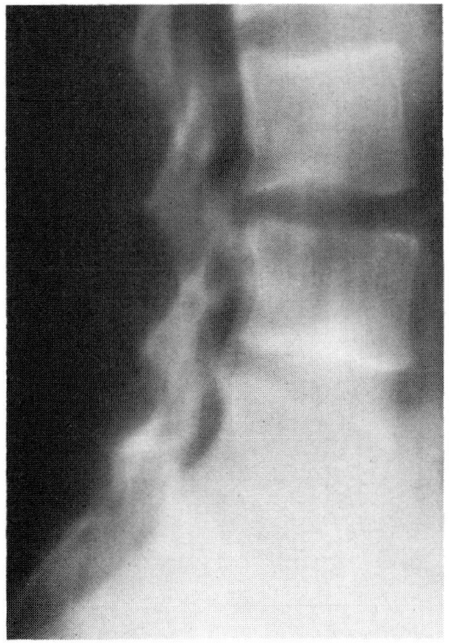

F

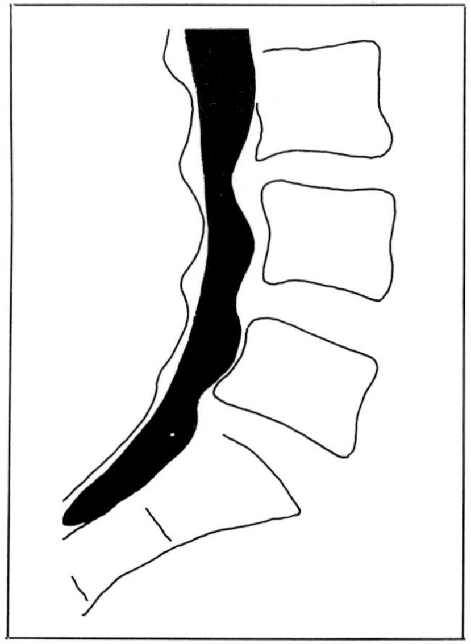

G

FIGURE 8–43 *A*. Position of patient for lumbar puncture and cervical myelography. (From Southworth et al.: Am. J. Roentgenol., *104*:487, 1969.) *B*. and *C*. Normal cervical cord. *D*. and *E*. Normal thoracic cord. *F* and *G*. Protruding disk at L4–L5. (*B, C, D, E, F, and G* from Wende, S., and Beer, K.: Am. J. Roentgenol., *104*:213–218, 1968.)

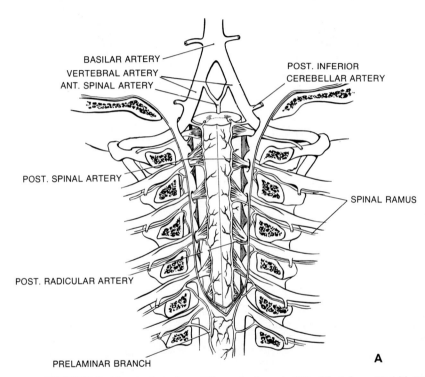

BASILAR ARTERY
VERTEBRAL ARTERY
ANT. SPINAL ARTERY

POST. INFERIOR
CEREBELLAR ARTERY

POST. SPINAL ARTERY

SPINAL RAMUS

POST. RADICULAR ARTERY

PRELAMINAR BRANCH

A

FIGURE 8–44 *A*. Arteries of the spinal cord. (Modified from Vakili, H.: The Spinal Cord. New York, Intercontinental Medical Book Corp., 1967.)

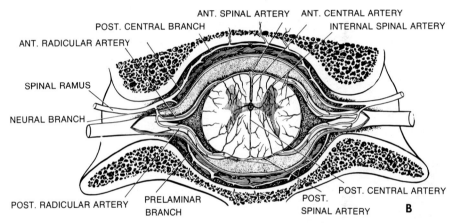

ANT. SPINAL ARTERY   ANT. CENTRAL ARTERY
POST. CENTRAL BRANCH
INTERNAL SPINAL ARTERY
ANT. RADICULAR ARTERY

SPINAL RAMUS

NEURAL BRANCH

POST. RADICULAR ARTERY   PRELAMINAR
BRANCH

POST. CENTRAL ARTERY

POST.
SPINAL ARTERY   B

FIGURE 8–44 *B*. Arteries of the spinal cord diagrammatically shown in horizontal section. (Modified from Vakili, H.: The Spinal Cord. New York, Intercontinental Medical Book Corp., 1967.)

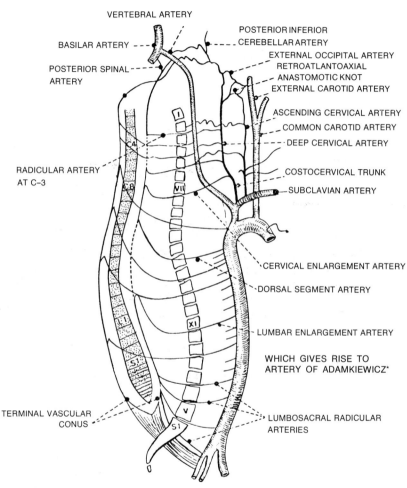

FIGURE 8–45 Drawing of the blood supply of the spinal cord. (Modified from Djindjian, R.: Am. J. Roentgenol., *107*:461–478, 1969.)

*The artery of Adamkiewicz becomes extremely important when it is the major blood supply of the spinal cord at or below its level. Spasm, or occlusion (as might occur from angiographic study in this immediate vicinity), may give rise to significant complications in the patient.

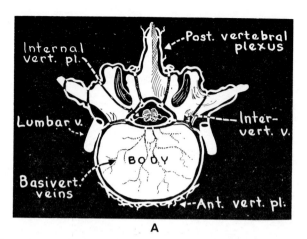

FIGURE 8–46 *A.* Diagrammatic representation of the vertebral plexuses at the lumbar level (seen from above). The external plexuses include anterior components in front of the vertebral bodies and posterior components, which surround the spinous and transverse processes. The internal plexuses include the dural and spinal veins; the longitudinal sinuses; and the basivertebral veins, which drain the vertebral bodies. The internal and external plexuses communicate with the intervertebral veins, which terminate in the lumbar veins. The lumbar veins are connected both with the inferior vena cava and the ascending lumbar veins. (From Abrams, H. L.: Angiography, 2nd ed. Vol. 1. Boston, Little, Brown & Co., 1971.)

Figure continued on opposite page.

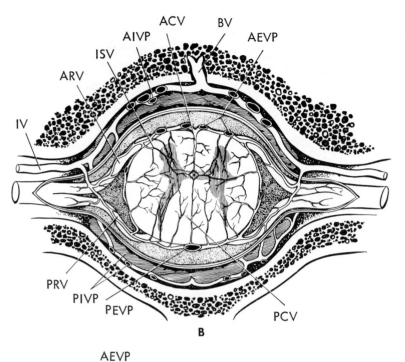

B

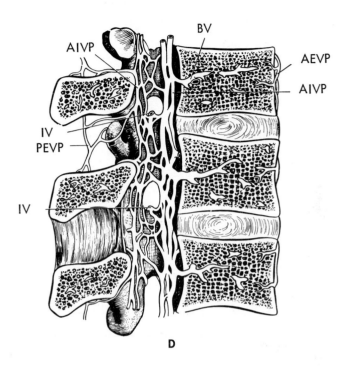

D

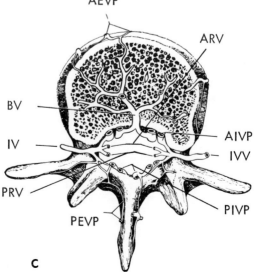

C

FIGURE 8–46 *Continued. B.* (IV) intervertebral vein, (ARV) anterior radicular vein, (ISV) internal spinal vein, (AIVP) anterior internal vertebral plexus, (ACV) anterior cerebral veins, (BV) basivertebral vein, (AEVP) anterior external vertebral plexus, (PRV) posterior-radicular vein, (PIVP) posterior internal vertebral plexus, (PEVP) posterior external vertebral plexus, (PCV) posterior central vein.

C. (AEVP) anterior external vertebral plexus, (BV) basivertebral vein, (IV) intervertebral vein, (PEVP) posterior external vertebral plexus, (ARV) anterior radicular vein, (PRV) posterior radicular vein, (PIVP) posterior internal vertebral plexus, (AIVP) anterior internal vertebral plexus, (IVV) internal vertebral vein. (Modified from Vakili, H.: The Spinal Cord. New York, Intercontinental Medical Book Corp., 1967.)

D. (AIVP) anterior internal vertebral plexus, (IV) intervertebral vein, (PEVP) posterior external vertebral plexus, (BV) basivertebral vein, (AEVP) anterior external vertebral plexus, (AIVP) anterior internal vertebral plexus. (Modified from Vakili, H.: The Spinal Cord. New York, Intercontinental Medical Book Corp., 1967.)

9

THE RESPIRATORY SYSTEM

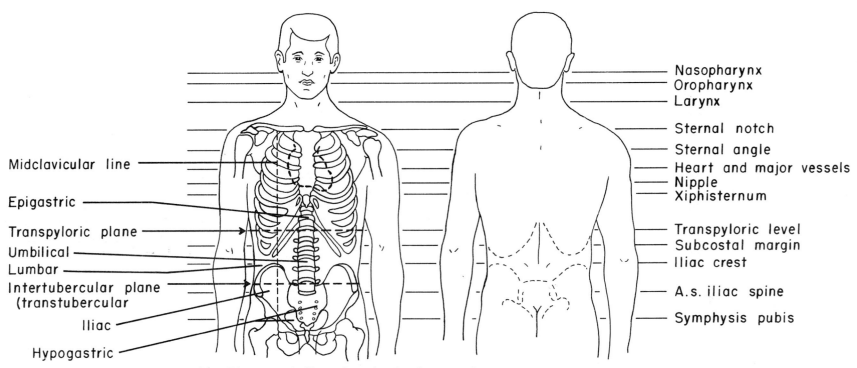

Midclavicular line

Epigastric

Transpyloric plane

Umbilical

Lumbar

Intertubercular plane
(transtubercular

Iliac

Hypogastric

Nasopharynx
Oropharynx
Larynx

Sternal notch

Sternal angle

Heart and major vessels
Nipple
Xiphisternum

Transpyloric level

Subcostal margin

Iliac crest

A.s. iliac spine

Symphysis pubis

FIGURE 9–1 Diagrammatic illustrations showing the anatomic correlation between surface and internal anatomy of the thorax and abdomen.

The respiratory tract can be conveniently subdivided for purposes of discussion into: (1) the upper air passages, (2) the larynx, (3) the trachea and bronchi, (4) the lung parenchyma, (5) the vascular supply, venous drainage, and lymphatics of the respiratory tract, (6) the lung hili, and (7) the thoracic cage, pleura, and diaphragm.

THE UPPER AIR PASSAGES

The upper air passages are usually amenable to direct and indirect inspection to such a great extent that radiography need not often be employed. Nevertheless, because considerable useful information can be obtained by fluoroscopic and radiographic methods, a consideration of this subject is worthwhile.

The nasal and upper air passages are referred to anatomically as the pharynx. This, in turn, consists of three fundamental areas: (1) the nasopharynx, which extends from the nasal cavity anteriorly and the base of the skull superiorly to the tip of the uvula and margin of the soft palate below; (2) the oropharynx, which extends from the soft palate above to the epiglottis and its pharyngoepiglottic folds, opposite the hyoid bone; and (3) the laryngeal pharynx, which extends from the hyoid bone above to the upper boundary of the esophagus below, opposite the sixth cervical vertebra (posterior to the larynx). The larynx itself is considered separately.

The pharynx is approximately 12 cm. in length. It communicates with the nasal cavity, the oral cavity, the middle ear via the auditory (eustachian) tube, the esophagus, and the trachea. The vital structures on either side of the pharynx are: the carotid arteries, the jugular veins, the ninth, tenth, eleventh, and twelfth cranial nerves, the cervical sympathetic chain, important lymph nodal chains, and important fascial planes which may extend into the mediastinum.

Nasopharynx (Fig. 9–2). The anterior boundary of the nasopharynx is formed by the choanae, with the vomer of the nasal septum between them. The posterior wall lies above the level of the anterior arch or tubercle of the atlas of the cervical spine and usually contains considerable lymphatic tissue, which is continuous with a ring of lymphatic tissue around the circumference of the pharynx. The lateral nasopharyngeal walls are concave outward or sigmoidal in contour, due to the soft tissue prominence surrounding the nasopharyngeal opening of the eustachian tube, the *torus tubarius*. Posterolateral to the torus tubarius is the fossa of Rosenmüller or pharyngeal recess. The normal nasopharyngeal air shadow on basal projection does not project beyond the bony pterygoids owing to muscular structures in its lateral walls as well as its attachment to the skull base. These structures are indicated radiographically in Figure 9–2 *A* and *B*. The shadows of the oropharynx and pyriform sinuses may be superimposed upon the nasopharyngeal air column (Fig. 9–2 *C*); they may project behind the anterior arch of C1 or extend beyond the bony pterygoids, usually presenting a convex border laterally. The uvula is often identified as a nodular structure surrounded by oropharyngeal air (Fig. 9–2 *C*).

The adenoids of children are composed of the lymphatic tissue on the posterior wall of the nasopharynx, which tends to become atrophic in adults. As a result, the soft tissue width of the nasopharyngeal posterior wall is considerably greater in children than in adults, and tends to swell forward and downward toward the soft palate in the very young. The extent of this swelling is readily visualized on the lateral radiograph of the child's neck and furnishes an accurate means of evaluating the extent of adenoid hypertrophy.

Oropharynx. The oropharynx is the common passageway of both the digestive tract (mouth to esophagus) and the respiratory tract (nasopharynx to larynx). It is bounded anteriorly by the posterior third of the tongue, which contains lymphoid follicles, and posteriorly by the soft tissue covering of the upper three cervical spine segments.

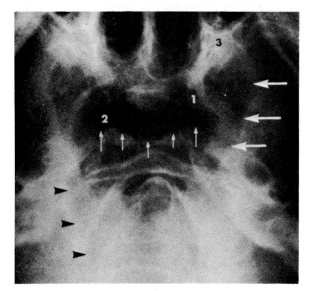

A

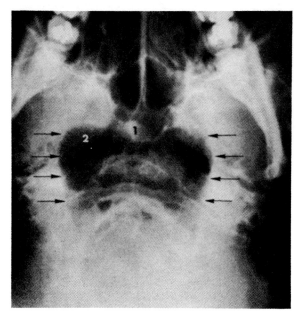

B

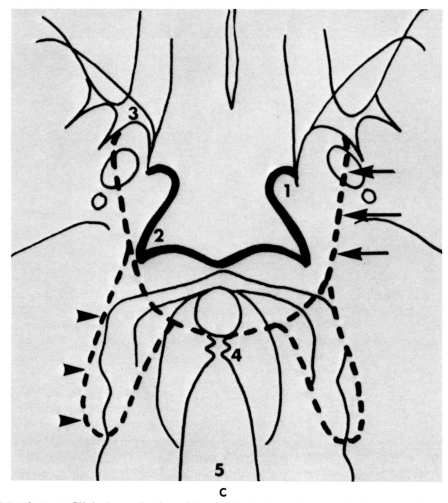

C

FIGURE 9–2 *A*. Clinical examination of the skull in the base view clearly demonstrating the outline of the nasopharynx. (1) Torus tubarius; (2) fossa of Rosenmüller; (3) pterygoid process; vertical arrows, posterior wall.

The oropharynx is convex outward and laterally situated (horizontal arrows). Arrowheads define piriform sinus.

B. Clinical radiograph in the base view. The oropharyngeal air shadow (horizontal arrows) is seen with its convex lateral margins projecting beyond the lateral pterygoid processes. The uvula (1) is surrounded by oropharyngeal air. The lateral concavity formed by the torus tubarius (2) is outlined by nasopharyngeal air and is seen apart from the more inferiorly related oropharynx.

C. Composite schematic drawing of *A* and *B*. (1) Torus tubarius; (2) fossa of Rosenmüller; (3) pterygoid process; (4) vocal cords; (5) trachea; bold line, nasopharynx; arrows, oropharynx; arrowheads, piriform sinus. (From Rizzuti, R. J., and Whalen, J. P.: Radiology, *104*:537–540, 1972.)

On each lateral wall of the oropharynx is the tonsillar fossa with its anterior and posterior pillars. Embedded between these pillars is the palatine or faucial tonsil.

Laryngeal Pharynx (Fig. 9–3). The laryngeal pharynx connects with the oropharynx above and the esophagus below. It is bounded posteriorly by the soft tissues overlying the fourth, fifth, and sixth cervical vertebrae, and anteriorly by the posterior wall of the larynx. The posterior wall of the larynx contains the arytenoid cartilages and the lamina of the cricoid cartilage. The lateral walls of this area are attached to the thyroid cartilage and to the hyoid bone. The epiglottis is situated anteriorly and superiorly, in the median plane, with the aryepiglottic folds extending posteriorly and inferiorly from the epiglottis to the arytenoids. Beneath the level of these folds on each side are the pyriform sinuses. The valleculae are hollow pockets situated between the epiglottis and the dorsal aspect of the tongue just lateral to the median plane.

THE LARYNX

The cartilaginous framework is illustrated in Figure 9–3. This consists of three large single cartilages: the thyroid, cricoid, and epiglottis; and three paired cartilages: the corniculate, cuneiform, and arytenoids.

The thyroid cartilage is composed of two wings or laminae, and two superior and two inferior horns or cornua. The superior margins of the two wings are convex and meet at the superior thyroid notch at an angle of 90 degrees in the male and 120 degrees in the female, which explains the greater laryngeal prominence in the male.

The cricoid cartilage attaches to and rests upon the first cartilaginous ring of the trachea, below the thyroid cartilage. It has the shape of a signet ring, being expanded posteriorly. This broad posterior aspect, or lamina, has a ridge centrally for attachment to the esophagus, an

upper elliptical surface for attachment to the arytenoid cartilages, and inner impressions for attachment of the cricoarytenoid muscles. The inferior horns of the thyroid cartilage articulate with the lateral aspect of the cricoid ring.

The arytenoid cartilages are paired pyramidal cartilages surmounting the laminae of the cricoid posteriorly, while the corniculate cartilages are mounted superiorly on the arytenoids. The cuneiform cartilages are embedded in the aryepiglottic folds.

The epiglottic cartilage is situated behind the root of the tongue above the thyroid cartilage and behind the body of the hyoid bone. It lies in front of and above the superior opening of the larynx and acts to deflect the swallowed bolus of food to either side into the pyriform fossae. The aryepiglottic folds act as a sphincter, preventing the food bolus from entering the larynx and trachea.

The thyroid, cricoid, and the greater part of the arytenoid cartilages are composed of hyaline cartilage that tends to calcify late in life and may be transformed into bone. The rest of the cartilages are composed for the most part of fibrocartilage, and do not calcify. The calcification may be irregular, and these open spaces must not be misinterpreted as erosion of the cartilage. Also, these areas of calcification must not be misinterpreted as foreign bodies in the esophagus or larynx. This distinction is readily made if barium is administered to the patient and the barium column is then seen to go behind the larynx.

Cavity of the Larynx. The laryngeal aditus or superior laryngeal aperture or inlet is readily identified on the soft tissue films of the larynx (Fig. 9–5) as an opening bounded by the epiglottis in front and the aryepiglottic folds on each side. The pyriform recess or sinus is identified just outside the aditus on either side, between the aryepiglottic fold and the inner wall of the thyroid cartilage.

The vestibule or upper laryngeal compartment of the larynx extends from the laryngeal aditus to the ventricular folds (false vocal cords). The narrow opening between the ventricular folds is the vestibular slit.

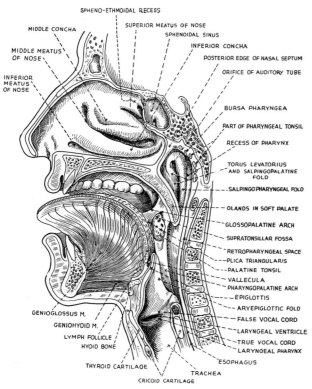

FIGURE 9-3 Sagittal section of the head and neck demonstrating the structure of the nasopharynx and larynx.

TABLE 9-1. Measurements Shown in Figure 9-4

		Range (in mm.)	Mean (in mm.)	Standard Deviation (in mm.)
A-B	Posterior wall of nasopharynx	12–24	18.4	2.5
C-D	Roof of nasopharynx	2–10.5	5.9	2.2
F-G	Postpharyngeal space	1.5–4.5	3.1	0.7
H-I	Post-tracheal space	8–17	12.4	1.9
J-H	Anteroposterior diameter of trachea (male)	15–23.5	19.2	1.8
	Anteroposterior diameter of trachea (female)	11.5–18	14.5	1.3

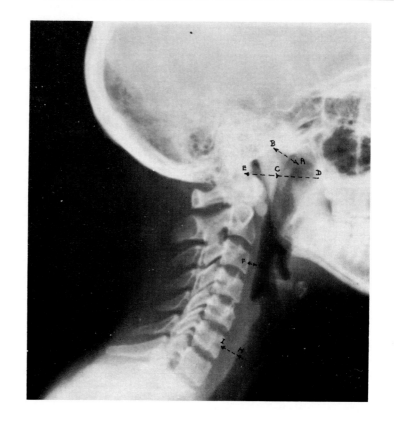

FIGURE 9-4 Measurements of the posterior wall of the nasopharynx, roof of the nasopharynx, postpharyngeal space, post-tracheal space, and the trachea itself in adults. (See also Table 9-1.) Comparative measurements for children are described in the text.

The middle laryngeal compartment is situated between the ventricular folds above and the vocal folds (true vocal cords) below. The ventricular folds are indented on each side by a small lateral outpouching forming the laryngeal ventricle.

The "rima glottidis" is an elongated slitlike opening between the true vocal folds. This is the narrowest part of the laryngeal cavity.

The portion of the laryngeal cavity below the level of the vocal folds is the lower laryngeal compartment and is the inferior entrance to the glottis. It changes from a slit to a rounded cavity surrounded by the cricoid cartilage below and is continuous with the trachea. This portion is a favorable site for the development of edema because of its loose connective tissue.

Articulations of the Laryngeal Cartilages. The cricothyroid articulation is lined with synovial membrane and is a typical arthrodial joint. As such it is subject to all of the diseases of the synovial joints and is of particular importance in rheumatoid arthritis or collagen diseases in which cricothyroid articular disease may occur, with esophageal cricothyroid pseudobulbar palsy and adjoining esophageal spasm. The cricoarytenoid articulation is also a typical arthrodial joint.

Position of the Larynx in the Neck. In fetal and infantile life the larynx is situated high in the neck, descending in later life. In a fetus of 6 months, the organ is in a position two vertebrae higher than in the adult. The larynx in general follows the thoracic viscera in their subsidence, which continues until old age.

At birth the space between the hyoid bone and the thyroid cartilage is relatively small and increases but little during early life.

Comparison of Width of the Retrolaryngeal Space with the Retrotracheal Space. The measurements of the nasopharynx, retropharyngeal space, post-tracheal space, and the trachea itself are shown in Figure 9–4. They are given by range, mean, and standard deviation.

These measurements tend to vary considerably with age, being larger, relatively, in the retropharyngeal and retrolaryngeal areas in the child than in the adult. A good base line for comparison in the child is the anteroposterior measurement of the C4 vertebra. Up to the age of 1 year, the postpharyngeal measurement is 1.5 times this length, and the postlaryngeal measurement is 2.0 times this measurement. From 1 year to 2, it is 0.5 and 1.5 times, respectively. From 2 years to 3, it is 0.5 and 1.2 times C4. From 3 years of age to adolescence, it is 0.3 and 1.2 times C4. In adults, it is 0.3 and approximately 0.6 or 0.7 of C4, respectively.

Eller et al.* carried out a careful statistical study of the nasopharyngeal soft tissues in males and females and plotted these against age with upper and lower tolerance limits. It was clear from this study that the amount of nasopharyngeal soft tissue in adults decreased with age and varied slightly between the sexes. However, the range of variation was so great that these investigators found this knowledge of little practical significance. It was also suggested that the involution of nasopharyngeal tissue was not complete by age 25 but continued throughout life. They recommended that other features of the nasopharynx should be regarded as more important than the measurements of the nasopharyngeal soft tissues. For example, there were two consistent features: (1) the roof thickness of the nasopharynx was always less than the thickness of the posterior wall (with one exception in which they were equal); and (2) there was a smooth concave contour of the soft tissue outline of the nasopharynx. Changes in these relationships should be regarded as significant.

---

*Eller, J. L., Roberts, J. F., and Ziter, F. M. H., Jr.: Normal nasopharyngeal soft tissue in adults: a statistical study. Am. J. Roentgenol., *112*:537–541, 1971.

Radiographic Methods of Study

The air passages are moderately well demonstrated by the fluoroscope and radiograph.

In addition to identifying the anatomic structures already described, the *fluoroscopic adjunct permits visualization of the movement of the vocal cords* in the anteroposterior projection, with phonation.

Soft Tissue Lateral Film of the Neck (with and without Barium) (Fig. 9–5). Visualization of the larynx is enhanced if the hypopharynx is distended with air by an effort at expiration with the mouth and nostrils closed. It is also helpful to extend the tongue. The technique is very similar to that employed for demonstration of the cervical spine, except that a "soft exposure" technique is employed. Barium may or may not be employed in the pharynx, as desired.

The pyriform sinuses and vallecula are best studied with the aid of Dionosil oily in the pharynx.

Xeroradiography has proved to be particularly helpful in the study of the soft tissues of the neck. The vocal cords, cartilage, soft tissues, bone, and tumors, if present, have a slightly different appearance of density in this method of representation (Fig. 9–6).

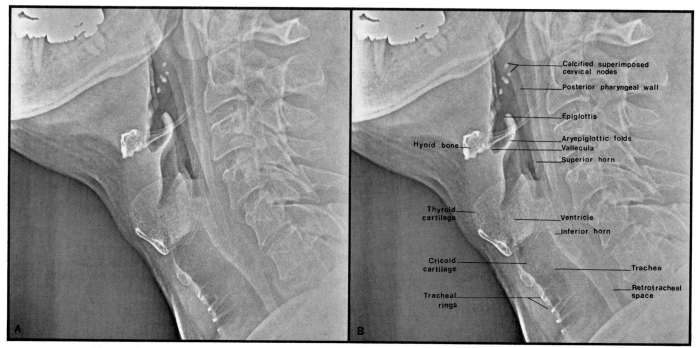

FIGURE 9–5 Normal larynx and trachea of a 55-year-old man is shown by (A) with structures of same xeroradiogram identified by (B). (From Xeroradiography, published by Xerox Corporation, Pasadena, California 91107. Courtesy of Dr. P. Holinger.)

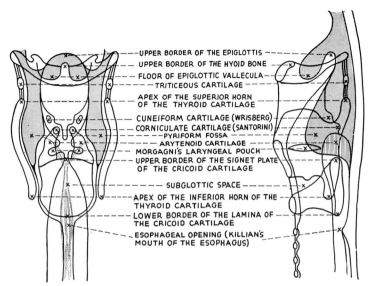

FIGURE 9–6 General schematic representation of the roentgen anatomy of the larynx and pharynx.

Labels on Figure 9–6:
- UPPER BORDER OF THE EPIGLOTTIS
- UPPER BORDER OF THE HYOID BONE
- FLOOR OF EPIGLOTTIC VALLECULA
- TRITICEOUS CARTILAGE
- APEX OF THE SUPERIOR HORN OF THE THYROID CARTILAGE
- CUNEIFORM CARTILAGE (WRISBERG)
- CORNICULATE CARTILAGE (SANTORINI)
- PYRIFORM FOSSA
- ARYTENOID CARTILAGE
- MORGAGNI'S LARYNGEAL POUCH
- UPPER BORDER OF THE SIGNET PLATE OF THE CRICOID CARTILAGE
- SUBGLOTTIC SPACE
- APEX OF THE INFERIOR HORN OF THE THYROID CARTILAGE
- LOWER BORDER OF THE LAMINA OF THE CRICOID CARTILAGE
- ESOPHAGEAL OPENING (KILLIAN'S MOUTH OF THE ESOPHAGUS)

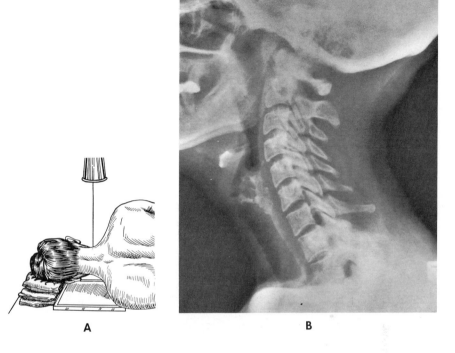

A

B

FIGURE 9–7 Lateral soft tissue film of the neck. *A*. Position of patient. *B*. Radiograph. *C*. Labeled film of *B*.

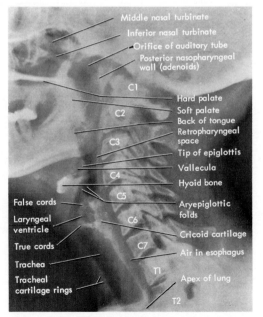

Labels on Figure 9–7 C:
- Middle nasal turbinate
- Inferior nasal turbinate
- Orifice of auditory tube
- Posterior nasopharyngeal wall (adenoids)
- C1
- Hard palate
- Soft palate
- C2
- Back of tongue
- Retropharyngeal space
- C3
- Tip of epiglottis
- Vallecula
- C4
- Hyoid bone
- False cords
- C5
- Aryepiglottic folds
- Laryngeal ventricle
- C6
- True cords
- Cricoid cartilage
- Trachea
- C7
- Air in esophagus
- Tracheal cartilage rings
- T1
- Apex of lung
- T2

C

Soft Palate Movement Studies with Phonation (Fig. 9–8). Soft palate movements with phonation can be studied in considerable detail to assist in analysis of speech defects. In its simplest form, these studies consist of four views, all in the lateral projection centering over the soft palate: (1) the resting state with normal breathing and no phonation; (2) the patient making the sound "ssss"; (3) the patient speaking the long vowel "eeeee"; and (4) the patient speaking the long vowel "ōoo." These views can, of course, be supplemented by cineradiographic studies and special film examinations of the swallowing function, although this extra radiation exposure is a disadvantage. Videotape studies at the time of image-amplified fluoroscopy require less radiation exposure and may prove to be just as helpful.

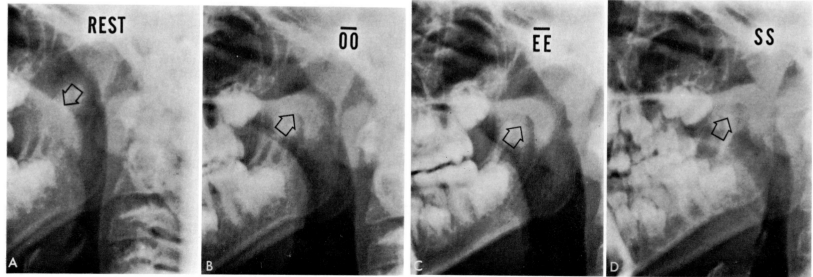

FIGURE 9–8 Phonation studies showing good mobility of the soft palate. *A*. Resting state. *B*. Oo. *C*. Ee. *D*. Ss. Note the complete approximation of the soft palate with the posterior nasopharyngeal wall in *D*.
These studies may be supplemented by cineradiographic examination and by an associated study of the swallowing function.

Anteroposterior Body Section Radiographs of the Larynx (Fig. 9–9). If a section through the middle of the larynx in the coronal plane is obtained, the vestibule and the "zeppelin-shaped" laryngeal ventricle are clearly demonstrated, along with the true and false vocal cords. Ordinarily, such radiographs are obtained with the larynx at rest (Fig. 9–9 *E*) and during phonation (Fig. 9–9 *A* and *D*).

The laryngogram (Fig. 9–10) contributes significantly to the management of malignant laryngeal tumors by permitting an accurate classification of the lesion.*

*Lehman, Q. H., and Fletcher, G. H.: Contribution of the laryngogram to the management of malignant laryngeal tumors. Radiology, *83*:486–500, 1964.

FIGURE 9–9 *A–C*. Body section radiographs of the larynx. *D* and *E*. Labeled tracing of larynx in phonation and at rest. *A. Tomogram:* The laryngopharyngeal walls, formed by the thin aryepiglottic fold above and the thicker false cord below, separate the vestibule from the pyriform sinuses. The vocal cords, approximating in the midline, delineate the ventricles above from the subglottic space below. The air-filled valleculae and midline glossoepiglottic fold can be seen above the hyoid bone. *B*. Radiograph of larynx at rest. *C. Lateral Soft-Tissue View:* The hyoid bone divides the epiglottis into supra- and infrahyoid portions. The vertical position of the epiglottis during phonation may cause bulging of its lower portion, which should not be mistaken for a tumor. Air contrast outlines the valleculae, the free margin of the aryepiglottic folds, the laryngeal ventricle, and the subglottic space. Thyroid cartilage calcification and pre-epiglottic soft tissue are readily studied. (*A* and *C* from Lehmann, Q. H., and Fletcher, G. H.: Radiology, *83*:486–500, 1964.)

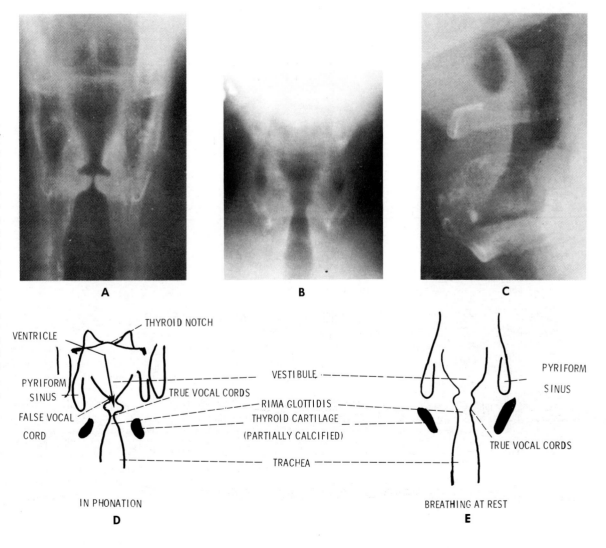

Laryngograms. Laryngograms may also be obtained using opaque media with and without phonation. In this procedure, a topical anesthetic such as 0.5 per cent Dyclone is sprayed onto and into the pharynx and larynx, and 10 to 20 ml. of Dionosil oily is dropped slowly over the tongue during quiet inspiration. Frontal and lateral spot film radiographs are made while the patient performs nasal inspiration and pho-

nation, strains down against a closed glottis, and breathes in against a closed glottis (Fig. 9–10). Powdered tantalum has also been utilized as a medium for human laryngography.*

*Zamel, N., et al.: Powdered tantalum as a medium for human laryngography. Radiology, 94:547–553, 1970.

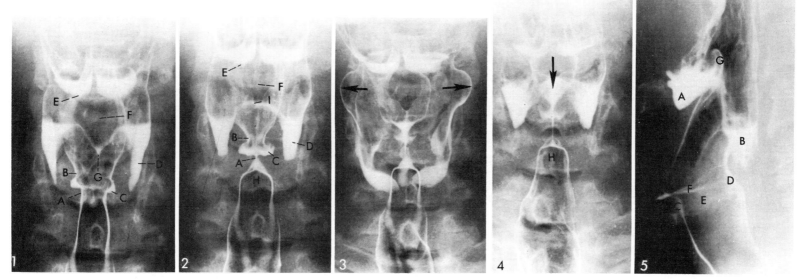

FIGURE 9–10 Laryngograms of a normal larynx employing Dionosil oily after local anesthesia of the pharynx and larynx: 1, Inspiration. 2, Phonation. 3, Modified Valsalva maneuver (forceful blowing against the cheek with lips closed as for blowing a horn). 4, True Valsalva maneuver (straining down against the closed glottis). 5, Lateral view in inspiration.

In parts 1, 2, 3, and 4: (*A*) true cords; (*B*) false cords; (*C*) collapsed ventricles; (*D*) pyriform sinuses; (*E*) valleculae; (*F*) laryngeal vestibules; (*G*) arytenoid groove; (*H*) subglottic angle; (*I*) postcricoid line. In 3, arrows point to lateral pharyngeal walls that balloon outward. In 4, arrow points to contrast material pooling above the contracted vestibule and pyriform sinuses.

In part 5, lateral view: (*A*) valleculae; (*B*) pyriform sinuses; (*C*) anterior commissure; (*D*) posterior commissure; (*E*) vocal cords; (*F*) collapsed ventricle; (*G*) epiglottis. (From Fletcher, G. H., and Jing, B-S.: The Head and Neck. Chicago, Year Book Medical Publishers, 1968. Courtesy of Dr. Bao-Shen Jing, Department of Diagnostic Radiology, University of Texas; M. D. Anderson Hospital and Tumor Institute, Houston, Texas.)

THE TRACHEA AND BRONCHI

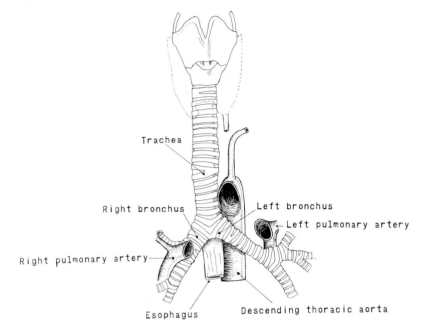

FIGURE 9–11   Relationships of tracheobronchial tree to the main ramifications of the pulmonary artery.

The angle which the two bronchi form with the trachea varies according to the age of the individual (Kobler and Hovorka, quoted in Miller)* as follows:

Age	Right Bronchus	Left Bronchus
Newborn	10–35 degrees	30–65 degrees
Adult male	20 degrees	40 degrees
Adult female	19 degrees	51 degrees

*Miller, W. S.: The Lung. 2nd ed. Springfield, Ill., Charles C Thomas, Publisher, 1950.

No effort will be made to describe in detail the anatomy of the chest; for this information, the student is referred to the authors' companion volume, *An Atlas of Anatomy Basic to Radiology*. The illustrations dealing with the anatomy of this region will be self-sufficient from a practical point of view.

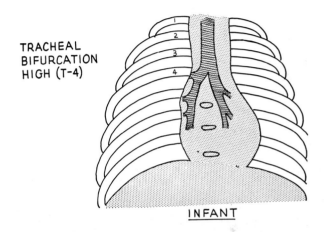

TRACHEAL BIFURCATION HIGH (T-4)

INFANT

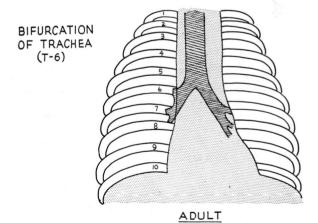

BIFURCATION OF TRACHEA (T-6)

ADULT

FIGURE 9–12   Comparison of level of bifurcation of trachea in adult and child. (After Pediatric X-ray Diagnosis, 6th ed., by Caffey, J. Copyright © 1972 by Year Book Medical Publishers, Inc., Chicago. Used by permission.)

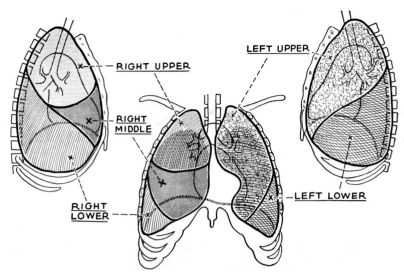

FIGURE 9–13 The lung: lobes and fissures.

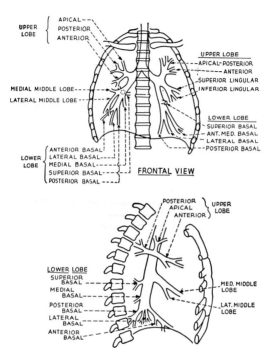

FIGURE 9–14 Bronchial distribution of the lung.

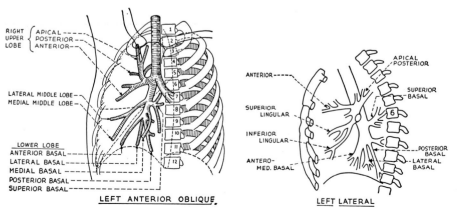

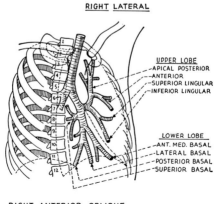

BRONCHOGRAPHY

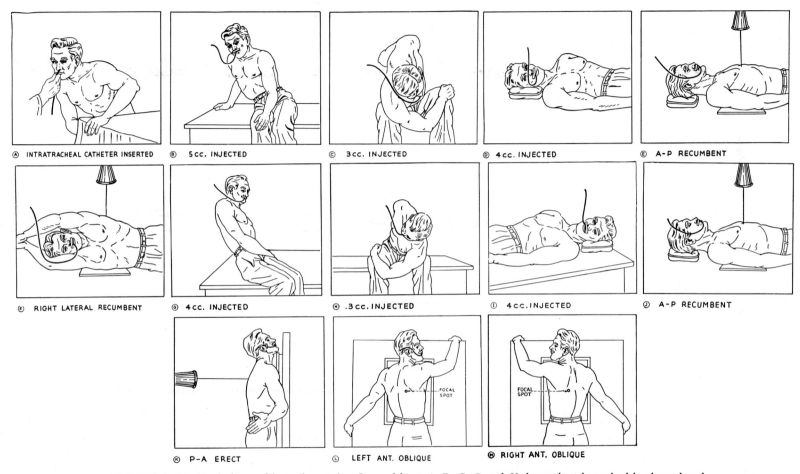

(A) INTRATRACHEAL CATHETER INSERTED

(B) 5 CC. INJECTED

(C) 3 CC. INJECTED

(D) 4 CC. INJECTED

(E) A-P RECUMBENT

(F) RIGHT LATERAL RECUMBENT

(G) 4 CC. INJECTED

(H) .3 CC. INJECTED

(I) 4 CC. INJECTED

(J) A-P RECUMBENT

(K) P-A ERECT

(L) LEFT ANT. OBLIQUE

(M) RIGHT ANT. OBLIQUE

FOCAL SPOT

FIGURE 9–15 Technique of bronchography. In positions *A, B, C, G* and *H* the patient is rocked backward and forward, still maintaining the general position as indicated in the diagram. In positions *D* and *I*, the patient is rolled slightly from side to side, likewise still maintaining the general position as indicated in the diagram. This rocking or rolling motion is efficacious in obtaining a better distribution of the iodized oil medium in the bronchi.

Segmental or lobar bronchography (or unilateral study) may be performed under fluoroscopic injection control and "spot film" radiography by selective catheterization and injection.

Our own preference at this time is Dionosil in oil suspension, although admittedly this is not ideal in either contrast or benignity of reaction.

The following film studies are obtained after the injection of the contrast media:

1. Anteroposterior recumbent and lateral views of the side first injected, immediately after injection and before the second side is injected (Fig. 9–17 A, and B or E).

2. An anteroposterior view of the chest after both sides are injected.

3. An erect posteroanterior view of the chest after both sides are injected (Fig. 9–17).

4. Both oblique views after both sides are injected (stereoscopic views may be obtained if desired) (Fig. 9–17 C and F).

The above study may be combined with fluoroscopy, if a good spot-film apparatus is available that will give detail as good as the conventional studies. One advantage of the fluoroscopic examination is that it permits visualization of the filling as it occurs, so that the examiner knows immediately whether or not further filling is required. Moreover, a concept of the physiologic function of the bronchial tree is also thereby acquired. Balanced against this great advantage, however, is the fact that spot films are seldom as satisfactory in minute detail as are conventional long distance and small focal spot-film studies. The examiner must therefore adapt the technique to his requirements.

Ordinarily, both sides of the lung are injected at the same examination if the patient's respiratory capacity will permit it. In many patients, injection of only one side at a single sitting is possible.

The radiographic anatomy of the bronchi and their distribution have been illustrated in previous diagrams (see Fig. 9–14).

BRONCHIAL BRUSH BIOPSY AND SELECTIVE BRONCHOGRAPHY. A bronchial abrasion technique for cytologic study of peripheral bronchial lesions was described some years ago (MacLean, 1958a).* In more recent times controllable brushes, telescoping catheters, and fibroscopes have provided a means not only for obtaining microbiopsies or cytologic study of peripheral lesions, but also for segmental bronchography of these regions (Fennessy, 1967; Sovak, Bean et al., 1968; Wilson and Eskridge).* A nonfiberoptic bronchoscopic technique, advocated by Willson and Eskridge, is carried out as follows: The patient is given a topical anesthetic as for bronchography. The outside larger catheter of a telescoping catheter (a 45 cm. No. 16 French radiopaque polyvinyl tube) is positioned with the tip in the trachea just above the carina. Through it is inserted a specially molded telescoping bronchial catheter of radiopaque polyethylene with a precurved tip to fit the desired lobar bronchus. A controllable guidewire is used to guide this catheter into the correct position under fluoroscopic control. Once the inner catheter is in position a special brush is passed through it to the desired location under fluoroscopic control and moved in a clockwise direction so that a scraping of the bronchial mucosa or a specimen of the lesion in question is obtained. This brush is then withdrawn back into the telescoping catheter and removed. Various specimens may be obtained by this method, including: (1) a smear of the tissue on a slide, (2) a microbiopsy specimen, or (3) cultures.

Following the procurement of satisfactory specimens, selective bronchography is carried out by injection through the catheter into the desired areas of lung, and spot films are taken of the areas in question.

FIBEROPTIC BRONCHOSCOPY (Schoenbaum et al.; Kahn).* A flexible bronchofiberscope was introduced by Ikeda in 1968. This instrument was inserted originally through a bronchoscope or an endotracheal tube under general anesthesia, but since that time commercial flexible fiberoptic bronchoscopes have become available.†

---

*References may be obtained in Meschan, I.: An Atlas of Anatomy Basic to Radiology, Chapter 10. Philadelphia, W. B. Saunders Co., 1975.

*References may be obtained in Meschan, I.: An Atlas of Anatomy Basic to Radiology, Chapter 10. Philadelphia, W. B. Saunders Co., 1975.

†Olympus Bronchofiberscope, Type 5 B; Olympus Bronchofiberscope, Type 5 B2, Olympus Corporation of America, 2 Nevada Drive, New Hyde Park, New York 11040; Fiber-Bronchoscope FBS-6T with associated instruments, American Optical Machida Company, Southbridge, Mass.

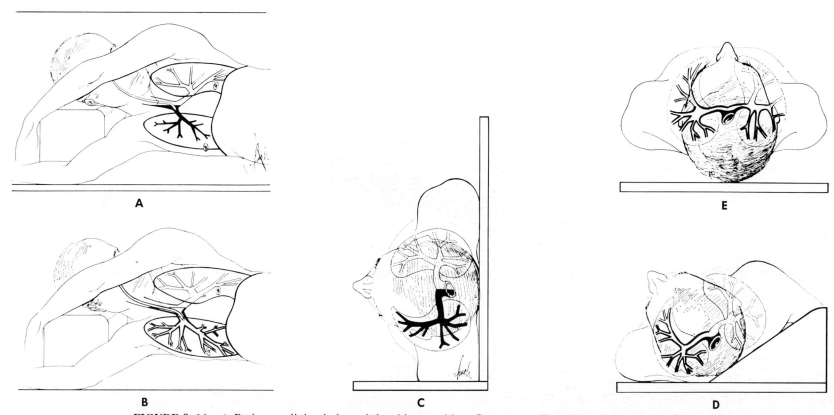

FIGURE 9–16 *A*, Patient reclining in lateral decubitus position. Contrast medium injected during forceful expiration allows filling of all proximal radicles with a single bolus injection. Orifices of all major bronchi are occluded by contrast medium, but distal radicles are not filled.

B. Following inhalation, the air pushes the contrast medium into peripheral radicles, resulting in double contrast visualization.

Spot-films and first overhead films made in lateral decubitus position (*C*) to be followed by posterior oblique (*D*). Last film made in supine position may result in spillage of contrast medium into contralateral lung, which is not objectionable in this view (*E*). (From Amplatz, K., and Haut, G.: Radiology, *95*:439–440, 1970.)

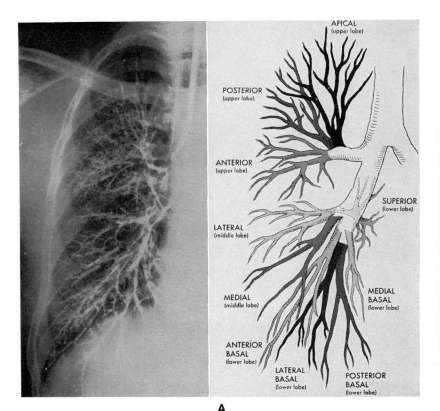

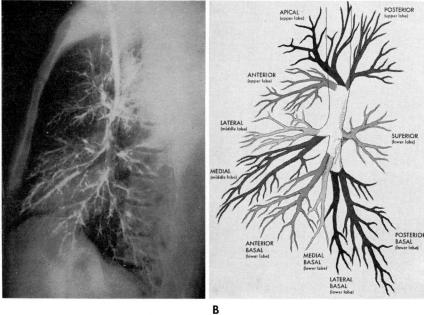

A

B

FIGURE 9–17 The normal human bronchial tree. *A*. Right posteroanterior projection. *B*. Right lateral projection (From Lehman, J. S., and Crellin, J. A.: Medical Radiology and Photography, *31*, 1955.)

Figure continued on opposite page

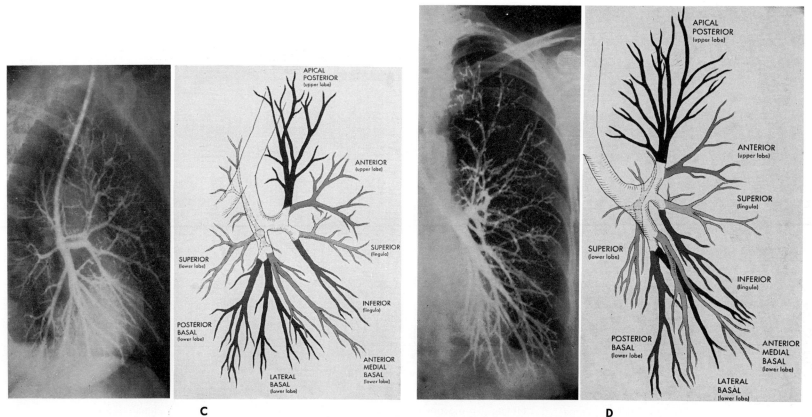

FIGURE 9–17 *Continued.* *C.* Right anterior oblique projection. *D.* Left posteroanterior projection.

Figure continued on following page

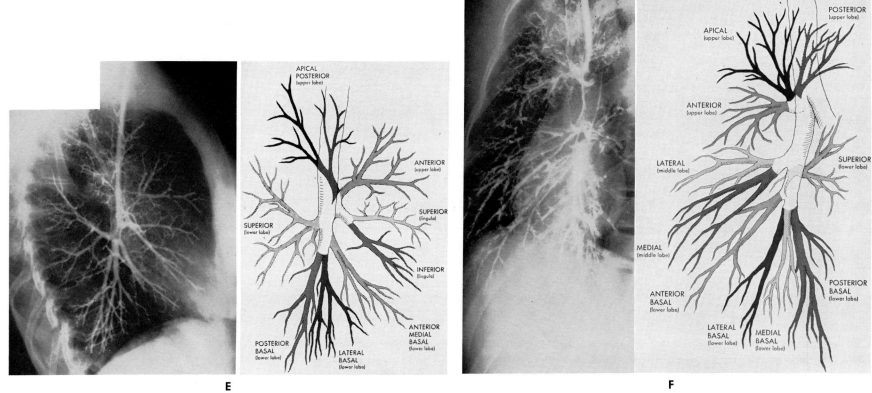

E

F

FIGURE 9–17 *Continued. E.* Left lateral projection. *F.* Left anterior oblique projection. (*C to F* from Lehman, J. S., and Crellin, J. A.: Medical Radiography and Photography, *31*, 1955.)

These instruments vary somewhat, but generally consist of a flexible tube which contains numerous bundles of thread-size glass fibers as image and light guides. The hard tip at the end of this scope has an outer diameter of 5.2 mm. and its bending section is flexible through an angle of 160 degrees. The angle is controlled by a lever in the handle or control unit. The outer diameter of the bending section is 5.4 mm., and the flexible tube has an outer diameter of 5.7 mm. and a working length of 600 mm. A biopsy forceps or a cytology brush can be inserted through the hollow suction channel from the control unit on the handle. Photographs may be taken with the attachable Olympus camera. Various other attachments are available for teaching and evaluation by groups of two or more physicians.

Patients are given premedication with a suitable sedative, atropine, and topical anesthesia. A No. 36 French nasopharyngeal airway is passed through the nose into the oropharynx and, in most instances, the fiberoptic bronchoscope is then passed through the airway into the trachea under direct visualization.

Biopsies may be made of centrally located lesions, which may be brushed under direct visualization through the scope. The specimen obtained is smeared on a slide coated with egg albumin and immersed immediately in 70 per cent alcohol, and is then sent for cytologic examination together with washings from the appropriate area. Biopsy specimens may be immersed in formalin and sent for histologic examination.

The fiberoptic bronchoscope may be guided to a lesion under suspicion by image-amplified fluoroscopy; bronchial brush biopsy, smears, and cultures may thereby be obtained. If a bronchogram is indicated, the fiberoptic bronchoscope is exchanged under fluoroscopic control over an appropriate angiographic guidewire for a polyethylene tube, the bronchogram then being obtained through the polyethylene catheter.

Generally, patients with heart failure, chronic obstructive pulmonary disease, asthma, pneumonia, or other pulmonary problems may be studied only after careful arterial blood gas samples have been analyzed. Even the premedication should not be given to patients with borderline pulmonary functions, hypoxemia requiring oxygen, or respiratory failure.

The control handle of the instrument cannot be immersed in any liquid sterilization substance since damage may result, but the flexible section of the scope may be sterilized by soaking it in Betadine and then rinsing in isopropyl alcohol 70 per cent followed by sterile water. Cold gas sterilization may also be used, but unfortunately this procedure takes 17 to 24 hours and is not practical when more than one patient must be examined in a day.

THE LUNG PARENCHYMA; THE AIR SPACES

The Primary Lobule (Fig. 9–20). The bronchi continue to ramify until a point is reached when the walls no longer contain cartilage, forming the tubular respiratory bronchioli. Eventually the tubular character changes, and small projections appear on all sides of the bronchiolus known as alveolar ducts. At the distal end of each alveolar duct, there are three to six spherical cavities called atria. These atria, in turn, communicate with a variable number of larger and more irregularly shaped cavities called air sacs. Projecting from the wall of each air sac and atrium there are a number of smaller spaces called pulmonary alveoli. This entire group of structures from the respiratory bronchiole distally, together with the accompanying blood vessels, lymph vessels, and nerves, forms a primary lobule. The primary lobules are grouped into bronchial segments, in accordance with the pattern previously described.

The primary lobule is too small to be seen radiographically.

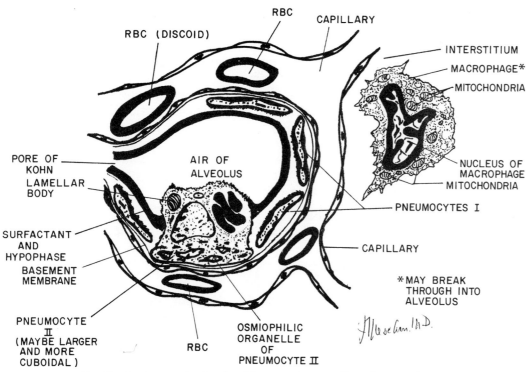

FIGURE 9–18 Anatomic sketch of the constituent cells and parts of an alveolus.

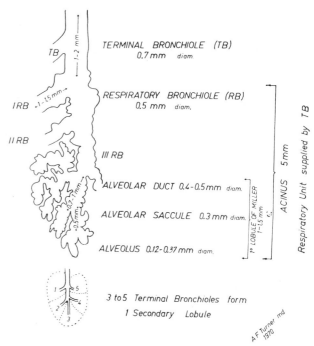

FIGURE 9–19 Anatomic drawing of terminal bronchiole and components of one acinus. (From Sargent, E. N., and Sherwin, R.: Am. J. Roentgenol., *113*:660–679, 1971.)

The Alveolus (Fig. 9–18). The *pulmonary alveolus* is a saccular structure arranged in a cluster around an *atrium,* connected by *air ducts* to *terminal bronchioles* (Fig. 9–19). The alveolus is a complex structure in which air exchange occurs and various surfactant-hypophasic compounds are manufactured to maintain a low-surface tension so that the alveoli may remain distended; in addition, macrophages reside within the alveolus to act as scavengers to remove debris cephalad from the alveoli. The lining of the alveolus contains flattened cells called *pneumocytes I,* which are said to manufacture the mucopolysaccharides of the hypophase; *pneumocytes II,* which are larger, more cuboidal cells with large nuclei and said to manufacture the lecithins (especially dipalmitol lecithin, or DPL), which are the main constituents of the surfactants; and immediately beneath the basement membrane of this lining, or protruding into the air-sac are the *macrophages,* or large scavenger cells (Fig. 9–18). Capillaries, connective tissue, lymphatics, and other blood constituent cells may also be found surrounding the alveolus, as well as nerve tissue.

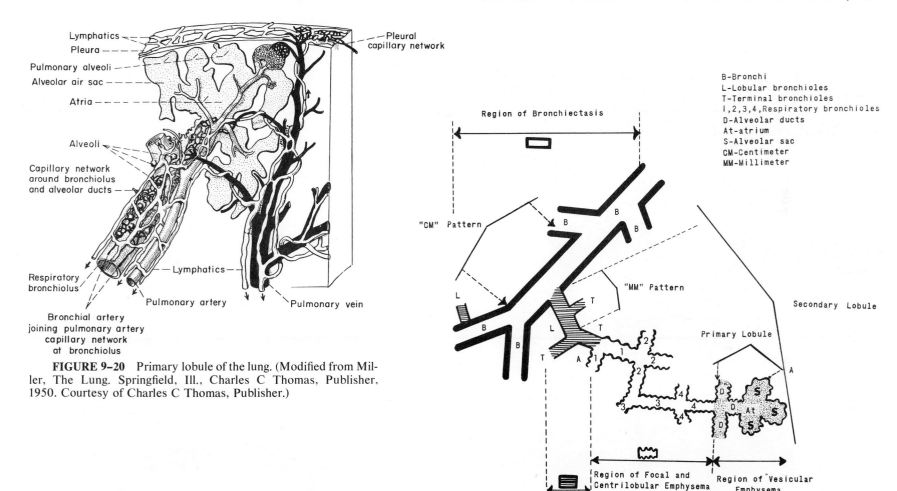

FIGURE 9–20 Primary lobule of the lung. (Modified from Miller, The Lung. Springfield, Ill., Charles C Thomas, Publisher, 1950. Courtesy of Charles C Thomas, Publisher.)

B–Bronchi
L–Lobular bronchioles
T–Terminal bronchioles
1,2,3,4,Respiratory bronchioles
D–Alveolar ducts
At–atrium
S–Alveolar sac
CM–Centimeter
MM–Millimeter

FIGURE 9–21 Diagrammatic view of the "secondary lobule."

Pores of Kohn are small perforations in the alveolus that allow an "air drift" between alveoli—just as the *canals of Lambert,* to be described shortly, allow an air drift between secondary lobules.

A

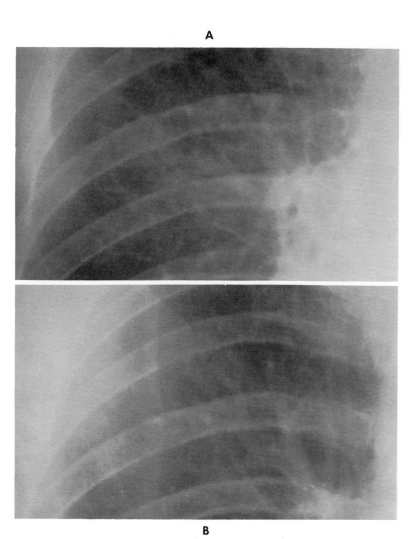

B

FIGURE 9–22 *A* and *B*. Magnified view of air space consolidation in acute pulmonary edema before and after diuresis. Some discrete acinar shadows are shown before diuresis.

A

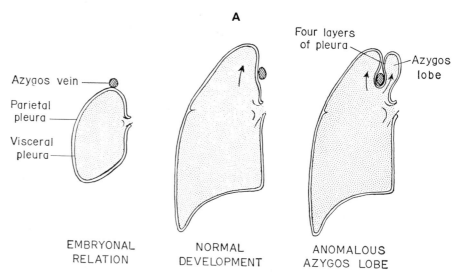

Azygos vein

Parietal pleura

Visceral pleura

Four layers of pleura

Azygos lobe

EMBRYONAL RELATION

NORMAL DEVELOPMENT

ANOMALOUS AZYGOS LOBE

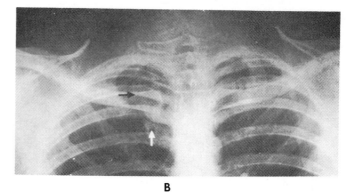

B

FIGURE 9–23 *A*. Anatomic concept of the "azygos" lobe. Normally the azygos vein migrates into its normal superhilar position by moving "around" the apex of the right upper lobe. In some cases, it takes a shorter route and indents both the parietal and visceral pleura, producing the anomalous "fissure." Unlike a true interlobar fissure, this one consists of four mesothelial layers—two from the parietal and two from the visceral pleura. The true interlobar fissure consists of only two layers of visceral pleura. *B*. Radiograph of chest showing position and appearance of the azygos lobe.

The epithelium of the alveoli, like that of the bronchi and bronchioli, rests upon a network of reticulum, which is of some importance in connection with interstitial disease processes of the lungs.

The interchange of gases takes place in the alveoli, and the entire structure of the lungs is subservient to this end.

Secondary Lobule. When a bronchial pathway is followed to its end, a point is reached where branching of parallel walls of the pathway occurs about every 0.5 to 1.0 cm. After three or four such branchings an abrupt transition takes place after which the branching patterns occur much more frequently—at 2 to 3 mm. intervals. Reid and Simon have called these the centimeter and millimeter patterns respectively. The centimeter pattern represents small bronchi and bronchioles; the millimeter pattern represents terminal bronchioles. A cluster of 3 to 5 terminal bronchioles in this millimeter pattern, together with the respiratory tissue that they supply, constitutes one *secondary lobule*. Generally, a secondary lobule is a unit with a diameter of about 1.0 to 1.5 cm., allowing 2 mm. as the distance between terminal bronchiolar branches and 5 mm. as the depth of respiratory tissue beyond the terminal bronchiole.

This concept of the secondary lobule is different from that of a lung unit demarcated by septal connective tissue passing into the lung from the pleura (Miller; VonHayek).*

The secondary lobule as defined by Reid and Simon is morphologically recognizable on films, particularly following bronchographic study, or when this sector of the lung contains a water density material. A "mulberry-like" shadow is produced (Fig. 9–22 *A* and *B*).

The *acinus* represents that portion of the lung parenchyma encompassing all the tissues distal to one terminal bronchiole, i.e., all of the respiratory bronchioles, alveolar ducts, and alveoli (Fig. 9–19). Thus, a secondary lobule contains a cluster of three to five terminal bronchioles supplying three to five acini. An acinus probably measures 5 to 7 mm. in diameter, in contrast to a secondary lobule which is approximately 1.0 to 1.5 cm. in diameter.

Each alveolar duct, in contrast, supplies a family of approximately 20 to 25 alveoli. The primary lobule of Miller comprises only the air spaces supplied by one alveolar duct and is probably 1.0 to 1.5 mm. in diameter; it is not to be confused with the much larger secondary lobule recognizable macroscopically.

Various histologic measurements of airway passages and alveoli are given for reference (Davies; Weibel; Pump).*

The secondary pulmonary lobule furnishes a practical concept for interpretation of both normal and abnormal chest radiographs (Heitzman et al.).*

Canals of Lambert. In the distal portions of the bronchiolar tree there are a number of epithelium-lined tubular communications that apparently provide an accessory route for the passage of air directly from the bronchioles into the alveoli. These are known as the *canals of Lambert* (Lambert).*

Alveolar Pores (the Pores of Kohn). These pores in the alveoli are openings or discontinuities of the alveolar wall that measure about 10 to 15 microns in diameter. These apparently permit the transfer of gases, fluids, or particulate matter between lobules. They exist only between segments of a lobe; the total lobe remains an isolated unit with no collateral channel communications with adjacent lobes. However, if segmental or subsegmental bronchial occlusion exists, ventilation of the occluded segment may be brought about through these collateral channels. Hence, this is known as "collateral air drift." McLean has suggested that the positive pressure of expiration produces a collapse of the pores of Kohn and that this causes a check-valve mechanism to operate at each of these collateral pathways. Reich and co-workers have referred to this as "an interalveolar air drift," and represent this as an integral part of the mechanism of coughing. They have discussed these anatomic structures in relation to various pathologic entities (Fig. 9–22) (Macklin).*

---

*References may be obtained in Meschan, I.: An Atlas of Anatomy Basic to Radiology, Chapter 10. Philadelphia, W. B. Saunders Co., 1975.

VASCULAR SUPPLY, VENOUS DRAINAGE, AND LYMPHATICS OF THE RESPIRATORY TRACT

Blood Vessels of the Lungs. PULMONARY ARTERY. The pulmonary artery (Fig. 9–24) follows closely the subdivisions of the bronchial tree. It arches over the right main-stem bronchus and lies dorsal and slightly lateral to the bronchus. The artery diminishes more rapidly in size than the bronchus it accompanies, and by the time it reaches the primary lobule, it is about one-fourth or one-fifth the size of the alveolar duct. It finally ends in a capillary network surrounding the alveolus. The pulmonary vein takes origin from the latter capillary network.

The common pulmonary artery divides into right and left pulmonary arteries (Fig. 9–25). The right pulmonary artery passes under the aortic arch below the tracheal bifurcation and crosses in front of the right bronchus between its upper lobe and lower division branches. It divides into three branches, two going to the upper lobe, and one supplying the middle and lower lobes. Each of the branches of these subdivisions follows the corresponding branches of the bronchial tree rather closely, with the artery lying along the upper side of the bronchus most of the way. The left pulmonary artery is seen just below the aortic knob as it arches posteriorly into the left lung, forming the crescentic shadow of the left hilus above the downward curving left bronchus. It enters the hilus as three branches and then subdivides into nine principal branches, five of which go to the upper lobe and four to the lower lobe following corresponding bronchial branches. (The relationships of the heart, major vessels, and other structures of the mediastinum will be discussed in greater detail in Chapter 10.)

CAPILLARIES. The network of capillaries is situated in the walls of the alveoli, and each capillary is common to two alveoli. The mesh of capillaries in the walls of the alveoli situated beneath the pleura is much coarser than that within the lung. The same holds true for the capillaries situated near the fibrous septa and larger blood vessels.

PULMONARY VEINS. Unlike the pulmonary artery, which is virtually in the same sheath as the bronchus, the more peripheral pulmonary veins are situated far removed from the corresponding bronchus in the septa that unite several lobules. The pulmonary veins have four sources of origin: (1) the capillary network of the pleura, which is derived from the bronchial artery; (2) the capillary network of the alveoli; (3) the bronchopulmonary veins, which are situated on either side of the junction of two bronchi or bronchioli; and (4) the capillary network in the alveolar ducts, which gives origin to two venous radicles, one on either side of the duct.

The veins and arteries come closer together at about the fourth bronchial bifurcation, the veins lying anterior to and below the arteries. As they approach the hilum, they again become dissociated, the veins lying below and anterior to the arteries and diverging from them to enter the left atrium.

BRONCHIAL ARTERIES. The bronchial arteries vary in number and origin. They may arise from the aorta (in over 90 per cent of cases), or from any of the first three intercostal subclavian or internal mammary arteries.

BRONCHIAL VEINS. True bronchial veins are found only at the hilus of the lung. These arise from the first or first two dividing points of the bronchial tree, and receive branches from part of the pleura close to the hilus. These bronchial veins empty into the azygos, the hemiazygos, or one of the intercostal veins.

Lymphatics of the Lungs (Figs. 9–28 and 9–29). The lung is provided with a great abundance of lymphatics, more than the liver, spleen, or kidney.* They may be divided grossly into a superficial set and a

---

*Miller, W. S.: The Lung. 2nd ed. Springfield, Ill., Charles C Thomas, Publisher, 1950.

deep set. The superficial lymphatics are situated in the pleura; the deep group are situated along the pulmonary artery, veins, and bronchi, and form a dense network between the secondary lobules in the connective tissue septa. These two sets of lymphatics communicate with one another at the pleura and in the hilus. The pleural lymphatics have unusually large diameters and are arranged in the form of irregular polyhedral rings. Numerous valves, 1 to 2 mm. apart, direct the flow of lymph in both pleural and intrapulmonary lymphatics.

Normal lymph nodes may be found in the substance of the lung far from the hilum.*

LYMPHATICS OF THE BRONCHI. The larger bronchi have two sets of lymphatics which intercommunicate with one another, but the smaller bronchi have only a single plexus of lymphatics which terminates at the alveolar ductules. Here they join the lymphatics accompanying the pulmonary veins that form at this point.

There are no lymphatics in the walls of the air spaces distal to the alveolar ductules.

LYMPHATICS OF THE PULMONARY ARTERY. The larger branches of the pulmonary artery are accompanied by two lymph channels, one of which is situated between the artery and its accompanying bronchus. These intercommunicate freely by means of a rich plexus. The smaller arterial branches are accompanied by only single lymph channels. Communications between the periarterial and peribronchial lymphatics occur in many places but predominantly in the region of bifurcations and at the distal end of the alveolar ductules.

LYMPHATICS OF THE PULMONARY VEINS. As in the case of the arteries and bronchi, lymph channels accompany all of the veins, except in the region of the alveolar sacs.

LYMPHATICS OF THE PLEURA. There is only a single plexus of lymphatics in the pleura, arranged in polyhedral rings. There are smaller rings within these larger ones, with smaller lymph channels.

DIRECTION OF LYMPH FLOW. The valves situated in the hilus, pleura, and at the junction of the deep and superficial systems permit flow in one direction only. *The flow in the peribronchial, periarterial, and perivenous lymphatics is toward the interior of the lung* or hilus.

---

*Trapnell, D. H.: Recognition and incidence of intrapulmonary lymph nodes. Thorax, *19*:44–50, 1964.

The *valves situated just beneath the pleura permit flow of lymph toward the pleura.* In the subpleural region, the pleural lymphatics occasionally dip into the lung and then return to the surface to become pleural again.*

In the presence of an obstructed lymph channel, a reversal of lymph flow can occur. These obstructed and distended lymphatics appear linear and stellate in relation to hilar lymph nodes.

LYMPHOID TISSUE. Lymphoid tissue may occur in the form of lymph nodes, lymph follicles, or small masses of lymphoid tissue. Lymph nodes in the normal lung are associated with the larger divisions of the bronchi, and are situated at the places where branching takes place (Fig. 9–30). There is in old age a definite increase in the lymphoid tissue independent of that produced by disease, but dependent to a great extent on the amount of irritating particles inhaled (such as carbon). In the normal lung, lymph nodes are not present in the pleura.

---

*Trapnell, D. H.: The peripheral lymphatics of the lung. Br. J. Radiol., *36*:660–672, 1963.

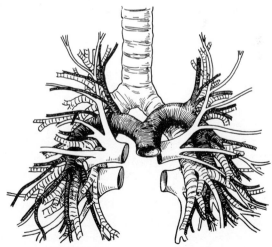

FIGURE 9–24 Relationship of major ramifications of pulmonary artery and tracheal bronchial tree to one another, also showing the relationship to major pulmonary veins. Note that the left pulmonary artery is slightly more cephalad than the right.

THE RESPIRATORY SYSTEM

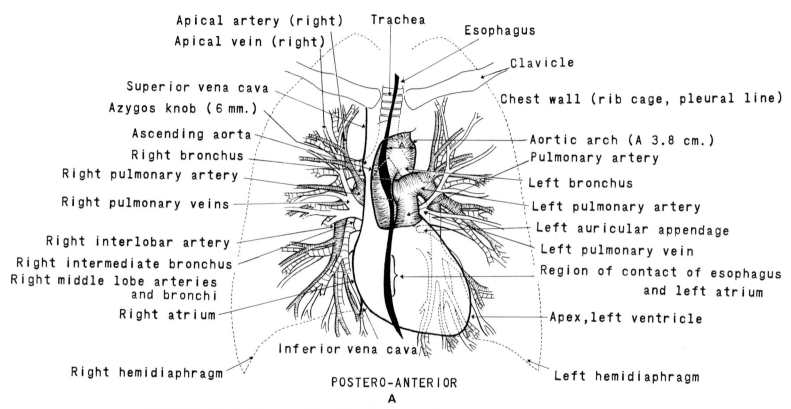

FIGURE 9–25 *A.* Diagram of chest film showing arteries, veins, and relationships to bronchi.

Figure continued on opposite page

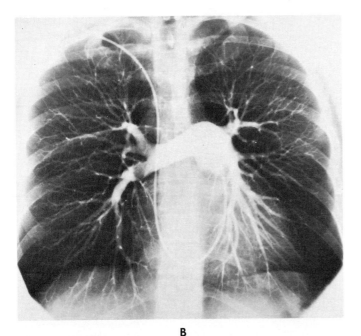

B

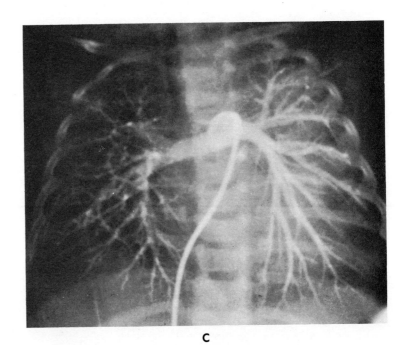

C

FIGURE 9–25 *Continued.* *B.* Pulmonary arteriogram, arterial phase. *C.* Pulmonary arteriogram in an infant, arterial phase.

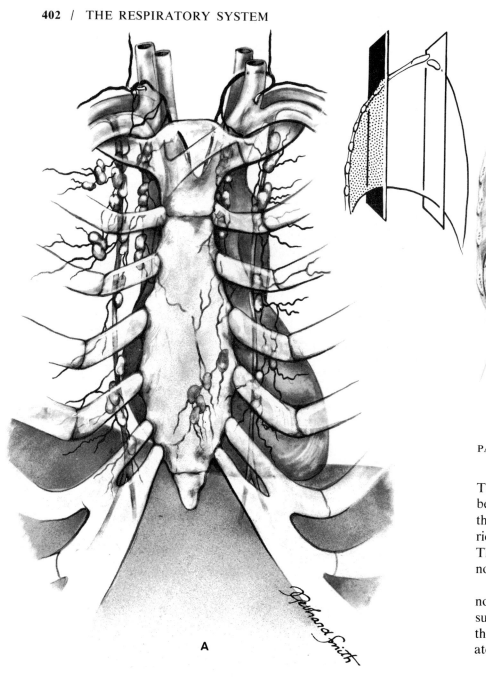

A

FIGURE 9–26 *A.* Anterior mediastinal lymph nodes. The nodes illustrated are chiefly those of the anterior parietal group (shown by the black and dotted plane in the inset), scattered along the internal mammary arteries and behind the anterior intercostal spaces and costal cartilages bilaterally. The prevascular (visceral) group relate to the superior vena cava and innominate vein on the right and to the aorta and carotid artery on the left. (From Fraser, R. G., and Paré, J. A. P.: Diagnosis of Diseases of the Chest. Philadelphia, W. B. Saunders Co., 1970.) *B.* The anatomy of the internal mammary lymph nodes. From Cunningham's Textbook of Anatomy, 10th ed. London, Oxford University Press, 1964.)

B

GROUP 1: LYMPH NODES OF THE ANTERIOR MEDIASTINAL COMPARTMENT (FIG. 9–26 *A* AND *B*)

(1) *The sternal, anterior parietal, or internal mammary group.* This group of nodes is distributed along the internal mammary arteries behind the anterior costochondral cartilages bilaterally. They drain the upper anterior abdominal wall, the anterior thoracic wall, the anterior portion of the diaphragm, and the medial portions of the breast. They communicate with a visceral group of anterior mediastinal lymph nodes and cervical nodes.

(2) *The anterior mediastinal lymph node group.* These are visceral nodes, lying posterior to the sternum in the lower thorax, along the superior vena cava and innominate vein on the right and in front of the aorta and carotid artery on the left. Some of these nodes are situated anterior to the thymus.

GROUP 2: THE POSTERIOR MEDIASTINAL LYMPH NODES (FIG. 9–27)

This group of lymph nodes lies posteriorly in the intercostal spaces and in paravertebral areas. They drain the parietal pleura and vertebral column. This group consists of parietal nodes and mediastinal visceral nodes, which communicate with each other. The posterior mediastinal group of visceral nodes lie along the lower esophagus and descending aorta, and drain the posterior portion of the diaphragm, the pericardium, the esophagus, and the lower lobes of the lungs.

The lymph from the anterior mediastinal nodes flows into the right lymphatic duct or bronchomediastinal duct, and the thoracic duct on the left. The posterior mediastinal lymph nodes drain into the thoracic duct and the cisterna chyli from the lower thoracic region. They also communicate with the visceral mediastinal lymph nodes draining mainly via the thoracic duct.

FIGURE 9–27 Posterior mediastinal lymph nodes. The intercostal (posterior parietal) group lies laterally, in the intercostal spaces, and medially, in the paravertebral areas adjacent to the heads of the ribs. The visceral group of posterior mediastinal nodes is situated along the lower esophagus and descending aorta. (From Fraser, R. G., and Paré, J. A. P.: Diagnosis of Diseases of the Chest. Philadelphia, W. B. Saunders Co., 1970.) (The plane and volume of tissue included are shown by the stippled and black area in the inset.)

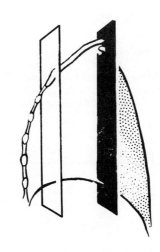

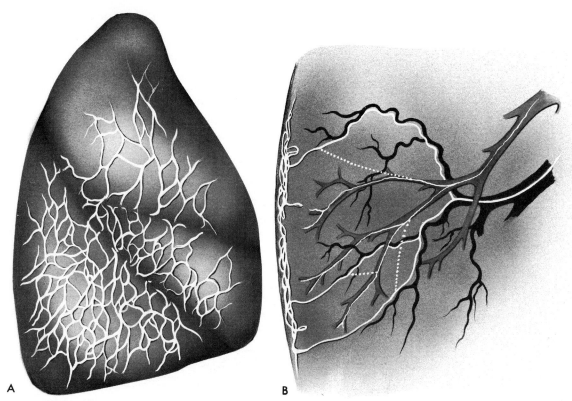

FIGURE 9–28 The lymphatic drainage of the pleura and lungs. *A.* A drawing of the lateral aspect of the right lung shows the pleural lymphatics to be much more numerous over the lower half of the lung than over the upper. *B.* In a coronal section through the midportion of the lung, lymphatic channels from the pleura enter the lung at the interlobular septa and extend medially to the hilum along venous radicals (dark shaded vessels); lymphatic channels originating in the peripheral parenchyma extend medially in the bronchovascular bundles (light shaded vessels). Communicating lymphatics (dotted lines) extend between the peribronchial and perivenous lymphatics. (From Fraser, R. G., and Paré, J. A. P.: Diagnosis of Diseases of the Chest. Philadelphia, W. B. Saunders Co., 1970.)

GROUP 3: THE MIDDLE MEDIASTINAL LYMPH NODES (FIG. 9–30)

The parietal group of lymph nodes in this chain are located mainly around the pericardial attachment to the diaphragm, whereas the visceral group consists mainly of the tracheobronchial and bifurcation nodes and bronchopulmonary nodes.

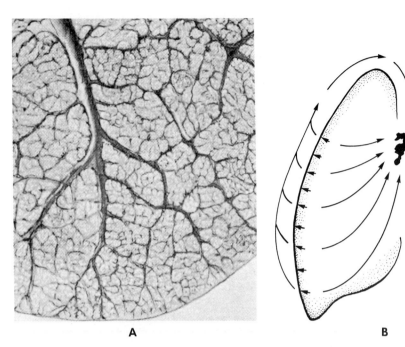

FIGURE 9–29 *A*. Drawing of lower surface of middle lobe showing lymphatic vessels outlining the lobules and acini of the lung parenchyma. (From Twining, E. W.: A Textbook of X-Ray Diagnosis. H. K. Lewis & Co., Publishers.) *B*. Diagrammatic illustration of the drainage of the lymphatics of the lungs. The superficial lymphatics are situated in the pleura and drain into the pleural space and around to the hili thereby. The deep lymphatics follow along the pulmonary arterial branches, veins, and bronchi and drain toward the hilus. The two sets of lymphatics communicate with one another immediately adjoining the pleura and in the region of the hilus, but are otherwise separate.

The middle mediastinal lymph nodes communicate with anterior mediastinal and posterior nodes, and also drain into the bronchomediastinal trunk on the right and the thoracic duct on the left (Rouviere). The bronchomediastinal trunk receives the lymph from the right lung and empties via the right lymphatic duct into the beginning of the innominate vein. Near their terminations, both thoracic ducts lie close to the lower deep cervical lymph nodes.

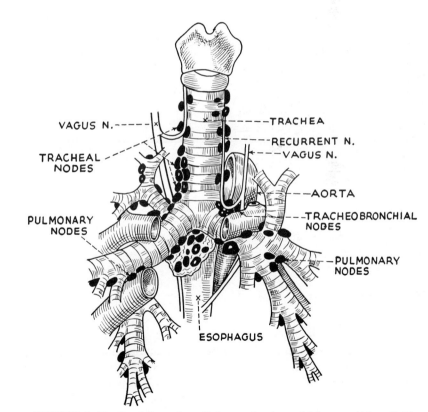

FIGURE 9–30 Lymph nodes of the tracheobronchial tree. (After Sukienikow.)

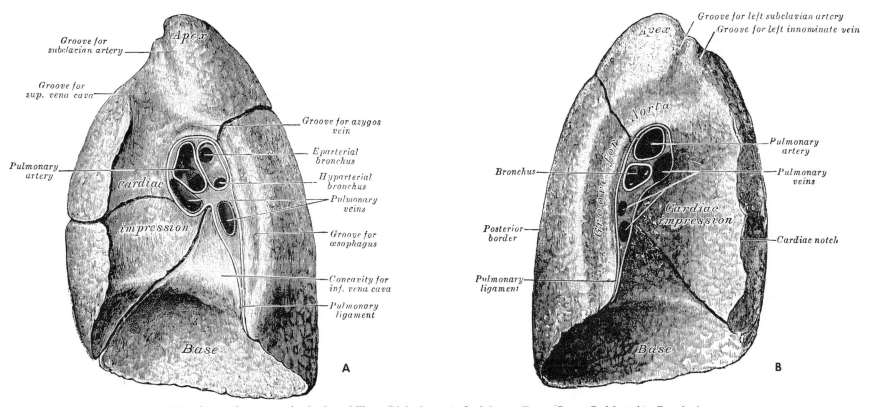

FIGURE 9–31 Structures in the lung hili. *A*. Right lung. *B*. Left lung. (From Goss, C. M. (ed.): Gray's Anatomy of the Human Body, 29th ed. Philadelphia, Lea & Febiger, 1973.)

THE LUNG HILI

The hilus of the lung (Fig. 9–31) is a wedge-shaped depressed area on the mediastinal surface of the lung above and behind the pericardial impression on the lung, within which the blood vessels, lymph vessels, nerves, and bronchi enter and leave the lung. Bronchial lymph nodes are located among those structures. The hilus is surrounded by the reflection of the pleura from the surface of the lung on to the pulmonary root. The mediastinal surface of the lung presents the pericardial im-pression produced by structures in the posterior mediastinum and the superior mediastinum in addition to the hili.

The term "root of the lung" is, strictly speaking, applied to a number of structures that enter and leave the lung on its mediastinal surface. It constitutes a pedicle that attaches the lung to the mediastinal wall of the pleural cavity. The large structures forming the pulmonary root are: (1) the two pulmonary veins, (2) the pulmonary artery, (3) the bronchus, (4) bronchial arteries and veins, (5) pulmonary nerves, and (6) lymph vessels and some lymph nodes (bronchial).

THE THORACIC CAGE, PLEURA, AND DIAPHRAGM

There are several important component parts of the thoracic cage, all of which may be visualized to some extent radiographically. These are: (1) the soft tissue structures of the thoracic wall, such as the skin, breasts, and muscular tissues; (2) the bony structures of the thoracic cage, consisting chiefly of ribs, costal cartilage, sternum, and thoracic spine; (3) the pleura, both visceral and parietal; and (4) the diaphragm.

Soft Tissue Structures of the Thoracic Wall

Skin and Subcutaneous Tissues. The skin and subcutaneous tissues of the thoracic cage cannot be entirely ignored in the consideration of the radiographic anatomy of the chest. Normally, these tegmental layers are seen only over the clavicle (Fig. 9–32) and as outlining shadows of the thoracic cage; abnormally, shadows contained within the skin and subcutaneous tissues can produce very dense shadows that must be differentiated from pulmonary constituents. Free air in the skin and subcutaneous tissues also produces its individual appearance. The fact that structures contained within the skin have radiographic significance must not be overlooked.

The Breasts. The breasts are situated in the superficial fascia covering the anterior aspect of the thoracic cage, and in the female usually extend from the level of the second or third rib to the level of the sixth. The hemispherical shadow of the female breast is cast over that of the pectoralis major muscle (Fig. 9–32), and together they form a notable haziness that may obscure to a great extent the lung substance proper. At the level of the fourth or fifth rib, the nipple, in turn, may cast an even denser shadow than that of the breast and has the appearance of a rather dense nodule. Occasionally the areola around the nipple may also be distinguished. Of course, the size and shape of the breasts vary occasionally among both women and men, and will vary in the same woman according to the physiologic state of the breast.

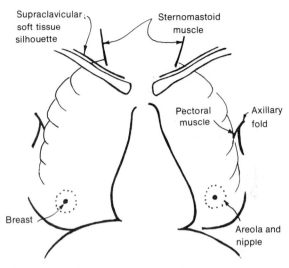

FIGURE 9–32   Soft tissues of the thoracic cage as seen radiographically.

The breast may be investigated radiographically in several ways: (1) soft tissue study tangential to the breast (Figs. 9–33 and 9–34); (2) study of the breast following injection of CO_2 into tissues around the breast; (3) injection of opaque media into the lactiferous ducts; and (4) by ultrasound.

The main purpose of these studies is to demonstrate abnormal mass lesions within the breast.

Muscular Tissues. The following muscles of the thoracic cage may produce a shadow upon the radiograph: (1) the pectoralis major and minor; (2) the sternocleidomastoid; (3) the serratus anterior; and (4) the intercostal muscles (may be seen on oblique views of the ribs and chest). Their importance lies chiefly in the recognition of their absence following radical mastectomy.

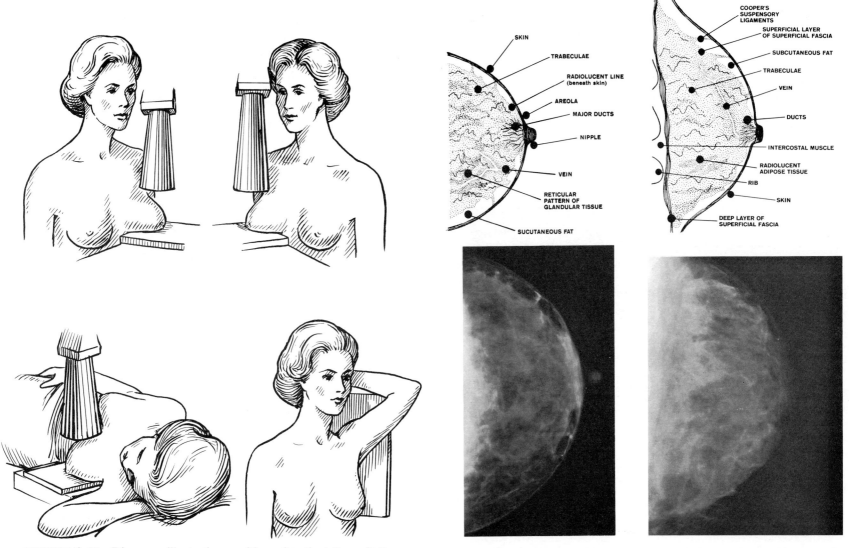

FIGURE 9–33 Diagrams illustrating position of patient for soft tissue mammography.

FIGURE 9–34 Representative mammograms in the craniocaudad (*left*) and mediolateral (*right*) projections and labeled line drawings of each. (From Egan, R. L.: Mammography. Springfield, Ill., Charles C Thomas, Publisher, 1964. Courtesy of Charles C Thomas, Publisher.)

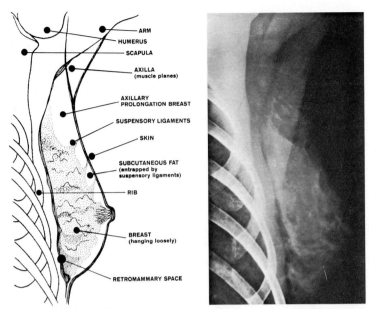

FIGURE 9–35 Representative mammogram in the axillary projection with labeled line drawing. (From Egan, R. L.: Mammography. Springfield, Ill., Charles C Thomas, Publisher, 1964. Courtesy of Charles C Thomas, Publisher.)

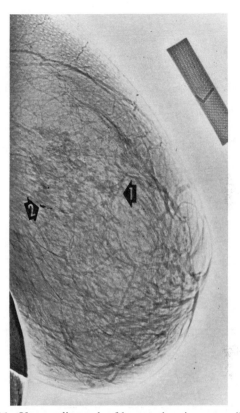

FIGURE 9–36 Xero-radiograph of breast showing a possible small malignancy deep in the breast with faint, flaky areas of calcification (arrow 1). The coarse calcification (arrow 2) is of no pathologic significance.

Mammography

General Principles of Technique. The principal factors in mammography are: (1) proper coning, (2) minimal kilovoltage adequate for penetration, (3) increased milliamperage seconds to give adequate exposure, (4) no intensifying screens, (5) minimal filtration of the x-ray beam combined with the kilovoltage used, and (6) short object-to-film distance. A fine grain emulsion with the necessary contrast range, comparable to the double emulsion Kodak Industrial Type "M" film must be used.* It is important that the *nipple be in profile,* if at all possible.

*Egan, R. L.: Mammography. Springfield, Ill., Charles C Thomas, Publisher, 1964.

Xeroradiography of the breast and the use of *vacuum cassettes* have enhanced the detail and accuracy of mammography by allowing us simultaneous visualization of both the internal lactiferous portions of the breast and the skin. *Computed axial tomography* of the breast is being tested at this writing and may allow the attainment of even greater accuracy.

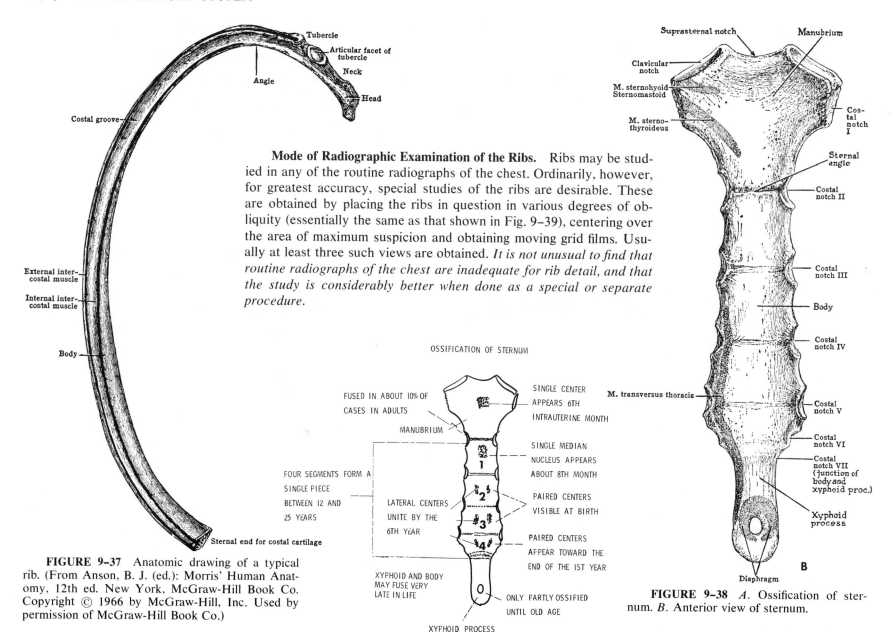

Mode of Radiographic Examination of the Ribs. Ribs may be studied in any of the routine radiographs of the chest. Ordinarily, however, for greatest accuracy, special studies of the ribs are desirable. These are obtained by placing the ribs in question in various degrees of obliquity (essentially the same as that shown in Fig. 9–39), centering over the area of maximum suspicion and obtaining moving grid films. Usually at least three such views are obtained. *It is not unusual to find that routine radiographs of the chest are inadequate for rib detail, and that the study is considerably better when done as a special or separate procedure.*

OSSIFICATION OF STERNUM

FUSED IN ABOUT 10% OF CASES IN ADULTS

MANUBRIUM

FOUR SEGMENTS FORM A SINGLE PIECE BETWEEN 12 AND 25 YEARS

LATERAL CENTERS UNITE BY THE 6TH YEAR

XYPHOID AND BODY MAY FUSE VERY LATE IN LIFE

SINGLE CENTER APPEARS 6TH INTRAUTERINE MONTH

SINGLE MEDIAN NUCLEUS APPEARS ABOUT 8TH MONTH

PAIRED CENTERS VISIBLE AT BIRTH

PAIRED CENTERS APPEAR TOWARD THE END OF THE 1ST YEAR

ONLY PARTLY OSSIFIED UNTIL OLD AGE

XYPHOID PROCESS

A

FIGURE 9–37 Anatomic drawing of a typical rib. (From Anson, B. J. (ed.): Morris' Human Anatomy, 12th ed. New York, McGraw-Hill Book Co. Copyright © 1966 by McGraw-Hill, Inc. Used by permission of McGraw-Hill Book Co.)

FIGURE 9–38 *A.* Ossification of sternum. *B.* Anterior view of sternum.

Oblique View of Sternum and Ribs

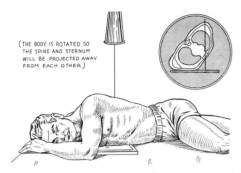

(THE BODY IS ROTATED SO THE SPINE AND STERNUM WILL BE PROJECTED AWAY FROM EACH OTHER.)

10" × 12" CASSETTE IN BUCKY TRAY

POINTS OF PRACTICAL INTEREST ABOUT FIGURE 9–39

1. At best, it is difficult to visualize the sternum with sufficient clarity in this view. Under these circumstances, body-section radiography is recommended. The best technique for this is as follows:

(a) A mobile cart is placed at right angles to the x-ray table, and the patient lies prone on the cart with his chest overlapping the table so that he is as nearly as possible *perpendicular to the x-ray table.*

(b) *The long axis of the sternum is therefore in contact with the surface of the x-ray table but at right angles to the long axis of this table.*

(c) The cassette is placed in the tray so that its long axis corresponds to that of the sternum.

(d) The body-section study is then made in the usual manner, and two or three "cuts" may be made.

2. Either of the oblique views may be utilized as shown. The long axis of the sternum is centered to the midline of the table.

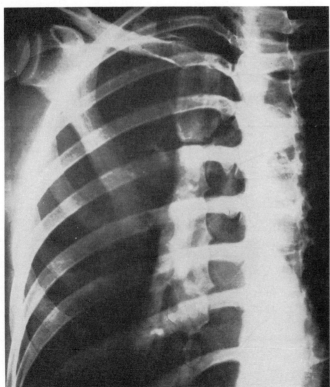

FIGURE 9–39 Oblique view of sternum and sternal clavicular joints (also ribs) to project the sternum away from the spine and heart.

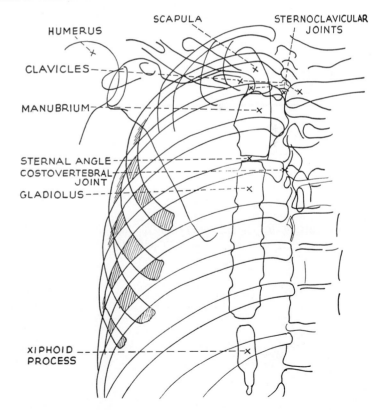

HUMERUS

SCAPULA

STERNOCLAVICULAR JOINTS

CLAVICLES

MANUBRIUM

STERNAL ANGLE

COSTOVERTEBRAL JOINT

GLADIOLUS

XIPHOID PROCESS

Lateral Projection of the Sternum (Fig. 9–40)

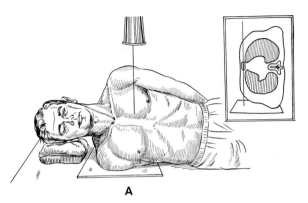

A

THE LONG AXIS OF THE STERNUM IS
PARALLEL TO THE TABLE AND CENTERED
TO ITS MIDLINE. THE ARMS ARE EITHER
UP OR BEHIND TO AVOID PROJECTION
OVER THE STERNUM. THE CENTRAL RAY
IS OVER THE MIDSTERNUM.

FIGURE 9–40 Lateral projection of sternum. *A*. Position of patient. *B*. Radiograph obtained. *C*. Labeled tracing of *B*.

POINTS OF PRACTICAL INTEREST ABOUT FIGURE 9–40

1. This view gives us maximum clarity of the sternum but unfortunately has the following disadvantages:

(a) When the sternum is depressed at all, it is concealed behind the costal cartilages and some lung in this projection. This is especially true of the condition called "pectus excavatum."

(b) Abnormalities which do not affect the entire width of the sternum may be obscured by the unaffected portion. Body-section radiographs are helpful when this is suspected.

(c) The various segments of the sternum must be recognized, and differentiated from other abnormalities which may be simulated at the costosternal junctions.

2. The retrosternal mediastinal and pleural shadows should always be examined very carefully. This is also true of the shadows which are superficial to the sternum. The clue to abnormality is often found here where it may escape detection by inspection of the sternal shadow only.

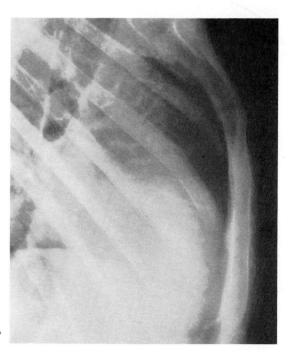

B

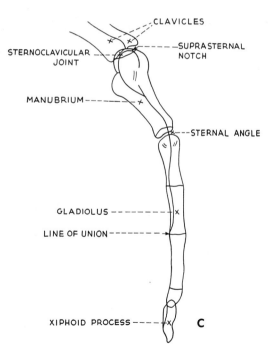

CLAVICLES

STERNOCLAVICULAR JOINT

SUPRASTERNAL NOTCH

MANUBRIUM

STERNAL ANGLE

GLADIOLUS

LINE OF UNION

XIPHOID PROCESS

C

Sternoclavicular Joints (Fig. 9–41)

The sternoclavicular joint is a two-chambered synovial or diarthrodial joint with an articular disk between the two chambers. Each chamber is usually distinct and separate from the other, unless the articular disk happens to be unusually thin (as in the case of the temporomandibular joint).

These joints are usually demonstrated on oblique projections such as are employed for the sternum proper, except that the tube is centered over the joint. *A comparison film of the opposite side is always obtained so that the two sternoclavicular joints can be compared in the same patient.*

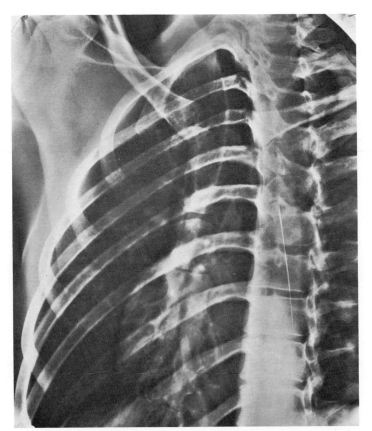

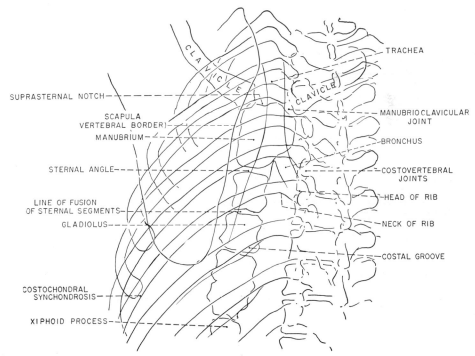

FIGURE 9–41 Oblique view of sternum and sternoclavicular joints (also ribs).

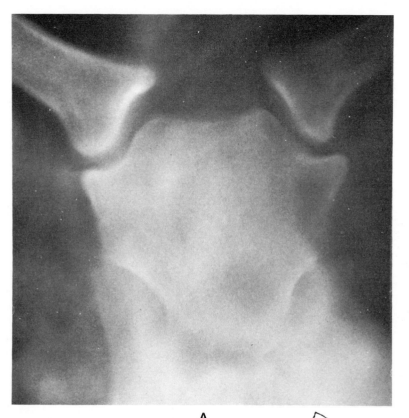

A

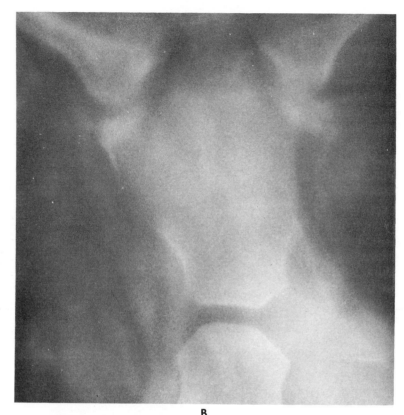

B

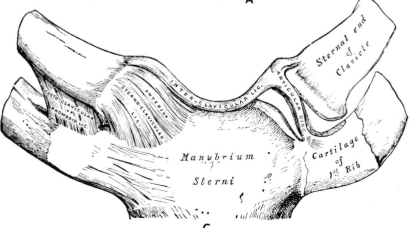

C

FIGURE 9–42 Tomographs of manubrium. *A.* Frontal projection. *B,* Oblique projection, including the manubriosternal junction. *C.* Gross anatomy of sternoclavicular joint. (From Goss, C. M. (ed.): Gray's Anatomy of the Human body. 29th ed. Philadelphia, Lea & Febiger, 1973.)

The Pleura

Gross Anatomic Features as Applied to Radiographic Anatomy. The pleura lines the entire thoracic cavity and invests the entire lung, and invaginations of the pleura form the interlobar fissures. That portion lining the thoracic cavity is called the *parietal pleura,* and that investing the lung is called the *visceral pleura.* The interlobar fissures are formed by invagination into the lung of two closely approximated layers of visceral pleura.

The lines of pleural reflection do not accurately correspond on the two sides of the thorax. These lines of reflection also vary in different subjects, depending upon body habitus.

The pleura is composed of a layer of endothelial cells resting on a membrane of connective tissue, within which are situated blood vessels, lymphatics, and nerves.

There is a thin layer of serous fluid between the two opposing layers of pleura ordinarily, with a slow and steady filtration and absorption occurring normally. The visceral pleural blood supply is obtained from the bronchial arteries as previously indicated, whereas the parietal pleura is supplied by systemic arteries that are branches of the subclavian artery and thoracic aorta. Also, the reader is referred to the previous discussion of the lymphatics in connection with the lung. The superficial lymphatics drain the visceral pleura outward, and communicate by means of short tributaries with the deep lymphatics that drain in the opposite direction toward the lung hilus. The parietal lymphatics do not drain directly into the hilar lymph nodes but rather into the lymph trunks at the junction of the internal jugular and subclavian veins.

Ordinarily, the pleura does not cast a significant radiographic shadow, except perhaps minimally in the costophrenic angles. When the pleural shadow can be identified, it is usually indicative of an abnormality.

There are usually small blebs or ruptured alveoli at the lung apices that cast a shadow on the chest radiograph.* This may simulate pleural disease and must not be confused with an abnormal appearance of the pleura or lungs in this location.

Ordinarily, the costophrenic angles are sharply delineated, and any significant degree of blunting is indicative of previous pleural disease; since these areas represent the most dependent portions of the pleura, disease is readily seen in these locations.

The cardiophrenic angles, however, vary considerably in appearance, and although the reflection of the pleura is normally sharp in this location also, a greater variability exists in the appearance of the pleural shadow here. An increased acuity of the appearance of this angle is of significance in detecting excessive fluid within the pericardial space, and thus an accurate conception of these angles must be constantly borne in mind.

---

*Cunningham, D. J.: Manual of Practical Anatomy. 12th ed. London, Oxford University Press, 1958.

The Diaphragm

Composition and Normal Attachments of the Diaphragm. The diaphragm consists of a peripheral muscular portion that completely surrounds an aponeurotic membrane and arches over the abdominal contents, separating the abdomen from the chest. There is extensive peripheral attachment to the xiphoid process, the lower six costal cartilages, the ribs, the first three lumbar vertebrae on the right side, and the first two on the left side. With varying degrees of curvature, the fibers arch centrally and end in the central tendon. This latter tendon is more anterior than posterior and thus is not truly central. It is incompletely divided into three lobes or leaflets. The middle one is anterior and intermediate in size, whereas the right lateral one is the largest and the left lateral the smallest. The crura of the diaphragm are two elongated musculotendinous bundles that arise on each side of the aorta and are partly separated from the lumbar vertebrae by the upper lumbar arteries, but are firmly attached to the upper three vertebrae on the right and the upper two on the left. There is a tendency for the cupola of the diaphragm to descend with age (Fig. 9–43).

Normal Openings in the Diaphragm (Fig. 9–45). The diaphragm is pierced by numerous structures: the superior epigastric artery, the musculophrenic artery, the splanchnic nerves, and the sympathetic trunks behind; the aorta, azygos vein, and thoracic duct passing between the crura; the inferior vena cava, and small branches of the right phrenic nerve passing through the foramen venae cavae; and the esophageal opening, transmitting the esophagus and two vagus nerves.

Three-Dimensional Concept of the Diaphragm (Fig. 9–43). The posterior attachment of the diaphragm is considerably lower than the anterior, and there is much lung substance and diaphragm which cannot be seen from the posteroanterior projection.

Moreover, much of the pleural space is likewise obscured from view by virtue of the attachments of the diaphragm. For that reason, it is important to attempt to visualize the structures behind it and frequently to obtain lateral and oblique projections.

Occasionally, the diaphragm may have a slightly irregular appearance, and by projection, a structure which actually lies beneath the diaphragm will be projected above a portion of it. Every effort must be made to obviate such projection phenomena and understand them when they occur.

Tenting and Scalloping of the Diaphragm. Occasionally, the contour of the diaphragm is broken into two or more arches, the outlines appearing as a scalloped margin (Fig. 9–44). This is usually caused by an irregular contraction of the diaphragmatic musculature, and usually these irregularities become less evident in expiration.

Occasionally, several peaks are present on the diaphragmatic surface that are likewise due to the rib attachments of the diaphragm. Occasionally, these are due to abnormal pleurodiaphragmatic adhesions, and the two processes must not be confused. This is spoken of as "tenting" of the diaphragm.

Overlapping Shadows Due to Diaphragm, Liver, and Heart Anteriorly (Fig. 9–47). The anteromedian part of the diaphragmatic dome, the heart shadow, and the anterior margin of the liver overlap one another in the lateral projection, producing a triangular shadow that may be confused with an interlobar effusion or consolidation of the inferior portion of the right middle lobe. Care must be exercised not to make this error of interpretation.

Diaphragmatic Movements. On quiet breathing, the range of motion of the diaphragm is about 1 to 2 cm. On deep breathing it will increase to 3 to 5 cm., or even somewhat more. There is usually an accompanying flare of the ribs upward and outward. Occasionally, half of the diaphragm will move somewhat more than the other, or in slightly different sequence, but marked differences in any area of the diaphragm or inequalities between the two sides are of definite pathologic significance.

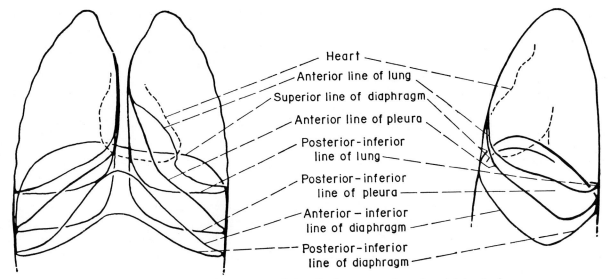

Heart
Anterior line of lung
Superior line of diaphragm
Anterior line of pleura
Posterior-inferior line of lung
Posterior-inferior line of pleura
Anterior-inferior line of diaphragm
Posterior-inferior line of diaphragm

FIGURE 9-43 Isometric concept of the diaphragm on frontal and lateral views.

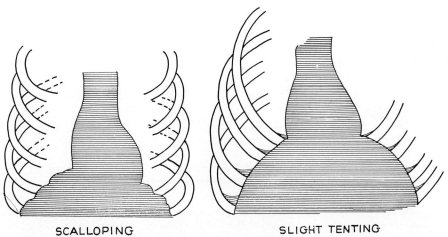

SCALLOPING   SLIGHT TENTING

FIGURE 9-44 Diagrammatic illustration of the scalloping and tenting of the diaphragm.

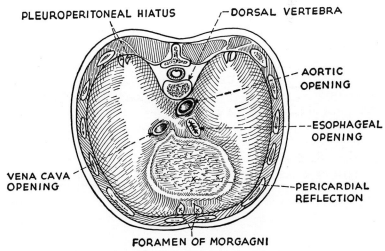

PLEUROPERITONEAL HIATUS   DORSAL VERTEBRA
AORTIC OPENING
ESOPHAGEAL OPENING
VENA CAVA OPENING
PERICARDIAL REFLECTION
FORAMEN OF MORGAGNI

FIGURE 9-45 Normal openings of the diaphragm.

ROUTINE POSITIONS IN THE RADIOGRAPHY OF THE CHEST

Posteroanterior Projection of the Chest (Fig. 9–46)

POINTS OF PRACTICAL INTEREST ABOUT FIGURE 9–46

1. Exposure is made at the end of full inhalation, without straining.
2. The slightest degree of motion will make the examination inadequate.
3. The central ray is centered over the sixth thoracic vertebra.
4. A film in expiration is occasionally required to show air trapping, or swaying of the mediastinum.
5. Barium may or may not be employed to delineate the esophagus.
6. The scapulae must be rotated enough that they do not obscure the lung fields.

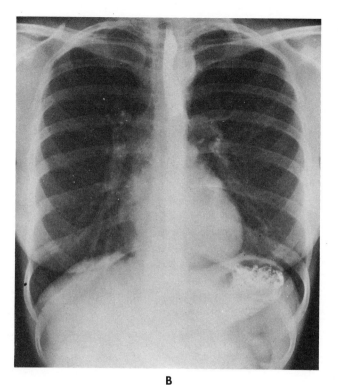

B

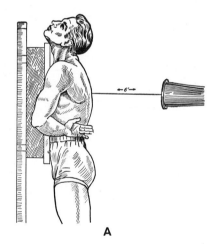

A

FIGURE 9–46 Posteroanterior projection of the chest. *A*. Position of patient. *B*. Radiograph (female).

FIGURE 9–46 *E–G*. Diagram illustrating changes in appearance of mediastinum with position of patient: *E*. Upright; *F*. lying on right side; *G*. lying on left side.

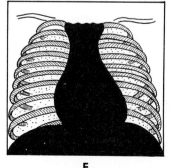

E

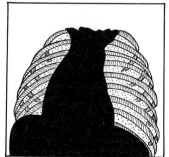

F

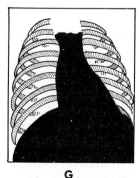

G

Figure continued on opposite page

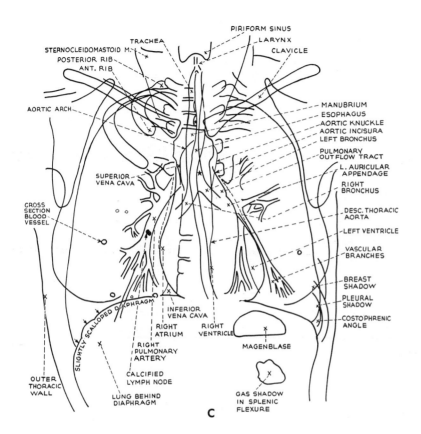

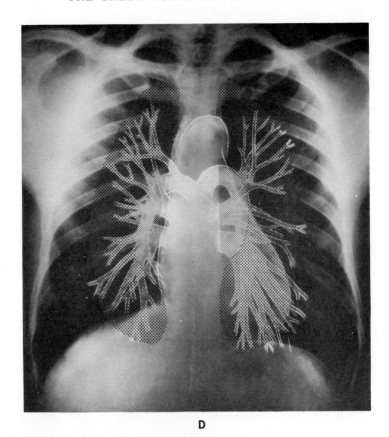

FIGURE 9–46 *Continued.* *C.* Labeled tracing of B. *D.* Normal radiographic chest showing three zones of study in the parenchyma.

Gross Subdivisions of the Lung Fields (Fig. 9–46). Arbitrarily one can subdivide the lung fields into three zones, depending on the size of the vascular radicles. The vascular branches gradually assume a smaller caliber proceeding from the hilus to the lung periphery. The inner one-third zone contains the largest channels; the middle one-third zone contains vessels of intermediate size; and the peripheral one-third zone usually has vessels that are 1 mm. or less in diameter. This arbitrary subdivision permits the radiologist to attribute definite significance to shadows that are inordinately large in diameter or size, particularly in the middle and outer zones. (See final section in this chapter: Methods of Studying Radiographs of the Chest.)

Lateral Projection of the Chest (Fig. 9–47)

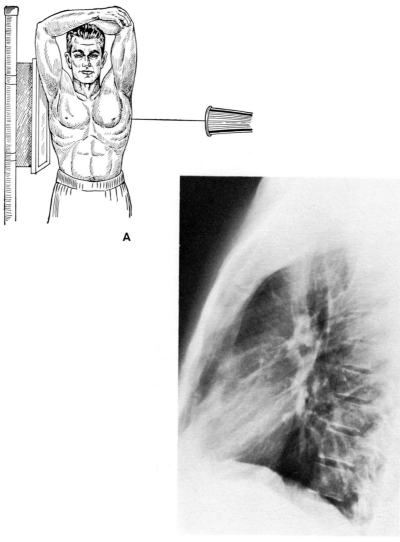

A

B

1. The central ray is directed to the level of the sixth thoracic vertebra. The exposure time is 4 or 5 times that of the PA projection.

2. At a 6-foot target-to-film distance, both sides of the chest are clearly seen. In order to visualize one side more clearly than the other, the side in question is placed next to the film, and the film-to-target distance is reduced to 36 inches; a focused grid must be employed.

3. The right lateral is routinely preferred. A left lateral may also be employed.

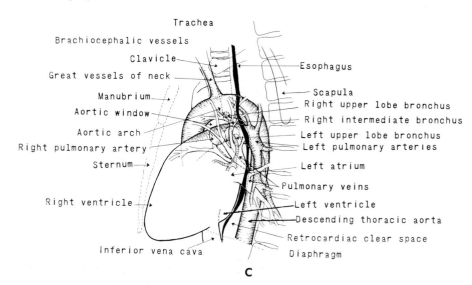

C

POINTS OF PRACTICAL INTEREST ABOUT FIGURE 9–47

1. The following areas are of particular interest and value for identification:

(a) The relationship of the right ventricle to the posterior margin of the sternum. With enlargement of the right ventricle, its shadow "rises" higher on the sternum.

(b) The degree of clarity of the anterior mediastinal clear space.

(c) The relationship of the left ventricle posteriorly to the shadow of the inferior vena cava. This will allow early and accurate detection of enlargement of the left ventricle.

(d) The relationship of the esophagus to the left atrium.

(e) The relative prominence of the pulmonary arteries. This requires considerable experience, but is very valuable from the standpoint of detecting abnormalities of lymph node origin, or tumor masses.

FIGURE 9–47 Lateral projection of chest. *A*. Position of patient. *B*. Radiograph. *C*. Lateral view of chest with anatomic parts labeled.

Left Posteroanterior Oblique Projection of the Chest (Fig. 9–48)

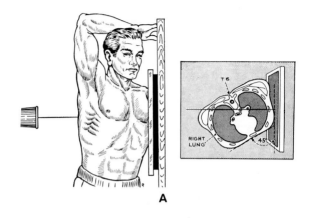

A

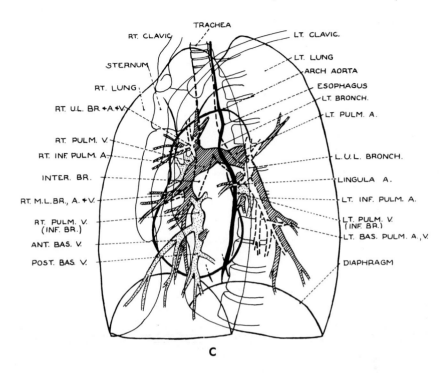

C

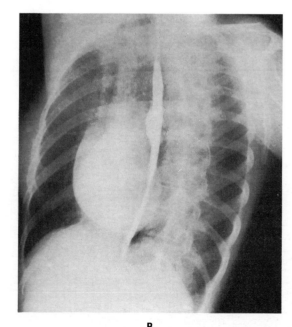

B

FIGURE 9–48 Left posteroanterior oblique projection of chest. *A*. Position of patient. *B*. Radiograph. *C*. Labeled tracing of *B*.

POINTS OF PRACTICAL INTEREST ABOUT FIGURE 9–48

1. The 45-degree obliquity may be increased to 50 or 55 degrees on occasion, to obtain maximum clearance of the spine.

2. Ordinarily the left ventricle clears the spine, and the right ventricle forms a smooth uninterrupted convexity with the ascending portion of the arch of the aorta.

3. This projection gives maximum clarity of the bifurcation of the trachea, the arch of the aorta, and the posterior basilar portion of the left ventricle. Pulsations are ordinarily of maximum amplitude in this portion of the cardiac silhouette.

4. Although the right ventricle is seen very adequately in most instances in this projection, the straight lateral is preferable, since the relationship of the right ventricle to the retrosternal space is more informative. Likewise, the left ventricle is more accurately evaluated in the straight lateral projection by noting its relationship to the shadow of the inferior vena cava. It should not normally project more than 5 or 6 mm. beyond this shadow in the lateral projection.

Right Posteroanterior Oblique Projection of the Chest (Fig. 9–49)

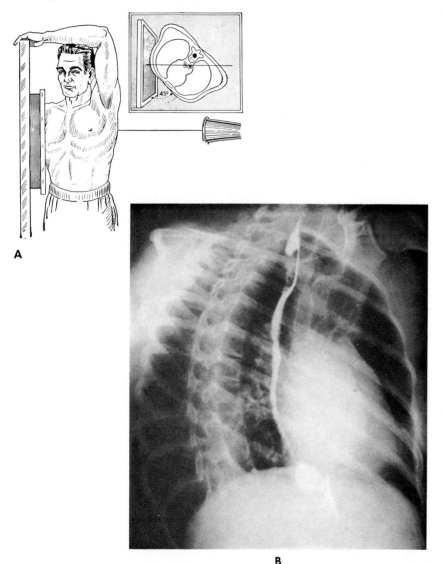

A

B

FIGURE 9–49 Right posteroanterior oblique projection of chest with barium in the esophagus. *A*. Position of patient. *B*. Radiograph. *C*. Labeled tracing of *B*.

POINTS OF PRACTICAL INTEREST ABOUT FIGURE 9–49

1. The patient's right shoulder is placed against the film and the body turned approximately 45 degrees from the film, resting the left arm in a convenient position, away from the body.

2. The central ray is directed just medial to the scapula nearest the x-ray tube at approximately the level of the sixth or seventh thoracic vertebra.

3. The patient is placed in proper position and then barium paste is administered. He is instructed to swallow and then take a deep breath and hold it while the x-ray exposure is made.

4. The maximum area of the right lung field is demonstrated in this projection but it is partially obscured by the shadow of the spinal column.

5. This projection is most advantageous for demonstration of the left atrium and its possible enlargement, since any slight enlargement will cause a significant impression upon the esophagus as indicated.

6. This projection is also of value for demonstrating the anterior apical portion of the left ventricle which is most significantly involved in anterior apical myocardial infarction, a rather common disease entity.

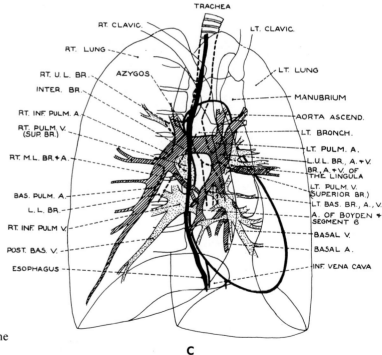

C

Anteroposterior Projection of the Chest (Fig. 9–50)

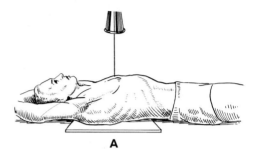

A

POINTS OF PRACTICAL INTEREST ABOUT FIGURE 9–50

1. Although it is difficult to obtain a view of the upper lung fields in this projection because of the shadows of the scapulae, considerable improvement will result if the patient crosses his arms above his head, thus rotating the scapulae outward.

2. The clavicles, on the other hand, are projected above the lung apices sufficiently so that this area of the lungs may be more clearly shown.

3. Analysis of the cardiac silhouette is not.as favorable in this projection in the adult, because of the straightening of the left margin and broadening of the base.

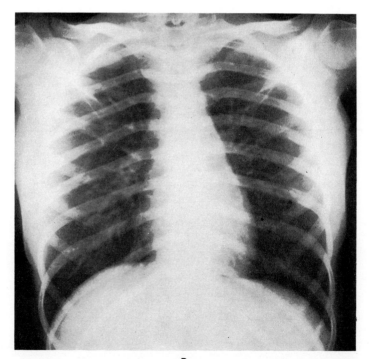

B

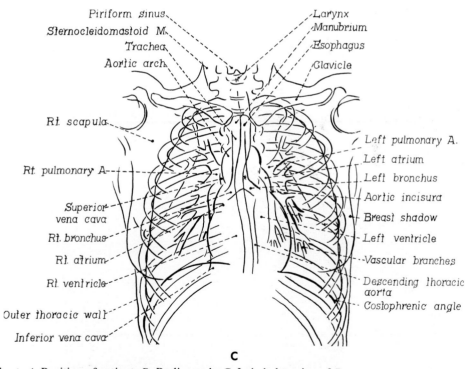

Piriform sinus
Sternocleidomastoid M.
Trachea
Aortic arch
Larynx
Manubrium
Esophagus
Clavicle
Rt. scapula
Left pulmonary A.
Left atrium
Rt. pulmonary A.
Left bronchus
Aortic incisura
Superior vena cava
Breast shadow
Rt. bronchus
Left ventricle
Rt. atrium
Vascular branches
Rt. ventricle
Descending thoracic aorta
Costophrenic angle
Outer thoracic wall
Inferior vena cava

C

FIGURE 9–50   Anteroposterior projection of chest. *A*. Position of patient. *B*. Radiograph. *C*. Labeled tracing of *B*. The main differences between Figures 9–46 and 9–50 are as follows: (1) the projection of the clavicles; (2) the scapulas are projected over the lung fields in the anteroposterior projection; (3) the superior mediastinal structures appear somewhat fuller in the anteroposterior projection; and (4) the obliquity of the ribs is different.

Apical Lordotic Projection (Fig. 9–51). This projection is particularly useful for clear demonstration of the lung apices and subapical areas. It also has its application in demonstrating the anterior mediastinum tangentially. Distortion of the lower chest areas is maximum in this projection.

POINTS OF PRACTICAL INTEREST ABOUT FIGURE 9–51

1. By standing the patient approximately 1 foot in front of the vertical cassette stand and then having him lean directly backward, a proper obliquity of the chest is obtained. The hands are placed palms outward on the hips in order to rotate the scapula as much as is feasible.

2. The top of the cassette is adjusted so that the upper border of the film is about 1 inch above the shoulders.

3. The central ray passes through the region of the manubrium. Occasionally a slight angle of 5 degrees toward the head may prove to be of advantage in demonstrating the apices more clearly.

4. This projection gives a very distorted picture of the lung fields and mediastinum, but is particularly valuable in showing more clearly: (1) the apices; (2) the interlobar areas of the lungs; and (3) the region of the pulmonary sector of the cardiac shadow.

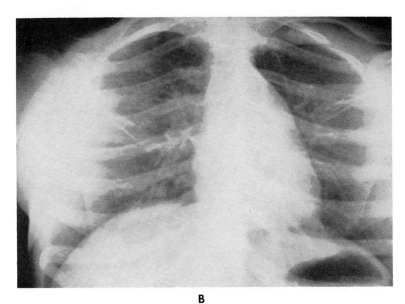

B

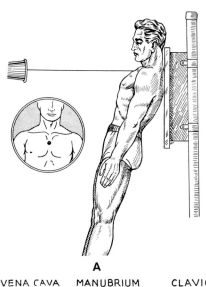

A

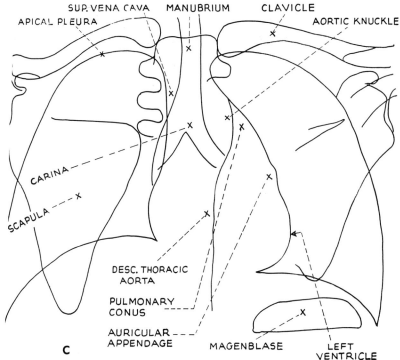

C

FIGURE 9–51 Apical lordotic projection of chest. *A.* Position of patient. *B.* Radiograph. *C.* Labeled tracing of *B.* (The tube may have to be angled cephalad 10°.)

Air Gap Technique. The air gap technique provides a positioning frame that displaces the patient's chest 6 to 10 inches from the cassette (Fig. 9–52). This has two advantages: (1) The air gap of 6 to 10 inches acts as a filter for secondary radiation, making this procedure a "gridless technique." There are no grid lines to interfere with the interpretation of the film.*† The air gap roentgenogram is considered by some to be of greater value than the over-penetrated grid roentgenogram on this basis. The kilovoltage is raised to 120 Kv., since lower values are found to give inadequate penetration. Also, the use of these higher voltages reduces the patient's dose‡. (2) The air gap roentgenogram may be considered a midchest laminagram since the structures in the midchest are seen in greatest detail, whereas the anterior and posterior chest regions are perhaps diminished in sharpness. Ideally, the distance of the tube-target from the film should be 10 feet for optimum results (3.05 meters).

Most adults require an exposure of 1000 Ma., 120 Kv., and one-40th of a second. Infants and children require an exposure of at least 300 Ma., 110 Kv., and one-60th of a second.

The disadvantage of this technique is that soft pulmonary infiltrates and small densities tend to be obscured. Moreover, a patient with a wide chest is most difficult to fit on the frame, unless the cassette is placed crosswise to the beam. If the anteroposterior position is utilized, it is important to move the scapulae out of the way by special positioning of the patient.

*Watson, W.: Gridless radiography at high voltage with air gap technique. X-ray Focus (Ilford), 2:12, 1958.

†Jackson, F. I.: The air gap technique: An improvement by anteroposterior positioning for chest roentgenography. Am. J. Roentgenol., 92:688–691, 1964.

‡Trout, E. D., et al.: High kilovoltage radiography. Radiology, 52:669–683, 1949.

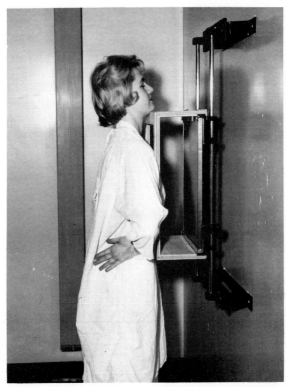

FIGURE 9–52 The patient is positioned against the frame for a posteroanterior air gap roentgenographic study. (From Jackson, F. I.: Am. J. Roentgenol. 92:688–691, 1964.)

Positive Pressure Radiography. The Valsalva maneuver may be utilized in radiologic diagnosis to increase intrathoracic pressure and lower the effective filling pressure of both cardiac ventricles. This maneuver requires the patient to blow against the closed mouth and nose to aid in diagnosis and therapy. Whitley and Martin have utilized this procedure as a diagnostic tool in chest disease. A mercury column is positioned so that it is superimposed over the edge of the posteroanterior film of the chest, and thus an instantaneous record of the pressure at the moment the film is made is obtained. The exposure is made approximately 5 to 6 seconds after initiation of the patient's positive pressure effort. This timing is important because after 8 to 10 seconds there is a return to normal pressures and cardiac output. The minimum level of intrabronchial pressure to assume a consistent response has been estimated to be between 30 and 40 mm. of mercury. A precise level in any individual is determined by his lung compliance, venous pressure, and vasomotor tone. In the overshoot or post-Valsalva maneuver phase following the release of the pressure, the visualization of the enlarged left atrial appendage is improved, as might occur in mitral stenosis. The overshoot phenomenon is best determined approximately 8 to 10 seconds after the cessation of the Valsalva maneuver. During the manuever, there is a diminution in cardiac size and intrapulmonary vasculature, since cardiac output has been lowered temporarily and visualization of the pulmonary vascular bed and the aorta and its principal branches has been improved by increased aeration of surrounding lung and diminished size of vasculature.

The Valsalva maneuver, as utilized above, has been found useful in the following circumstances: (1) differentiation of enlarged hilar vessels from hilar lymphadenopathy; (2) differentiation of hyperemia, both isolated and associated with other abnormalities, from infiltration and fibrosis of the lung; (3) differentiation of pulmonary arteriovenous fistula from solid tumors; (4) visualization of the miliary and small nodular pulmonary densities; (5) differentiation of focal nodular areas of hyperemia and infiltration from ill-defined tumor nodules.

METHOD OF STUDYING RADIOGRAPHS OF THE CHEST (Fig. 9–53)

1. Localize the abnormal shadow with respect to the chest wall, pleura, lung parenchyma, or mediastinum. If localized in the lung, determine the exact lobe or segment involved if possible.

2. Study the level of the diaphragm on each side, noting its general contour and position and any abnormalities contiguous with it.

3. Study the costophrenic and cardiophrenic sinuses in relation to their clarity and sharpness for indication of pleural disease.

4. Survey the lung fields. First compare the two sides in relation to one another. Second, divide the lung fields into three zones as shown in Figure 9–46. The innermost zone contains hilar blood vessels of large caliber, the intermediate or middle zone contains the medium-sized blood vessels, and the outer zone contains the very small blood vessels, usually so small that only minimal detection is obtained in the usual radiographs. When any shadows that are extraordinary in any respect appear, therefore, in any of these zones, they are immediately suspicious of abnormality.

5. Note the lung apices particularly, and take care to look "under the bones" so that no actual pulmonary markings of unusual character are overlooked.

6. Study the hilar blood vessels and mediastinum. The position of the trachea and its major ramifications should be noted. The trachea is ordinarily located near the midline. A further analysis of the mediastin-

um will follow in later chapters; here, it is enough to say that a study of the mediastinum cannot be separated from a study of the respiratory system.

The major hilar blood vessels should be traced so that arteries and veins are distinguished, especially in the lung apices and the lung bases. Is there a "deflection" or "cephalization-of-flow" phenomenon in the upright position so that venous distention is noted? Is there an accentuation of the interstitial pattern? Is there arterial distention?

7. Study the thoracic cage, tracing each rib carefully. The widths and symmetry of the intercostal spaces are evaluated simultaneously. The clavicle, scapulae, and visible bony structures of the neck should be noted. Although the skeletal structures of the dorsal spine are not seen adequately enough for careful diagnosis, it can be noted whether or not there is a scoliosis or other significant spine deformity which may affect the radiographic diagnosis of chest lesions. Is there a sternal depression or deformity, pectus excavatum, or pectus carinatum?

8. Study the soft tissue structures of the thoracic cage (Fig. 9–32). Identify the breasts, nipples, areoli, muscular shadows, particularly the pectoralis major and minor, and the sternocleidomastoids, which very often cast a significant soft tissue shadow across the medial aspect of the lung apices. A tegmental shadow, ordinarily seen above the superior border of the clavicle, must be identified and distinguished from the abnormal.

9. Any unusual pleural shadows are identified. The pleura does not ordinarily cast a significant visible shadow, except occasionally the posterior mediastinal (paraesophageal) stripe to a minimal degree in the costophrenic sinuses and overlying the lung apices. In the region of the lung apices, small blebs may occur normally. They are without pathologic significance and must be identified and distinguished from a pathologic process.

10. Identify structures underlying the diaphragm. A posteroanterior erect chest film offers a very good opportunity for visualizing free air under the diaphragm. Dense areas of calcification such as calcified cysts of the liver are also identified. The distance of the stomach (fundal air bubble or Magenglase) from the left hemidiaphragm should be noted. Is there a filling defect in the fundus? Is the spleen enlarged?

11. In the lateral projection of the chest it is particularly important to identify the *mediastinal shadow* and to form in the mind's eye a concept of the normal in this regard. Identify the left and right pulmonary artery, the trachea, and the bifurcations. We find the lateral projection extremely valuable in detecting abnormal lymphadenopathy or tumor masses in the central mediastinum.

12. In the lateral view identify the *anterior mediastinal clear space* which is just anterior to the cardiac silhouette and underlies the sternal shadow. On occasion the lateral is the only projection in which the clear space is obliterated in the presence of a space-occupying lesion in the anterior superior mediastinum.

13. In the lateral projection, *the pleural reflection over the internal mammary vessels should be studied.* Metastases will at times produce detectable masses in this location.

14. In the oblique projections, further care must be exercised to identify the trachea and bronchial structures which can be seen to excellent advantage. The oblique projections are also particularly valuable in analysis of the cardiac silhouette, especially when barium delineates the esophagus (this will be described in Chapters 10 and 11).

15. Study the clear pneumonic space in the posterior mediastinum and identify the relationship it has with the posterior margin of the left ventricle and the reflection of the inferior vena cava especially.

16. Study the dorsal spine.

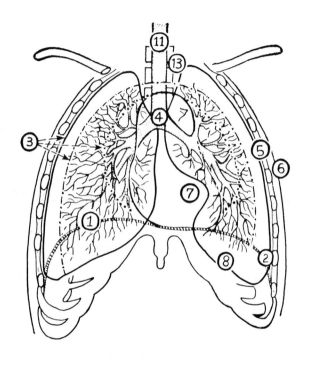
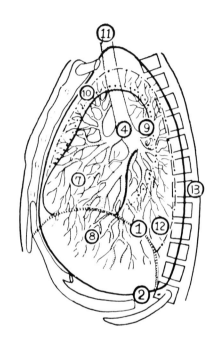

1. DIAPHRAGM
2. COSTOPHRENIC SINUSES
3. ZONES OF LUNG FIELDS
4. TRACHEA IN THORAX
   AND HILI
5. RIBS AND PLEURA
6. THORACIC WALL
7. HEART
8. UNDER DIAPHRAGM
9. HILI ON LATERAL VIEW
10. ANT. MEDIASTINUM
11. TRACHEA IN NECK
12. POST. MEDIASTINUM
13. VERTEBRA

FIGURE 9–53 A suggested routine to be followed in examining radiographs of the chest.

10

THE MEDIASTINUM
AND THE HEART

BASIC ANATOMY

Mediastinal Boundaries

The mediastinum is that compartment of the thoracic cage that is bounded laterally by the parietal pleural reflections along the medial aspects of both lungs, superiorly by the thoracic inlet, inferiorly by the diaphragm, anteriorly by the sternum, and posteriorly by the anterior surfaces of the thoracic vertebral bodies.

Arbitrary Compartments of the Mediastinum (Figure 10–1). Classically, the mediastinum is divided into *superior* and *inferior* compartments, as shown in Figure 10–1. The inferior compartment, in turn, is divided into three further subdivisions: (a) *anterior*, (b) *middle*, and (c) *posterior*.

These subdivisions are particularly useful in defining the nature of the pathology, when such is recognized, because of the statistical incidence of certain abnormalities within each of these compartments.

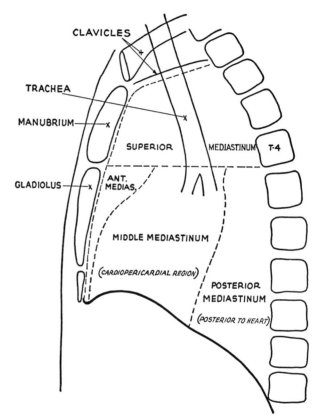

FIGURE 10–1   Compartments of the mediastinum.

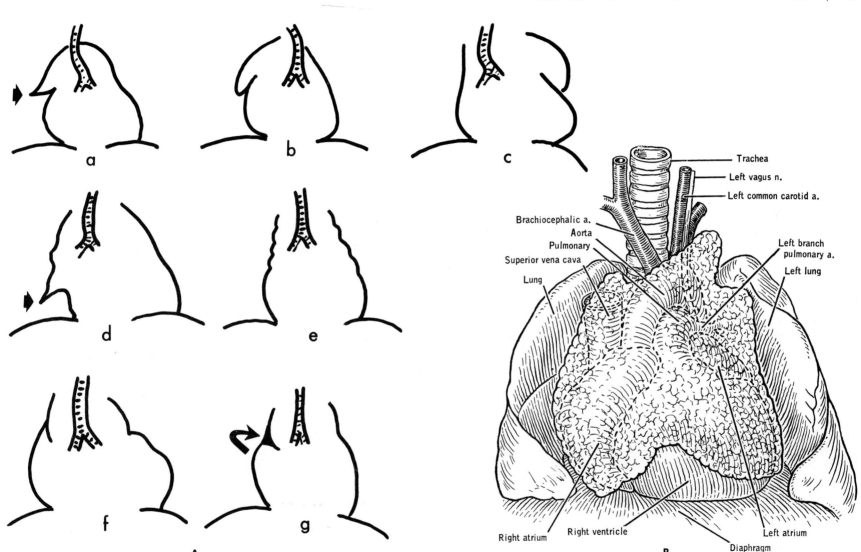

FIGURE 10–2 *A*. Variations in shape of the thymus gland in the newborn infant. (Modified from Tausend, M. E., and Stern, W. Z.: Am. J. Roentgenol., *95*:125–130, 1965.) *B*. Thymus of a full-term stillborn infant to show its relation to subjacent structures in the superior and anterior mediastinum prior to inflation of the lungs. Right and left lungs have been retracted laterally. (From Anson, B. J. (ed.): Morris' Human Anatomy, 12th ed. New York, McGraw-Hill Book Company, 1966. Copyright © 1966 by McGraw-Hill, Inc. Used by permission of McGraw-Hill Book Company.)

FIGURE 10–3 *A.* Diagram illustrating a view of the mediastinum from its right aspect (left lung removed).

Figure continued on opposite page.

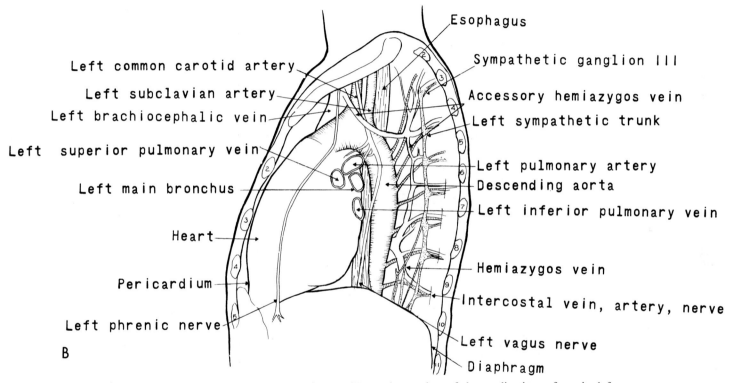

FIGURE 10–3 *Continued.* *B*. Diagram illustrating a view of the mediastinum from its left aspect (right lung removed). (After Pernkopf, E.: Atlas of Topographical and Applied Human Anatomy, Vol. 2. Philadelphia, W. B. Saunders Co., 1964.)

BASIC ANATOMY OF THE CARDIOVASCULAR SYSTEM

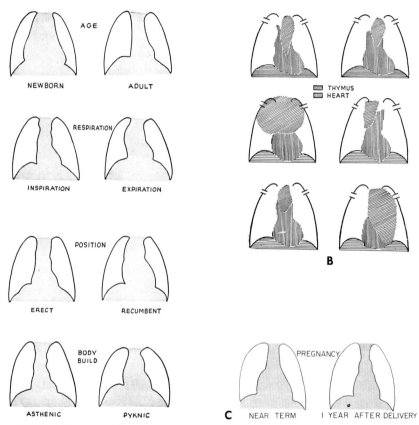

FIGURE 10–4 *A.* Normal factors causing variation in the supracardiac shadow and cardiac contour. *B.* Variations in size and position of supracardiac thymic shadow in the infant, which must be considered when measuring the infant's heart. *C.* Changes in cardiac size and contour which occur in hypervolemia of pregnancy.

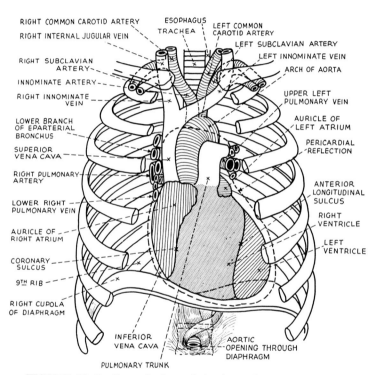

FIGURE 10–5 Frontal view of the heart in the thoracic cage with lung and rib structures removed.

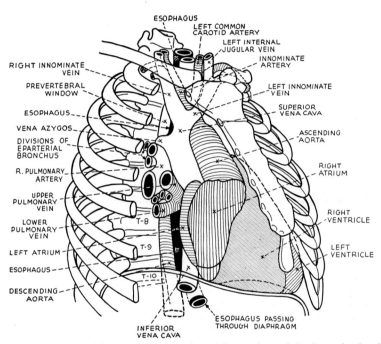

FIGURE 10-6   Right posteroanterior oblique view of the heart in the thoracic cage with lung and rib structures removed.

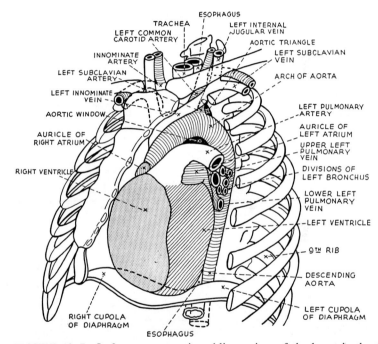

FIGURE 10-7   Left posteroanterior oblique view of the heart in the thoracic cage with lung and rib structures removed.

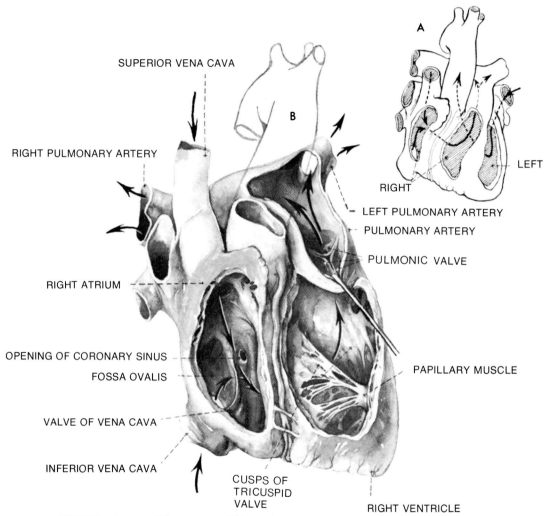

FIGURE 10–8 *A*. The course of blood through the chambers of the heart. *B*. The right atrium and right ventricle opened up for view, along with the outflow tract from the right ventricle to the pulmonary artery. (From Anson, B. J.: An Atlas of Human Anatomy. Philadelphia, W. B. Saunders Company, 1968.)

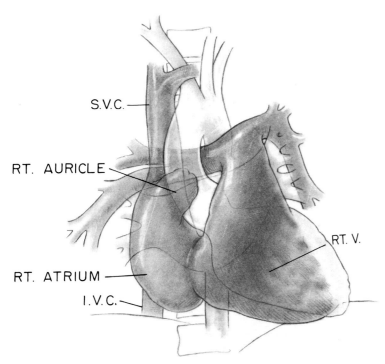

FIGURE 10–9 Frontal view of the heart showing the relationship of inflow and outflow tracts to the right cardiac chambers. (I.V.C.) inferior vena cava, (S.V.C.) superior vena cava, (RT.V.) right ventricle. (After Schad, N., et al.: Differential Diagnosis of Congenital Heart Disease. New York, Grune & Stratton, 1966. Used by permission of Grune & Stratton.)

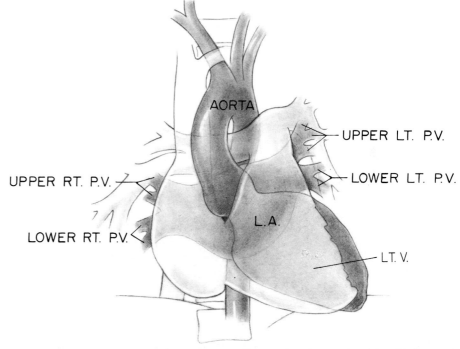

FIGURE 10–10 Frontal view of the heart showing the relationship of inflow and outflow tracts to the left cardiac chambers. (RT. P.V.) right pulmonary veins, (L.A.) left atrium, (LT. V.) left ventricle (shaded), (LT. P.V.) left pulmonary veins. (After Schad, N., et al.: Differential Diagnosis of Congenital Heart Disease. New York, Grune & Stratton, 1966. Used by permission of Grune & Stratton.)

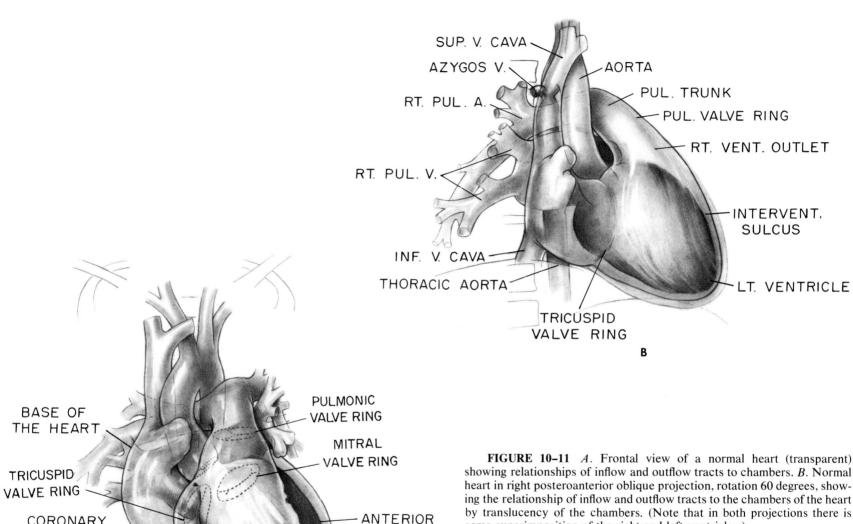

FIGURE 10–11 *A.* Frontal view of a normal heart (transparent) showing relationships of inflow and outflow tracts to chambers. *B.* Normal heart in right posteroanterior oblique projection, rotation 60 degrees, showing the relationship of inflow and outflow tracts to the chambers of the heart by translucency of the chambers. (Note that in both projections there is some superimposition of the right and left ventricles.)

Figure continued on opposite page.

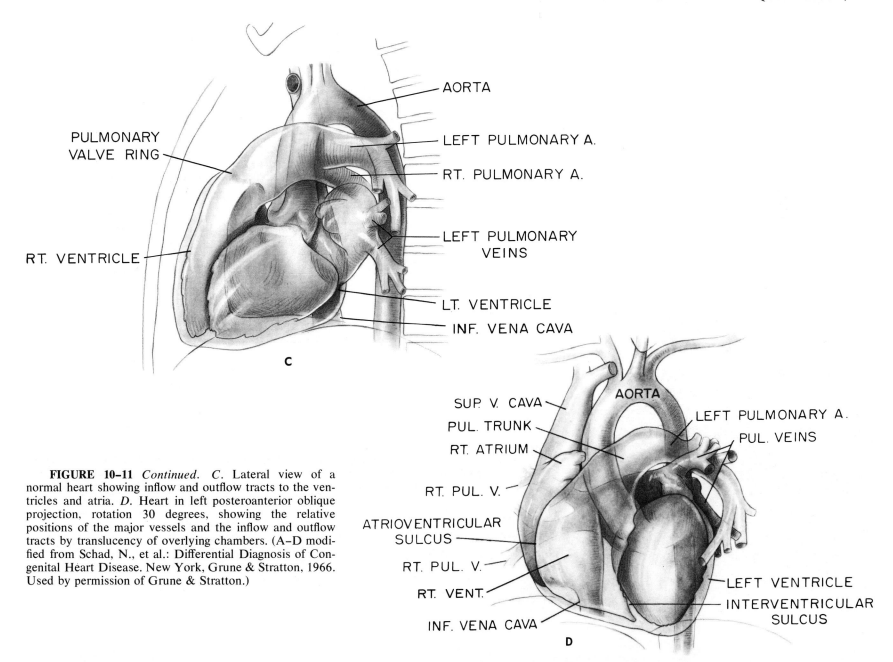

AORTA

PULMONARY
VALVE RING

LEFT PULMONARY A.

RT. PULMONARY A.

LEFT PULMONARY
VEINS

RT. VENTRICLE

LT. VENTRICLE

INF. VENA CAVA

C

FIGURE 10–11 *Continued. C.* Lateral view of a normal heart showing inflow and outflow tracts to the ventricles and atria. *D.* Heart in left posteroanterior oblique projection, rotation 30 degrees, showing the relative positions of the major vessels and the inflow and outflow tracts by translucency of overlying chambers. (A–D modified from Schad, N., et al.: Differential Diagnosis of Congenital Heart Disease. New York, Grune & Stratton, 1966. Used by permission of Grune & Stratton.)

SUP. V. CAVA

AORTA

PUL. TRUNK

LEFT PULMONARY A.

PUL. VEINS

RT. ATRIUM

RT. PUL. V.

ATRIOVENTRICULAR
SULCUS

RT. PUL. V.

RT. VENT.

LEFT VENTRICLE

INTERVENTRICULAR
SULCUS

INF. VENA CAVA

D

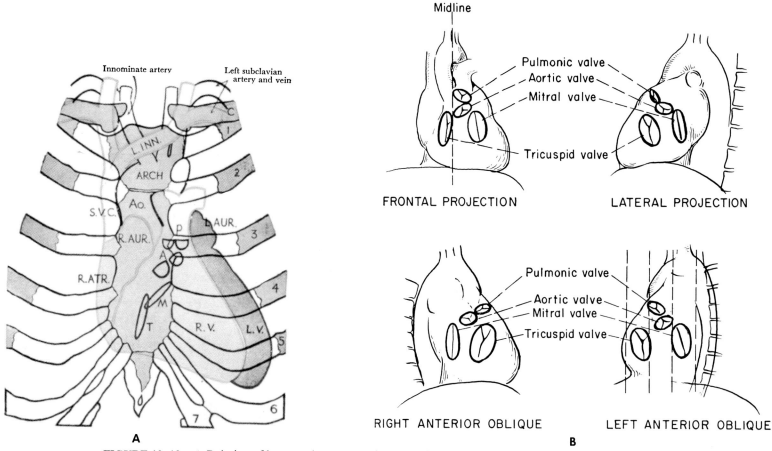

FIGURE 10–12 *A*. Relation of heart and great vessels to anterior wall of thorax. (1 to 7) Ribs and costal cartilages, (A) aortic orifice, (Ao) ascending aorta, (C) clavicle, (L.V.) left ventricle, (M) mitral orifice, (P) pulmonary orifice, (R.V.) right ventricle, (S.V.C.) superior vena cava, (T) tricuspid orifice. (From Brash, J. C. (ed.): Cunningham's Manual of Practical Anatomy, 12th ed., Vol. 2. London, Oxford University Press, 1958.) *B*. Views of cardiac valves obtained in routine radiographic projections. (Right anterior oblique = right posteroanterior oblique projection. Left anterior oblique = Left posteroanterior oblique projection.)

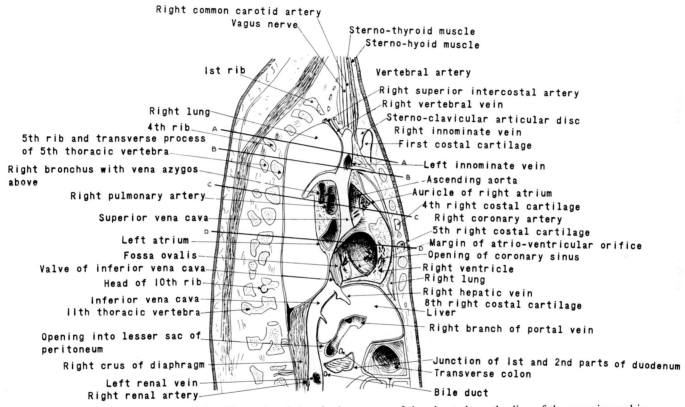

Right common carotid artery
Vagus nerve
Sterno-thyroid muscle
Sterno-hyoid muscle

Ist rib
Vertebral artery
Right superior intercostal artery
Right vertebral vein
Right lung
Sterno-clavicular articular disc
4th rib
Right innominate vein
5th rib and transverse process
of 5th thoracic vertebra
First costal cartilage
Left innominate vein
Right bronchus with vena azygos
above
Ascending aorta
Auricle of right atrium
Right pulmonary artery
4th right costal cartilage
Right coronary artery
Superior vena cava
5th right costal cartilage
Left atrium
Margin of atrio-ventricular orifice
Fossa ovalis
Opening of coronary sinus
Valve of inferior vena cava
Right ventricle
Head of 10th rib
Right lung
Inferior vena cava
Right hepatic vein
11th thoracic vertebra
8th right costal cartilage
Liver
Opening into lesser sac of
peritoneum
Right branch of portal vein
Right crus of diaphragm
Junction of 1st and 2nd parts of duodenum
Left renal vein
Transverse colon
Right renal artery
Bile duct

FIGURE 10–13 Line drawing illustrating the sagittal anatomy of the chest along the line of the superior and inferior venae cavae. (Innominate vein = "brachiocephalic vein" in Nomina Anatomica, 1966.) (After Cunningham's Textbook of Anatomy, 6th ed. London, Oxford University Press, 1931.)

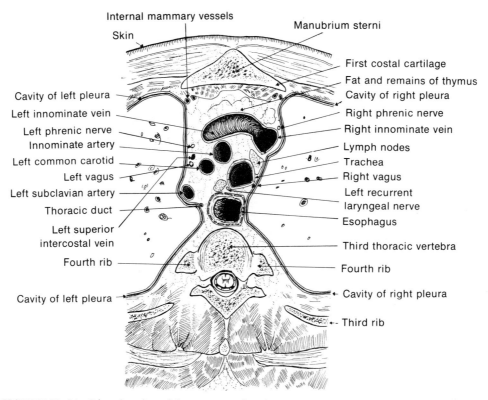

FIGURE 10–14 Line drawing of the cross-sectional anatomy of the chest at the level of the manubrium. (Innominate vein = brachiocephalic vein and innominate artery = brachiocephalic artery in Nomino Anatomica, 1966.) (Modified from Cunningham's Textbook of Anatomy, 6th ed. London, Oxford University Press, 1931.)

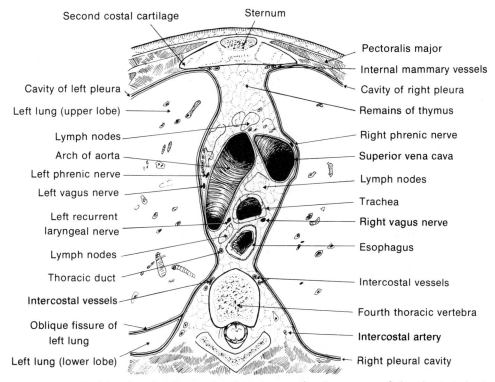

FIGURE 10–15 Line drawing illustrating the cross-sectional anatomy of the chest at the level of the fourth thoracic vertebra. (Modified from Cunningham's Textbook of Anatomy, 6th ed. London, Oxford University Press, 1931.)

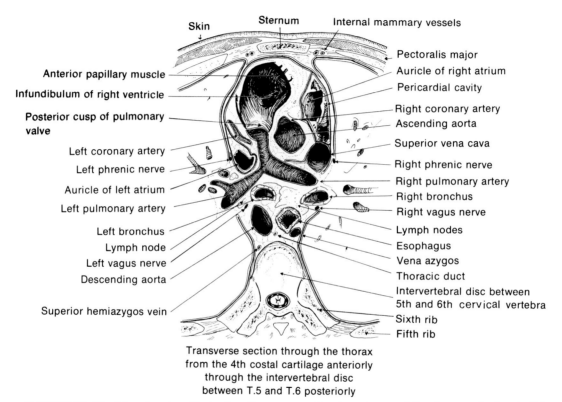

Skin Sternum Internal mammary vessels

Pectoralis major

Anterior papillary muscle

Auricle of right atrium

Infundibulum of right ventricle

Pericardial cavity

Posterior cusp of pulmonary valve

Right coronary artery

Ascending aorta

Left coronary artery

Superior vena cava

Left phrenic nerve

Right phrenic nerve

Auricle of left atrium

Right pulmonary artery

Left pulmonary artery

Right bronchus

Right vagus nerve

Left bronchus

Lymph nodes

Lymph node

Esophagus

Left vagus nerve

Vena azygos

Descending aorta

Thoracic duct

Intervertebral disc between 5th and 6th cervical vertebra

Superior hemiazygos vein

Sixth rib

Fifth rib

Transverse section through the thorax from the 4th costal cartilage anteriorly through the intervertebral disc between T.5 and T.6 posteriorly

FIGURE 10–16 Line drawing illustrating the cross-sectional anatomy of the chest at the level of the fifth thoracic vertebra, just below the inferior boundary of the superior mediastinum. (Modified from Cunningham's Textbook of Anatomy, 6th ed. London, Oxford University Press, 1931.)

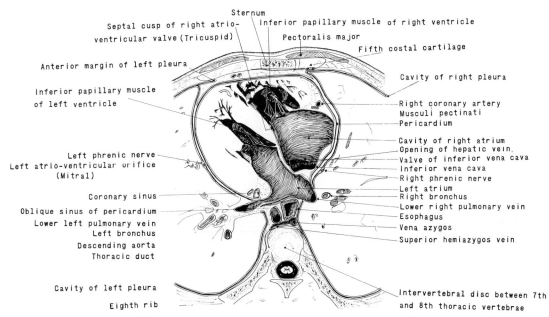

Sternum
Septal cusp of right atrio-
ventricular valve (Tricuspid)
Inferior papillary muscle of right ventricle
Pectoralis major
Fifth costal cartilage
Anterior margin of left pleura
Cavity of right pleura
Inferior papillary muscle
of left ventricle
Right coronary artery
Musculi pectinati
Pericardium
Left phrenic nerve
Left atrio-ventricular orifice
(Mitral)
Cavity of right atrium
Opening of hepatic vein
Valve of inferior vena cava
Inferior vena cava
Right phrenic nerve
Left atrium
Coronary sinus
Right bronchus
Oblique sinus of pericardium
Lower right pulmonary vein
Lower left pulmonary vein
Esophagus
Left bronchus
Vena azygos
Descending aorta
Superior hemiazygos vein
Thoracic duct

Cavity of left pleura

Eighth rib

Intervertebral disc between 7th
and 8th thoracic vertebrae

FIGURE 10–17 Line drawing illustrating the cross-sectional anatomy of the chest at the interspace between the level of the seventh and eighth thoracic vertebrae. (Modified from Cunningham's Textbook of Anatomy, 6th ed. London, Oxford University Press, 1931.)

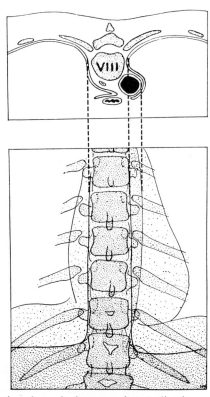

FIGURE 10–18 *Upper,* cross section through the posterior mediastinum at the level of the eighth thoracic vertebra. *Lower,* diagram taken from a roentgenogram depicting the posterior portions of the visceral or parietal pleura as lines along the vertebral column. Dotted lines indicate anatomic substrates of pleural lines and aortic lines in cross section. (From Lachman, E.: Anat. Rec., *83*:521, 1942.)

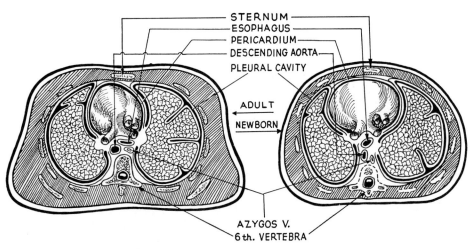

FIGURE 10–19 Differences in infantile and adult posterior mediastinal relationships. (Modified from Caffey.)

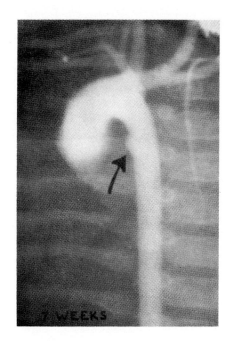

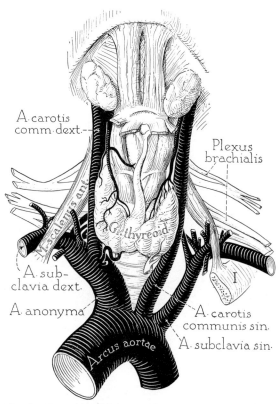

FIGURE 10–20 Branches of the aortic arch, shown in the usual schema. (A. carotis dext., right carotid artery; A. subclavia dext., right subclavian artery; A. anonyma, brachiocephalic artery; A. subclavia sin., left subclavian artery; A. carotis communis sin., left common carotid artery; Plexus brachialis, brachial plexus.) (From Anson, B. J.: An Atlas of Human Anatomy. Philadelphia, W. B. Saunders Company, 1963.)

FIGURE 10–21 Normal aorta. Seven weeks. The aortic arch and its great branches are clearly defined. The silhouette of the arch and the descending aorta resembles an inverted J. A localized bulge at the site of the ligamentum arteriosum (*arrow*) is present. This corresponds to the "ductus diverticulum," or "infundibulum" of the ductus. (From Abrams, H. L.: Angiography, 2nd ed., Vol. 1. Boston, Little, Brown & Co., 1971.)

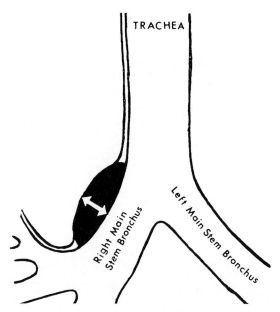

FIGURE 10–22 Method of measurement of azygos "knob" proposed by Keats et al. (From Keats, T. E., Lipscomb, G. E., and Betts, C. S., III: Radiology, *90*:990–994, 1968.)

TABLE 10–1. Average Values for Azygos Vein Shadow Width*

Investigator	Conditions of Measurement	Normal Range
Fleischner and Udis, 1952	Upright posteroanterior teleroentgenogram	Up to 6 mm.
Doyle et al., 1961	Supine anteroposterior tomograms	14.2 ± 2.6 mm.
Felson, 1967	Upright anteroposterior teleroentgenograms	Up to 10 mm.
Keats et al., 1968	Erect teleroentgenogram	3–7 mm.
	AGE	MEAN ± 1 STANDARD DEVIATION
Wishart, 1972	Birth to 6 months	3.5 ± 1.3 mm.
	6 to 24 months	4.1 ± 1.0 mm.
	2 to 7 years	4.8 ± 1.2 mm.
	8 to 14 years	5.1 ± 1.6 mm.

*Modified from Wishart, D. L.: Normal azygos vein width in children. Radiology, *104*:115–118, 1972.

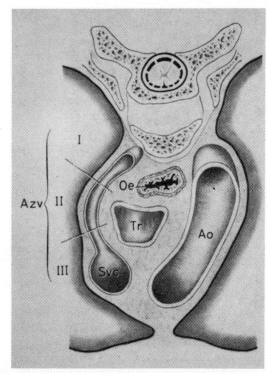

FIGURE 10–23 Drawing (modified from Andreassi) of a transverse section of thorax at the level of the fourth dorsal vertebra illustrates how the arch describes a medially concave curve, first passing laterally from the point of origin (I, posterior segment), then in a forward direction (II, intermediate segment), and finally, turning inward and downward (III, terminal segment). (Ao, aorta; Azv, azygos vein; Oe, esophagus; Svc, superior vena cava; Tr. trachea.) (From Tori, G., and Garusi, G. F.: Am. J. Roentgenol., *87*:238, 1962.)

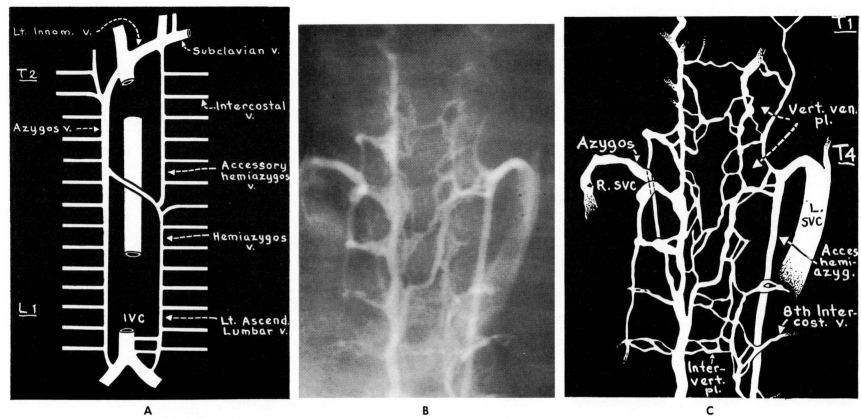

FIGURE 10–24 *A,* Diagrammatic representation of the azygos venous system. The segmental lumbar veins are joined to each other by a longitudinal vessel, the ascending lumbar vein. The right ascending lumbar vein as it enters the thorax becomes the azygos vein, and the left ascending lumbar vein is continuous with the hemiazygos vein. The hemiazygos vein crosses in front of the vertebral column at the level of the eighth or ninth thoracic vertebra to join the azygos vein. The accessory hemiazygos vein is continuous with the hemiazygos, receives the upper thoracic veins on the left, and joins the left superior intercostal vein above.

B and *C*. The vertebral veins at the upper thoracic level. The vertebral venous plexuses are opacified following the injection of the opaque medium into the left saphenous vein. The primitive paired arrangement of both the azygos and the superior vena cava veins is preserved, the accessory hemiazygos emptying into the left superior vena cava and the azygos emptying into the right superior vena cava. The medial portions of the intercostal veins are opacified. (R.SVC, right superior vena cava; L.SVC, left superior vena cava.) (Courtesy of Dr. Franz P. Lessman, Rothswell Park Memorial Institute, Buffalo, New York.) (Reproduced from Abrams, H. L.: Angiography, 2nd ed. Boston, Little, Brown & Co., 1971.)

Radiologic Methods Used in the Roentgen Cardiac Examination

1. **The Posteroanterior (PA) Teleroentgenograms of the Chest** (6 foot target-to-film distance), preferably with barium outlining the esophagus (Fig. 9–46).

2. **The Right Posteroanterior Oblique Projection with Esophagram.**

3. **The Left Posteroanterior Oblique Projection with Barium in the Esophagus.**

4. **The Anteroposterior Recumbent Study of the Cardiopericardial Shadow (Fig. 9–50).**

5. **The Lateral View of the Chest with Barium in the Esophagus (Fig. 9–47).**

6. **Fluoroscopy.** Fluoroscopy with image amplification should precede the film studies. The following outline is recommended.

THE HEART AND MEDIASTINAL STRUCTURES ARE STUDIED IN THE FRONTAL PERSPECTIVE. (1) The pulsations along the left cardiac border are investigated and the radiologist proceeds around the periphery of the mediastinum, studying carefully the pulsations of the pulmonary arteries, aorta, and right atrium. (2) The cardiac position is carefully noted, both in inspiration and expiration, and changes with respiration are detected.

THE PATIENT IS THEREAFTER TURNED IN THE RIGHT POSTERO-ANTERIOR OBLIQUE PROJECTION. (1) Once again the cardiac contour and pulsations are carefully noted. The pulsations in the apex of the left ventricle are particularly important, since this area is prone to suffer from coronary vascular impairment. (2) The pulmonary outflow tract is observed, since this projection is particularly suited for this purpose. (3) The anterior margin of the ascending aorta is then studied. (4) Thereafter the posterior mediastinal space is viewed. Normally this space is clear, because it is occupied by structures of lesser opacity such as the esophagus, aorta, and veins. The prominence of the left atrium in relation to the posterior mediastinum is particularly noteworthy. Its relationship to the esophagus (barium-filled) is particularly important.

THE PATIENT IS THEN TURNED IN THE LEFT POSTEROANTERIOR OBLIQUE PROJECTION. (1) In this position the posterior basilar portion of the left ventricle is studied. The pulsations here are usually of greater amplitude than elsewhere. Some concept of left ventricular size can be obtained from the fact that in the 45 degree obliquity the left ventricle normally clears the spine. (2) The anterior margin of the heart in this projection is formed by the right ventricle usually. A fairly straight line is formed by the anterior margin of the right ventricle and the ascending aorta in this projection. Any unusual convexities, either in the right ventricle or in the ascending aorta, are of pathologic significance. (3) This position affords the most accurate means of studying the arch of the aorta in relation to the left pulmonary artery, which lies beneath it. There is ordinarily a clear space known as the "aortic window" between the aortic arch and the pulmonary artery. Any enlargement of a contiguous structure will cause its obliteration.

SIZE OF FLUOROSCOPIC FIELD. By carefully restricting the size of the fluoroscopic field, the cardiac shadow is surveyed for any areas of calcification and hyperlucency. (1) Care must be exercised to insure that the calcification is projected within the heart in every view and pulsates synchronously with the heart, since calcified mediastinal lymph nodes can cause occasional confusion. (2) The heart normally does not contain calcification, but the following cardiopericardial structures may contain calcium abnormally: (a) the pericardium, (b) the coronary vessels, (c) the myocardium, (d) the endocardium, (e) the papillary muscles, (f) the cardiac valves, and (g) the rings at the base of the cardiac valves and (h) the aortic sinus of Valsalva.

The position of the cardiac valves in various projections is indicated in Figure 10–12. Calcified valves may be differentiated by their characteristic "dance," which is synchronous with the cardiac pulsations. The motion is jerky and steplike.

DETERMINATION OF RELATIVE CARDIAC VOLUME (Amundsen)*

The physical factors employed are (1) a target-to-film distance on frontal view of 2 meters, and (2) a target-to-film distance on lateral view of 1.5 meters.

Basic Formula. Volume = K × L × B × D (Fig. 10–25), where K = 0.42 (standard deviation 7.4 per cent) based on 45 cases, comparing calculated value with autopsy-determined value.

Relative heart volume is defined as the volume per square meter of surface area using the DuBois nomograms for calculation of surface area from body height and weight. Thus, the formula for *relative heart volume* is:

$$\frac{0.42 \times L \times B \times D}{\text{Body surface area in square meters}}$$

A difference of 90 ml. per square meter or more between two successive examinations of the same patient indicates a significant change in relative heart volume.

The mean volume per square meter for adult males is 420 ± 40 cc., and for adult females it is 370 ± 40 cc. The second or third standard deviation indicates a strong suspicion of cardiomegaly, and above this limit there is only a 3 per cent chance of a normal heart size.

The second to third standard deviation above the mean is:

Female adults	450–490 ml. per sq. m.
Male adults	500–540 ml. per sq. m.
Birth to 3 months	284–311 ml. per sq. m.
3 months to 2 years	334–371 ml. per sq. m. •

*Amundsen, P.: The diagnostic value of conventional radiological examination of the heart in adults. Acta Radiol. (Suppl.), *181*:1–87, 1959.

The greatest internal diameter of the chest has a poor correlation with cardiac frontal area.

The right and left cardiac margins must be delineated as separate and distinct from the pericardial fat pads in the cardiophrenic angles.

In infants, Lind's technique calls for carefully centered antero-posterior *supine* films.

Nomograms for the determination of body surface area of children and adults are appended for use.

Normal Heart Volumes in Children (Table 10–2; Fig. 10–26). These values may be utilized along with those of Amundsen and Lind.

Relative heart volume calculation is now considered the method of choice for daily practice for both children and adults.

TABLE 10–2. Normal Heart Volumes in Children*

Age	Volume per Square Meter of Body Surface (Relative Heart Volume)	Standard Error of the Mean
0–30 days	196	22.6
30–90 days	217.8	33.9
90–360 days	282	35.8
1–2 years	295	30.4
2–4 years	304	41.5
4–7 years	310	36.2
7–9 years	324	28.6
9–12 years	348	33.6
12–14 years	369	53.8
14–16 years	398	61.9

*Adapted from Mannheimer, in Keats, T. E., and Enge, I. P.: Radiology, *85*:850, 1965.

CARDIAC MENSURATION

1. UNGERLEIDER AND GUBNER NOMOGRAM METHOD
(FOR INDIVIDUALS 56-80" HT.; 95-300# WT.)

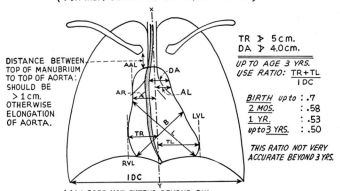

DISTANCE BETWEEN TOP OF MANUBRIUM TO TOP OF AORTA: SHOULD BE > 1 cm. OTHERWISE ELONGATION OF AORTA.

TR > 5 cm.
DA > 4.0 cm.

UP TO AGE 3 YRS.
USE RATIO: $\dfrac{TR+TL}{IDC}$

BIRTH up to	: .7
2 MOS.	: .58
1 YR.	: .53
up to 3 YRS.	: .50

THIS RATIO NOT VERY ACCURATE BEYOND 3 YRS.

AAL : DOES NOT EXTEND BEYOND RVL.
RVL : DOES NOT EXTEND BEYOND MEDIAL 1/3 of DIAPHRAGM.
LVL : DOES NOT EXTEND BEYOND MEDIAL 1/2 of DIAPHRAGM.

1. $A = \dfrac{\pi}{4}\, L \times B = .7854 \times L \times B$

2. GREATEST TRANSVERSE DIAMETER (GTD) OF HEART: TR + TL

3. COMPARE MEASURED AND CALCULATED VALUES FOR A and GTD WITH VALUES ANTICIPATED FROM BODY HEIGHT AND WEIGHT. NORMAL RANGE IS VALUE ANTICIPATED ± 10%

4. MEASURED AORTIC VALUE : AR + AL
ANTICIPATED AORTIC VALUE :

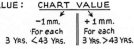

CHART VALUE	
−1 mm. ·For each 3 YRS. < 43 YRS.	+1 mm. For each 3 YRS. > 43 YRS.

A

2. USE SIMILAR MEYER'S TABLES FOR CHILDREN 3-16 YRS. OF AGE EXCEPT A = .68 × L × B.

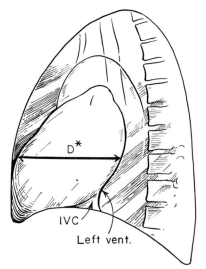

LATERAL VIEW OF NORMAL HEART

*D = Greatest anterior-posterior measurement of heart

B

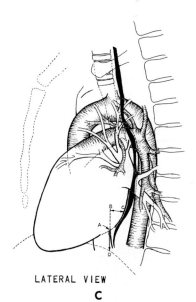

LATERAL VIEW

C

FIGURE 10–25 *A*. Cardiac mensuration by the Ungerlieder and Gubner technique. *B*. Lateral view of the normal heart showing the method of obtaining measurement D, the greatest anteroposterior measurement of the heart in calculation of cardiac volume. *C*. Important measurements on lateral view of heart. Point A is the crossing of the inferior vena cava and left ventricle. Point B is 2 cm. cephalad to A. Line BC parallels the plane of the dorsal vertebrae. Line AD is the vertical distance to the left hemidiaphragm. Left ventricular enlargement is present when BC is greater than 18 mm. Left ventricular hypertrophy is suspect when AD is less than 0.75 cm.

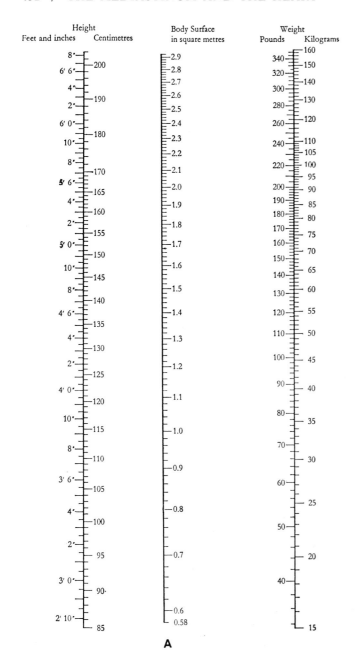

Height — Feet and inches / Centimetres
Body Surface in square metres
Weight — Pounds / Kilograms

A

FIGURE 10–26 *A.* Nomogram for the determination of body surface area of adults and children (by Du Bois). *Key:* The body surface area is given by the point of intersection with the middle scale of a straight line joining the height and weight. *B.* Summary of concepts of relative heart volume determination and roentgenologic heart volume in infants according to Amundsen and Lind, respectively. Mannheimer's values for children are presented in Table 10–2.

Relative Heart Volume Determination (Amundsen)

Predicted Heart Volume (PHV) = $0.4^* \times L \times B \times D$
(P-A view, TSD = 2 m.; lateral view, 1.5 m.)

Relative Heart Volume (RHV) = $\dfrac{PHV}{Body\ surface\ area}$ (BSA in m.²)

	RHV (ml./m.²)
Significant difference between sequential exams	90 or more
Female adults (maximum normal)	450–490
Male adults (maximum normal)	500–540
Birth to 3 months (maximum normal)†	284–311
3 months to 2 years (maximum normal)†	334–371

Roentgenologic Heart Volume in Infants (Lind)

Actual volume preferred as determined by nomogram.
Heart Volume (HV$_{RTG}$; *BD* = B above; *LD* = L above; DD$_H$ = D above.
For nomogram see Figure 22–10.
  * Varies, as noted in text, by different investigators.
  † Antero-posterior recumbent, at least 3 hours after eating.

B

SPECIAL STUDIES OF THE HEART AND MAJOR BLOOD VESSELS

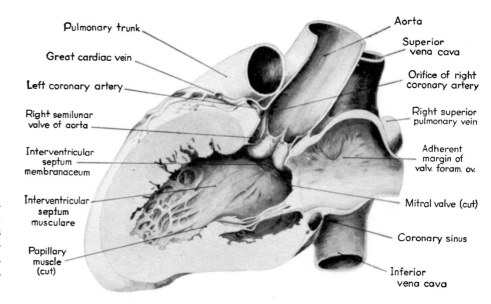

Pulmonary trunk

Great cardiac vein

Left coronary artery

Right semilunar
valve of aorta

Interventricular
septum
membranaceum

Interventricular
septum
musculare

Papillary
muscle
(cut)

Aorta

Superior
vena cava

Orifice of right
coronary artery

Right superior
pulmonary vein

Adherent
margin of
valv. foram. ov.

Mitral valve (cut)

Coronary sinus

Inferior
vena cava

FIGURE 10–27 Left side of the heart opened in a plane approximately parallel to the septa, to show the interior of the left atrium and left ventricle. A segment of the anterior leaflet of the mitral valve has been cut away to expose more fully the region of the membranous portion of the interventricular septum and the aortic orifice. (From Gould, S. E. Pathology of the Heart, 2d ed. Springfield, Ill., Charles C Thomas, Publisher, 1959. Courtesy of Charles C Thomas, Publisher.)

CATHETERIZATION OF THE HEART

Cardiac Catheterization. In view of the great technical advances made by cardiac surgeons in relation to open heart surgery and repair of defects, the roentgen examination of the heart and its inflow and outflow tracts has become much more exacting. The surgeon must know the answers to many questions, such as the size and extent of a defect or stenosis, the degree of overriding of the aorta, and the appearance of the pulmonary arteries, veins, and systemic arteries.

In recent years, the technique of cardiac catheterization has been increasingly applied and developed in this direction. Passing a catheter into the right heart and then sequentially into the pulmonary artery provides the physician with the following opportunities: (1) blood samples may be obtained from any of these areas or all of them, and *gas analysis* may be performed on the samples to determine the site of shunt formation; (2) the *volume of blood shunting* may be calculated; (3) *pulmonary blood flow* may be readily calculated; (4) *pressures* in the various chambers may be recorded and evaluated in relation to the dynamics of the cardiac circulation; (5) if the catheter takes an *abnormal route,* a defect may be recognized directly—for example, a patent interatrial septum; (6) at the end of these procedures, one may selectively inject into any region a quantity of opaque media under sufficient pressure to visualize carefully a given area without too much interference from adjoining areas. This latter technique is called "selective angiocardiography," in contrast to the previously described venous angiocardiography.

Selective Angiocardiography. There are different types of catheters used for this purpose, each with its own advocates. A mechanical pressure device for the injection must usually be employed to provide a satisfactory jet of contrast media within 1/2 to 1 second. A number of

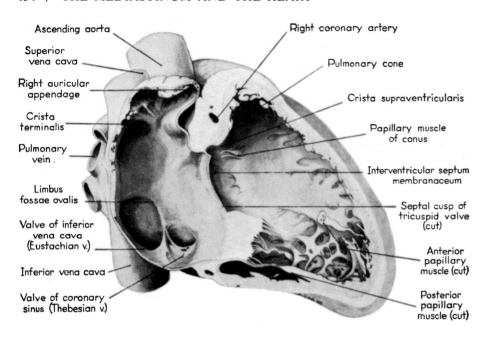

Ascending aorta
Superior vena cava
Right auricular appendage
Crista terminalis
Pulmonary vein
Limbus fossae ovalis
Valve of inferior vena cava (Eustachian v.)
Inferior vena cava
Valve of coronary sinus (Thebesian v.)
Right coronary artery
Pulmonary cone
Crista supraventricularis
Papillary muscle of conus
Interventricular septum membranaceum
Septal cusp of tricuspid valve (cut)
Anterior papillary muscle (cut)
Posterior papillary muscle (cut)

FIGURE 10–28 Right side of the heart opened in a plane approximately parallel to the septa, to show the interior of the right atrium and the right ventricle. A segment of the septal leaflet of the tricuspid valve has been cut away to expose more fully the region of the membranous portion of the interventricular septum. (From Gould, S. E. Pathology of the Heart, 2d ed. Springfield, Ill., Charles C Thomas, Publisher, 1959. Courtesy of Charles C Thomas, Publisher.)

these are available commercially, varying in complexity and cost from several hundred dollars to several thousand. Injection directly into the right ventricle is by far the most common procedure, and the injection is followed by serial films taken as rapidly as 12 per second (simultaneously in two planes), or by 16 or 35 mm. cineradiographs for cinema depiction. Care must be exercised to locate the catheter tip accurately, lest the injection be made into a coronary vein.

The projection planes most frequently employed are the straight frontal (anteroposterior), right posteroanterior oblique, and lateral. Usually, a simultaneous biplane technique is desirable.

CORONARY ARTERIOGRAPHY AND VENOGRAPHY

Basic Anatomy. Two coronary arteries supply the heart. The *left coronary* originates from the left aortic sinus at the level of the free edge of the valve cusp. Its short common stem bifurcates or trifurcates

about 0.5 to 2 cm. from its origin (Figs. 10–33; 10–34). The *anterior interventricular or descending branch* courses downward in the anterior interventricular groove just to the right of the apex of the heart and may ascend a short distance up the posterior interventricular groove. There are branches to the adjacent anterior right ventricular wall and septal branches, supplying the anterior two-thirds of the apical portion of the septum. The anteroapical portions of the left ventricle ordinarily have several branches. The second branch of the left coronary artery, the *circumflex,* runs in the left atrioventricular sulcus, giving off branches to the upper lateral left ventricular wall and left atrium. When there is a third branch of the left coronary artery, it originates between the anterior interventricular and circumflex branches and supplies the left ventricle.

The *right coronary artery* arises from the right anterior sinus of Valsalva (aortic sinus) and courses along the right atrioventricular sulcus. It rounds the acute margin of the right ventricle to reach the crux (junction of the posterior interventricular sulcus and the posterior atrioventricular groove). It gives off branches to the anterior right ventricu-

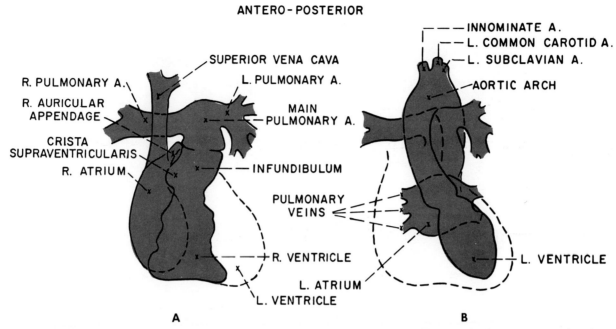

ANTERO-POSTERIOR

FIGURE 10–29 *A* and *B*. Major structures visualized in venous angiocardiograms in the anteroposterior view. *A*. Lesser circulation phase. *B*. Greater circulation phase. (Innominate a. = "brachiocephalic" artery.)

Figure continued on following page.

lar wall; the branch along the acute margin of the heart and another supplying the posterior interventricular branch are usually well developed. The posterior papillary muscle of the left ventricle usually has a dual supply from both the left and the right coronary arteries. One branch, which originates from the right coronary artery, ascends along the anteromedial wall of the right atrium and supplies the *superior vena caval branch or nodal artery,* posterior and to the left of the superior vena caval ostium. It then rounds this ostium to the sinoatrial node.

Variations in the branching pattern of the coronary artery are frequent. In about two-thirds of the cases, the right coronary artery is dominant, crossing the crux and supplying part of the left ventricu-

wall and the ventricular septum. In 15 per cent of cases the left coronary artery is dominant and its circumflex branch crosses the crux, supplying the posterior interventricular branch and all of the left ventricle, the ventricular septum and part of the right ventricle. In 18 per cent of cases both coronary arteries reach the crux and this is the so-called "balanced coronary arterial pattern."* In about 40 per cent of cases, a large anterior atrial branch of the left coronary artery courses toward the superior vena cava rather than the anterior atrial branch of the right

*Netter, F. H.: Ciba Collection of Medical Illustrations, Vol. 5. Ciba Pharmaceutical Division of Ciba-Geigy Corporation, 1969.

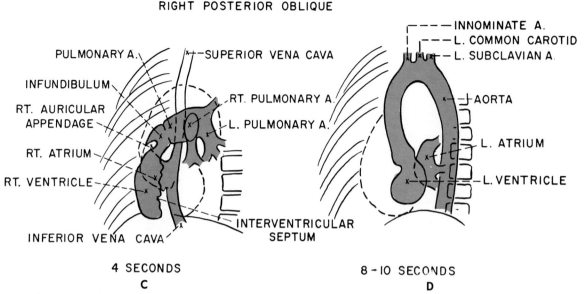

RIGHT POSTERIOR OBLIQUE

FIGURE 10–29 *C* and *D*. Major structures visualized in venous angiocardiograms in the right postero-anterior oblique projection. *C*. Lesser circulation phase. *D*. Greater circulation phase. (Innominate a. = "brachiocephalic" artery.)

Figure continued on opposite page.

coronary artery. It is also quite common for the first, second, and even third branches of the right coronary artery to originate independently from the right aortic sinus rather than from the right coronary artery proper.

Oblique projections of the right and left coronary arteries are shown diagrammatically in Figure 10–34.

The two largest veins are the *great cardiac vein* in the anterior interventricular groove along with the left coronary artery, and the *middle cardiac vein* in the posterior interventricular groove, along with the posterior interventricular branch of the right coronary artery. There may also be a large *posterior left ventricular vein* as well. Small valves may be present in each of these larger veins. The oblique vein of the left atrium enters the coronary sinus near its junction with the great cardiac vein and it does not have a valve. The small cardiac vein may enter the coronary sinus as shown (Fig. 10–35), or it may enter the right atrium independently. There are anterior cardiac veins that do almost always enter the right atrium independently. As shown in the illustration, there are veins in the inferior interventricular groove and the atrioventricular groove along the right border that appear to flow into the small cardiac vein and thence into the coronary sinus. Small veins situated in the atrial septum and ventricular walls that enter the cardiac chambers directly are called the *Thebesian* veins.

LEFT POSTERIOR OBLIQUE

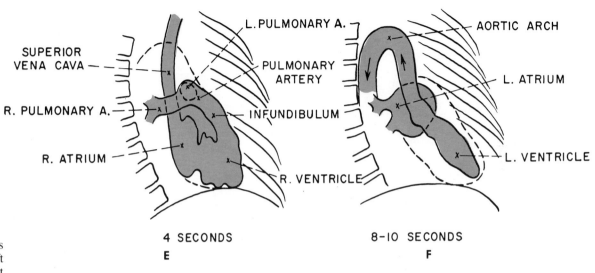

4 SECONDS
E

8-10 SECONDS
F

FIGURE 10–29 *E* and *F*. Major structures visualized in venous angiocardiograms in the left posteroanterior oblique projection (same as right anteroposterior oblique view). *E*. Lesser circulation phase. *F*. Greater circulation phase. *G* and *H*. Major structures visualized in venous angiocardiograms in the right lateral view. *G*. Lesser circulation phase. *H*. Greater circulation phase. (Innominate a. = "brachiocephalic" artery.)

RIGHT LATERAL

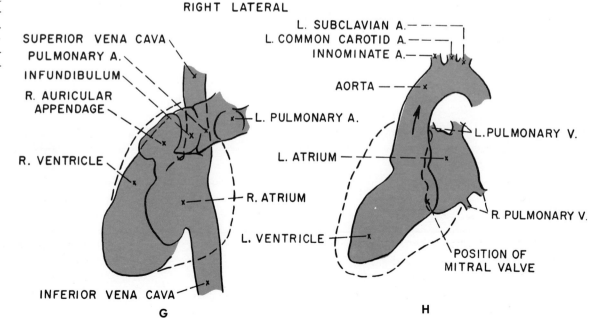

G

H

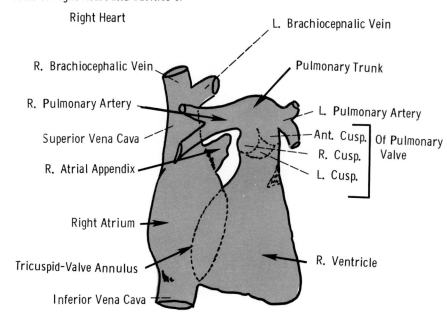

Ant. Post. Projection of Inflow and Outflow
Tracts of Right Heart and Cavities of
Right Heart

A

L. Brachiocepnalic Vein

R. Brachiocephalic Vein

Pulmonary Trunk

R. Pulmonary Artery

L. Pulmonary Artery

Superior Vena Cava

Ant. Cusp.
R. Cusp.
L. Cusp.
Of Pulmonary Valve

R. Atrial Appendix

Right Atrium

Tricuspid-Valve Annulus

R. Ventricle

Inferior Vena Cava

FIGURE 10–30 *A.* Anteroposterior and lateral views of inflow and outflow tracts of the right heart and cavities of the right heart, also showing the relative positions of the cusps of the pulmonary valve.

Figure continued on opposite page.

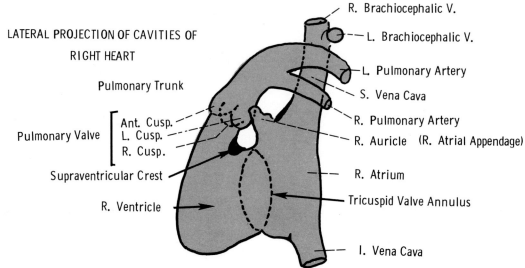

LATERAL PROJECTION OF CAVITIES OF
RIGHT HEART

Pulmonary Trunk

R. Brachiocephalic V.

L. Brachiocephalic V.

L. Pulmonary Artery

S. Vena Cava

R. Pulmonary Artery

Pulmonary Valve
Ant. Cusp.
L. Cusp.
R. Cusp.

R. Auricle (R. Atrial Appendage)

Supraventricular Crest

R. Atrium

R. Ventricle

Tricuspid Valve Annulus

I. Vena Cava

Ant. Post. Projection Left Heart and Aorta

as seen in Angiography

B

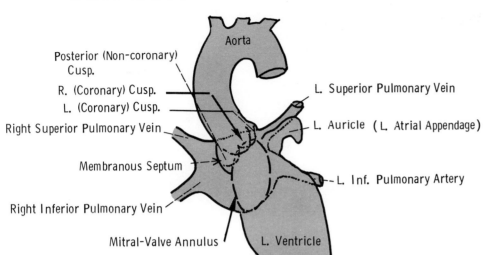

Posterior (Non-coronary) Cusp.

R. (Coronary) Cusp.

L. (Coronary) Cusp.

Right Superior Pulmonary Vein

Membranous Septum

Right Inferior Pulmonary Vein

Mitral-Valve Annulus

Aorta

L. Superior Pulmonary Vein

L. Auricle (L. Atrial Appendage)

L. Inf. Pulmonary Artery

L. Ventricle

FIGURE 10–30 *Continued.* *B.* Anteroposterior and lateral views of the cavities of the left heart and the outflow tracts, also showing the relative positions of the cusps of the aortic valves.

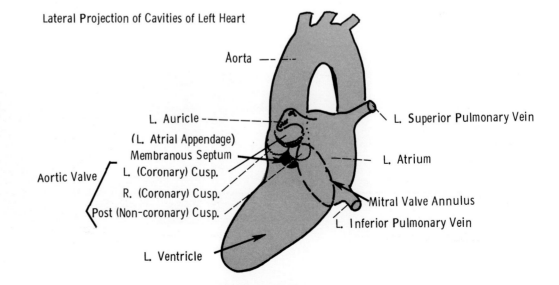

Lateral Projection of Cavities of Left Heart

Aorta

L. Auricle

(L. Atrial Appendage)

Membranous Septum

Aortic Valve

L. (Coronary) Cusp.

R. (Coronary) Cusp.

Post (Non-coronary) Cusp.

L. Superior Pulmonary Vein

L. Atrium

Mitral Valve Annulus

L. Inferior Pulmonary Vein

L. Ventricle

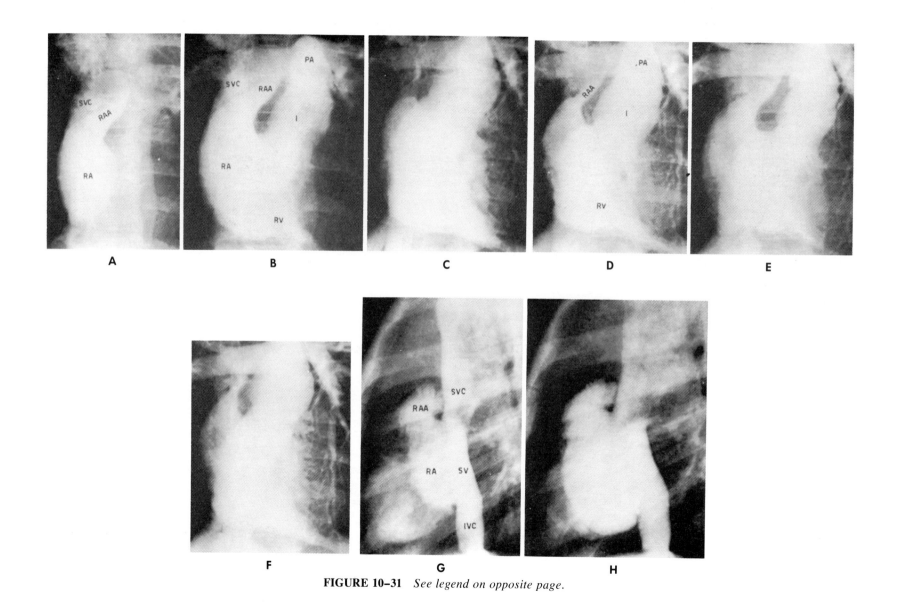

FIGURE 10–31 *See legend on opposite page.*

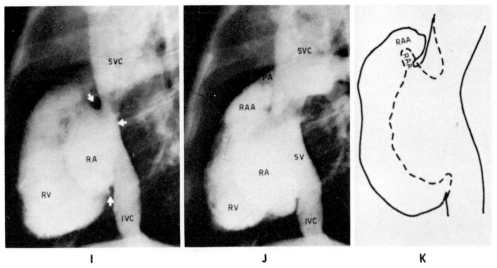

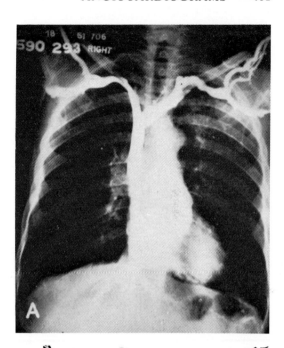

FIGURE 10–31 Representative angiocardiograms. *A–F.* Lesser circulation phase, frontal view. Right auricular appendage lies directly to the right of the infundibulum and the right ventricle and lower part of the pulmonary artery which, consequently, in lateral view, are overlapped by the appendage. (AO) Aorta, (I) infundibulum, (IVC) inferior vena cava, (LA) left atrium. (LV) left ventricle, (PA) pulmonary artery, (RA) right atrium, (RAA) right auricular appendage, (RV) right ventricle, (SV) sinus venosus, (SVC) superior vena cava. *G–K.* Lesser circulation phase, lateral view. During atrial systole, the atrioventricular border is shifted dorsally, while the dorsal wall of the atrium remains in the same position. The crista terminalis presses into the lumen like a membrane *(I, lower arrow).* Sphincter mechanism of the venae cavae is clearly visible. *K.* Collective picture of appearance of atrium in late diastole (solid line) and late systole (broken line). (From Diagnosis of Congenital Heart Disease, 2d ed., by Kjellberg, Sven R., et al. Copyright © 1959 by Year Book Medical Publishers, Inc., Chicago, Used by permission.)

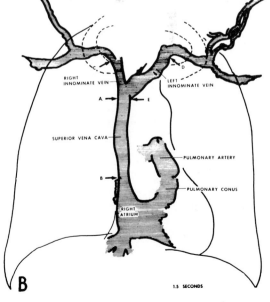

FIGURE 10–32   The superior vena cava and innominate veins as visualized by venous angiocardiography. (Innominate = "brachiocephic" in Nomina Anatomica, 1966.) (From Roberts, D. J., Jr., Dotter, C. T., and Steinberg, I.: Am. J. Roentgenol., *66:*341–352, 1951.)

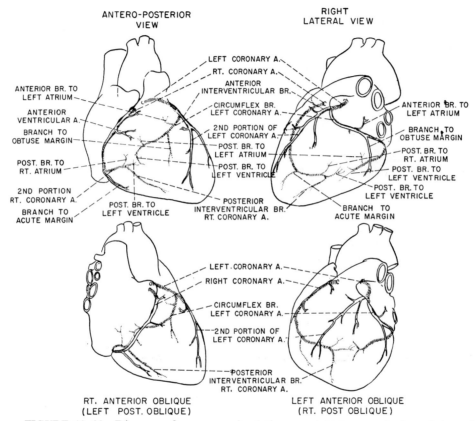

ANTERO-POSTERIOR
VIEW

RIGHT
LATERAL VIEW

LEFT CORONARY A.
RT. CORONARY A.
ANTERIOR
INTERVENTRICULAR BR.
CIRCUMFLEX BR.
LEFT CORONARY A.
2ND PORTION OF
LEFT CORONARY A.
POST. BR. TO
LEFT ATRIUM
POST. BR. TO
LEFT VENTRICLE

ANTERIOR BR. TO
LEFT ATRIUM
ANTERIOR
VENTRICULAR A.
BRANCH TO
OBTUSE MARGIN
POST. BR. TO
RT. ATRIUM
2ND PORTION
RT. CORONARY A.
BRANCH TO
ACUTE MARGIN
POST. BR. TO
LEFT VENTRICLE
POSTERIOR
INTERVENTRICULAR BR.
RT. CORONARY A.

ANTERIOR BR. TO
LEFT ATRIUM
BRANCH TO
OBTUSE MARGIN
POST. BR. TO
RT. ATRIUM
POST. BR. TO
LEFT VENTRICLE
POST. BR. TO
LEFT VENTRICLE
BRANCH TO
ACUTE MARGIN

LEFT CORONARY A.
RIGHT CORONARY A.
CIRCUMFLEX BR.
LEFT CORONARY A.
2ND PORTION OF
LEFT CORONARY A.
POSTERIOR
INTERVENTRICULAR BR.
RT. CORONARY A.

RT. ANTERIOR OBLIQUE
(LEFT POST. OBLIQUE)

LEFT ANTERIOR OBLIQUE
(RT. POST OBLIQUE)

FIGURE 10–33 Diagram of coronary circulation as might be seen in frontal, lateral, and oblique views. (Modified from Guglielmo and Guttadauro: Acta Radiol., Supp. 97:1952.)

RIGHT CORONARY ARTERY—BOTH OBLIQUE PROJECTIONS

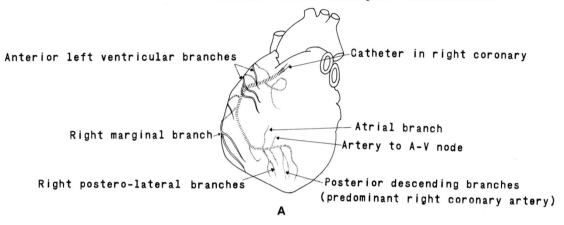

Anterior left ventricular branches

Catheter in right coronary

Right marginal branch

Atrial branch

Artery to A-V node

Right postero-lateral branches

Posterior descending branches
(predominant right coronary artery)

A

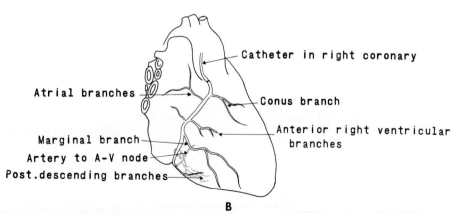

Catheter in right coronary

Atrial branches

Conus branch

Anterior right ventricular
branches

Marginal branch

Artery to A-V node

Post.descending branches

B

FIGURE 10–34 Oblique projections of the coronary arteries individually considered. *A.* Right coronary artery in left posteroanterior oblique projection. *B.* Right coronary artery in right posteroanterior oblique projection.

Figure continued on following page.

LEFT CORONARY ARTERY—BOTH OBLIQUE PROJECTIONS

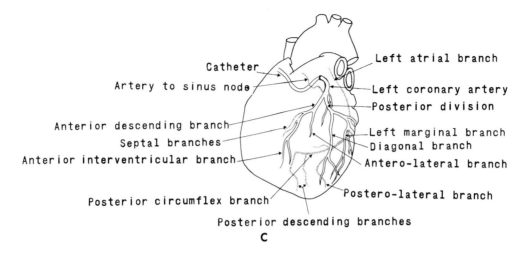

C

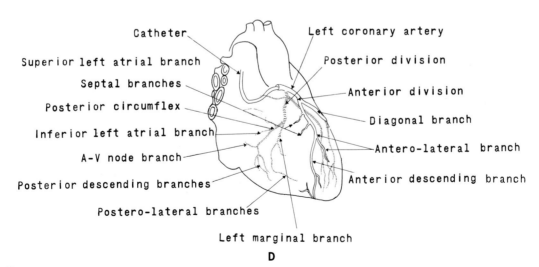

D

FIGURE 10–34 *C.* Left coronary artery in left posteroanterior oblique projection. *D.* Left coronary artery in right posteroanterior oblique projection.

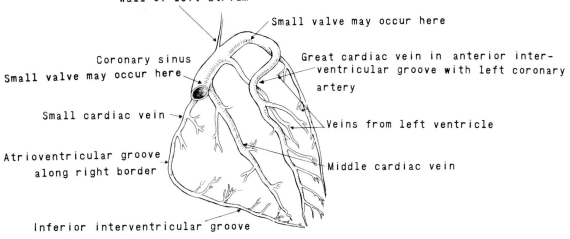

Oblique vein over posterior
wall of left atrium

Small valve may occur here

Coronary sinus

Small valve may occur here

Great cardiac vein in anterior interventricular groove with left coronary
artery

Small cardiac vein

Veins from left ventricle

Atrioventricular groove
along right border

Middle cardiac vein

Inferior interventricular groove

FIGURE 10–35 Lateral erect view of the veins of the heart.

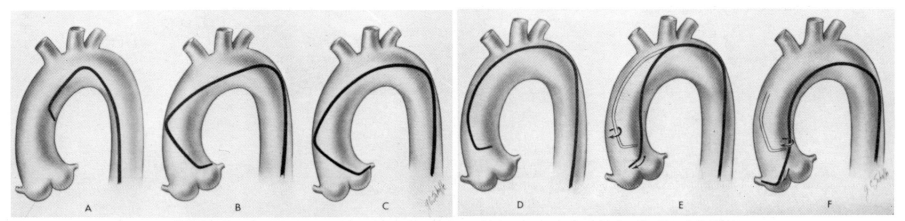

FIGURE 10–36 *A, B,* and *C.* Diagrammatic illustrations of left coronary catheterization. *D, E,* and *F.* Diagrammatic illustrations of right coronary catheterization (see text). (From Judkins, M. P.: Radiol. Clin. North Am., 6:467 - 492, 1968.)

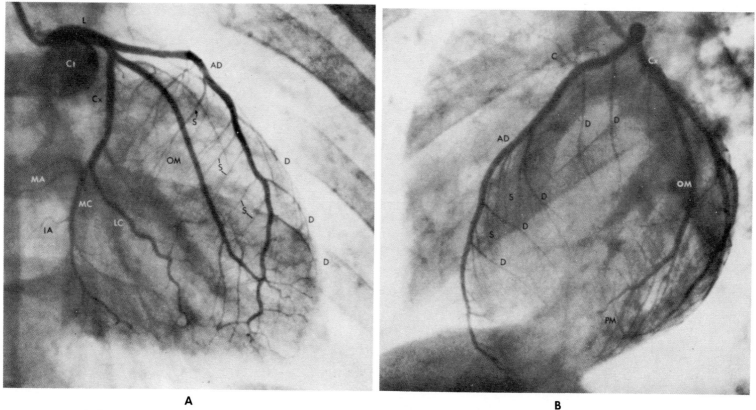

FIGURE 10–37 *A–C.* High-resolution normal left selective coronary arteriography. *A.* Right anterior oblique view 20°. *B.* Left anterior oblique view 70°. Contrast agent injections of each coronary artery are filmed in three projections (right anterior oblique, left anterior oblique, and lateral) by both cinéfluorography and high-resolution serial techniques. L, left main; AD, anterior descending; D, diagonal; S. septal; C, conus branches; Cx, circumflex; OM, obtuse marginal; LC, lateral circumflex; MC, medial circumflex; AC, atrial circumflex; MA, middle arterial; IA, inferior atrial; PM, papillary muscle artery; Ct, contrast material in the sinus of Valsalva.

Figure continued on opposite page.

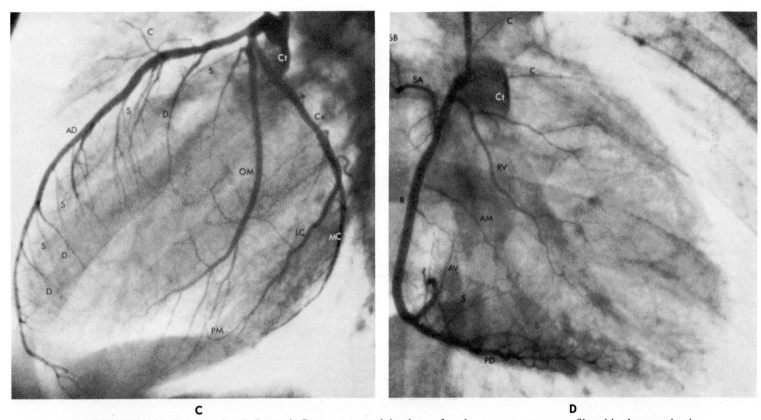

C   **D**

FIGURE 10–37 *Continued.*   *C.* Lateral. Contrast agent injections of each coronary artery are filmed in three projections by both cinéfluorography and high-resolution serial techniques. Projections *A, B,* and *C* were selected because they uncover and give dimension to all parts of the coronary tree. In each, the heart is projected free of the spine. *D–F,* High-resolution normal right selective coronary arteriography. *D.* Right anterior oblique view, 20°. R, Right main; C, conus branch; RV, right ventricular artery; SA, sinus node artery; SB, sinus node branch; PA, posterior atrial branch; AS, atrial septal branch; AM, acute marginal; PD, posterior descending; AV, atrioventricular node artery; PL, posterior lateral arteries; MA, middle atrial; IA, inferior atrial; S, septal; Ct, contrast material in the sinus of Valsalva.

Figure continued on opposite page.

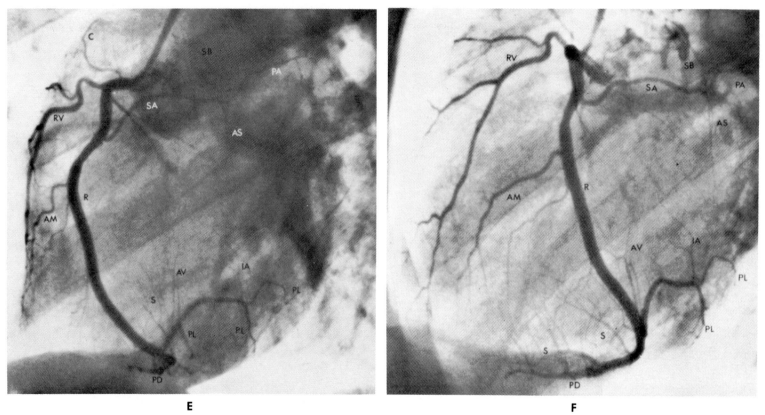

E

F

FIGURE 10–37 *Continued.* *E*. Left anterior oblique view, 70°. *F*. Lateral film in normal right selective coronary arteriography. (*A–F* from Judkins, M. P.: Radiol. Clin. North Am., *6*:467–492, 1968.)

11

THE ABDOMEN AND PERITONEAL SPACE

GROSS ANATOMY OF THE ABDOMINAL CAVITY AND ABDOMINAL WALL

Introduction and Brief Review of Basic Diagrams. (For a more complete description of those aspects of basic morphologic anatomy having a close relationship to radiology, the reader is referred to the companion text, An Atlas of Anatomy Basic to Radiology.)

In this abbreviated compendium and format, the first section is composed of the following:

1. The peritoneal folds and relationships of the anterior folds to what may be seen radiographically, particularly in pneumoperitoneum in infants (Fig. 11–1).

2. The fatty and muscular layers of the flank portion of the abdominal wall laterally, which may be altered, particularly in accumulations of fluid from inflammation or tumor (Fig. 11–2).

3. The splenic and hepatic angles, which may be obliterated early in inflammatory states particularly (Fig. 11–3).

4. The posterior peritoneal reflections, particularly in relation to the mesenteries and potential spaces contained within the peritoneal cavity (Figs. 11–4*A* and 11–5*B*).

5. The mesenteric insertions around the cecum and the variations in the positions of the appendix (Fig. 11–4*B* and *C*).

6. The lesser omental bursa and its relationship to the liver and stomach anteriorly (Fig. 11–5*B*).

7. Transverse sections of the abdomen at various levels, especially at the level of the lesser omental sac and lower down at the fourth lumbar region, showing the relationship of the mesentery of the small intestine to the greater sac (Fig. 11–6C).

8. The most frequent locations where pockets of purulent material may accumulate in the peritoneal cavity (Fig. 11–7).

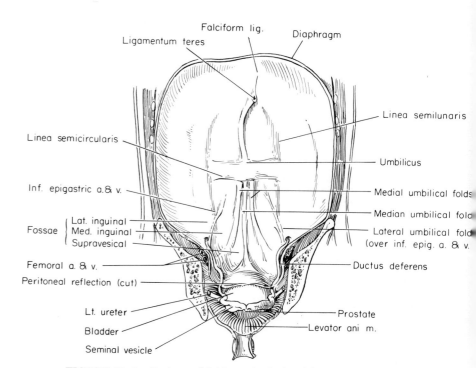

FIGURE 11–1 Peritoneal folds and relationships to the anterior (dorsal) abdominal wall.

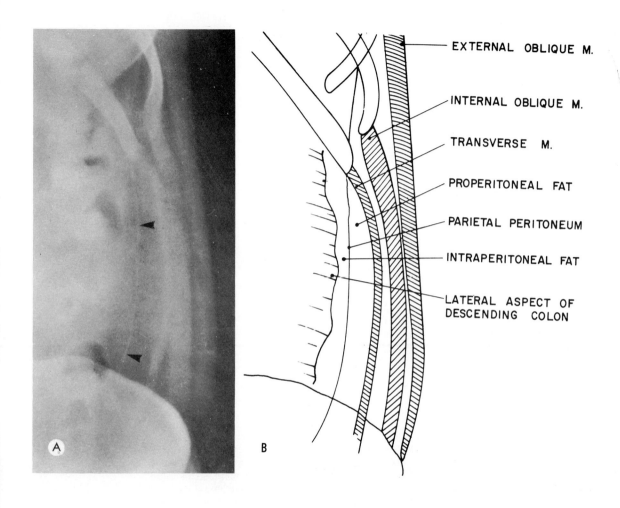

EXTERNAL OBLIQUE M.

INTERNAL OBLIQUE M.

TRANSVERSE M.

PROPERITONEAL FAT

PARIETAL PERITONEUM

INTRAPERITONEAL FAT

LATERAL ASPECT OF
DESCENDING COLON

FIGURE 11–2 *A.* Normal roentgenographic anatomy in the flank. There is unusually extensive visualization of the parietal peritoneum (arrows). *B.* Diagram of roentgenogram. (From Budin, E., and Jacobson, G.: Am. J. Roentgenol., *99:*62, 1967.)

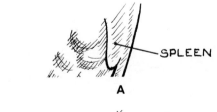

SPLEEN

A

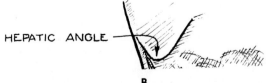

HEPATIC ANGLE

B

FIGURE 11–3 *A* and *B*. Diagrams demonstrating hepatic and splenic angles.

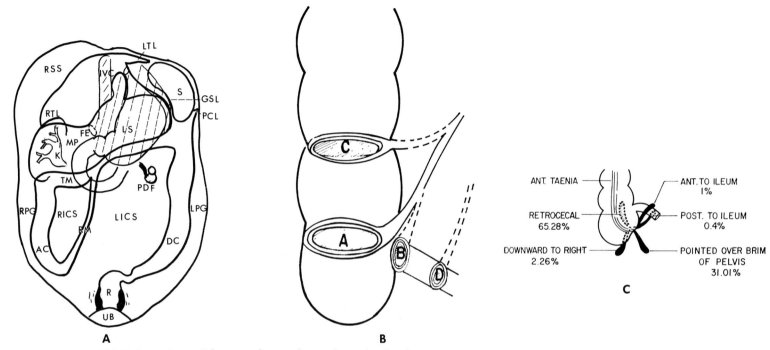

FIGURE 11–4 *A.* Diagram of posterior peritoneal reflections and recesses. *(S)* Spleen, *(LS)* lesser sac, *(IVC)* inferior vena cava, *(FE)* foramen epiploicum, *(K)* right kidney, *(R)* rectum, *(UB)* urinary bladder, *(AC)* attachment of peritoneal reflections of ascending colon, *(RPG)* right paracolic gutter, *(RM)* root of mesentery, *(RICS)* right infracolic space, *(TM)* root of transverse mesocolon, *(MP)* area of Morrison's pouch, *(RTL)* right triangular ligament, *(RSS)* right subphrenic space, *(LTL)* left triangular ligament, *(GSL)* gastrosplenic ligament, *(PCL)* phrenicocolic ligament, *(LICS)* left infracolic space, *(PCL)* phrenicocolic ligament. *(LPG)* left paracolic gutter, *(DC)* attachment of peritoneal reflections of descending colon, and *(PDF)* paraduodenal fossae.

B. Diagram showing variations in the insertion of the lower end of the small-bowel mesentery. The commonest insertion is at the cecocolic junction *(A),* but possible variations include the ileocecal valve *(B),* the ascending colon *(C),* or the terminal ileum *(D).* (After Testut and Latarjet.)

C. Diagram showing the incidence of variations in position of the appendix, as determined by Wakeley. The majority of the retrocecal appendices are also intraperitoneal. *(A, B,* and *C* from Meyers, M. A.: Radiology, 95:547–554, 1970.) (A modified.)

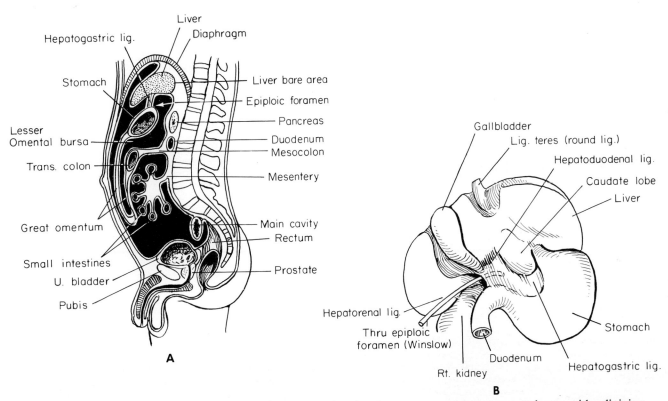

FIGURE 11–5 *A*. Sagittal section of abdominal cavity showing greater and lesser omental sacs with adjoining mesenteric attachments. *B*. View of hepatogastric ligament and epiploic foramen into lesser omental bursa, with adjoining structures.

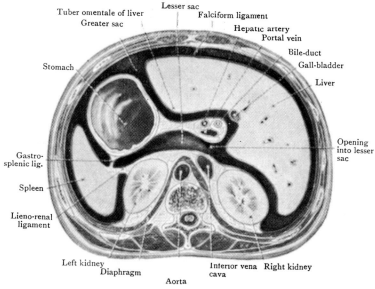

Tuber omentale of liver
Lesser sac
Greater sac
Falciform ligament
Hepatic artery
Portal vein
Bile-duct
Gall-bladder
Stomach
Liver
Opening into lesser sac
Gastro-splenic lig.
Spleen
Lieno-renal ligament
Left kidney
Diaphragm
Aorta
Inferior vena cava
Right kidney

A

Lesser sac
Stomach
Falciform ligament
Duodenum, 1st part
Greater sac
Liver
Gastro-duod. artery
Greater sac
Gastro-splenic lig.
Lieno-renal lig.
Bile-duct
Greater sac
Left kidney
Pancreas
Left suprarenal gland
Aorta
Portal vein
Inferior vena cava
Right kidney
Right suprarenal gland

B

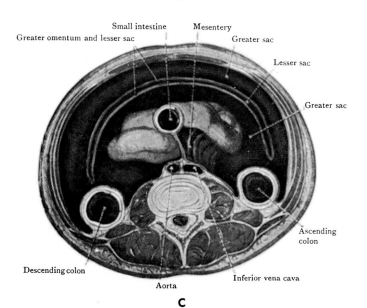

Small intestine
Mesentery
Greater omentum and lesser sac
Greater sac
Lesser sac
Greater sac
Ascending colon
Descending colon
Aorta
Inferior vena cava

C

FIGURE 11–6 *A.* Transverse section of abdomen to show the arrangement of peritoneum at the level of the opening into lesser sac. *B.* Transverse section of abdomen to show the arrangement of the peritoneum immediately below the opening into the lesser sac. *C.* Transverse section of abdomen through the fourth lumbar vertebra, to show the arrangement of the peritoneum. (From Cunningham's Manual of Practical Anatomy, 12th ed. London, Oxford University Press, 1958.)

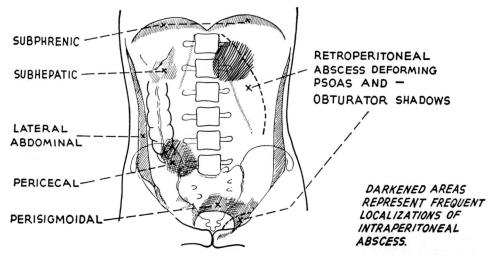

SUBPHRENIC

SUBHEPATIC

LATERAL
ABDOMINAL

PERICECAL

PERISIGMOIDAL

RETROPERITONEAL
ABSCESS DEFORMING
PSOAS AND —
OBTURATOR SHADOWS

DARKENED AREAS
REPRESENT FREQUENT
LOCALIZATIONS OF
INTRAPERITONEAL
ABSCESS.

FIGURE 11–7 Diagram illustrating the various localizations of intraperitoneal and retroperitoneal abscesses.

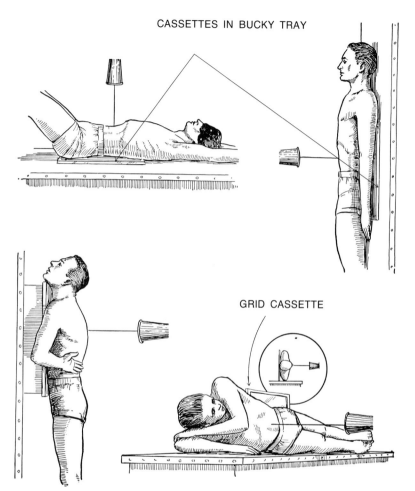

CASSETTES IN BUCKY TRAY

GRID CASSETTE

FIGURE 11–8 Position of patient for routine film studies required for plain film survey of abdominal disease. Note that a posteroanterior chest film is part of this routine. (Decubitus left lateral may be preferable.)

RADIOGRAPHIC STUDY OF THE ABDOMEN

The basic positions for study of the abdomen are (Fig. 11–8):
1. Anteroposterior film of the abdomen, recumbent (also called KUB film, the letters standing for kidney, ureter and bladder areas).
2. Anteroposterior film of the abdomen, erect.
3. Patient supine; horizontal x-ray beam.
4. Patient on one side or other; horizontal x-ray beam.
5. Posteroanterior film of chest, including upper abdomen for areas just beneath the diaphragm.

It is best, if time permits, to prepare patients for this examination by thorough cleansing of the gastrointestinal tract, best accomplished by prescribing a cathartic such as 2 ounces of castor oil (or X-Prep Liquid) on the evening prior to the examination and allowing approximately 10 or 12 hours for action. On the morning of the examination, this may be supplemented by enemas until returns are clear.

Air which has escaped from the gastrointestinal tract into the peritoneal space as the result of rupture of a portion of the gut, will rise to the uppermost part of the abdomen—usually beneath the diaphragm. It is absolutely important that the diaphragm be motionless when this film is taken; hence a very rapid exposure technique is essential.

In general, since most of the organs gravitate to the lower abdomen in the erect position, this film is not as good as the recumbent one for best anatomic detail. It is essential, however, that fluid levels, bowel wall thickness, properitoneal fat lines, and fascial planes around kidneys and psoas muscles be clearly shown (Fig. 11–9).

Anteroposterior Projection of the Abdomen, Patient Supine (Fig. 11–9)

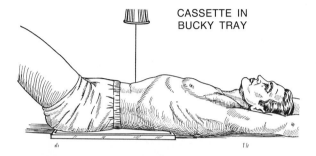

CASSETTE IN BUCKY TRAY

1. The midline of the body is aligned to the midline of the table.
2. The cassette in the Bucky tray is centered to the iliac crest and includes the pubic symphysis.
3. A compression band may be employed. The film is taken in expiration.
4. This technique is chosen to show the abdominal, retroperitoneal, and organ structures.
5. For differences between *supine* and *prone* projections of the abdomen, see Figure 11–14.

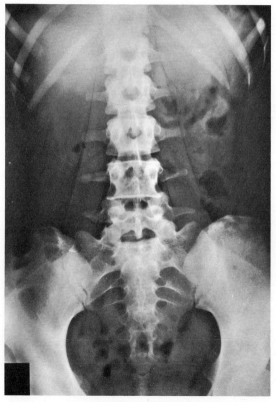

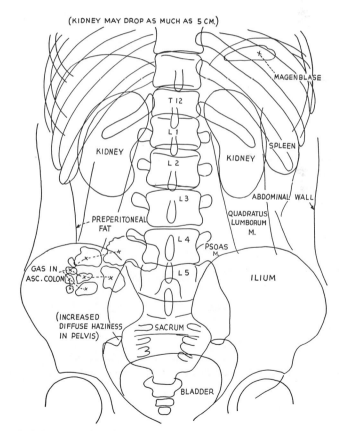

(KIDNEY MAY DROP AS MUCH AS 5 CM.)

MAGENBLASE

T 12

L 1

KIDNEY

SPLEEN

L 2

KIDNEY

ABDOMINAL WALL

L 3

PREPERITONEAL FAT

QUADRATUS LUMBORUM M.

L 4

PSOAS M.

GAS IN ASC. COLON

L 5

ILIUM

(INCREASED DIFFUSE HAZINESS IN PELVIS)

SACRUM

BLADDER

FIGURE 11–9 Anteroposterior projection of abdomen (KUB film).

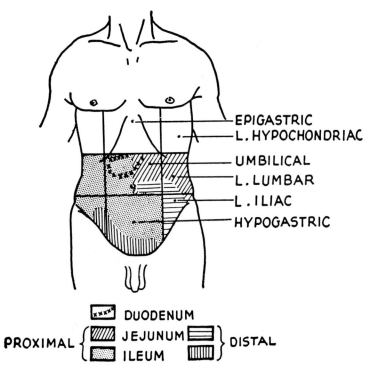

EPIGASTRIC
L. HYPOCHONDRIAC
UMBILICAL
L. LUMBAR
L. ILIAC
HYPOGASTRIC

⊠⊠ DUODENUM

PROXIMAL { ▨ JEJUNUM ▤ } DISTAL
          { ▦ ILEUM ▥ }

FIGURE 11-10 Approximate distribution of the small intestine within the abdomen.

CHANGES IN APPEARANCE OF
GAS-CONTAINING STOMACH

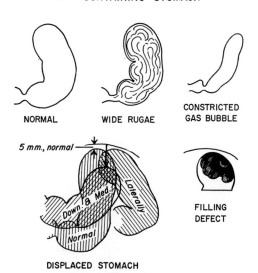

NORMAL   WIDE RUGAE   CONSTRICTED
                                    GAS BUBBLE

5 mm., normal

Down. & Med.   Laterally

Normal

FILLING
DEFECT

DISPLACED STOMACH

FIGURE 11-11 Changes in appearance of gas-containing stomach.

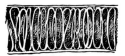

JEJUNUM
(NO INDENTED SEROSA;
COILED SPRING APPEARANCE)

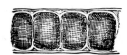

ILEUM
(NO INDENTED SEROSA)

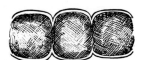

COLON
(NOTE INDENTED SEROSA BY
HAUSTRA)

FIGURE 11-12 Schematic illustration of distended bowel, showing differences between jejunum, ileum, and colon.

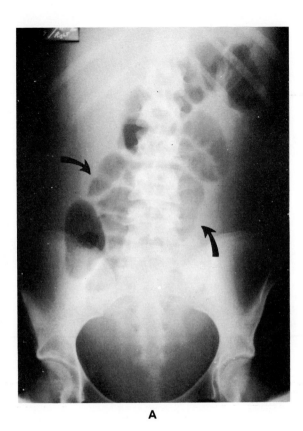

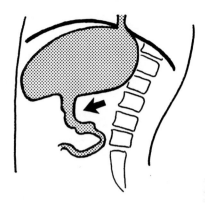

CAUDATE LOBE OF LIVER ENLARGEMENT

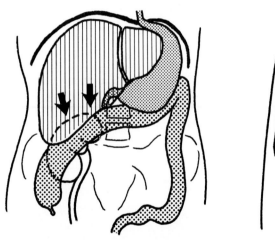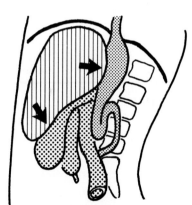

FIGURE 11–13 *A*. Anteroposterior projection of the abdomen: hepatoma with ascites and floating loops of bowel. *B*. Diagrams show changes with enlargement of the right lobe and caudate lobe of the liver.

RIGHT LOBE OF LIVER ENLARGEMENT

DISPLACEMENT OF STOMACH TO LEFT AND POSTERIORLY
DOWNWARD DISPLACEMENT OF RIGHT KIDNEY
NO DISPLACEMENT OF SECOND PART OF DUODENUM
DOWNWARD DISPLACEMENT OF TRANSVERSE COLON
DOWNWARD AND POSTERIOR DISPLACEMENT OF HEPATIC FLEXURE
NO DISPLACEMENT OF DUODENOJEJUNAL FLEXURE

B

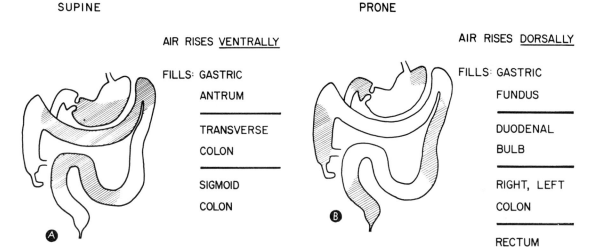

FIGURE 11–14 *A.* Diagram of supine abdomen showing localization of air. Note obscuration of renal areas, leading to confusion of the transverse and sigmoid colon with the small bowel. *B.* Diagram of prone abdomen showing shift of air with resultant clearing of the renal areas, and improved separation of the colon gas from the small bowel gas. (From Bendon, W. B., Baker, D. H., and Leonidas, J.: Am. J. Roentgenol., *103*:444, 1968.)

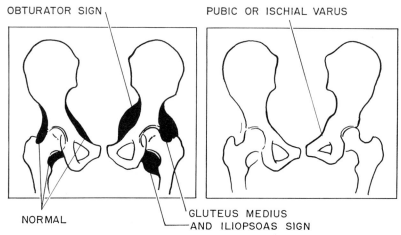

FIGURE 11–15 Diagram illustrating the normal and abnormal obturator and iliopsoas fascial planes of the pelvis and hips.

Blood Supply of the Abdomen

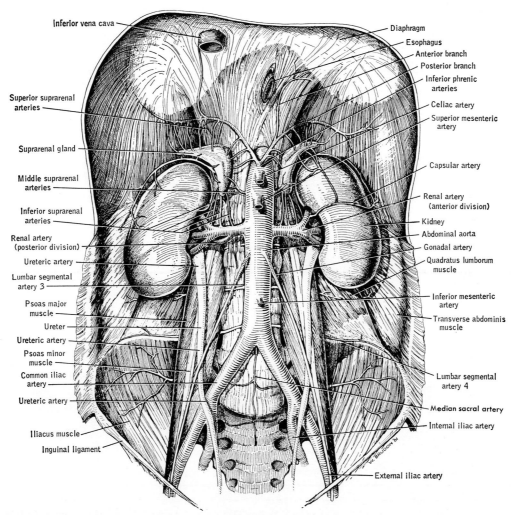

FIGURE 11–16 Abdominal aorta and its branches. (From Anson, B. J. (ed.): Morris' Human Anatomy. 12th ed. New York, McGraw-Hill Book Co., 1966. Copyright © 1966 by McGraw-Hill, Inc. Used by permission of McGraw-Hill Book Co.)

TABLE 11–1. Arterial Supply of the Abdomen*

Distribution	Artery	Origin	Distribution	Artery	Origin
Phrenic Artery, Right and Left			Spleen, pancreas, stomach, greater omentum	Splenic	Celiac
Right crus of diaphragm, central tendon of diaphragm	Inferior phrenic (right and left)	Abdominal	Left portion, greater curvature of stomach	Short gastric	Splenic
Anastomoses with left phrenic, internal mammary and pericardiophrenic arteries	Anterior branch (right and left)	Phrenic			
Anastomoses with intercostals	Posterior branch (right and left)	Phrenic	*Superior Mesenteric Artery*		
			Pancreas, duodenum	Inferior pancreaticoduodenal	Superior mesenteric
Suprarenal gland, branches to vena cava, liver and pericardium	Superior suprarenal (right and left)	Phrenic	Ileum, jejunum	Intestinal	Superior mesenteric
			Transverse colon	Middle colic	Superior mesenteric
			Ascending colon	Right colic	Superior mesenteric
Suprarenal Arteries, Right and Left			Cecum, appendix, ascending colon	Ileocolic	Superior mesenteric
Suprarenal gland (right and left)	Middle suprarenal (right and left)	Aorta	Mesentery of vermiform appendix	Appendicular	Ileocolic
Lumbar Arteries, I, II, III, IV			*Renal Arteries, Right and Left*		
Bodies of vertebrae and ligaments	Vertebral	Lumbar	Kidney	Renal	Abdominal aorta
Psoas, quadratus lumborum, oblique muscles of abdomen	Muscular	Lumbar	Suprarenal gland	Inferior suprarenal	Renal
			Kidney capsule and perirenal fat	Capsular	Renal
			Upper end of ureter	Ureteral	Renal
Longissimus dorsi and multifidus spinae	Dorsal	Lumbar	Kidney	Terminal branches	Renal
Multifidus	Lateral branch	Dorsal	*Internal Spermatic and Ovarian Arteries*		
Sacrospinalis	Medial branch	Dorsal	Testis	Internal spermatic	Abdominal aorta
Vertebral canal	Spinal	Dorsal	Ureter, adjacent retroperitoneal tissue	Ureteral	Internal spermatic
Celiac Axis			Cremaster muscle	Cremasteric	Internal spermatic
Esophagus, lesser curvature of stomach	Left gastric	Celiac	Epididymis	Epididymal	Internal spermatic
			Terminal branches to testis	Testicular	Internal spermatic
Anastomoses with branches from thoracic aorta	Esophageal branches	Left gastric	Ovary, ureter, uterus, tubes	Ovarian	Abdominal aorta
Stomach, greater omentum	Left gastroepiploic	Splenic	*Inferior Mesenteric Artery*		
Pancreas	Pancreatic	Splenic	Lower half of descending colon, sigmoid, rectum	Inferior mesenteric	Abdominal aorta
Stomach, pancreas, liver, duodenum	Common hepatic	Celiac	Descending colon	Left colic	Inferior mesenteric
Lesser curvature of stomach	Right gastric	Hepatic	Sigmoid flexure of colon	Sigmoid	Inferior mesenteric
Right lobe of liver	Right hepatic	Hepatic proper	Upper part of rectum	Superior hemorrhoidal	Inferior mesenteric
Left lobe of liver	Left hepatic	Hepatic proper			
Gallbladder, undersurface of liver	Cystic	Hepatic proper			
Stomach, duodenum, pancreas	Right gastroepiploic	Gastroduodenal			

*From Bierman, H. C.: Selective Arterial Catheterization. Springfield, Ill., Charles C Thomas, 1969. Table 11.1. Courtesy of Charles C Thomas, Publisher.

TABLE 11–2. Average Age and Diameter in Mm. of Abdominal Aorta at Sites Measured*

Sex	No. of Cases	Age	At 11th Rib	Above Renal Arteries	Below Renal Arteries	At Bifurcation of Aorta	Difference between 11th Rib and Bifurcation of Aorta
Male	29	53.9 ± 13.7	26.9 ± 3.96	23.9 ± 3.92	21.4 ± 3.65	18.7 ± 3.34	8.14 ± 2.14
Female	44	56.9 ± 14.3	24.4 ± 3.45	21.6 ± 3.16	18.7 ± 3.96	17.5 ± 2.52	6.80 ± 4.54

*From Steinberg, C. R., Archer, M., and Steinberg, I.: Measurement of the abdominal aorta after intravenous aortography in health and arteriosclerotic peripheral vascular disease. Amer. J. Roentgenol., *95*:703, 1965.

Element of magnification not indicated. Target-film distance is 48 inches.

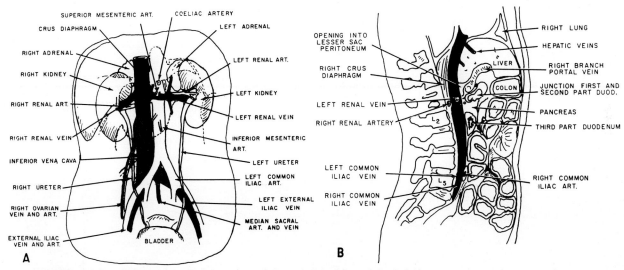

FIGURE 11–17 Schematic representation of the relationships of the inferior vena cava (shown in black) with the surrounding anatomic structures. *A.* In the anteroposterior view notice the relationships of the vena cava to the course of the external iliac vein and artery, the right ureter, and the relation of the right renal artery, as it crosses from the aorta behind the vena cava, to the right kidney. *B.* In the lateral view the compression of the vena cava by the right renal artery is demonstrated at the level of the interspace between L-1 and L-2. A slight anterior indentation at the lower end of the vena cava caused by anterior compression from the right common iliac artery is also shown. The pancreas and third portion of the duodenum lie just anterior to the vena cava. (From Hillman, D. C., Tristan, T. A., and Bronk, A. M.: Radiology, *81*:416, 1963.)

Diagnostic Criteria for Normal Lymph Nodes

ARCHITECTURE OF NODES. Lymph nodes generally have a very fine reticular internal architecture. They should normally have no significant filling defects. In the presence of some of the lymphomas (malignant lymphosarcomas), a lymph node often will take on a marked foaminess in its architecture—this must be regarded as abnormal. Moreover, the replacement of more than one-third of a lymph node by a filling defect is an indicator of abnormality.

LYMPHATIC CHANNELS. The persistence of multiple channels on the 24 hour film is an indicator of lymphatic obstruction. Moreover, excessive filling of channels is sometimes an indicator of partial obstruction.

MEASUREMENTS. Abrams* has advocated three measurements to aid diagnosis of normal lymph nodes. The right lateral spine-to-node distance is the measurement from the right lateral border of a lumbar vertebral body at its midpoint to the most lateral border of the right juxtacaval node group. Another measurement is the left lateral spine-to-node distance similarly obtained. A third measurement is obtained from the lateral view and represents the distance to the most anterior margin of the lymph node chain from the twelfth to the second lumbar vertebrae.

Single lymph nodes were also measured for size, care being taken not to measure clusters but rather isolated nodes. The 95 per cent confidence limit for the maximum size of a lymph node is shown to be 2.7 cm. The third measurement should not exceed 3 cm.; the other two measurements should not exceed 2 cm. Although the original study was based upon 60 normal and 60 abnormal cases, these measurements are generally used merely as guides to further interpretation of such factors as architecture, filling defects, and filling or lack of filling.

Lymphographic Technique. A superficial lymphatic vessel on the medial aspect of the dorsum of the foot is cannulated and the contrast material, usually Ethiodol, is slowly injected over a period of approximately 2 hours. (Ethiodol is the ethyl ester of poppyseed oil and contains approximately 37 per cent iodine.) Usually 5 cc. (but as much as 10 cc. can be used on occasion) is injected on each side by a special pumping device.

Generally, 6 to 24 hours after the injection, the Ethiodol concentrates in the lymph nodes, and disappears from the lymphatic channels proper. The lymph nodes retain the contrast material for several months.

Roentgenograms are taken immediately after the injection and then 24 and 48 hours later. The roentgenograms obtained are the anteroposterior, oblique, and lateral projections as well as a posteroanterior view of the chest. At times, at the 24 or 48 hour period it may be desirable to combine this study with intravenous pyelograms. Pelvic arteriograms or venograms may be obtained following the lymphograms for better topographic evaluation.

---

*Abrams, H. L. (ed.): Angiography, Vol. 2. 2nd ed. Boston, Little, Brown & Co., 1971.

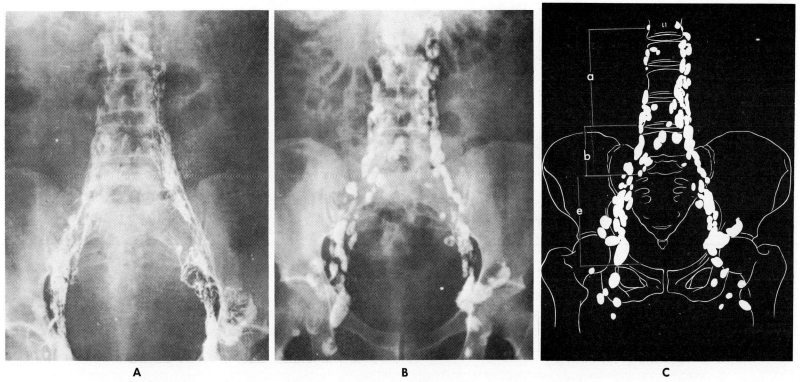

A   B   C

FIGURE 11–18 *A*. Anteroposterior projection made immediately after completion of injection of contrast medium. Lymphatic channels are primarily filled, while the lymph nodes are incompletely opacified.

B. Anteroposterior projection showing the lymph nodes, taken 24 hours after.

C. Tracing of *B*, illustrating the major node groups. (a) Juxta-aortic, (b) common iliac, (e) external iliac. (From Herman, P. G., Benninghoff, D. L., Nelson, J. H., Jr., and Mellins, H. Z.: Radiology, *80*:82–193, 1963.)

Figure 11–18 continued on following page

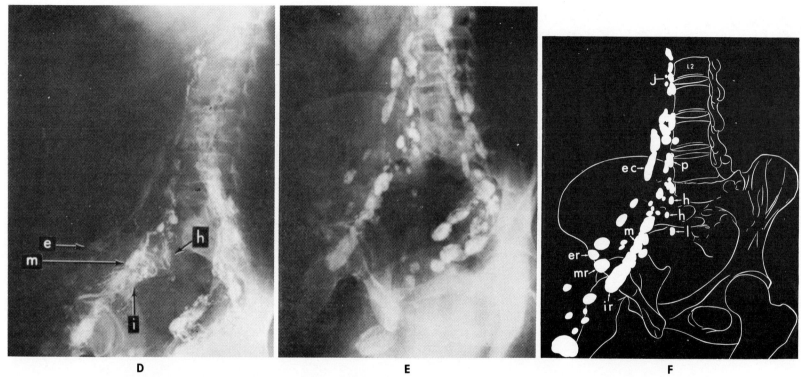

D   **E**   **F**

FIGURE 11–18 *Continued.* *D.* Right posterior oblique projection made immediately after completion of injection. Lymphatic channels are filled, while the lymph nodes are incompletely opacified. (e) External chain of the external and common iliac groups, (m) middle chain of the external and common iliac groups, (i) internal chain of the external and common iliac groups, (h) channels connecting hypogastric with external and common iliac groups.

E. Right posterior oblique projection showing lymph nodes as they appeared 24 hours after *D.*

F. Tracing of *E.* (er) External retrocrural node, (mr) middle retrocrural node, (ir) internal retrocrural node, (m) middle node of the internal chain, (l) lateral sacral node of the hypogastric group, (h) hypogastric nodes, (j) juxtaaortic nodes, (p) node of the promontory, (ec) common iliac node. (From Herman, P. G., Benninghoff, D. L., Nelson, J. H., Jr., and Mellins, H. Z.: Radiology, *80*:82–193, 1963.)

Figure 11–18 continued on opposite page

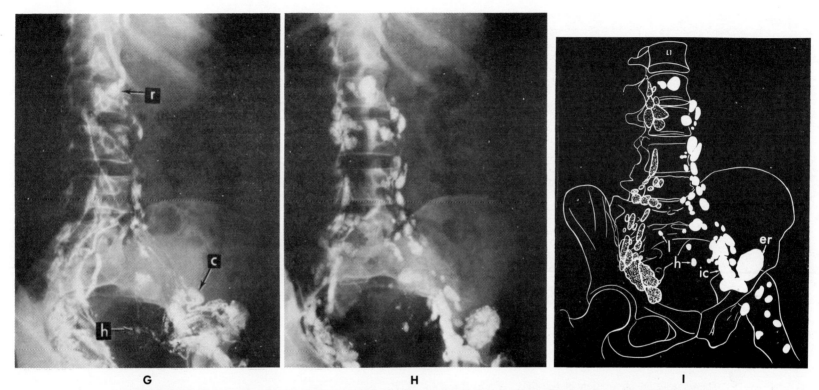

G   H   I

FIGURE 11–18 *Continued.*   *G.* Left posterior oblique projection made immediately after completion of injection. Lymphatic channels again dominate the picture, while the nodes are incompletely filled. (h) Hypogastric tributaries connecting with the external and common iliac chains, (c) communications between external and middle chains of the external iliac group, (r) receptaculum chyli (cisterna chyli).

H. Left posterior oblique projection showing lymph nodes as they appear 24 hours after K.

I. Tracing of *H.* (er) External retrocrural node, markedly enlarged, (ic) internal chain, represented by a closely packed group of nodes, (h) hypogastric nodes, (l) lateral sacral nodes of hypogastric group. (From Herman, P. G., Benninghoff, D. L., Nelson, J. H., Jr., and Mellins, H. Z.: Radiology, *80*:182–193, 1963.)

Special Radiographic Study of the Liver

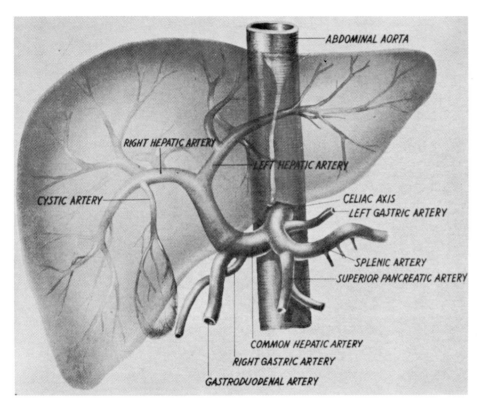

FIGURE 11–19 Classic arterial circulation of the liver. (From Bierman, H. R.: Selective Arterial Catheterization. Springfield, Ill., Charles C Thomas, Publisher, 1969. Courtesy of Charles C Thomas, Publisher.)

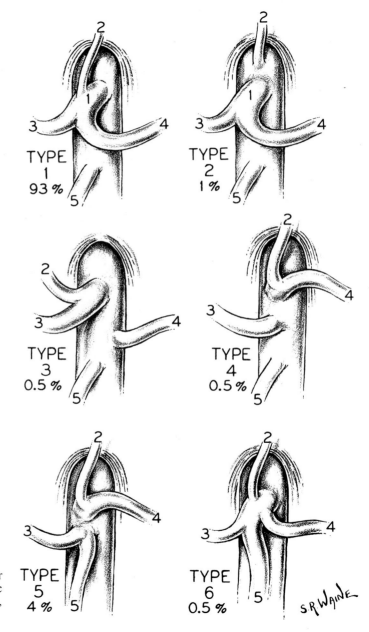

FIGURE 11–20 Variations in origin of the celiac and its branches as well as in the superior mesenteric artery. *(1)* Celiac trunk, *(2)* left gastric artery, *(3)* common hepatic artery, *(4)* splenic artery, *(5)* superior mesenteric artery. (From Ruzicka, F. F., and Rossi, P.: N.Y. State J. Med., *23*:3032–3033, 1968; reproduced with permission.)

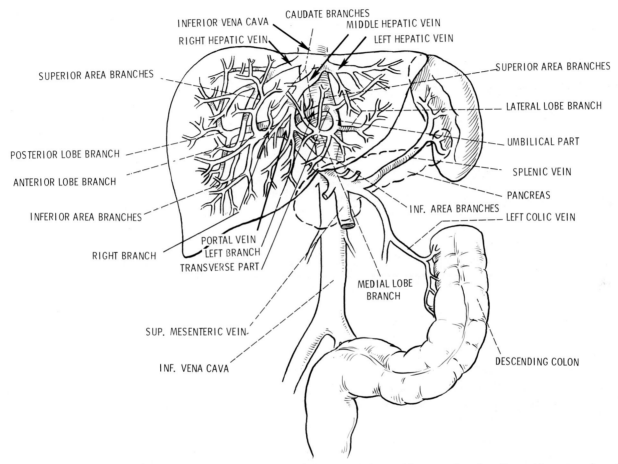

FIGURE 11–21 Scheme of portal system of veins and its connections with systemic veins. It must be remembered that the systemic blood carried by the hepatic artery also enters the capillaries of the liver, and the hepatic veins contain, therefore, both portal and systemic blood.

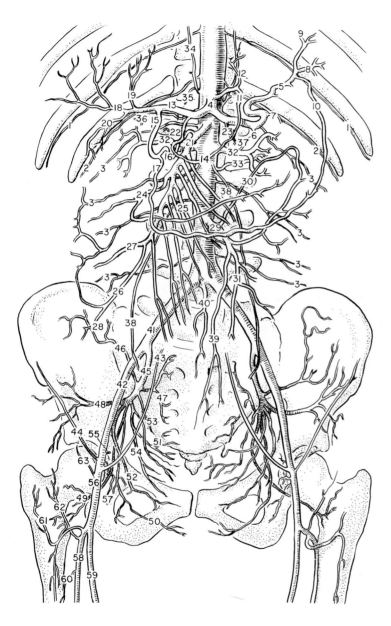

FIGURE 11–22 The arteries of abdomen, pelvis and thigh: 1, Intercostal; 2, subcostal; 3, lumbar; 4, celiac axis; 5, splenic; 6, dorsal pancreatic; 7, great pancreatic; 8, terminal branches to spleen; 9, short gastric branches; 10, left gastroepiploic; 11, left gastric; 12, esophageal branches; 13, common hepatic; 14, right gastric; 15, gastroduodenal; 16, anterior superior pancreaticoduodenal; 17, right gastroepiploic; 18, right hepatic; 19, left hepatic; 20, cystic; 21, superior mesenteric; 22, inferior pancreaticoduodenal; 23, inferior pancreatic; 24, middle colic; 25, intestinal branches; 26, ileocolic; 27, right colic; 28, appendiceal; 29, inferior mesenteric; 30, left colic; 31, sigmoid; 32, renal; 33, accessory renal; 34, inferior phrenic; 35, superior suprarenal; 36, middle suprarenal; 37, inferior suprarenal; 38, internal spermatic (or ovarian); 39, superior hemorrhoidal; 40, middle sacral; 41, common iliac; 42, external iliac; 43, inferior epigastric; 44, deep circumflex iliac; 45, hypogastric; 46, iliolumbar; 47, lateral sacral; 48, superior gluteal; 49, inferior gluteal; 50, internal pudendal; 51, middle hemorrhoidal; 52, obturator; 53, uterine; 54, vesical; 55, superficial epigastric; 56, common femoral; 57, superficial external pudendal; 58, deep femoral (profunda); 59, superficial femoral; 60, perforating muscular branches; 61, lateral femoral circumflex; 62, medial femoral circumflex; 63, superficial circumflex iliac. (Modified from Muller, R. F., and Figley, M. M., Am. J. Roentgenol. 77, 1957.)

THE SPLEEN

Special Radiographic Study of the Spleen

The spleen lies in the left upper quadrant posterior to the stomach and immediately under the diaphragm. It varies in size considerably, but ordinarily does not project significantly below the horizontal plane at the level of the left costal margin. The diaphragm separates it from the ninth, tenth, and eleventh ribs on the left. The medial surface of the spleen is in contact with the tail of the pancreas (Fig. 11–6), and the lower pole of the spleen is in contact with the splenic flexure of the colon. The anteromedial portion of the spleen is in contact with the greater curvature of the stomach.

The spleen is supported by *three main ligamentous attachments:* (1) the *phrenicosplenic* ligament, which is a reflection of the peritoneum running from the diaphragm and ventral aspect of the left kidney to the hilum of the spleen, and which contains splenic vessels; (2) the *gastrosplenic* (or gastrolienal), which is actually a dorsal mesentery between the spleen and the stomach and contains the short gastric and left gastroepiploic artery; and (3) the *phrenicocolic* ligament, which lies beneath the caudal end of the spleen.

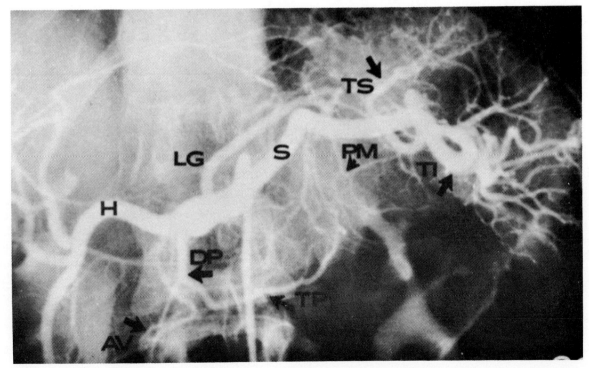

FIGURE 11–23 Normal splenic arterial anatomy. This 40-year-old female patient was investigated for abdominal pain. Hepatic artery *(H)*; left gastric artery *(LG)*; splenic trunk *(S).* Superior terminal *(TS)* and inferior terminal *(TI)* vessels supply numerous branches to the splenic parenchyma. The dorsal pancreatic branch *(DP)* is well visualized originating from the proximal splenic and divides into the transverse pancreatic *(TP)* and anastomotic vessels *(AV)* which supply the head of the pancreas and anastomose with the pancreaticoduodenals. The pancreatica magna *(PM)* originates from the second segment of the splenic trunk. (From Abrams, H. L.: Angiography, 2d ed. Vol. 2. Boston, Little, Brown & Co., 1971.)

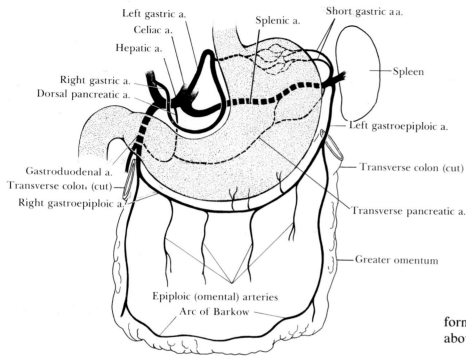

Left gastric a.
Celiac a.
Hepatic a.
Splenic a.
Short gastric a a.
Right gastric a.
Dorsal pancreatic a.
Spleen
Left gastroepiploic a.
Gastroduodenal a.
Transverse colon (cut)
Right gastroepiploic a.
Transverse colon (cut)
Transverse pancreatic a.
Greater omentum
Epiploic (omental) arteries
Arc of Barkow

FIGURE 11–24 Line drawing representing celiac arterial axis as related to stomach and greater omentum and splenic artery. (Modified from Ruzicka, F. F., Jr., and Rossi, P.: Radiol. Clin. N. Am., *8*:3–29, 1970.)

The Spleen in the Anteroposterior Film of the Abdomen. The splenic shadow can usually be identified along the left upper lateral aspect of the stomach as a tonguelike structure, the tip of the tongue normally extending to the left costal margin (Fig. 11–9). Only the inferior one-half or one-third of the spleen is visible radiographically on a plain film of the abdomen. Small 3 to 5 mm. calcific tubercles or phleboliths may frequently be recognized within the spleen. Rarely, the splenic capsule itself is calcified. In older age groups, the splenic artery is often seen as a tortuous calcific aneurysmal structure arising from the celiac trunk medial to the spleen and projected over the stomach.

Measurement of Splenic Size. The caudal tip of the splenic shadow forms a good basis for measurement. Measurement of the spleen 2 cm. above its tip should not exceed 3.5 cm.*

Whitley et al.† have demonstrated by means of a computer approach to the prediction of splenic weight from routine films, that the parameters L and W, as indicated on a routine film, provide the most accurate basis for predicting the weight of the spleen (Fig. 11–25). L is estimated by a vertical line from the tip of the spleen to the intercept with the diaphragm, and W is the width of the spleen at the midpoint of L or as close to this point as this measurement can be made. In their study, the measurement of the spleen 2.5 cm. above the tip was the least accurate and has the lowest correlation coefficient. The product of L and W alone offered a fairly accurate first approximation of splenic weight. Actually, the measurement of L alone is in itself quite accurate and was the single best indicator found by these investigators: "On a routine abdominal film in an average sized adult, an L of more than 11.3 cm. can give a 70

*Wyman, A. C.: Traumatic rupture of the spleen. Am. J. Roentgenol., *72*:51–63, 1954.
†Whitley, J. E., et al.: A computer approach to the prediction of spleen weight from routine films. Radiology, *86*:73–76, 1966.

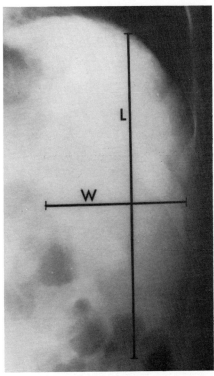

FIGURE 11-25 Anteroposterior radiograph of the left upper abdomen illustrating the parameters L and W superimposed on the image of the spleen. (From Whitley, J. E., Maynard, C. D., and Rhyne, A. L.: Radiology, *86*:73–76, 1966.)

The *splenic vein* emerges from the hilum of the spleen, runs in a groove on the dorsum of the pancreas below the splenic artery, and usually joins the superior mesenteric vein behind the neck of the pancreas to form the portal vein (see Chapter 15).

The *lymphatics of the spleen* drain into the pancreaticosplenic lymph nodes.

The splenic artery and vein run in the phrenicolienal ligament to the hilus and, as noted previously, the artery's course is often tortuous.

To summarize, the significant branches from the splenic artery and vein are: (1) a *left gastroepiploic,* which may or may not anastomose with the right gastroepiploic; (2) *pancreatic branches;* and (3) *short branches to the stomach;* and all of these may provide collateral circulation for the spleen. Because of the endorgan relationship of the arteries, the spleen is subject to infarction.

Ordinarily, the spleen creates a slight impression upon the splenic flexure of the colon and the greater curvature of the stomach.

Calcification is frequent in the region of the spleen, and this may be due to phleboliths, tubercles, calcified infarcts, splenic artery aneurysms, and certain cysts (hydatid), but this subject is outside the scope of this text. Subcapsular calcification may also occur, but this is also most likely a pathologic degenerative change.

Apart from lobulation, accessory spleens are not infrequently found. These are usually in the neighborhood of the main organ but sometimes they may be distributed elsewhere in the abdominal cavity.

A congenital absence of the spleen may also occur, particularly in relation to some types of congenital heart disease.

Techniques of Examination. The usual techniques of visualization of the spleen are: (1) *plain film studies,* especially anteroposterior or posteroanterior views of the left upper quadrant; (2) *contrast visualization* of the *stomach, kidneys,* or *splenic flexure* of the colon; (3) *pneumoperitoneum;* (4) *splenic angiography;* (5) *splenoportography;* (6) *radioisotopic techniques;* and (7) *computed axial tomography.*

Pancreas. To be discussed with the stomach and duodenum (see Chapter 14).

Suprarenal Glands (Adrenal Glands). To be discussed with the urinary tract (see Chapter 12).

Liver. To be discussed with the hepatobiliary tract (see Chapter 15).

per cent probability, and an L above 15 cm., a 98 per cent probability of the spleen being enlarged. . . .

"If the product of L and W is obtained, correcting for magnification: if this product is 50 or more, the probability is 75 per cent that the spleen's weight is more than 200 grams; and if this product is 75 or more, the probability is 98 per cent that the spleen's weight is more than 200 grams."

12

THE URINARY TRACT

CORRELATED GROSS AND MICROSCOPIC ANATOMY OF THE URINARY TRACT

The Kidneys

Normal Kidney Size.

TABLE 12–1. Normal Adult Renal Size (The Mean Plus or Minus Two Standard Deviations)[a] (Modified after Moell)

Male:	Right kidney	Vertical: 11.3–14.5 cm.
		Width: 5.4– 7.2 cm.
	Left	Vertical: 11.6–14.8 cm.
		Width: 5.3– 7.1 cm.
Female:	Right kidney	Vertical: 10.7–13.9 cm.
		Width: 4.8– 6.6 cm.
	Left	Vertical: 11.1–14.3 cm.
		Width: 5.1– 6.9 cm.

[a]Standard deviation = 0.8 cm. for vertical dimension.

Kidney Mobility. There is considerable mobility of the kidneys during respiration. Normally, the range of movement is about 3 cm. less on the right side than on the left and is somewhat larger for women than for men. However, on deeper inspiration, excursion up to 10 cm. may be recorded.

A maximum excursion of 5 cm. (or 1½ vertebral bodies) occurs in the change from the recumbent to the erect position.

Gondos has recommended that measurements of the kidneys be made from a film taken with the patient prone, suggesting that in this position renal rotation is reduced or eliminated.

Renal Shape. Normally, the kidney is bean-shaped. Fetal lobulation (Fig. 12–2), however, is frequently encountered in children and tends to occur in three basic patterns (Cooperman and Lowman):[*] (1) there may be a local bulge of the lateral border of the left kidney; (2) the left kidney may be triangular, and somewhat enlarged; (3) there may be a diffuse multilobulated form that is either unilateral or bilateral.

Relationship of the Kidney to Other Retroperitoneal Structures. Each kidney is retroperitoneal alongside the last thoracic and upper three lumbar vertebrae, the left usually being higher than the right.

Longitudinal Section Through the Kidney (Coronal Section) (Fig. 12–3). The substance of the kidney as revealed by this section has three main parts: an external cortex, an internal medulla, and the renal tubules. The *external cortex* is approximately 12 mm. thick and contains numerous renal corpuscles, convoluted tubules, and minute vessels. The cortex is actually composed of two portions: (1) a *peripheral layer,* the cortex proper; and (2) processes called *"renal columns"* which dip inward between renal pyramids to reach the bottom of the sinus of the kidney.

---

*Cooperman, L. R., and Lowman, R. M.: Fetal lobulation of the kidneys. Am. J. Roentgenol., *92*:273, 1964.

RADIOGRAPHIC SIZE OF THE KIDNEY

Department of X-ray Diagnosis
University College Hospital
London, England

NORMAL MEASUREMENTS IN ADULTS AND CHILDREN

This chart is published in response to considerable demand by radiologists and clinicians for graphic data on the size of normal kidneys as determined from radiographs. The size of a normal kidney varies widely from person to person, depending on the number and distribution of calyces and the actual shape of the organ, making accurate estimation of the size of an individual kidney difficult. However, knowledge that a kidney is larger or smaller than average has considerable significance.

Good radiographic definition of the renal outline of a majority of patients is a simple matter, provided the patient is prepared properly.
Good definition of the renal outline of infants and bedridden patients is more difficult to obtain, however, and usually tomography or localized abdominal compression must be used.

The graphs have been found useful in the interpretation of radiographs, especially those of children. Statistically, the graphs are valid.
In particular, the one relating to children shows an unusually close relation between the length of the kidney and the height of the body throughout the period of growth. The simple relation of length of kidney to height of body or to age and sex was chosen because statistically this measurement is as satisfactory as others more complicated.[1,2]

TECHNICAL POINTS

A. The data were derived using a target-film distance of 36 inches (91.5 cm). Radiographs made at a target-film distance of 40 inches (101.8 cm) would show a 2 percent reduction in the size of the kidney.

B. For the normal kidney, 68 percent of the readings lie within the range of mean plus or minus 1 standard deviation; 99.5 percent lie within the range of mean plus or minus 2½ times the standard deviation.

REFERENCES

1. Karn, M. N.: Radiographic Measurements of Kidney Section Area. **Ann. Hum. Genet.**, 25:379-385, May, 1962.

2. Hodson, C. J.; Drewe, J. A.; Karn, M. N., and King, A.: Renal Size in Normal Children. A Radiographic Study During Life. **Arch. Dis. Child.**, 37:616-622, December, 1962.

BIBLIOGRAPHY

Hodson, C. J.: Radiology of the Kidney. In Black, D. A. K. (editor): **Renal Disease.** Published by F. A. Davis Company, Philadelphia, Pennsylvania, and Blackwell Scientific Publications, Oxford, England, 1962, pp. 388-417.

Moell, H.: Kidney Size and Its Deviation from Normal in Acute Renal Failure. A Roentgenographic Study. **Acta Radiol.**, Supp. 206, 1961, pp. 5-74.

Panichi, S., and Bonechi, I.: Il volume del rene in condizioni normali. **Boll. Soc. Medicochir. Pisa**, 26:611-614, November-December, 1958.

Vuorinen, P.; Anttila, P.; Wegelius, U.; Kauppila, A., and Koivisto, E.: Renal Cortical Index and Other Roentgenographic Renal Measurements. **Acta Radiol.**, Supp. 211, 1962, pp. 5-54.

EASTMAN KODAK COMPANY
Radiography Markets Division
Rochester, N.Y. 14650

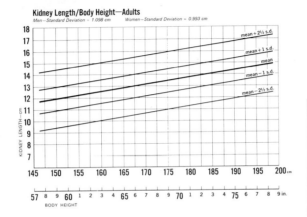

Kidney Length/Body Height—Adults
Men—Standard Deviation - 1.098 cm   Women—Standard Deviation - 0.993 cm

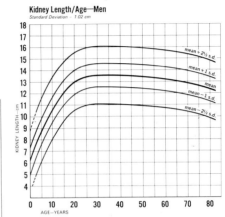

Kidney Length/Age—Men
Standard Deviation - 1.02 cm

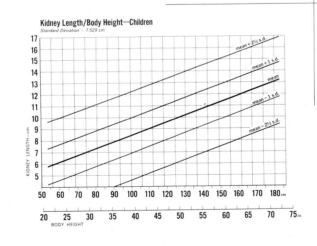

Kidney Length/Body Height—Children
Standard Deviation - 1.529 cm

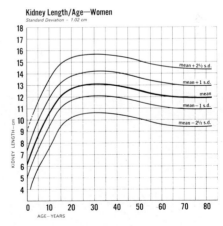

Kidney Length/Age—Women
Standard Deviation - 1.02 cm

M4-8A

3-67

FIGURE 12–1.

INFANT   ADULT

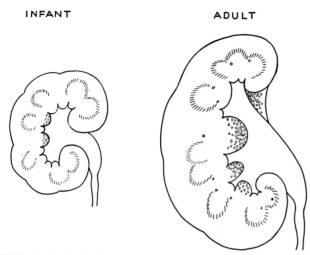

FIGURE 12-2 Infantile renal lobulation and its comparison with the adult renal contour. (After Caffey.)

Cortical substance
Medullary substance
Minor calyces

Hilum
Major calyx
Nephron

RENAL VEIN

PELVIS
Interlobular artery
and vein

URETER
Arcuate artery
and vein

Interlobar artery
and vein

Renal sinus   Pyramid

FIGURE 12-3 Longitudinal section through a normal kidney. (From Goss, C. M. (ed.): Gray's Anatomy of the Human Body, 29th ed. Philadelphia, Lea & Febiger, 1973.)

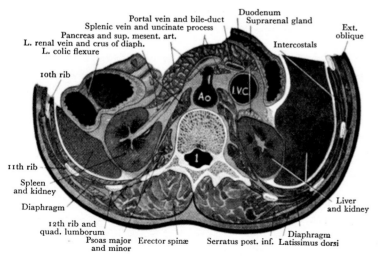

Duodenum
Portal vein and bile-duct   Suprarenal gland
Splenic vein and uncinate process
Pancreas and sup. mesent. art.   Ext.
L. renal vein and crus of diaph.   oblique
L. colic flexure   Intercostals

10th rib

Ao   IVC

11th rib

Spleen
and kidney

Diaphragm   Liver
and kidney

12th rib and
quad. lumborum   Diaphragm
Psoas major   Erector spinæ   Serratus post. inf. Latissimus dorsi
and minor

A

FIGURE 12-4 *A.* Transverse section through abdomen at the level of the first lumbar vertebra.

Figure 12-4 continued on opposite page

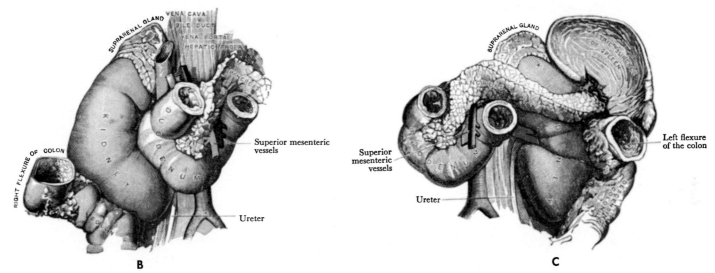

B **C**

FIGURE 12–4 *Continued.* *B*. Right kidney and duodenum. The relation of the duodenum and the right flexure to the kidney is not so extensive as usual. *C*. Relations of left kidney and pancreas. (From Cunningham's Manual of Practical Anatomy, 12th ed., Vol. 2. London, Oxford University Press, 1958.)

Blood Vessels of the Kidney

ARTERIES. The renal arteries arising from the aorta usually divide into *two main branches* directed anteriorly and posteriorly to the kidney (Fig. 12–5). The *posterior* or *dorsal* branch usually arises first and is somewhat smaller in caliber than the *anterior* or *ventral* branch. Secondary branches from the dorsal and ventral branches supply the *five main renal arterial segments* of the kidney as shown in Figure 12–9. The *apical segment* is usually supplied largely by the posterior or dorsal branch of the renal artery, whereas the *lower segment* is supplied mostly by the anterior or ventral branch. Furthermore, *upper and middle branches* of the anterior segment can usually be identified. The renal arteries thereafter branch into *interlobar arteries* between the pyramids (Fig. 12–3). At the bases of the pyramids, the interlobar arteries unite to form the *arcuate* arteries. The arcuate arteries, in turn, send branches into the cortex as the *interlobular arteries,* and these give rise to *afferent glomerular arteries* and some *nutrient* and *perforating capsular*

arteries. Arising out of the glomerulus are the *efferent glomerular arteries* which form a capillary network around the nephrons but also give rise to a few *arteriolae rectae,* which enter the medulla and run directly toward the pelvis.

VEINS. The renal veins (Fig. 12–7) begin in the plexuses around the tubules. Anastomoses between the renal and systemic vessels occur in the fat around the kidney. The renal veins terminate in the inferior vena cava. The *left* renal is longer than the right, crossing the ventral side of the aorta just below the superior mesenteric artery and opening into the inferior vena cava above the right renal vein. It receives as tributaries the *left inferior phrenic,* the *left internal spermatic,* and the *left suprarenal.* It usually lies above the level of the right renal vein, and dorsal to the renal vein, the body of the pancreas, and splenic vein; the inferior mesenteric vein crosses it ventrally. The *right* renal vein is short and lies in front of the renal artery with no extrarenal tributaries ordinarily.

RENAL ARTERY AND ITS SEGMENTAL BRANCHES

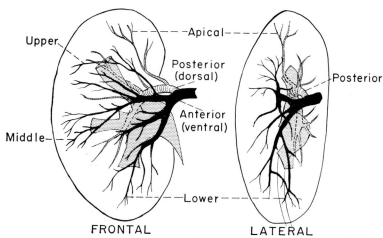

FIGURE 12–5 Diagram illustrating the renal artery and its segmental branches in frontal and lateral perspectives, showing the relationship to the pelvocalyceal system. (After Boijsen, E.: Acta Radiol. (Suppl.), *183*:51, 1959.)

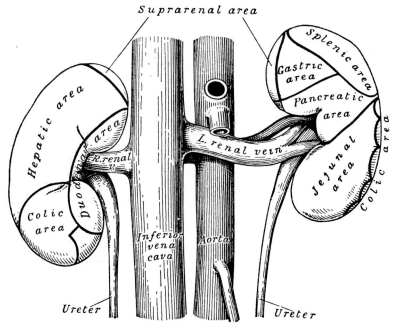

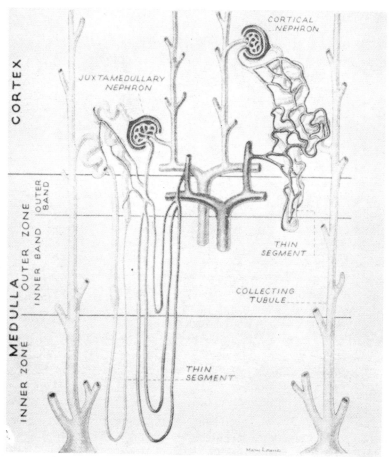

FIGURE 12–6 Diagram of the nephron showing those portions which are situated in the cortex as against those situated in the medulla. The cortical nephron and juxtamedullary nephron are separately shown. (From Smith, H. W.: Principles of Renal Physiology. New York, Oxford University Press, 1956.)

FIGURE 12–7 Gross relationships of renal veins to inferior vena cava and anterior surface relationships of the kidneys. (From Warwick, R., and Williams, P. L. (eds.): Gray's Anatomy, 35th British ed. London, Longman [for Churchill-Livingstone], 1973.)

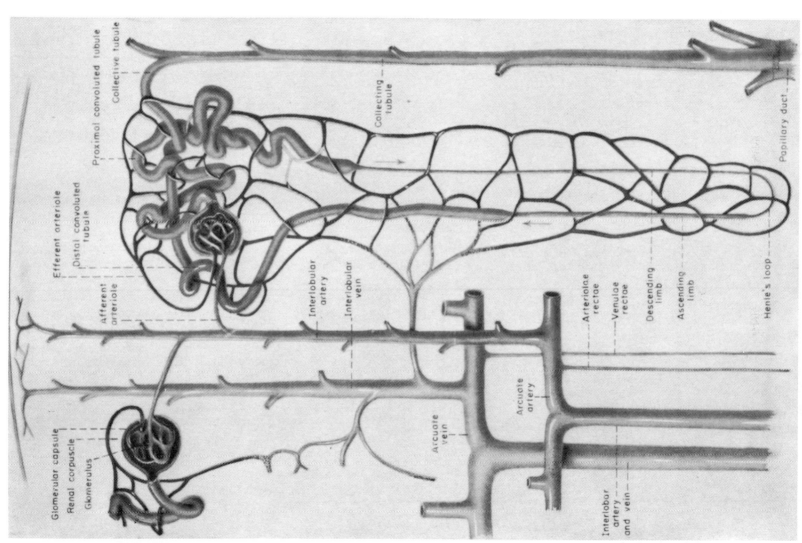

FIGURE 12–8 Diagram of the glomerular tuft and nephron of the kidney and the relationship to associated arteries and veins. (From Anson, B.J. (ed.): Morris' Human Anatomy, New York, McGraw-Hill Book Company. 12th ed. Copyright © 1966 by McGraw-Hill, Inc. Used by permission of McGraw-Hill Book Company.)

SEGMENTAL DISTRIBUTION OF RENAL ARTERY

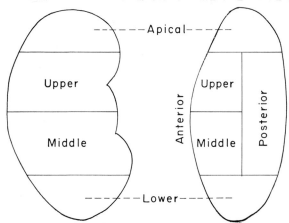

FIGURE 12–9 Diagram illustrating the segmental distribution of the renal artery. The apical segment is usually supplied largely by the posterior or dorsal branch of the renal artery, whereas the lower segment of the kidney is supplied by the anterior or ventral branch of the renal artery for the most part. (After Boijsen, E.: Acta Radiol. [Suppl.], *183*:10, 1959.)

Ureters (Fig. 12–10)

The *abdominal portions* of the ureters on both sides are embedded on the medial aspect of the psoas major muscles and pass ventral to the common or external iliac artery to enter the true pelvis. They lie ventral to the transverse processes of the third, fourth, and fifth lumbar vertebrae, and both are crossed by the spermatic or ovarian vessels. The right abdominal portion of ureter is covered by descending duodenum and is situated to the right of the inferior vena cava. It is crossed by right colic and ileocolic vessels, the mesentery, and terminal ileum. The left abdominal ureter is crossed by left colic vessels and sigmoid meso-

colon. The left ureter is ordinarily separated from the aorta by a space which ranges from 2.5 cm. cranially to 1.5 cm. opposite the bifurcation of the aorta.

The *pelvic portion* of the ureters must be described separately for males and females. In the *male,* this portion of the ureter begins at the pelvic brim, courses caudad close to the internal iliac artery along the ventral border of the greater sciatic notch. It lies medial to the obturator, inferior vesicle, and middle rectal arteries. It turns medially to reach the lateral angle of the urinary bladder at the level of the lower part of the greater sciatic notch. Here, it lies ventral to the seminal vesicles. The vas deferens crosses over it as it approaches the urinary bladder.

In the *female,* the pelvic ureter forms the dorsal boundary of the ovarian fossa. It runs medially and ventrally on the lateral aspect of the cervix and upper part of the vagina to the fundus of the urinary bladder. As it runs ventrally it passes inferior to the uterine artery.

At the level of the urinary bladder the two ureters on each side are about 5 cm. apart in both male and female.

The *intramural* portion of the ureters runs obliquely through the urinary bladder for a distance of approximately 2 cm. and opens into the urinary bladder through two slitlike apertures, the *ureteral ostia,* which are about 2.5 cm. apart in the empty bladder but may be as much as 5 cm. distant from each other when the bladder fills. The ureteral ostia together with the urethral opening of the urinary bladder constitute the *bladder trigone.* On occasion, reflux of urine from bladder to ureter probably takes place normally. Reflux is particularly important in the presence of recurrent infection, in which case pyelonephritis may ensue. The ureter is constantly undergoing peristalsis and hence its lumen is variable in size.

ARTERIES. The arteries of the ureter are branches of the renal, internal spermatic, superior, and inferior vesicle arteries.

The *veins* follow correspondingly named arteries and terminate in correspondingly named veins.

The *lymphatics* pass to the lumbar and internal iliac nodes (Fig. 12–11).

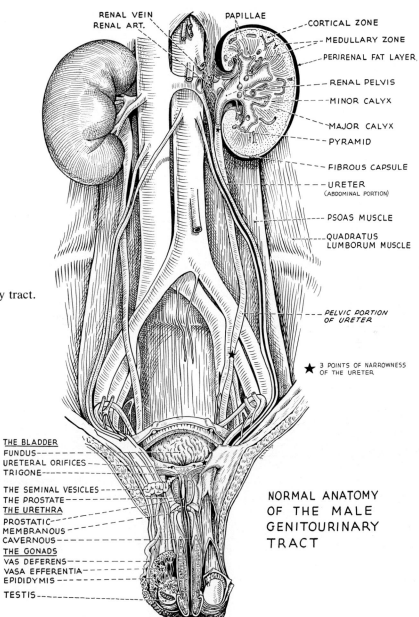

RENAL VEIN
RENAL ART.
PAPILLAE
CORTICAL ZONE
MEDULLARY ZONE
PERIRENAL FAT LAYER
RENAL PELVIS
MINOR CALYX
MAJOR CALYX
PYRAMID
FIBROUS CAPSULE
URETER
(ABDOMINAL PORTION)
PSOAS MUSCLE
QUADRATUS
LUMBORUM MUSCLE

PELVIC PORTION
OF URETER

★ 3 POINTS OF NARROWNESS
OF THE URETER

THE BLADDER
FUNDUS
URETERAL ORIFICES
TRIGONE

THE SEMINAL VESICLES
THE PROSTATE
THE URETHRA
PROSTATIC
MEMBRANOUS
CAVERNOUS
THE GONADS
VAS DEFERENS
VASA EFFERENTIA
EPIDIDYMIS

TESTIS

NORMAL ANATOMY
OF THE MALE
GENITOURINARY
TRACT

FIGURE 12–10 Gross anatomy of the urinary tract.

Ureteral Arterial Blood Supply

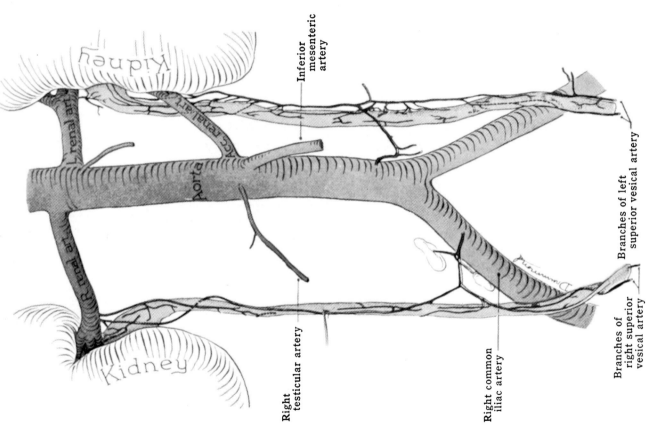

FIGURE 12–11 Blood supply to the ureter. The arterial system was injected with latex by way of the femoral artery. (Dissection by W. R. Mitchell.) (Reproduced by permission from J. C. B. Grant: An Atlas of Anatomy, 5th ed. Baltimore, Md., The Williams & Wilkins Company. Copyright © 1962, The Williams & Wilkins Company.)

The Urinary Bladder

Introduction. The urinary bladder is surrounded by extraperitoneal fatty tissue. In a *child,* even when empty, it is in contact with the abdominal wall, and is located almost entirely in the abdomen proper. By 6 years of age the greater part of the urinary bladder is ordinarily accommodated by the pelvis, but it is not wholly a pelvic organ until shortly after puberty.

In the male, the seminal vesicles and deferent ducts lie on the lower part of the *posterior surface* of the urinary bladder (Fig. 12–12). The bladder is separated from the rectum by the rectovesical septum, seminal vesicles, and vas deferens (bilaterally).

The *neck* of the urinary bladder is about 2 to 3 cm. behind the pubic symphysis, a little above its lower border. Pubovesical ligaments are attached in front and at the sides. In the female it narrows abruptly to become continuous with the urethra. In the male it is continuous with the prostate which surrounds the first part of the urethra, and posteriorly it is in contact with the commencement of the ejaculatory ducts.

The *inferolateral surface* of the bladder is separated from the pubis by a prevesical cleft and is spoken of as the *retropubic space of Retzius.*

In the female, the *fundus* of the urinary bladder is separated from the ventral surface of the uterus by a vesicouterine pouch below; behind, it is proximal to the cervix and the upper vaginal wall. The inferior surface of the bladder rests on pelvic and urogenital diaphragms.

Interior of Urinary Bladder. When the bladder is full its mucous coat is smooth. When empty, it is wrinkled except over the *trigone,* which is a smooth triangular area above the urethral orifice. The three points of reference for the trigone are the two *ureteric orifices* dorsolaterally and the *internal urethral orifice* ventrally. The base of the triangle is formed by the *interureteric ridge* between the orifices (Fig. 12–12 C). The internal urethral orifice, placed at the apex of the trigone, presents a very slight elevation, the *uvula vesicae,* caused by the middle lobe of the prostate (Fig. 12–12).

Vessels and Nerves. The arteries supplying the bladder are the superior, middle, and inferior vesical, which are derived from the anterior trunk of the hypogastric artery (Fig. 12–13). The obturator and inferior gluteal arteries also supply small visceral branches to the bladder. In the female additional branches are derived from the uterine and vaginal arteries.

The *veins* consist largely of a plexus on the inferolateral surface, the plexus communicating with the prostatic plexus. Several veins drain this plexus and pass into the internal iliac vein.

The Male Urethra

The male urethra extends from the internal urethral orifice of the urinary bladder to the external urethral orifice at the end of the penis. It is divided into three portions: *prostatic, membranous,* and *cavernous* (Fig. 12–14).

The Female Urethra

The *female urethra* is about 4 cm. long and extends from the internal to the external urethral orifice. Located behind the pubic symphysis and embedded in the wall of the vagina, it is approximately 6 mm. in diameter and perforates the urogenital diaphragm. Its external orifice is situated in front of the vaginal opening about 2.5 cm. from the glans of the clitoris. A prominent feature is a slight elevation or fold which is called the *urethral crest.* Many small urethral glands open into the urethra, the largest of which are the *paraurethral glands of Skene* (Fig. 12–15).

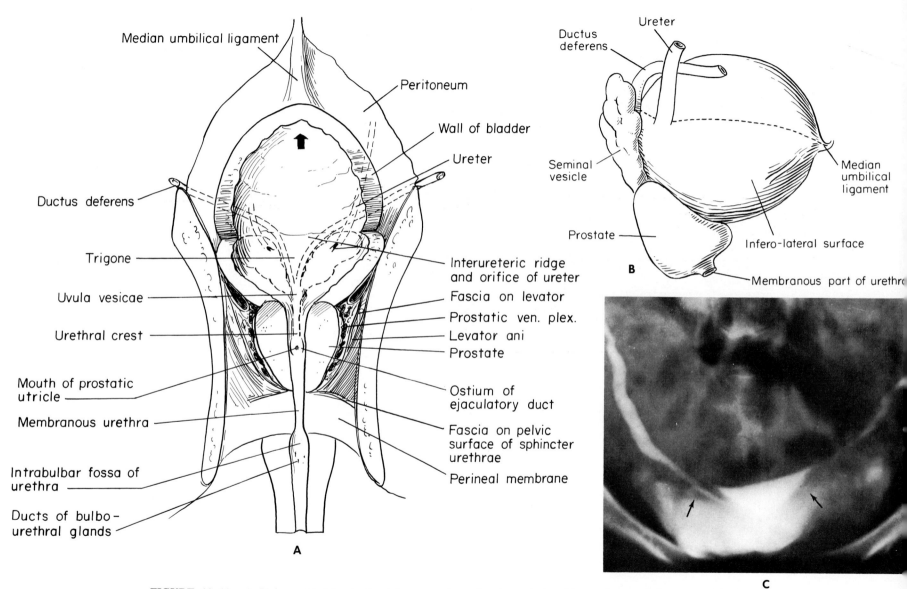

FIGURE 12–12 *A,* Urinary bladder in frontal perspective, showing relationship to ductus deferens, prostate, ureters, and male urethra. *B,* Urinary bladder hardened in situ showing relationship to ureters, ductus deferens, seminal vesicles, and prostate in lateral view. (From Cunningham's Manual of Practical Anatomy, 12th ed., Vol. 2. London, Oxford University Press, 1958.) *C,* Radiograph of urinary bladder cystogram showing interureteric ridge. (Accentuation of the interureteric ridge may occur from edema following recent passage of a ureteral calculus.)

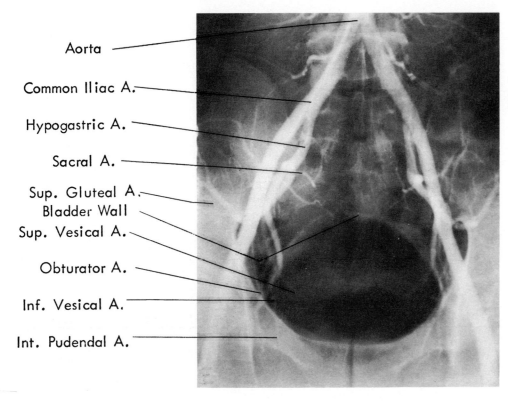

Aorta

Common Iliac A.

Hypogastric A.

Sacral A.

Sup. Gluteal A.
Bladder Wall
Sup. Vesical A.

Obturator A.

Inf. Vesical A.

Int. Pudendal A.

FIGURE 12–13 Triple contrast study of the urinary bladder, with air in the urinary bladder, air interstitially in the urinary bladder wall, and arterial angiograms for demonstration of the urinary bladder arterial blood supply.

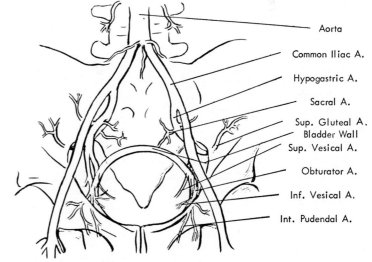

Aorta

Common Iliac A.

Hypogastric A.

Sacral A.

Sup. Gluteal A.
Bladder Wall
Sup. Vesical A.

Obturator A.

Inf. Vesical A.

Int. Pudendal A.

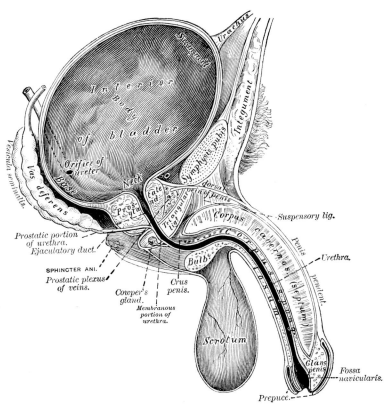

FIGURE 12–14 Vertical section of bladder, penis, and urethra. (From Lewis, W. H. (ed.): Gray's Anatomy of the Human Body, 24th ed. Philadelphia, Lea & Febiger, 1942.)

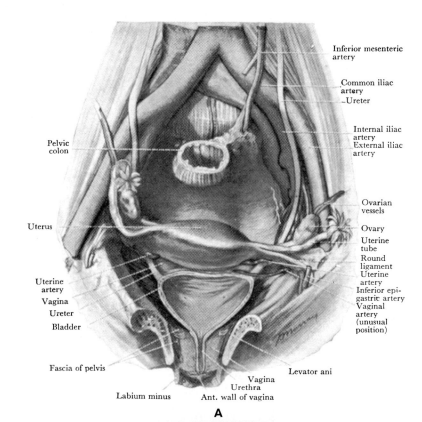

A

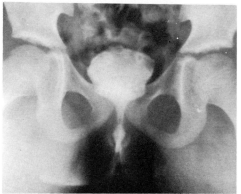

B

FIGURE 12–15 *A.* Dissection of pelvis of a multiparous female, showing the relations of bladder to uterus and vagina, of vagina to urethra and broad ligaments, and of ureters to broad ligaments and vagina. *B.* Normal female urethrogram. (*A* from Brash, J. C. (ed.): Cunningham's Manual of Practical Anatomy. 12th ed., Vol. 2. London, Oxford University Press, 1958.)

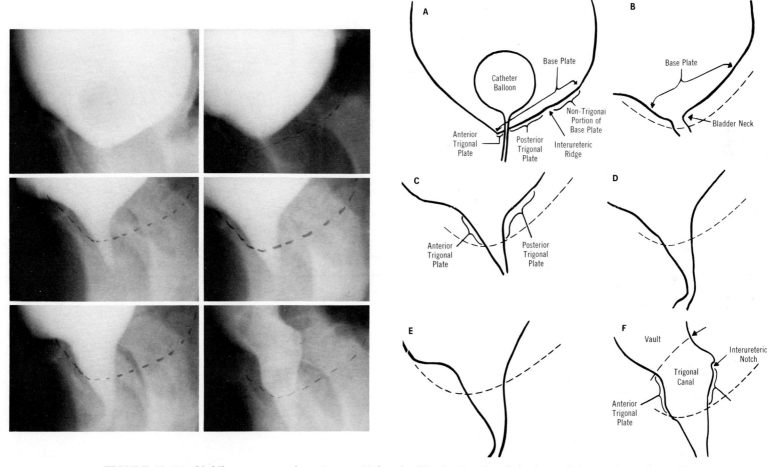

FIGURE 12–16 Voiding sequence in a 4-year-old female. The landmarks of the base plate are shown in *A*. The contraction ring in *F* indicates the division between the base plate below and the vault above. Progressive cephalic movement of the anterior and posterior trigonal plates creates the trigonal canal which is continuous with the posterior urethra. The contraction ring is above the interureteric ridge, indicating that the trigonal canal is formed by the entire base plate and not by the trigonal plates alone. (From Shopfner, C. E., and Hutch, J. A.: Radiology, *88*:209–221, 1967.)

R   L   R   L

Supine   Prone

Supine   Prone

FIGURE 12–17 Schematic drawings of arterial impressions on the renal collecting system. (From Weissleder, von H., Emmrich, J., and Schirmeister, J.: Fortschr. Geb. Roentgenstr. Nuklearmed., *97*:703–710, 1962.)

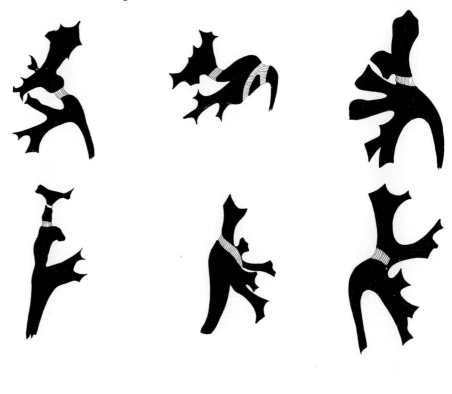

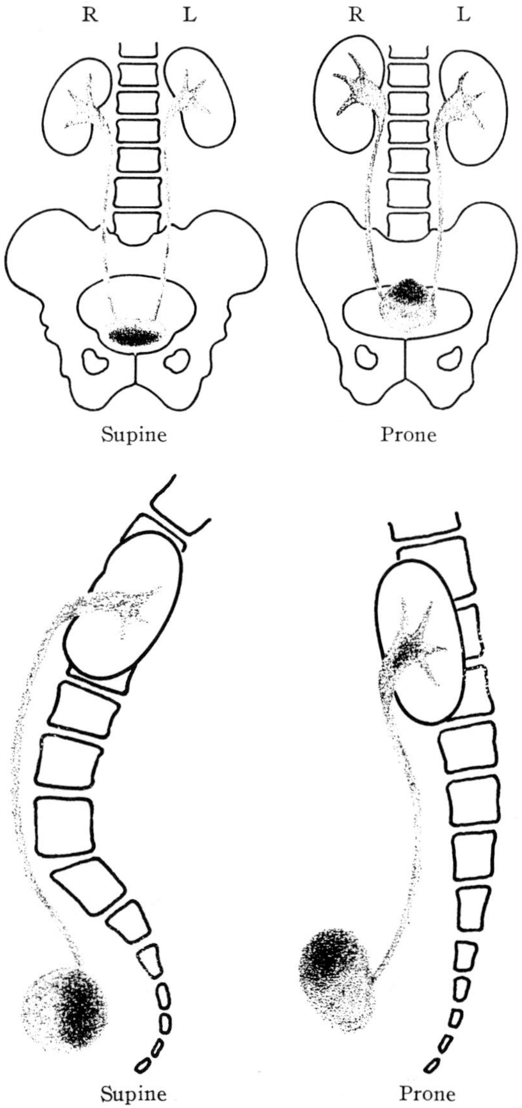

FIGURE 12–18 Summary of anatomic changes in the majority of cases. *Upper,* In the prone view both kidneys appear larger and are more parallel to the spine. The profile of the renal pelves is better, i.e., wider. Right kidney is higher and more medial, but the left kidney is slightly lower. Dome of the bladder is higher and more convex.

Lower, In the prone view the spine shows straightening of lumbar lordosis. Both kidneys are more parallel to the spine. There is a slight tendency to anterior movement. Pelves appear more true lateral. Bladder appears higher and more anterior. (From Riggs, W., Jr., Hagood, J. H., and Andrews, A. E.: Radiology, *94*:107–113, 1970.)

Basic Physiology of the Kidneys

Blood Supply. The basic blood supply of the kidney has already been described. Approximately 70 per cent of all kidneys are supplied by a single renal artery originating from the aorta; two or more arteries supply the remainder.

The Nephron. Figure 12–8 diagrammatically illustrates the nephron unit, consisting of the isolated glomerular tuft, its blood supply, and adjoining tubules.

Renal Function. The function of the kidney may be outlined as follows (Fig. 12–20):

1. *Filtration* of the blood plasma and removal of some of its solutes such as potassium chloride sulfate, sodium, urea, glucose, amino acid and the like.
2. *Selective tubular reabsorption.*
3. *Tubular synthesis and excretion.*
4. *Acid-base regulation.*
5. *Volume regulation* of the fluid environment of the body.
6. *Osmolality regulation.*
7. *Maintenance of a normal blood pressure.*
8. *Erythropoiesis.*

As a result of an effective filtration pressure gradient in the glomerulus, the walls of the glomerular capillaries act as a sieve, allowing particles of certain sizes to filter through and retaining larger ones.

The renal tubules, on the other hand, are primarily concerned with: (1) *water reabsorption* from the glomerular filtrate; (2) *reabsorption* of certain *threshold substances* and ions necessary for the equilibrium of the organism; (3) *excretion* of some organic and inorganic compounds in substances; (4) *synthesis* of certain metabolites; and (5) *excretion of the final waste products* into the collecting system, after an appropri-

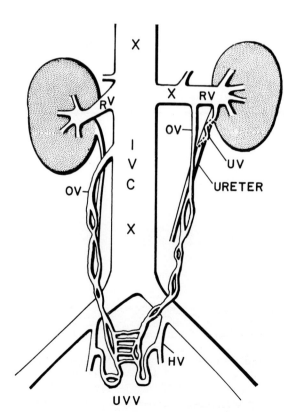

FIGURE 12–19 Sketch of abdominal, renal, and periureteric venous anatomy. The left gonadal vein (ovarian vein in the sketch) almost invariably empties into the left renal vein, while the right empties into the inferior vena cava below the right renal vein. The ureteral veins generally empty into the renal veins at a location peripheral to the site of gonadal emptying. Either of these two latter structures is capable of causing ureteral notching either of a serpentine nature or of a simple extrinsic pressure type. Free communication between them has been noted on multiple occasions. The ovarian veins are in free communication in the broad ligament with the uterine veins and therefore with the hypogastric and iliac veins. It will be seen therefore that occlusion or stenosis of the inferior vena cava above the renal veins, below the renal veins, or in the renal veins (sites marked X) is capable of altering flow in the gonadal or ureteric veins and thereby accounting for vascular notching. (RV) renal vein, (OV) ovarian (gonadal) vein, (UV) ureteral vein, (HV) hypogastric vein, (UVV) uterine veins, (X) sites of occlusion. (From Chait, A., Matasar, K. W., Fabian, C. E., and Mellins, H. Z.: Am. J. Roentgenol., *111*:729–749, 1971.)

ate regulation of acid-base balance and osmolality. It is probable that water is absorbed from both proximal and distal convoluted tubules.

In addition, approximately 14 per cent of water is reabsorbed in the collecting tubules under the control of an antidiuretic hormone derived from the pituitary gland (ADH). To some extent this reabsorption is accomplished by the hyperosmotic environment of the interstitial fluid in the medulla of the kidney involving and surrounding the loops of Henle. This is part of the so-called counter-current phenomenon.

Glomerular filtration and tubular secretion and excretion are the two renal functions especially identified by roentgenologic techniques. Contrast agents such as Hypaque, Miokon, and Renografin are in large measure excreted normally by glomerular filtration, much as is inulin. These compounds, therefore, offer the opportunity for physiologic tests of glomerular filtration. Para-aminohippurate and Hippuran are largely excreted (or secreted) via the tubules and are useful in measuring tubular secretion or excretion.

Sodium diatrizoate (Hypaque) is excreted at the rate of approximately 65 per cent in 2 hours and 88 per cent in 6 hours.

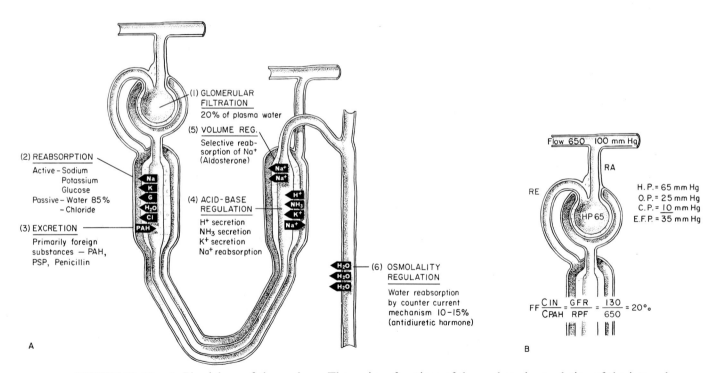

FIGURE 12-20 *A.* Physiology of the nephron. The various functions of the nephron in regulation of the internal environment of the body are diagrammatically illustrated. *B,* Diagrammatic illustration of glomerular hemodynamics in the maintenance of filtration pressure. (H.P.) Hydrostatic pressure, (O.P.) osmotic pressure, (C.P.) capillary pressure, (E.F.P.) effective filtration pressure, (RA) afferent arterioles, (RE) efferent arterioles, (FF) filtration fraction, (CIN) clearance of inulin, (CPAH) clearance of para-aminohippurate, (GFR) glomerular filtration rate. (RPF) renal plasma flow. (From Meschan, I.: Radiol. Clin. North Am., *3*:18, 1965.)

TABLE 12-2. Contrast Media Used in Urography and Angiography

Trade Name	Organic Compound	Per Cent Iodine W/V	Concentration of Drug in Commercially Available Solution	Manufacturer's Suggested Dosage			
				Adult Dose[f]	Children's Dose[f]	Subcutaneous Administration	Intramuscular Administration
Neo-Iopax[a]	Sodium iodomethamate	25.8 38.6	50% 75%	20 cc. of 50% 30 cc. of 50% 20 cc. of 75%	10 cc. of 50%	10% solution (dilute 14 cc. of 75% solution to 100 cc. with normal saline)[e]	Not recommended
Diodrast[b]	Iodopyracet, U.S.P.	17.5 (35% in 70% solution)	35% (70% also available)	20–30 cc. of 35%	0– 6 mo.: 5 cc. 7–12 mo.: 6– 7 cc. 1– 3 yr.: 7–10 cc. 4– 6 yr.: 10–16 cc. 7– 8 yr. 16–20 cc.	7% solution (dilute 20 cc. of 35% solution to 100 cc. with normal saline)[e]	35% solution Children: 10–20 cc. Adults: 20–30 cc.
Hippuran[c]	Sodium iodohippurate	7 (in 20% solution)	Powder only available. Mix 12 gm. with 60 cc. of distilled water to make 20% solution	60 cc. of 20%	0–12 mo.: 6 gm.+ 9.55 cc. water 1– 4 yr.: 8 gm.+ 12.5 cc. water 4– 8 yr.: 10 gm.+ 21 cc. water	Not recommended	Not recommended
Urokon[c]	Sodium acetrizoate, U.S.P.	19.74 (46.06% in 70% solution)	30% 70% for difficult cases only or aortography or nephrotomography	25 cc. of 30% 25 cc. of 70%	<4 yr.: 0.7 cc. of 30% solution >4 yr.: 25 cc. of 30% solution	Not recommended	Not recommended
Miokon[c]	Sodium diprotrizoate, U.S.P.	28.7	50%	20 cc. of 70% 25 cc. of 50% 30 cc. of 50%	<3 mo.: 6 cc. 3– 6 mo.: 6– 8 cc. 6–12 mo.: 8–10 cc. 1– 2 yr.: 10–15 cc. 2– 6 yr.: 15–20 cc. >6 yr.: 20–25 cc.	Not recommended	Not recommended
Hypaque-50[b]	Sodium diatrizoate, U.S.P.	30	50% for excretory urography	30 cc. of 50%	0– 6 mo.: 5 cc. 6–12 mo.: 6– 8 cc. 1– 2 yr.: 8–10 cc. 2– 5 yr.: 10–12 cc. 5– 7 yr.: 12–15 cc. 7–11 yr.: 15–18 cc. 11–15 yr.: 18–20 cc.	Dilute with equal quantities of distilled water[e]	Inject undiluted or diluted with equal parts distilled water
Hypaque-75[b]	Sodium diatrizoate, U.S.P.	39.3	75% 90% for nephrotomography	50 cc. or more	Infants: 5–10 cc. Older children: 15–20 cc.	Not recommended	Not recommended
Hypaque-90[b]	Sodium diatrizoate, U.S.P.	46	75% 90% for nephrotomography	50 cc. or more	Infants: 5–10 cc. Older children: 15–20 cc.	See text	See text

[a]Schering
[b]Winthrop Laboratories
[c]Mallinckrodt Pharmaceuticals
[d]E. R. Squibb and Sons
[e]Subcutaneous injections are given in divided doses over each scapula. Intramuscular injections are given in divided doses into each gluteal region. To increase the rate of absorption, the addition of hyaluronidase to the solution is recommended (150–200 turbidity units on each side for children, 500 for adults).
[f]See page 519 for higher doses usually employed with infusion excretory urography and nephrotomography, very widely used now.

Table continued on following page

TABLE 12–2.   Contrast Media Used in Urography and Angiography *(Continued)*

Trade Name	Organic Compound	Per Cent Iodine W/V	Concentration of Drug in Commercially Available Solution	Manufacturer's Suggested Dosage			
				Adult Dose	Children's Dose	Subcutaneous Administration	Intramuscular Administration
				Retrograde pyelograms:			
Renografin-30[d]	Diatrizoate methyl-glucamine, U.S.P.	15	30%	15 cc. (unilateral)	Proportionately smaller for children	Not used	Not used
Renografin-60[d]	Methylglucamine diatrizoate, U.S.P.	29	60%	25 cc. of 60% (over 15 yrs.)	Under 6 mo.: 5 cc. 6–12 mo.: 8 cc. 1– 2 yr.: 10 cc. 2– 5 yr.: 12 cc. 5– 7 yr.: 15 cc. 8–10 yr.: 18 cc. 11–15 yr.: 20 cc.	Not used	Not used
Renografin-76[d]	Diatrizoate methyl-glucamine	37	76%	20–40 cc. of 76% (over 15 yrs.)	Under 6 mo.: 4 cc. 6–12 mo.: 6 cc. 1– 2 yr.: 8 cc. 2– 5 yr.: 10 cc. 5– 7 yr.: 12 cc. 8–10 yr.: 14 cc. 11–15 yr.: 16 cc.	Not used	Not used
Renovist[d]	Sodium and methyl-glucamine diatrizoate	37	69%	25 cc. of 37% solution (over 15 yrs.)	Under 6 mo.: 5 cc. 6–12 mo.: 8 cc. 1– 2 yr.: 10 cc. 2– 5 yr.: 12 cc. 5– 7 yr.: 15 cc. 7–10 yr.: 18 cc. 10–15 yr.: 20 cc.	Not used	Not used
				Retrograde pyelography:			
Retrografin	Neomycin sulfate solution with methyl glucamine diatrizoate	15	25% neomycin 30% methylgluca-mine diatrizoate	15 cc. (unilateral)	Proportionately smaller for children	Not used	Not used
Ditriokon[c]	Sodium diprotrizoate and diatrizoate	40	68.1%	40–50 cc. (over 12 yrs.)	0.5–1 cc./kg. body weight	Not used	Not used
Conray-60[c]	Meglumine iothalamate	28.2	60%	25–30 cc. (14 yrs. and over)	Under 6 mo.: 5 cc. 6–12 mo.: 8 cc. 1– 2 yr.: 10 cc. 2– 5 yr.: 12 cc. 5– 8 yr.: 15 cc. 8–12 yr.: 18 cc. 12–14 yr.: 20–30 cc.	Not used	Not used
Conray–400[c]	Sodium iothalamate 66.8%	40	66.8%	40–50 cc. (over 14 yrs.)	0.5–1 cc./kg. under 14 yrs.	Not used	Not used

Normal Intrarenal Circulation Time. Circulation times of 6 to 8, 8 to 10, and 10 to 12 seconds have been published.* Generally, an intrarenal circulation time of less than 5 seconds is considered abnormal when a bolus of 8 ml. of contrast material is used, delivered in 1 second.

Gallbladder Visualization Following the Injection of Diatrizoate. Excretion of pyelographic agents via the bile and into the gallbladder with incidental opacification of the gallbladder may occur in unusual circumstances. As a general rule, when this phenomenon occurs with the diatrizoates, renal dysfunction with delayed excretion of contrast material occurs, and creatinine and blood urea nitrogen values are elevated.†

Contrast Media Used in Urography and Angiography

The most commonly used contrast media in urography and angiography are indicated in Table 12–2, with the manufacturer's suggested dosage. From a study of the physiologic evaluations of the dose of the contrast medium Urografin, the following conclusions may be drawn: (1) There is a good correlation between the dose of contrast medium and plasma concentration. This is initially largely independent of the renal function. (2) The minimum concentration of contrast agent in the glomerular filtrate necessary to produce an appreciable nephrogram is probably in the range of 70 mg. iodine per cent. This can apparently be attained with 20 cc. of Urografin 76 per cent in 1 to 2 seconds. If 140 cc. of Urografin-76 is infused slowly, levels well above this are maintained for well over 60 minutes.

The mean plasma concentration of Urografin occurs at identical rates regardless of the rapid intravenous injection of 20 cc. or the slow infusion of 140 cc. of Urografin.

If a contrast medium is injected slowly over 8 to 10 minutes, the peak plasma concentration is not reached until 15 minutes, and this should indeed be the period of maximum density of the nephrogram and optimum period of nephrotomography.

The contrast medium itself acts as a simple osmotic diuretic. The concentration of contrast medium in the urine is accurately reflected by the diuresis.

In patients with normal renal function who have been deprived of fluid for some 12 hours, the concentration of contrast medium in the urine continues to increase with increasing doses up to 140 cc. of Urografin-76, despite the increasing diuresis.

The better the dehydration of the patient, the higher will be the "optimal" dose for this patient. Maximum dehydration, however, is not achieved within the usual period of 8 to 12 hours of fluid restriction before urography. The optimal dose of contrast medium, or one which will produce no further increase in concentration of contrast medium in the urine, will depend on the state of hydration of the patient at the start of the procedure.

Even in high dose urography, dehydration will improve the concentration of contrast medium in the urine in patients with normal renal function. *Actually, however, drip infusion pyelography probably offers no advantage over high dose urography in which equivalent doses of the undiluted contrast medium are injected. A rapid injection usually causes a higher peak of the plasma concentration and a denser nephrogram than a slower injection.*

O'Connor and Neuhauser‡ described a method of total body opacification with relatively large doses of intravenously injected radiopaque contrast media—2 to 4 cc. per kilogram of body weight in infancy. The mechanism of this is thought to be opacification of the entire blood vascular compartment in less than 60 seconds. The added density of the various tissues is proportional to the blood supply. An avascular or hypovascular lesion will be radiolucent in contrast to the adjacent structures with a greater blood supply. The method is limited in differentiating a chronic or poorly vascularized neoplasm from a cyst, but it is particularly useful in defining cystic, hemorrhagic, and chronic lesions.

*Becker, J. A., Canter, I. E., and Perl, S.: Rapid intrarenal circulation. Am. J. Roentgenol., *109*:167–171, 1970.

†Segall, H. D.: Gallbladder visualization following the injection of diatrizoate. Am. J. Roentgenol., *107*:21–26, 1969.

‡O'Connor, J. F., and Neuhauser, E. B. D.: Total body opacification in conventional and high dose venous urography in infancy. Am. J. Roentgenol., *90*:63–71, 1963.

Apparently, untoward reactions are not dose-related in the dose ranges employed, but *it is probable that the intravenous injection of any such contrast media should not be performed when hyperbilirubinemia is present in the newborn.*

Generally, the use of higher volumes of the contrast material improves the quality of intravenous urograms significantly. It increases the diagnostic accuracy of the examination and reduces the need for retrograde pyelography with its attendant hazards.

TABLE 12–3. Dosage Schedule Tested for High-Volume Urography*

Body Surface Area (sq. meters)	Volume (ml.)
Less than 1.30	30
Less than 1.50	40
Less than 1.70	50
Less than 1.90	60
Less than 2.10	70
Less than 2.25	80
Less than 2.40	90
Greater than 2.40	100

*From Friedenberg, M. J., and Carlin, M. R.: Routine use of higher volumes of contrast material. Radiology, *83*:405–413, 1964.

RADIOLOGIC METHODS OF STUDY

Preparation of the Patient. The patient should have a small supper or no meal at all on the night prior to the examination, with nothing by mouth after this meal. Dehydration for at least 12 hours prior to the examination is highly desirable and enhances the concentration in the kidney with either single-dose or infusion techniques.

Catharsis with preparations such as 45 cc. of X-Prep liquid, 1 or 2 oz. of castor oil, or a full dose of magnesium citrate U.S.P. at approximately 6:00 P.M. on the evening prior to the examination is preferred. Some investigators have preferred cleansing enemas on the morning of the examination, but often this will introduce gas into the gastrointestinal tract that will interfere with the clarity of the examination. Suppositories to stimulate colonic evacuation on the morning of the examination may be employed. Aloin, cascara sagrada, or phenolphthalein may be utilized in lieu of the cathartics mentioned above.

Plain Film, Patient Supine (Fig. 12–21)
Single Injection Excretory Urogram (IVP) (Fig. 12–22)

Immediately before injection of any contrast medium the patient is instructed to *void.*

Contrast media which have been and are being used are listed in Table 12–2. The most commonly used at this time are: 50 per cent sodium diatrizoate; 60 per cent meglumine diatrizoate; 60 per cent meglumine iothalamate; and occasionally, 66.8 per cent sodium iothalamate.

The *usual intervals* for taking of films after intravenous injection of the opaque medium are: 4 to 5 minutes; 8 to 15 minutes; 25 to 40 minutes; 60 minutes; 90 minutes; 2 hours; and delayed urography at hourly intervals if necessary up to 8 hours following the intravenous injection if so indicated. If only four films are utilized in the entire examination (three films in addition to the plain film), the recommended time intervals for use with the diatrizoates are 4 minutes, 8 minutes, and 15 to 30 minutes. Nephrotomograms (with high dose, rapid injection urography) are obtained at 1 minute or less.

In some instances, *oblique films* will also be taken, and usually the best time for these is immediately following maximal visualization of the ureters (10 to 20 minutes).

If the lower ureters are not accurately visualized in the supine position the patient may then be turned in the *prone position* and a repeat study obtained at an optimum time interval.

KUB Film Preceding Excretory Urogram (Fig. 12–21)

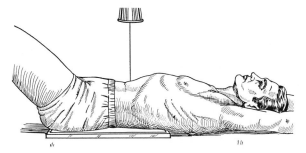

FILM IN
BUCKY
TRAY

POINTS OF PRACTICAL INTEREST ABOUT FIGURE 12–21

1. The technique is same as for KUB, with the patient in suspended respiration.

2. In children, the prone position may be preferred, or compression may be employed in the supine position.

3. Include diaphragm to the pubic symphysis.

4. This or another projection is usually taken in the erect position in the course of the entire study.

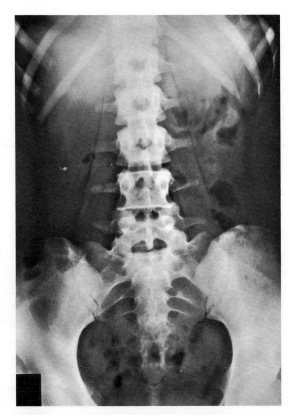

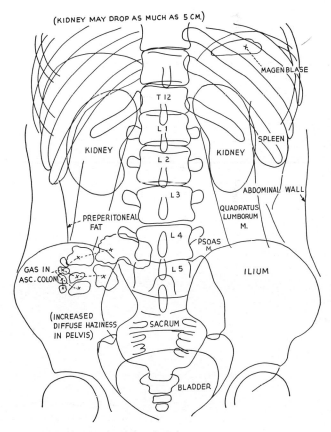

FIGURE 12–21 Radiograph and tracing show a posteroanterior view or anteroposterior projection of abdomen (KUB film).

Dose. Many radiologists employ doses larger than those suggested by the manufacturer as indicated in Table 12–2. For example, in infants 6 months or younger, 10 cc. of the diatrizoate are employed; in older children, a minimum dose of 2 to 3 cc. per pound is usually employed; in adults, the usual dose is often 1.5 cc. per pound or even greater, to a maximum of 150 cc. if necessary.

CYSTOGRAM AND VOIDING URETHROGRAM. If, in addition, a cystogram is desired by this excretory method, oblique studies of the urinary bladder are obtained. Urethrograms require an oblique study of the urethra while the patient is urinating into a suitable receptacle (voiding cystourethrogram). Usually it is more satisfactory to perform urethrograms following instillation of the medium directly into the bladder (Fig. 12–33 C).

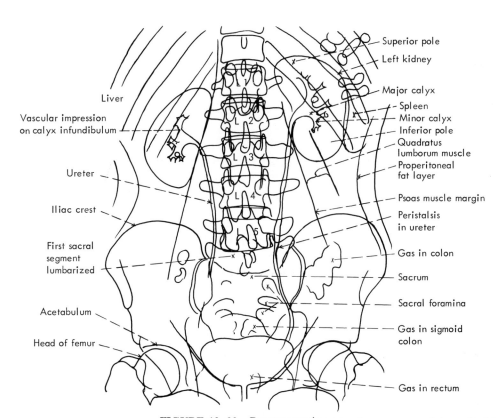

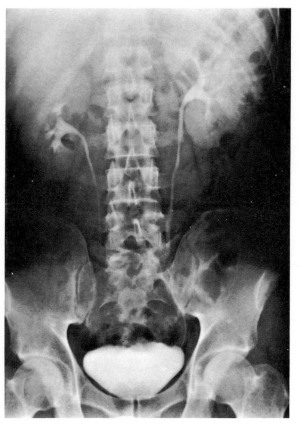

FIGURE 12–22 Representative excretory urogram (also called intravenous pyelogram) obtained 15 minutes after the intravenous injection of a suitable contrast agent.

RADIOLOGIC METHODS OF STUDY OF THE URINARY TRACT

1. Preparation of patient.
2. Plain film, patient supine (KUB).
   a. Prone film in infants.
3. Single injection excretory urogram.
4. Infusion excretory urogram.
5. Hypertension study pyelogram—rapid sequence dehydrated urogram, combined with a hydrated pyelogram.
6. Nephrotomography.
7. Retrograde pyelography.
8. Cystography and cystourethrography.
   a. With voiding urethrogram.
   b. Retrograde urethrogram.
   c. Cystogram (with excretory or retrograde pyelogram).
   d. With double contrast (air).
   e. Triple contrast—angiography plus pneumocystogram plus interstitial air in wall of urinary bladder.
   f. "Chain" cystourethrogram—investigation of stress incontinence.
9. Renal arteriography and aortography.
10. Phlebography and inferior vena cavography.
11. Roentgen evaluation of the surgically exposed kidney.
12. Cineradiography of the upper urinary tract and cystourethrography.
13. Perirenal air insufflation.
14. Seminal vesiculography.
15. Reactions to contrast media.

FIGURE 12–23

Infusion Excretory Urography. Infusion excretory urography is the technique of opacifying the urinary tract by means of a large amount of contrast medium introduced by continuous intravenous drip. The technique, described by Harris and Harris,* involves the intravenous infusion of 140 cc. of 50 per cent sodium diatrizoate (Hypaque) mixed with an equal amount of physiologic salt solution and allowed to run freely through a 19 gauge hypodermic needle. After 225 cc. has been introduced the infusion is slowed in order to maintain an open needle for the duration of the study. The first roentgenogram is made 20 minutes following commencement of the infusion. Thereafter, any other radiographs may be obtained as necessary.

A rapid infusion of 100 ml. of Renografin-76 plus 1 ml. of isotonic dextrose solution per pound of body weight may be similarly employed.

The main advantage of this technique is the increased clarity with which the collecting system and ureters may be identified, sometimes avoiding the necessity for retrograde pyelography (Fig. 12–25). Moreover, body section radiographs can be obtained when nephrotomography might be indicated, such as the differentiation of renal cysts and neoplasms.

The Rapid Sequence Dehydrated Excretion Urogram Combined with a Hydrated Pyelogram. The Hypertension Pyelogram (Fig. 12–24). At the onset of an excretory urogram, the patient is decidedly dehydrated. Normally, hydration of a patient undergoing an excretory urogram will produce a marked dilution of the contrast agent within a normal kidney and some dilatation of the calyces, so that the visualization of the calyces may be indistinct. In patients with renovascular hypertension, such dilution of the contrast agent does not ordinarily occur, and hydration may actually enhance the visualization of an otherwise poorly seen collecting system.

To facilitate hydration, urea diuresis has been recommended as follows: a slow-drip intravenous infusion of 40 grams of urea in 500 ml. of 5 per cent dextrose (rather than isotonic saline as in the Amplatz method) is begun through an 18 gauge needle. This is momentarily

*Harris, J. H., and Harris, J. H., Jr.: Infusion pyelography. Am. J. Roentgenol., *92:* 1391–1396, 1964.

clamped off and 50 cc. of 75 per cent Hypaque-M is introduced as rapidly as possible through this needle (within 30 seconds). Films are obtained immediately thereafter and then at 1 minute intervals for 6 minutes. The slow drip is continued only to keep the needle from being obstructed by a blood clot. An additional film is obtained at 8 minutes. Following exposure of the 8 minute pyelogram, at which time the renal collecting systems are usually at their peak of opacification, a more rapid infusion of the urea-dextrose mixture is begun so that the entire infusion occurs in 10 to 15 minutes. Thereafter films are obtained at 5 minute intervals for a total of 20 minutes. The best washout phenomenon appears on the 15 and 20 minute films ordinarily.

A 5 per cent solution of mannitol may be substituted for the urea-dextrose mixture to produce diuresis and is probably easier to manage than the urea (author's preference).

The first phase of this study has been called the minute pyelogram or rapid sequence intravenous pyelogram. The latter phase has been called the "washout" study. The latter is a radiologic adaptation of the Howard and Stamey tests.

Nephrotomography (Figure 12–25 *B*)

Retrograde Pyelography (Fig. 12–26). Patient preparation for retrograde pyelography is much the same as for intravenous pyelography.

This method requires that catheters be introduced into the ureters by cystographic manipulation. Most urologists prefer opaque ureteral catheters. Ordinarily the tip of the catheter is introduced well into the renal pelvis, but care must be exercised not to penetrate the renal calyces because local infarction may result.

It is customary to obtain a plain film of the abdomen after the introduction of the ureteral catheters and prior to the injection of the opaque medium. Oblique studies are taken if necessary, especially if ureteral calculi are suspected.

Following the initial studies, an opaque medium is injected through the ureteral catheter. This may be an organic iodide preparation such as Hippuran (sodium orthoiodohippurate dihydrate), Skiodan, or a 12 per cent solution of sodium iodide or bromide. Skiodan is combined with the antibiotic Neomycin in Retropaque as an antibacterial medium. The organic iodide media are preferred and 20 to 30 per cent solutions of any of these are quite satisfactory. Too great an opacity is undesirable since calculi may be obscured.

When the injection is made, overdistention of the pelvis and calyces should be avoided. A good method of introduction is by means of gravity or carefully controlled pressure (46 cm. of water). Ordinarily 5 to 10 cc. of medium will make a satisfactory pyelogram. Films are developed immediately to assure good filling and good visualization of the various anatomic structures. Special films may be taken as necessary following these exploratory studies.

Following this initial injection and after satisfactory visualization of the renal calyces and pelvis, a film is obtained while withdrawing the catheter, all the while injecting the opaque medium. This permits a complete visualization of the ureter as well as the pelvis and kidney calyces.

When ureteral obstruction is expected, a delayed pyelogram is sometimes desired. This may be obtained in the erect position to visualize the point of obstruction to better advantage.

THE SIMPLE RETROGRADE CYSTOGRAM (FIG. 12–31). The procedure is performed as follows: after the patient has completely voided, the urinary bladder is catheterized and the residual urine measured. Thereafter 150 to 200 ml. of a 10 to 30 per cent solution of any of the diiodinated or triiodinated compounds used for excretory urography are instilled in the urinary bladder through the catheter and the catheter is removed. The urinary bladder is filled within the limits of comfort to the patient. The views obtained are shown in Figure 12–31 and 12–32. The oblique and profile studies are necessary to distinguish diverticula

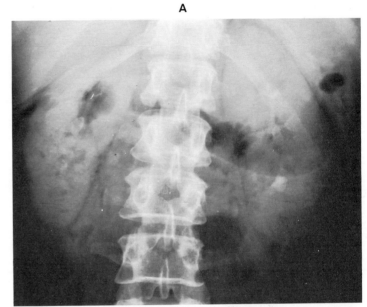

A

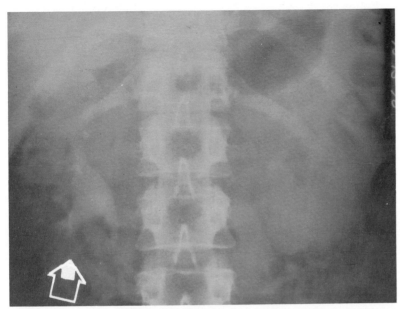

FIGURE 12–24   Renovascular hypertension with a positive washout test. Note the hyperconcentration of the right renal pelvis and calyces even after the left renal collecting system is completely washed out. The blood pressure in this patient was 190/120. The above film was obtained 15 minutes after the injection of a large volume diuretic (Mannitol).

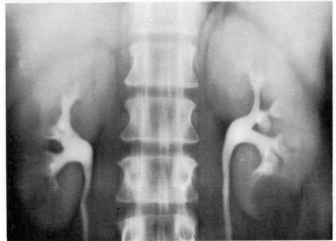

B

FIGURE 12–25   Value of drip-infusion urogram with tomogram. *A.* Routine low-dose excretory urogram, showing poor visualization of renal pelvis and calyces. *B.* Drip-infusion urogram with tomogram. Excellent visualization of renal parenchyma and collecting system. Previously unsuspected mass (simple cyst) is present in lower pole of left kidney. (From Emmett, J. L., and Witten, D. M.: Clinical Urography, 3rd ed., Vol. 1. Philadelphia, W. B. Saunders Co., 1971.)

or filling defects which otherwise might be obscured. Finally, the patient is encouraged to void as completely as possible, but if unable to void, the bladder is evacuated by catheter. The *postvoiding study* is of some value to demonstrate: (a) vesical diverticula, (b) filling defects caused by neoplasm, and (c) vesicoureteral reflux. The demonstration of the latter requires that a full 14 × 17 inch film be utilized to include both ureters and kidneys as well as the urinary bladder. Under normal conditions it is not unusual for 10 to 20 cc. to remain in the urinary bladder after the patient has apparently voided completely.

THE AIR CYSTOGRAM (FIG. 12–33 *D*). Approximately 100 to 200 cc. of air are introduced by catheter. Vesical tumors may produce a soft tissue density within the air cystogram. Air cystography may be enhanced by double contrast by using opaque media in addition to air. In the presence of a rupture of the urinary bladder air will enter the abdominal cavity or soft tissue space surrounding the urinary bladder. Fatal air embolism has been described as a complication of air cystography.*

THE TRIPLE-VOIDING CYSTOGRAM.† Voiding in three installments often permits better emptying of a large atonic bladder. The films obtained after each voiding are called the triple-voiding cystogram. Usually the patient is allowed to walk around for approximately 2 minutes after each voiding episode. This technique provides a mechanism for measuring residual urine as well as for demonstrating vesicoureteral reflux.

DELAYED CYSTOGRAPHY FOR CHILDREN. This method is of particular value in children in order to check urinary retention, particularly since children are often unable to void on command. Vesicoureteral reflux that has not been visible by other methods may be demonstrated thereby. Indeed, excretory urography and cystoscopy may be misleading, and this diagnosis may be missed without evidence from a delayed cystogram.

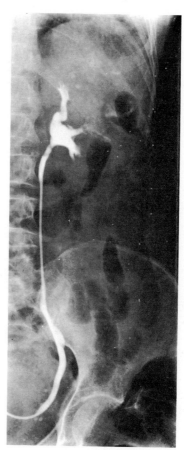

FIGURE 12–26 Representative retrograde pyelogram with ureteral catheter in situ.

---

*Emmett, J. L., and Witten, D. M.: Clinical Urography: An Atlas and Textbook of Roentgenologic Diagnosis. 3rd ed. Philadelphia, W. B. Saunders Co., 1971.

†Lattimer, J. K., Dean, A. L., Jr., and Furey, C. A.: The triple voiding technique in children with dilated urinary tracts. J. Urol., *76*:656–660, 1956.

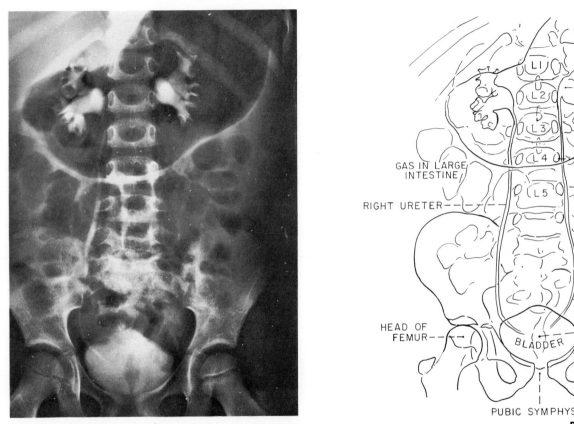

A

B

FIGURE 12–27 *A*. Intravenous pyelogram of a child. The upper urinary tract is demonstrated clearly through the gas-distended stomach. *B*. Corresponding tracing.

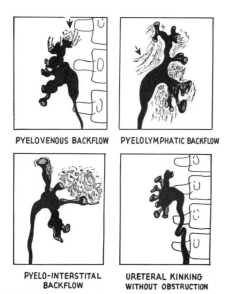

PYELOVENOUS BACKFLOW   **PYELOLYMPHATIC BACKFLOW**

PYELO-INTERSTITAL BACKFLOW   **URETERAL KINKING WITHOUT OBSTRUCTION**

FIGURE 12–28 Variations of normal collecting systems of urinary tract related to backflow phenomena and also ureteral kinking.

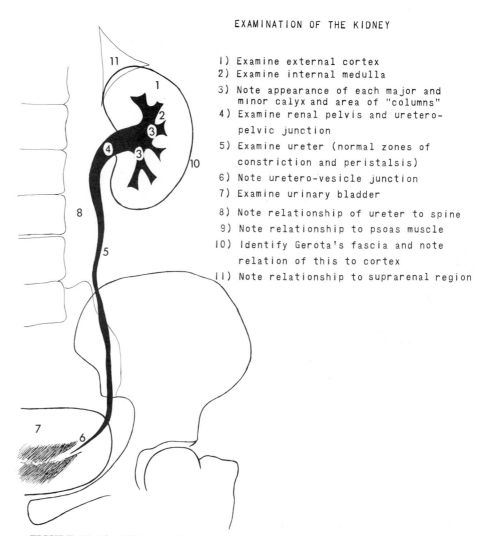

EXAMINATION OF THE KIDNEY

1) Examine external cortex
2) Examine internal medulla
3) Note appearance of each major and minor calyx and area of "columns"
4) Examine renal pelvis and uretero-pelvic junction
5) Examine ureter (normal zones of constriction and peristalsis)
6) Note uretero-vesicle junction
7) Examine urinary bladder
8) Note relationship of ureter to spine
9) Note relationship to psoas muscle
10) Identify Gerota's fascia and note relation of this to cortex
11) Note relationship to suprarenal region

FIGURE 12–29 Kidney collecting system with excretory urography: method of studying films.

TABLE 12–4. Advantages and Disadvantages of Excretory Urography as Opposed to Retrograde Pyelography

Excretory Urograms	Retrograde Pyelograms
Greater comfort to patient; no risk of infection.	Great discomfort and risk of infection
Does not require ureteral catheterization.	Requires ureteral catheterization.
Yields some information regarding renal function and may allow selectivity in retrograde study.	No information regarding renal function.
Probably of no value when BUN is elevated above 50 mg. per cent but may be tolerated when small doses of contrast agent are employed (Davidson et al.).	May precipitate anuria in some medical diseases such as pyelonephritis, glomerulonephritis, and arteriolar nephrosclerosis.
Detail fair when infusion pyelograms are employed but usually not as good as in retrograde study.	Structural detail optimal, but artificial distention of the collecting structures of the kidney usually occurs.
Safe in the presence of obstructing ureteral calculus.	Inadvisable to inject contrast medium above a point of obstruction, since a severe reaction in the patient may ensue.
Dangerous in cases with strong history of allergy or iodine sensitivity.	May be utilized with caution.
Possibly dangerous in patients with multiple myeloma and related disorders.	May be utilized with caution.
Should not be utilized when in vivo studies of thyroid by radioactive iodine are contemplated.	May be utilized.

Summary: Excretory and retrograde studies are complementary and supplementary. One does not exclude the utilization of the other.

It has been estimated that there has been an incidence of 6.6 deaths per million examinations.* Approximately 90 per cent of fatal reactions occurred during or immediately after injection, and hence it is vital that medications to counteract reactions be immediately available to the physician who performs the injection.

*Pendergrass, H. P., et al.: Reactions associated with intravenous urography: Historical and statistical review. Radiology, *71*:1–12, 1958.

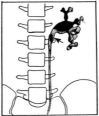 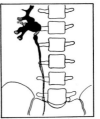

KINKING OF URETER WITHOUT OBSTRUCTION

ATYPICAL URETEROPELVIC JUNCTIONS NORMAL VARIANTS

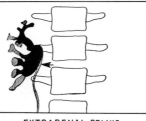 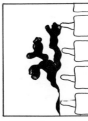 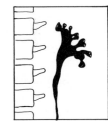

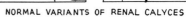

EXTRARENAL PELVIS

NORMAL VARIANTS OF RENAL CALYCES

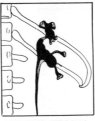 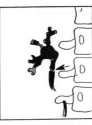 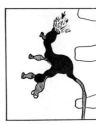 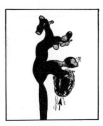

CALYCEAL NORMAL VARIANTS

PERISTALSIS IN URETER

PYELOTUBULAR BACKFLOW

PYELOSINOUS TRANSFLOW

FIGURE 12–30 Some confusing pyelographic appearances.

The Normal Cystogram

1. A 5- to 15-degree caudal tilt of the central ray may be used. This will project the pubic symphysis away from the base of the bladder.

2. A postvoiding cystogram is always obtained, preferably on a 14 × 17 inch film, since reflux may appear only after voiding.

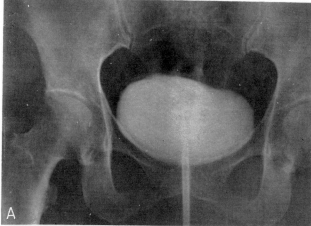

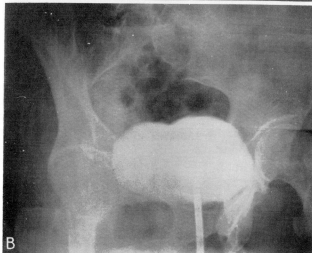

CASSETTE IN
BUCKY TRAY

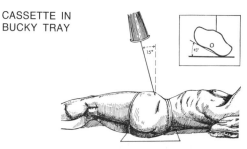

Position for opposite oblique is identical
with patient lying on left side

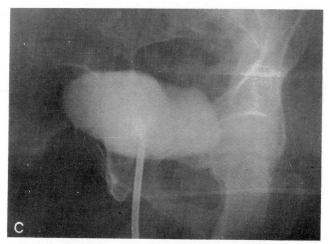

FIGURE 12–31 Representative normal cystograms: *A.* Anteroposterior projection. *B.* Left posterior oblique projection. *C.* Right posterior oblique projection. A lateral view may also be employed. The positions for other patients and central ray are shown in diagram.

Normal Cystogram *(continued)*

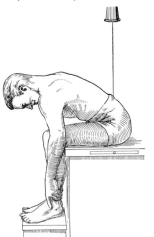

POINTS OF PRACTICAL INTEREST ABOUT FIGURE 12–32

1. The dynamic activity of the urinary bladder may be studied by obtaining films of the bladder area after voiding. This may show a residuum in the bladder (bladder retention) or reflux up the ureters.

2. The thickness of the bladder wall is also important, and may be gauged readily, particularly when the wall is hypertrophied in association with cystitis.

3. The patient is positioned so that the pubic symphysis is centered to the film and the central ray exits at this point.

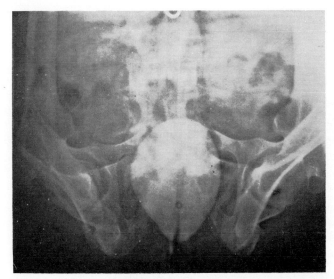

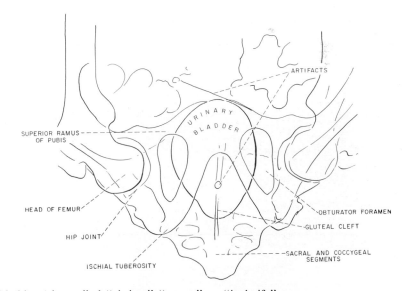

Figure 12–32 Chassard-Lapiné projection of urinary bladder (also called "sitting," "squat," or "jacknife" projection).

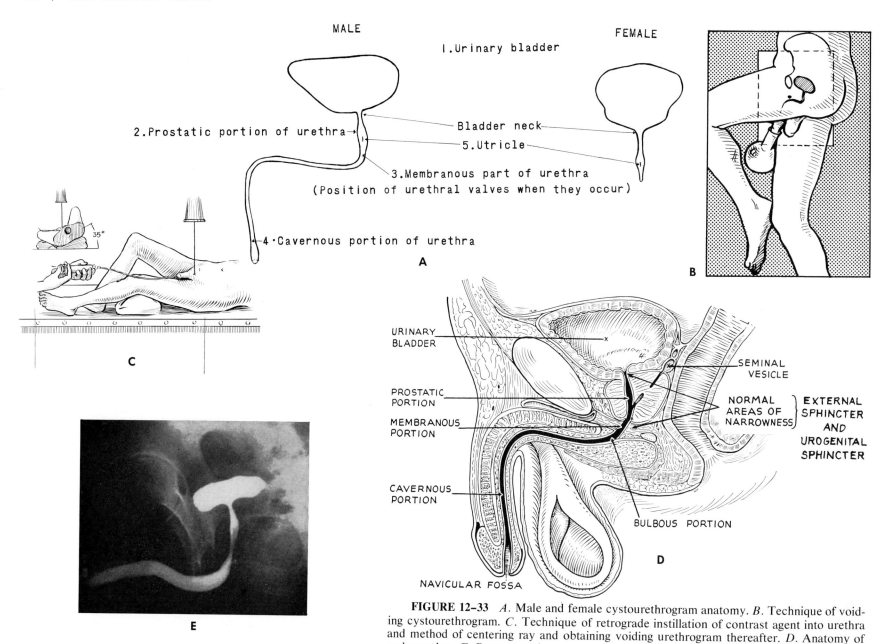

MALE

FEMALE

1. Urinary bladder

2. Prostatic portion of urethra

Bladder neck

5. Utricle

3. Membranous part of urethra
(Position of urethral valves when they occur)

4. Cavernous portion of urethra

A

35°

C

B

URINARY
BLADDER

PROSTATIC
PORTION

MEMBRANOUS
PORTION

CAVERNOUS
PORTION

SEMINAL
VESICLE

NORMAL
AREAS OF
NARROWNESS

EXTERNAL
SPHINCTER
AND
UROGENITAL
SPHINCTER

BULBOUS PORTION

NAVICULAR FOSSA

D

E

FIGURE 12–33 *A.* Male and female cystourethrogram anatomy. *B.* Technique of voiding cystourethrogram. *C.* Technique of retrograde instillation of contrast agent into urethra and method of centering ray and obtaining voiding urethrogram thereafter. *D.* Anatomy of male urethra. *E.* Representative cystourethrogram. (Reproduced with permission of Goodyear, Beard, and Weens and the publishers of Southern Medical Journal.)

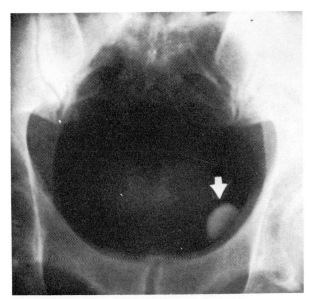

FIGURE 12–34 Air cystogram of the urinary bladder demonstrating a filling defect due to a small sessile bladder carcinoma.

MICTURITION CYSTOURETHROGRAM (VOIDING CYSTOURETHROGRAM) (FIG. 12–33 *B*). Voiding cystourethrogram usually distends the prostatic urethra sufficiently to demonstrate the external urethral sphincteric mechanism. The anterior urethra is also thereby visualized. In very young children, who cannot void on command, *expression cystourethrography* may be necessary under anesthesia.

THE RETROGRADE CYSTOURETHROGRAM (FIG. 12–33 *C*). The simple retrograde urethrogram is of less value than a voiding cystourethrogram for unimpeded visualization of the vesical neck and prostatic urethra. Voiding cystourethrography ordinarily permits a good visualization of the posterior as well as the anterior urethra. This procedure is of particular importance in children in whom valves of the urethra and vesicoureteral reflux are best demonstrated by voiding cystourethrography. Films in an oblique position with the patient standing are preferred if at all feasible.

Kjellberg et al.* have used simultaneous biplane sequential films with automatic filming at 3 to 5 second intervals, depending on the rate of micturition. Waterhouse,* on the other hand, has reduced the technique by making only one x-ray exposure with the patient lying in the right oblique posterior position, thus diminishing x-ray exposure. Cineradiography has also been extensively employed (Dunbar).*

Renal Arteriography and Aortography (Figs. 12–35 and 12–36). Visualization of the renal arteries, their major ramifications, nephrograms, renal collecting systems, and to a limited extent, renal veins, may be accomplished by (1) translumbar aortography, (2) percutaneous aortography by catheter techniques, and (3) selective renal arteriography (Colapinto and Steed).* Translumbar aortograms may be employed in patients with severe aortoiliac disease in whom retrograde catheterization may be impossible or hazardous. On the other hand, transbrachial or axillary artery catheterization may be attempted for selective catheterization in some of these cases. We have considered these techniques as special procedures outside the scope of this text and the student is referred to extensive monographs on these subjects (Schobinger and Ruzicka).*

Percutaneous transfemoral renal arteriography is probably the procedure of choice. Not only can the individual single or multiple renal arteries be selectively visualized, but midstream injection into the aorta may help determine the multiplicity of renal arteries for greatest accuracy. The use of a mechanical injector and rapid film sequencing equipment permits a dynamic study of the arterial blood supply of the kidney and allows an accurate assay of the pathology and physiology as well as anatomy.

Phlebography and Inferior Vena Cavography (Fig. 12–37). Generally, the techniques employed for selective phlebography are similar to those for renal arteriography, except that the bifid, trifid, or plexiform is quite short—1 to 2 cm. There are rarely any anastomotic veins adjoining it. It adjoins the inferior vena cava at an acute angle. The *left renal vein* is longer, 4 to 6 cm., and its junction with the inferior vena cava usually forms a right angle. A large *left ovarian* or *testicular vein* usually joins it. The inferior *left adrenal vein* and a number of anastom-

Text continued on page 531

*References may be obtained in Meschan, I.: An Atlas of Anatomy Basic to Radiology. Philadelphia, W. B. Saunders Co., 1975, Chapter 16.

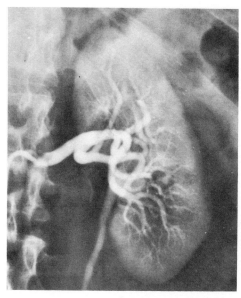

A

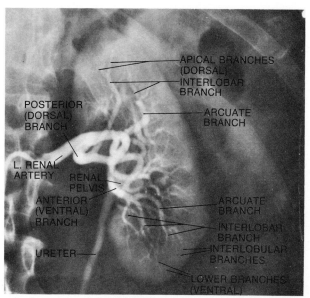

APICAL BRANCHES (DORSAL)

INTERLOBAR BRANCH

ARCUATE BRANCH

POSTERIOR (DORSAL) BRANCH

L. RENAL ARTERY

RENAL PELVIS

ANTERIOR (VENTRAL) BRANCH

ARCUATE BRANCH

INTERLOBAR BRANCH

INTERLOBULAR BRANCHES

URETER

LOWER BRANCHES (VENTRAL)

B

FIGURE 12–35 Normal selective renal arteriogram with anatomic parts labeled. *A* and *B*: Arteriogram phase. *C* and *D*: Venogram phase.

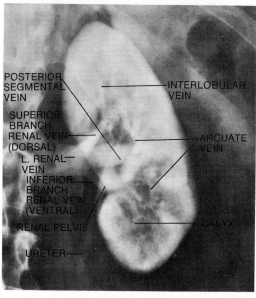

POSTERIOR SEGMENTAL VEIN

INTERLOBULAR VEIN

SUPERIOR BRANCH RENAL VEIN (DORSAL)

L. RENAL VEIN

ARCUATE VEIN

INFERIOR BRANCH RENAL VEIN (VENTRAL)

RENAL PELVIS

URETER

CALYX

C

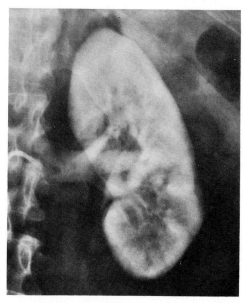

D

otic channels to the lumbar paraspinal plexus also join the left renal vein.

Apart from the utilization already mentioned, catheterization of the renal veins is useful in assessing the patency of splenorenal shunts and in estimation of renal blood flow, by measuring the rate of clearance of a contrast agent from the renal venous system.

INTRARENAL VENOUS STRUCTURES. The normal intrarenal venous anatomy is shown in Figure 12–37 *C*. The main renal vein may have three to four primary tributary veins and these in turn have two to three interlobar veins coursing between the calyces and medullary pyramids. The interlobar veins are linked by arcuate veins running between the cortex and medulla. Fine, parallel cortical veins drain the outer surface, flowing into the arcuate veins. There are a few sub-capsular stellate veins as well. The veins are not segmental end vessels, unlike the renal arteries. Communications between veins are free and numerous. Of interest is the distortion of the venous system by cysts in the kidney. The thickness of the renal cortex may also be measured accurately by virtue of the cortical veins (Sorby; Kahn).*

Implacements upon, deformity, or displacements of the inferior vena cava also have assumed greater importance in diagnosis, particularly in relation to malignancies which involve the central axis of the body (lymphomas or metastasizing carcinomas).

Triple Contrast Study of the Urinary Bladder (Fig. 12–13). This type of study consists of (1) oxygen or air injected into the perivesical tissue space; (2) air injected into the urinary bladder via catheter; and (3) serial arterial filming during retrograde femoral arteriography for visualization of the blood supply of the urinary bladder and, particularly, of any neoplasms it may contain. This technique assists materially in the staging of such neoplasms as a guide to appropriate treatment.

---

*References may be obtained in Meschan, I.: An Atlas of Anatomy Basic to Radiology. Philadelphia, W. B. Saunders Co., 1975, Chapter 16.

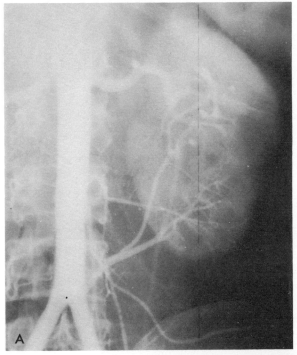

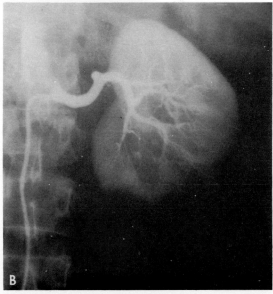

FIGURE 12–36 Selective arteriograms showing the appearance with a double renal artery supplying one kidney when both left renal arteries are filled *(A)*, and when only the upper is filled *(B)*.

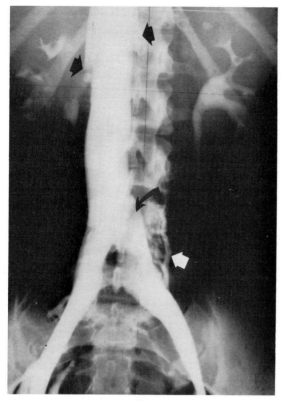

A

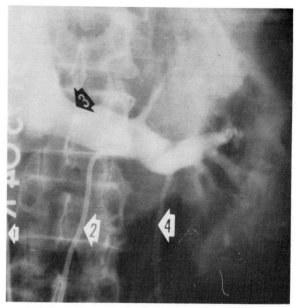

B

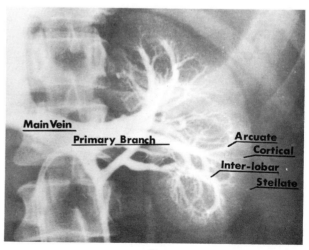

Main Vein

Primary Branch

Arcuate

Cortical

Inter-lobar

Stellate

C

FIGURE 12–37 *A*. Renal venogram and inferior vena cavagram (black curved arrow). Black straight arrows point to origin of renal veins. White arrow shows paravertebral veins. *B*. Left normal renal venogram. (1) Catheter in inferior vena cava. (2) catheter in aorta and left renal artery, (3) left renal vein, (4) left spermatic vein. (Courtesy of University of Iowa, Department of Radiology.) *C*. Normal renal venous anatomy. (*B* and *C* by kind permission of the Honorary Editor of Clinical Radiology. Sorby, W. A.: Renal phlebography. Clin. Radiol. *20*:166–172, 1969. Published by E. & S. Livingstone, Ltd.)

Roentgen Examination of the Surgically Exposed Kidney. Radiography of the surgically exposed kidney, particularly during removal of renal stones, may be accomplished by wrapping a suitably sized film in black paper and packing it in a sheet of sterile rubber to be placed next to the kidney during its radiography at the time of surgery. Sterile packs are commercially available for this purpose. The films may be placed in a sterile rubber glove at the time of radiography also. A special cassette utilizing intensifying screens has also been devised for this technique (Olsson).*

Cineradiography (Dux et al.).* Cineradiography of the excretory urogram may be readily accomplished with image amplification and cinematography. Urine is transported toward the urinary bladder as a result of the active coordinated contraction of muscle groups in the renal pelvis, major and minor calyces, and ureter. Emptying of the renal pelvis depends on its shape and size, on flow from individual calyceal groups, and on filling pressure (the pressure changes in the ureter). Peristalsis or antiperistalsis cannot ordinarily be demonstrated in the normal renal pelvis. In the ureter, on the other hand, urine transport appears to depend upon pure peristaltic contraction.

Cineradiography may also be employed as an adjunct to urethro-cystograms, but because of the greater radiation exposure of the gonads by this technique single or selected rapid film sequences on 70 to 105 mm. spot films are usually preferred.

Pneumograms of the Urinary Bladder and Pneumopyelograms. Air may be injected through a ureteral catheter for the latter purpose. Unfortunately, small bubbles of air will simulate calculi or small polypi, and hence the constancy of a finding must be interpreted with caution. Filling defects, however, are sometimes demonstrated to excellent advantage by this technique. The danger of air embolism must be considered.

Perirenal Air Insufflation (Figs. 12–38 and 12–40). Perirenal air insufflation, direct or by means of the introduction of presacral air, may be utilized (Cocchi).* When introduced presacrally, the air rises in the tela subserosa and follows along the fascial planes, giving rise to a delineation not only of the kidney but also of the suprarenal structures. This method is particularly useful for the delineation of suprarenal tumor masses. It is of special value when it is combined with intravenous or retrograde pyelograms and body section radiographs.

Seminal Vesiculography. Seminal vesiculography is a specialized procedure not frequently employed. It is utilized primarily to study the appearance of the seminal vesicles and the vas deferens, and occasionally in relation to prostatic carcinoma (Emmett et al.)* (Fig. 13–4).

Reactions to Contrast Media

General Comments. Reactions to the intravenous injection of contrast media are common. Mild reactions include warmth and flushing, nausea, vomiting, tingling, numbness, cough, and local pain in the arm, especially if the injection is carried out slowly. Serious reactions may include conjunctivitis, rhinitis, urticaria, facial edema, glottic edema, or even shocklike responses with dyspnea, convulsions, cyanosis, and shock. Other adverse effects include severe allergies, drug reactions, asthma, hay fever, sensitivity to iodine, previous reactions to excretory urography, and related conditions.

Although results are variable in relation to the prior administration of antihistamine drugs, it appears that the preliminary intravenous injection of antihistamines, 3 to 5 minutes prior to the injection of the contrast medium, may reduce the incidence or severity of a reaction. Fifty milligrams of Benadryl (diphenhydramine hydrochloride) or 20 milligrams of Chlor-Trimeton (chlorpropheniramine-maleate) are perhaps most widely used.

In treatment of reactions the following must be judiciously employed:

---

*References may be obtained in Meschan, I.: An Atlas of Anatomy Basic to Radiology. Philadelphia, W. B. Saunders Co., 1975, Chapter 16.

1. Immediate subcutaneous or intramuscular administration of 0.5 cc. of 1:1000 epinephrine; this may be repeated in 10 to 15 minutes. Blood pressure must be watched closely for hypotension and impending shock.

2. One hundred per cent oxygen may be administered immediately through a face mask. If there is inadequate airway, an anesthesiologist should be called to introduce an endotracheal tube. Artificial respiration then may be carried out as necessary.

3. If shock is profound, epinephrine may be administered slowly intravenously in a dose of 0.25 cc.

4. Benadryl (50 mg.) or hydrocortisone (100 mg.), or both, may be administered intravenously at once.

5. Asthma and pulmonary edema may be combatted with 0.5 grams of Aminophylline, given intravenously over a period of 5 to 20 minutes.

6. If the patient exhibits wheezing or hypotension, the drug of choice is epinephrine administered intravenously if possible, intramuscularly if not possible. Epinephrine 1:1000 is given in 0.5 to 1 cc. dose; if the dilution is 1:10,000, it is given in a 5 to 10 cc. dose. Oxygen may also be administered. Tracheal intubation may be used as a last resort, as may the intracardiac administration of epinephrine.

7. Convulsions should indicate the need to administer 100 per cent oxygen. Laryngospasm may be controlled with the intravenous injection of a barbiturate such as 2 to 3 cc. of 2.5 per cent solution of thiopental sodium. If the laryngeal edema cannot be controlled by tracheal intubation, an emergency tracheotomy may be performed.

RISK OF EXCRETORY UROGRAPHY IN MULTIPLE MYELOMA. It has been postulated that urinary contrast media may be a precipitating or existing factor which sets the stage for precipitation of hyaline casts in the kidney in patients with multiple myeloma. *It is thought that this may be obviated by alkalinization of the urine and adequate hydration.* A few reports of fatal anuria following excretory urography in patients with multiple myeloma have appeared.

THE ADRENAL GLANDS (SUPRARENALS)

Gross Anatomy. The adrenal glands are two small glands that lie upon the superior poles of each kidney, and are 3 to 5 cm. in height, 3 cm. in width, and 1 to 2 cm. in anteroposterior thickness. Each is composed of a thick cortex, a medulla of chromaffin tissue, and each lies within Gerota's capsule, which also surrounds the kidney.

The right adrenal is rather pyramidal in shape, having its anterior surface laterally in contact with the liver and with the inferior vena cava, its posterior surface with the diaphragm, and its base with the kidney below. Both of its sides are concave and its general appearance is that of a "cocked hat."

The left gland is more semilunar in shape. Anteriorly it is in contact with the stomach above, the pancreas below, and the diaphragm posteriorly; its base touches the left kidney below it. The left adrenal lies as much medial to the left kidney as above it, in contrast to the right adrenal, which caps the kidney. The amount of peritoneum covering the gland is variable. The right gland is more medial and lower in relation to the spine than the left.

The dimensions, weight, and area of the suprarenal gland as gathered from the literature are summarized in Table 12–5.

TABLE 12–5. Dimensions, Weight, and Area of the Suprarenal Gland

Reference	Length	Width	Thickness	Weight	Area Right	Left
Herbut	3–5 cm.	2–4 cm.	0.4–0.6 cm.	3.5–5 Gm.		
Soffer	4–6 cm.	2–3 cm.	0.2–0.8 cm.	3–5 Gm.		
Steinbach and Smith					2.0–7.8 (aver. 4.2) sq. cm.	2.0–8.7 (aver. 4.3) sq. cm.

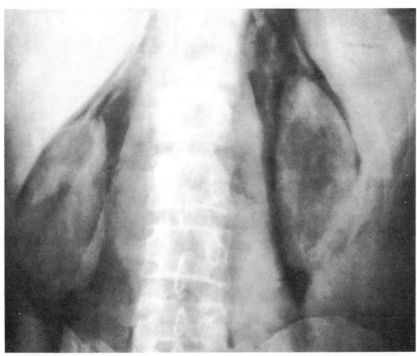

FIGURE 12–38 Normal retroperitoneal pneumogram. (From McLelland, R., Landes, R. R., and Ransom, C. L.: Radiol. Clin. North Am., *3*:115, 1965.)

With *retroperitoneal pneumography* the films recommended by Meyers* are: (1) both supine posterior obliques, (2) anteroposterior erect, (3) body section radiographic cuts at 1 cm. intervals between 6 and 12 cm. from the posterior, and (4) a 24-hour film if oxygen is used. If air or oxygen is used, a scout film centered over the suprarenals is obtained 2 hours after the injection and hourly thereafter until maximum visualization is obtained. Excretory urograms and nephrotomograms may be combined with this procedure at this time.

Adrenal Arteriography (Fig. 12–41). Although generally the three adrenal arteries already described represent the main blood supply of the adrenal gland, more than one adrenal branch arises directly from the aorta in approximately 30 per cent of cases. There are a number of other variations.† The *middle* adrenal artery traverses laterally to the posterior surface of the adrenal gland where it breaks up into a number of twigs (4 or 5) just barely visible on the radiograph. The *superior* adrenal arteries supply the upper pole of the adrenal gland and arise principally from the inferior phrenic arteries. These branch off the aorta just above the celiac axis usually. At times, however, the inferior phrenic arises below the celiac or even from the renal artery itself. The adrenal arteries are actually a number of twigs arising from the inferior phrenic and its posterior division. The inferior adrenal arteries arise from the renal arteries either directly or with the superior renal capsular branch. Other adrenal branches may arise from the gonadal arteries.

Adrenal Venography. Each adrenal gland drains by only one vein (Fig. 12–41).

There are no valves in adrenal veins. On the right side there are three main tributaries to the renal vein—inferolateral, ventromedial, and posterior. The junction of these three veins occurs near the top or the middle of the gland, thus forming the adrenal vein, usually about 3 mm. in diameter and rarely exceeding 10 mm. in length. The right adrenal vein usually drains into the inferior vena cava about 3 to 4 cm. above the right renal vein and near the T12 vertebra. This occurs in very close proximity to or in conjunction with the hepatic vein. On the left side there are four main venous trunks: inferolateral, ventral, medial, and posterior. The left adrenal vein is usually 20 to 40 mm. long, and it is joined by the left inferior phrenic vein about 15 to 20 mm. below the left adrenal gland. The left adrenal vein therefore empties into the left renal vein on its upper surface to the left of the aorta near the point at which the renal vein crosses the lateral border of the vertebral body.

---

*Meyers, M. A.: Diseases of the Adrenal Gland: Radiological Diagnosis. Springfield, Ill., Charles C Thomas, Publisher, 1963.

†Gagnon, R.: Middle suprarenal arteries in man: a statistical study of 200 human adrenal glands. Rev. Canad. Biol., *23*:461, 1964.

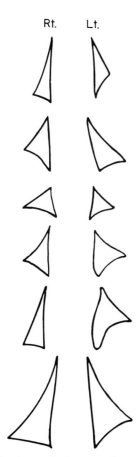

Rt.   Lt.

FIGURE 12–39 Tracings of six normal retroperitoneal pneumograms. (From McLelland, R., Landes, R. R., and Ransom, C. L.: Radiol. Clin. North Am., *3*:120, 1965.)

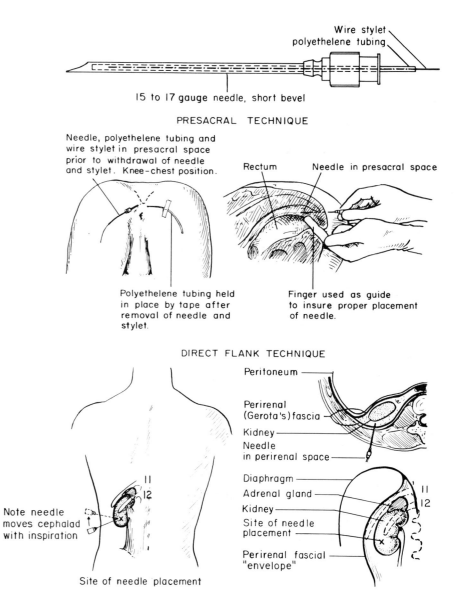

Wire stylet
polyethelene tubing

15 to 17 gauge needle, short bevel

PRESACRAL TECHNIQUE

Needle, polyethelene tubing and wire stylet in presacral space prior to withdrawal of needle and stylet. Knee-chest position.

Rectum   Needle in presacral space

Polyethelene tubing held in place by tape after removal of needle and stylet.

Finger used as guide to insure proper placement of needle.

DIRECT FLANK TECHNIQUE

Peritoneum

Perirenal (Gerota's) fascia

Kidney

Needle in perirenal space

Diaphragm
Adrenal gland
Kidney
Site of needle placement

Perirenal fascial "envelope"

Note needle moves cephalad with inspiration

Site of needle placement

FIGURE 12–40 Diagrams illustrating the direct flank and presacral techniques for retroperitoneal pneumography. (From McLelland, R., Landes, R. R., and Ransom, C. L.: Radiol. Clin. North Am., *3*:116, 1965.)

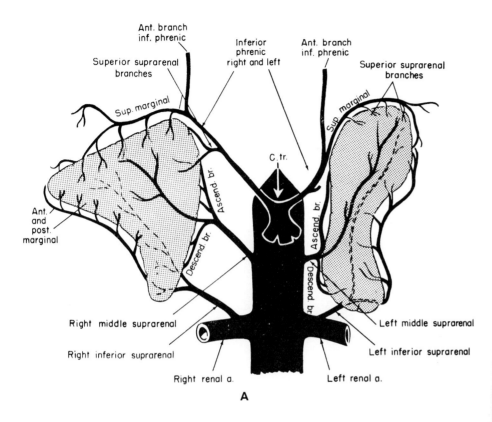

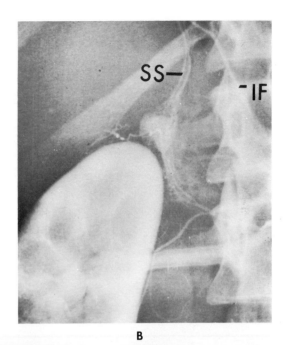

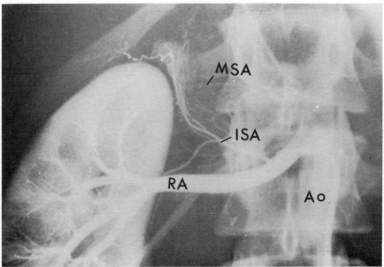

FIGURE 12–41 *A*. Schematic diagram of adrenal circulation. (After Gérard.) (From Kahn, P. C., and Nickrosz, L. V.: Am. J. Roentgenol., *101*:739–749, 1967.) *B* and *C*. Close-up views of adrenal arterial supply and capillary phase.

Figure 12–41 continued on following page

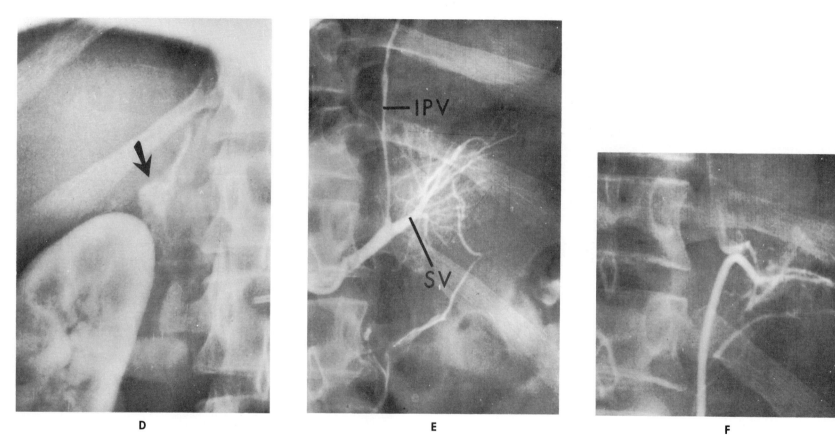

D   E   F

FIGURE 12–41 *Continued.*   *D.* Capillary phase. *E* and *F.* Close-up views of left (SV) suprarenal or adrenal vein.

13

THE GENITAL SYSTEM

THE MALE GENITAL SYSTEM

Related Gross Anatomy. Each *testis* (Fig. 13–1) is formed by numerous lobules each containing coiled tubules called seminiferous tubules. The spermatozoa are formed in these tubules. These lobules and tubules converge posteriorly toward the rete testis, which consists of a network of tubules which empty by coiled ducts into the head of the *epididymis*. Here the duct of the epididymis is formed and extends in very tortuous fashion to the tail of the epididymis where it becomes the *ductus deferens*. In the vicinity of the trigone of the urinary bladder it undergoes slight bulbous dilatation to form the *ampulla of the ductus deferens*. Near the lower margin of this ampulla, there is a diverticulumlike structure, the *seminal vesicle*. The continuation of the ampulla of the ductus deferens beyond the point of junction with

the seminal vesicle is called the *ejaculatory duct,* and this empties into the lower posterior aspect of the prostatic urethra, one opening on either side of the *prostatic utricle*. In its course, the ejaculatory duct traverses about two-thirds of the length of the prostate.

The *prostate gland* is a conical structure, its base directed craniad and in contact with the caudal surface of the urinary bladder, and its apex pointing caudad. Posteriorly it is separated from the rectum by fascia which is continued over the seminal vesicles and over the pelvis laterally.

The posterior surface is separated from the rectum by the *rectovesical septum*. The *urethra* enters the prostate near its anterior surface and descends almost vertically within it so that the greater part of the prostate is posterior to the urethra. Its midsagittal pattern and relationship to the bladder and urethra are shown in Figure 13–2. In

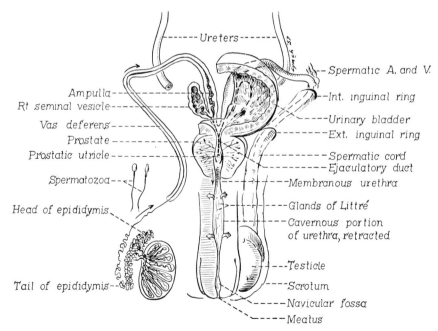

FIGURE 13–1 The male reproductive system. (Modified from Dickinson, R. L.: Atlas of Human Sex Anatomy. Baltimore, The Williams & Wilkins Co. 1949. © 1949 The Williams & Wilkins Co., Baltimore.)

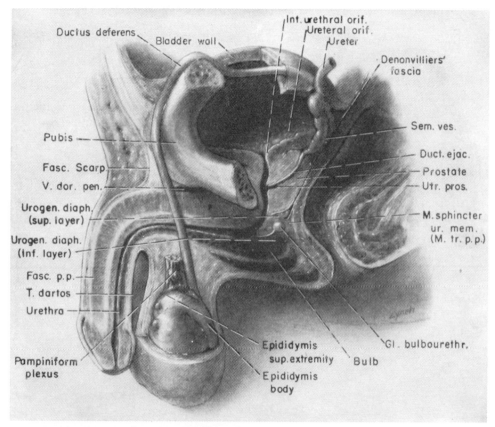

FIGURE 13–2 Midsagittal section of male pelvis. *Gl. bulbourethr.*, bulbourethral gland; *Fasc. p. p.*, deep perineal fascia; *T. dartos*, dartos tunic; *Duct. ejac.*, ejaculatory duct; *M. tr. p. p.*, m. sphincter urethrae membranaceae (m. transversus perinei profundus); *Fasc. Scarp.*, Scarpa's fascia; *Sem. ves.*, seminal vesicle; *Utr. pros.*, prostatic utricle; *V. dor. pen.*, v. dorsalis penis. (From Anson, B. J. (ed.): Morris' Human Anatomy, 12th ed. New York, McGraw-Hill Book Company, 1966. Copyright © 1966 by McGraw-Hill, Inc. Used by permission of McGraw-Hill Book Company.)

cross section the prostate gland has four lobes, the *lobes anterior and posterior* to the urethra, the *lateral lobes* on either side of the urethra, and the *middle lobe* lying between the posterior aspect of the urethra near its junction with the urinary bladder and the ejaculatory duct. The *anterior lobe* is small and nonglandular and lies in front of the urethra. The *lateral lobes* extend not only laterally but also anterior to the urethra. The *middle lobe* contains the subtrigonal and cervical glands (Albarran's glands). As shown previously, the prostatic urethra contains a longitudinal ridge on its dorsal wall called the *urethral crest,* depressions on the sides of the crest into which the prostatic ducts open called the *prostatic sinuses,* and a *seminal colliculus* that is the summit of the urethral crest on which the ejaculatory ducts open. This colliculus also contains a median blind-ending sac, the *prostatic utricle.*

The *seminal vesicles* are bilateral lobulated sacs consisting of irregular pouches. They lie against the fundus of the bladder ventrally, and their dorsal surfaces are separated from the rectum by rectovesical fascia. Superiorly they are closely related to the *vas deferens* and *ureters.* Inferiorly, the seminal vesicles join the vas deferens from either side on the posterior surface of the prostate (Figs. 13–2 and 13–3).

The course of the vas deferens and relationship to the pelvis and seminal vesicles are indicated in Figure 13–4.

The relationships of the *male urethra* with cross sections of the penis at different levels are shown in Figure 13–5. The urethra and its examination have been previously discussed with the urinary tract in Chapter 12.

The *bulbourethral glands* or *Cowper's glands* are two small glands that lie on each side of the membranous portion of the urethra (Fig. 13–5), embedded between the two fascial layers of the urogenital diaphragm. The duct from this gland traverses the substance of the *corpus spongiosum of the penis* and opens on the floor of the bulbar portion of the urethra. This gland can be clinically significant in that occasionally a cyst may occur or accessory glands may be demonstrated distal or proximal to the main ductal openings.

The most important lobes of the prostate clinically are the median lobe, enlargement of which leads to urinary tract obstruction with encroachment on the urethra; and the lateral lobes, hypertrophy of which causes urinary obstruction. It is the posterior lobe which is encountered by rectal digital examination.

Technique of Examination. There are only certain portions of the male genital system which can be examined radiographically by presently known methods. The examination is confined to a soft tissue study of the prostate, seminal vesicles, and scrotal contents, and the direct injection of opaque media into the lumen of the seminal vesicles, vas deferens, and ejaculatory duct via the vas deferens. (Computed tomography may yield additional information.)

Radiographic Appearances. On a plain radiograph the prostate may be visualized when enlarged as an impression directed upward at the base of the urinary bladder. Calculi may be seen within the prostate, but the outline of the gland cannot be delineated.

Using contrast material, one finds that the numerous racemose or diverticulumlike tubes of the seminal vesicles appear like an indefinite mass, and the ductus deferens may be seen as a tubular structure which conforms closely to the anatomic description just given (Fig. 13–4).

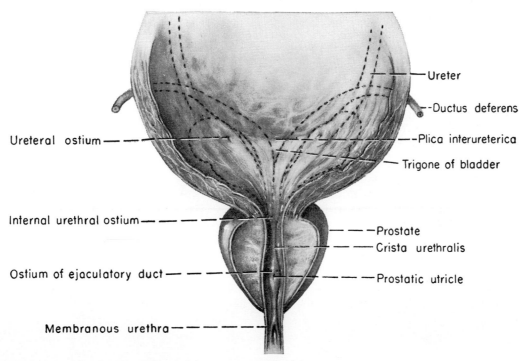

Ureter

Ductus deferens

Ureteral ostium

Plica interureterica

Trigone of bladder

Internal urethral ostium

Prostate

Crista urethralis

Ostium of ejaculatory duct

Prostatic utricle

Membranous urethra

FIGURE 13–3 Trigone of bladder and floor of prostatic urethra. (From Anson, B. J. (ed.): Morris' Human Anatomy. 12th ed. New York, McGraw-Hill Book Company, 1966. Copyright © 1966 by McGraw-Hill, Inc. Used by permission of McGraw-Hill Book Company.)

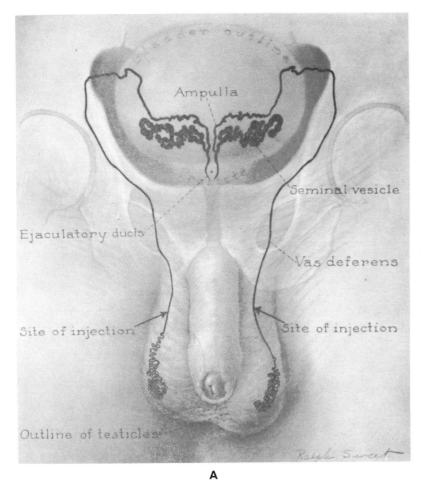
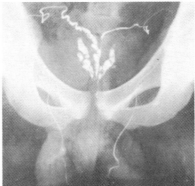
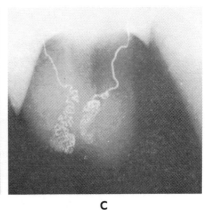

A

B

C

FIGURE 13-4 *A*. The male genital tract. The sites of exposure of the vas deferens are indicated, into which injections of the contrast media are made upward and frequently downward. *B*. Normal seminal vesiculogram. The distal segment of the right vas deferens is larger than that of the left. The right seminal vesicle is slightly better filled than the left. The injection of the left vas was made 24 hours before this film, and that of the right 4½ hours before this film. *C*. Same patient as above with filling of the distal portions of the epididymides achieved at the same time as *B*. Greater filling has been obtained on the right than on the left. (From Tucker, A. S., Yanagihara, H., and Pryde, A. W.: Am. J. Roentgenol., *71*:490–500, 1954.)

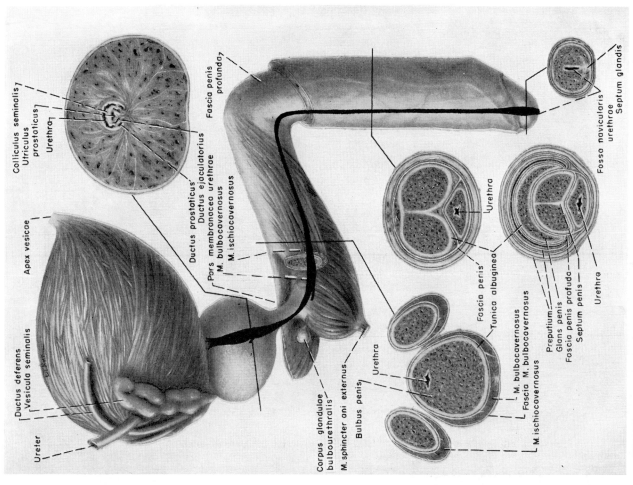

FIGURE 13–5 Relations of the male urethra with cross sections of the penis at different levels. Semidiagrammatic. (From Anson, B. J. (ed.): Morris' Human Anatomy, 12th ed. New York, McGraw-Hill Book Company, 1966. Copyright © 1966 by McGraw-Hill, Inc. Used by permission of McGraw-Hill Book Company.)

THE FEMALE REPRODUCTIVE SYSTEM

The soft tissue structures of this system will be described first and then a brief account will be given of the bony pelvis and its anatomic variations.

Soft Tissues. The organs of the female genital system consist of two *ovaries*, two *oviducts*, the *uterus*, the *vagina*, and the *external genitalia*. The suspensory and supplementary structures are the *broad ligaments* (and *mesosalpinx*) on either side, the *round ligament*, the *mesovarium*, and the *mesometrium* (Fig. 13–6).

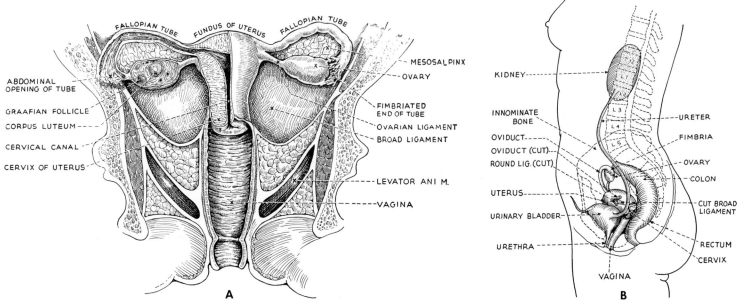

FIGURE 13–6 *A*. Gross anatomy of female reproductive system; frontal view. *B*. Lateral view.

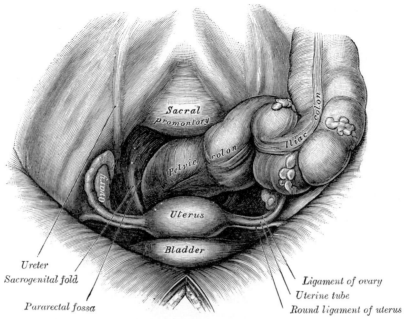

FIGURE 13–7 Female pelvis and its contents, seen from above and in front. (From Goss, C. M. (ed.): Gray's Anatomy of the Human Body, 29th ed. Philadelphia, Lea & Febiger, 1973.)

Pelvic Architecture of the Female

Bony Pelvis. In addition to the normal anatomic landmarks of the pelvis described previously, certain areas should receive the attention of the radiologist as having an influence on the course of labor. Differences characteristic of male and female types should be borne in mind. These areas are as follows:

1. THE SUBPUBIC ARCH (Fig. 13–9). Note should be made of the bones of the pubic rami, whether they are delicate, average, or heavy; whether the pubic angle is wide and curved (female) or narrow and straight (male), and whether the side walls of the forepelvis are divergent, straight, or convergent. The configuration of the pelvic arch is a guide to the capacity of the true pelvis.

2. THE ISCHIAL SPINES. These are classified as sharp, average, or anthropoid. Sharp spines are definitely a male characteristic and when present, direct the attention to the necessity for a more detailed examination of the pelvis, as they may be associated with converging side walls of the forepelvis. The anthropoid spines are blunt and shallow.

3. THE SACROSCIATIC NOTCH AND SACRUM. The capacity of the posterior pelvic inlet is related to the width of the sacrosciatic notch and the configuration of its apex. The male pelvis shows a long narrow notch with a high rounded apex and the female a wide notch with a blunt apex.

The inclination of the sacrum directly affects the capacity of the birth canal since a forward tilt will offer a barrier to normal delivery.

If the forepelvis is wide and divergent, compensation occurs but if convergent a funnel pelvis will result. The female sacrum is wide and short compared with that of the male.

The curvature of the sacrum on the lateral projection is also important. Normally the sacrum is concave anteriorly. When this curvature is absent owing to any developmental aberration, the midpelvis is diminished and the progress of labor is impeded. The absence of this curvature will be readily apparent from measurements to be described later.

4. THE PELVIC INLET. The pelvic inlet with its variations can be classified into four major types (Fig. 13–8):

The inlet of the anthropoid pelvis is relatively long in anteroposterior measurements and narrow in transverse diameter.

The gynecoid pelvis is the average type as seen in the human female. The inlet is round or slightly oval, the pubic angle is wide, and the sacrosciatic notch is also wide. The cavity of the pelvis is ample in all directions.

The android pelvis refers to a female pelvis which has marked masculine characteristics. These include what is described as a blunt heart-shaped or wedge-shaped inlet with narrow forepelvis, and the widest diameter is close to the sacral promontory. A narrow masculine type of sciatic notch is present and the sacrum is set forward in the pelvis. The pubic arch is usually narrow.

The platypelloid or flat pelvis is characterized by an inlet with a transversely oval shape. The anteroposterior diameter is short and the greatest transverse diameter is wide—this diameter occurring well in front of the sacrum. The angle of the forepelvis is wide also, but the sacrosciatic notch and subpubic angle vary in size.

It should be stated that gradations between all types are seen and individual variations should be described as they appear on the radiograph.

The reader is referred to the work of Caldwell and Moloy on this subject.*

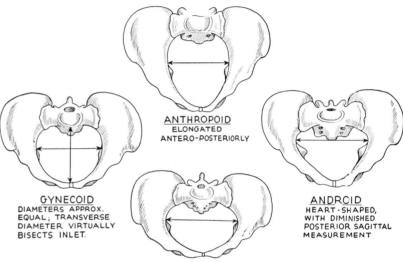

DIFFERENT PELVIC TYPES
(PELVIC INLET VIEW)

ANTHROPOID
ELONGATED
ANTERO-POSTERIORLY

GYNECOID
DIAMETERS APPROX.
EQUAL; TRANSVERSE
DIAMETER VIRTUALLY
BISECTS INLET.

ANDROID
HEART-SHAPED,
WITH DIMINISHED
POSTERIOR SAGITTAL
MEASUREMENT

PLATYPELLOID (FLAT)
ELONGATED TRANSVERSELY

FIGURE 13–8 Variations in size and shape of the pelvic inlet. (From Golden, R.: Diagnostic Roentgenology, Vol. 2. Baltimore, The Williams & Wilkins Co., 1963–1969. © 1969 The Williams & Wilkins Co., Baltimore.)

---

*Caldwell, W. E., and Moloy, H. C.: Anatomical variations in the female pelvis and their effect in labor with a suggested classification. Am. J. Obstet. Gynecol., *26*:479–503, 1933.

A

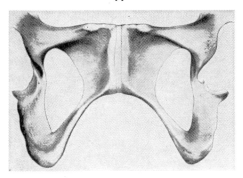

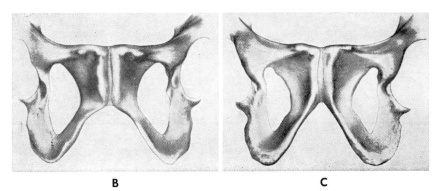

B   **C**

FIGURE 13–9 *A.* Well-curved, wide-angled, and delicate. *B.* Average moderate angle, average curvature. *C.* Masculine-type narrow angle, heavy boned.

Methods of Study of the Female Genital System

In the entire description below of the applications and usefulness of radiographic techniques in investigation of obstetrical and gynecologic problems, the student must bear in mind those aspects of radiologic protection which pertain here (see Chapter 3). The information to be gained must justify the exposure of the patient (and the fetus, if one is present). *In any case, radiation exposure of the patient and the fetus in*

the first trimester of pregnancy is to be avoided unless the problem at hand is a critical one.

Direct Radiography and Its Applications.   Anteroposterior, lateral, and "inlet" views of the pelvis (Fig. 13–12) are obtained and a considerable amount of information is available from these views (Fig. 13–15).

The purposes of roentgen study of the female patient in obstetrics and gynecology may be outlined as follows:

1. *The study of the female pelvis and abdomen* (apart from pregnancy), including (a) the determination of an extrauterine fetus; (b) the study of pelvic soft tissues outside the uterus, particularly to determine if interference to parturition might result; (c) pelvic mensuraion and description as a guide to determination of possible cephalopelvic disproportion; and (d) all those anatomic and pathologic possibilities in the abdomen and pelvis that exist regardless of the sex of the patient.

2. *Special gynecologic study of the nonpregnant female* for: (a) hysterosalpingography, or the detailed study of the uterine cavity and oviducts and determination of the patency of the latter; (b) pelvic pneumography—the study of the pelvic peritoneal space by introduction of gas into the space; (c) a combination of these; and (d) pelvic angiography.

3. *A study of the pregnant mother in respect to the fetus* for the purpose of: (a) determining the presence of a fetal skeleton *in utero* or intra-abdominally; (b) determining the presence of multiple fetuses; (c) determining fetal normalcy, age, and development; (d) determining fetal viability or death; or (e) describing the accurate presentation of the fetus. (Where ultrasonic examinations are adequate and available for this purpose, they are to be preferred. A discussion of this application is outside the scope of this text.)

4. *A study of the pregnant uterus apart from the fetus,* including: (a) the placenta—its size, position, and density; (b) the amniotic space (the amniotic space may be entered to withdraw fluid for special study, or may serve as a guide to fetal transfusion); or (c) general uterine density and normalcy of appearance.

5. *Genitography of the abnormal infant or child* (intersex problems).

Study of the Female Pelvis and Abdomen

Introductory Comments. The study of the pregnant woman for intra-abdominal abnormalities outside the uterus lies outside the scope of this text. The features of the extrauterine fetus, for example, tubal pregnancy, and the implantation of a placenta anywhere in the abdominal cavity are subjects which have been discussed in our companion text, *Analysis of Roentgen Signs,* and the student is referred for brief discussion to this reference. This applies to a consideration of the ruptured uterus also.

Study of Pelvic Soft Tissue Structures Outside the Uterus (especially to determine if interference to parturition may result). This, too, involves abnormalities in the retroperitoneal space such as tumors of the sacrum, inflammatory swellings, or urinary tract abnormalities. Similarly, abnormalities of the intestine may be considered here. These are outside the scope of this text and the student is referred to *Analysis of Roentgen Signs* for further discussion.

Cephalopelvic Disproportion and Pelvic Measurement. Many methods of measurement of the maternal pelvis and the fetal head have been proposed. These include such adjuncts as special rulers or grids which are projected over the pelvis in its midsection, special tables and graphs which provide for determination of the extent of magnification, special slide rules which facilitate determination of magnification, nomograms which help resolve the extent of magnification if the basic factors are known, and teleroentgenograms which minimize the extent of magnification to the point where the degree of accuracy possible is related largely to the degree of accuracy of the actual measurement.

In all these proposed methods the *basic concepts and objectives are to measure the important diameters of the pelvis and head,* eliminating as much as possible the elements of magnification and distortion; *to describe the pelvic architecture* as accurately as possible from the standpoint of parturition; and *to describe any other factors* in relation to the pelvis, fetus, or placenta such as have been previously indicated in this section.

It is important for the student to adopt that method of correction for magnification and distortion that is most feasible in his particular installation and to learn that method thoroughly rather than to be attracted to one proposal or another by various authors. If it is possible to obtain at least 72 inch target-to-film distance films (teleroentgenograms), one may assay the size of the pelvis and fetal head without difficulty, since a maximum magnification on the order of 10 per cent is thereby feasible. For those measurements such as the interischial spinous diameter, to be obtained in the middle of the pelvis, the magnification is on the order of only 5 per cent. Moreover, when nonengagement of the fetal head occurs in a pendulous abdomen, the distance between head and inlet is not as significant in the teleroentgenogram as in other proposed techniques. Fetal head and pelvic measurements are more easily obtained with breech presentations when teleroentgenograms are employed, since distortion is minimal.

Templeton has utilized high kilovoltage pelvimetry with a teleroentgenographic technique and a target-to-film distance of 10 feet; by using 150 Kv. and a 1 mm. focal spot, he was able to obtain antero posterior and lateral roentgenograms with the patient standing against a grid cassette (100 lines per inch). He employed an angulation of 20 degrees toward the feet for the anteroposterior roentgenogram. Comparison of radiation exposure to the fetus and maternal pelvis was made using a pelvic phantom. Whereas the conventional kilovoltage technique averaged a total of 1020 milliroentgens to the midpelvis, this high kilovoltage technique averaged a total of 60 milliroentgens. Also, the teleroentgenograms made magnification correction unnecessary. All obstetric measurements were made readily on the two upright roentgenograms.

If methods other than the teleroentgenographic technique are employed, it is important to obtain both the lateral and anteroposterior views without moving the patient. This is important because the lateral view is employed to correct for magnification on the anteroposterior projection, and similarly the anteroposterior projection is employed to obtain certain measurements which are applied to the lateral view. If there is a difference in the position of the fetal head, for example, in these two views, the correction factors are much more complex and virtually nullified.

For this reason erect films are preferred by some. When the patient is standing, the position of the fetus with respect to the maternal pelvis is not apt to change when the patient moves from the anteroposterior to the lateral position. The erect standing film may also be preferred in order to obtain maximum gravitational effect of the fetus above the maternal pelvis.

Evaluation of Pelvicephalography in the Light of Radiation Hazard. Considerable confusion has resulted with respect to the indications and contraindications for the radiologic study of the female pelvis and fetal skull in pregnancy. While radiation is not the only genetic hazard in our environment which can result in increased mutations, every effort should be made to reduce this particular hazard as much as possible. Although it has not been absolutely proved in mammals, it is generally accepted that genetic aberrations from exposure to radiation can occur at virtually any dose level.

The reader is referred to Chapter 3 for a more detailed consideration of the many aspects of radiation protection. From these discussions, however, we may derive the following conclusions:

1. Roentgen pelvic encephalometry should not be considered a routine procedure. It must be employed only after thorough obstetrical examination and evaluation, and the information to be obtained must be of critical value. Nevertheless, this procedure must be undertaken with the full understanding that the radiologist cannot and should not by himself attempt to predict the outcome of delivery. The data obtained should permit a thorough study of the maternal pelvis in all its aspects and should provide some idea of the relative size, shape, and position of the fetal skull in relation to the maternal pelvis.

2. All precautions should be employed to minimize radiation exposure. These must include high kilovoltage techniques, fast films, fast screens, collimation, additional filtration, increased target-to-film distance, and superior darkroom processing so that repeated exposures are unnecessary.

3. The optimal time for roentgen pelvic encephalometry is during the last 2 weeks of pregnancy. Under these circumstances, with a cephalic presentation the fetal gonads may actually lie outside the primary beam of radiation if one concentrates on the maternal pelvis.

4. Although information regarding the fetus, including fetal maturity, age, and development, may be obtained, fetal weight predictions have proved inaccurate and unsatisfactory since no relationship has been established between fetal skull measurements and body weight.

Pelvic and Fetal Measurements in Use. Regardless of the method employed for correction for magnification and distortion, the measurements that are most valuable are indicated in Figure 13–10. These are measurement of the pelvic inlet in both the anteroposterior and transverse diameters, measurement of the midpelvis in its anteroposterior diameter, the interischial spinous diameter, the posterior sagittal measurement of the midpelvis, the intertuberous diameter as a measurement of the pelvic outlet, and the two largest perpendicular diameters of the fetal head in both the anteroposterior and lateral projections (it is well to add approximately 4 mm. to the average diameter in consideration of the scalp soft tissues).*†

We have elected to describe in great detail one technique with which we have considerable experience, rather than to give a brief, cursory description of the many techniques which are available for the purposes of pelvicephalometry. This technique has been modified by the author for teleroentgenography, in which erect films are not as essential as they would be for shorter film-to-target distances.

---

*Ball, R. P., and Golden, R.: Roentgenographic obstetrical pelvicephalometry in the erect posture. Am. J. Roentgenol., *49*:731–741, 1943.

†Schwarz, G. S.: A simplified method of correcting roentgenographic measurements of the maternal pelvis and fetal skull. Am. J. Roentgenol., *71*:115–120, 1954.

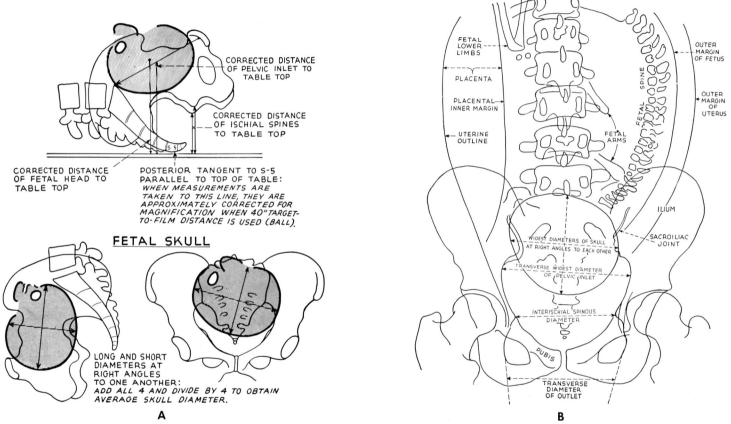

FIGURE 13–10 *A.* Diagrams illustrating the various measurements of the fetal head which are obtained and compared with the pelvic measurements. *B.* Anteroposterior (position same as KUB film) with measurements of the fetal head and pelvis indicated.

Figure continued on page 553

Having obtained the various measurements, one may utilize the following procedure (modification of Ball method; Schwarz's classification):

All four diameters of the fetal head are averaged together, and an average fetal head diameter is obtained. From this average fetal head diameter, an average fetal head volume (computed from the formula $4/3 \, \pi \, r^3$, where r is the average radius of the fetal head). Figure 13–14 may be used for these purposes.

The greatest transverse and anteroposterior diameters of the pelvic inlet are averaged together; utilizing this as a diameter, the volume of a sphere is obtained.

The anteroposterior diameter of the midpelvis and the interischial spinous diameter are averaged together and again the volume of a sphere is obtained, using this average diameter. Another method of finding midpelvis sphere volume is to double the posterior sagittal midpelvic index and to average this with interischial spinous diameter. This becomes the average diameter of the midpelvis, and the volume of the associated sphere is thereby determined.

Thus, the volume of the fetal head, the volume of a sphere with an average diameter equivalent to the average diameter of the pelvic inlet, and the volume of a sphere having as its diameter the average diameter of the midpelvis have been computed. These three spheres are thereafter compared in volume. If the midpelvic and inlet volumes each exceed the volume of the fetal head, no further computation is necessary. This group would be considered as "no disproportion demonstrated," and the incidence of cesarean section, regardless of reason, would be about 4 per cent. Incidence for cephalopelvic disproportion in this group would prove to be about 1 per cent, based upon 350 patients (Schwarz).*

A "borderline disproportion" group may be differentiated, in which the fetal head volume exceeds the volume capacity of the inlet by 70 cc. or less, or the volume capacity of the bispinous diameter by 50 to 220 cc. (In the latter instance, anything less than 50 cc. would fall into the "no disproportion" category.) Incidence of cesarean section in this group would prove to be about 33 per cent.

The "high disproportion" group consists of those patients with fetal head volumes exceeding the volume capacity of the inlet by more than 70 cc., or the bispinous diameter volume capacity by more than 220 cc. The incidence of cesarean section in this group would prove

to be about 80 per cent for any reason, and the incidence of "difficult delivery" 87 per cent. "Difficult" is defined as applying to deliveries requiring cesarean section, high or midforceps, or to infant death resulting from proved brain injury (Schwarz).*

In all of these computations it is important to remember this basic principle: *Under no circumstances do any of these measurements indicate that spontaneous delivery will or will not occur.* These measurements are for purposes of comparison only. It is impossible by these measurements to predict the intensity of labor contractions, uterine atonia, and a host of other factors in the individual case which have not been reduced to mathematical terms.

---

*Additional references may be obtained in Meschan, I.: An Atlas of Anatomy Basic to Radiology. Philadelphia, W. B. Saunders Co., 1975, Chapter 17.

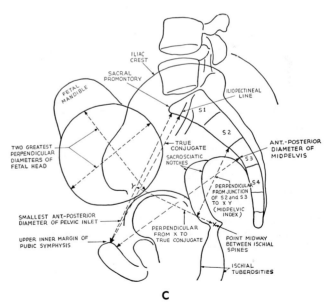

C

FIGURE 13–10 *C.* Tracing of radiographs routinely used in pelvicephalometry (lateral view).

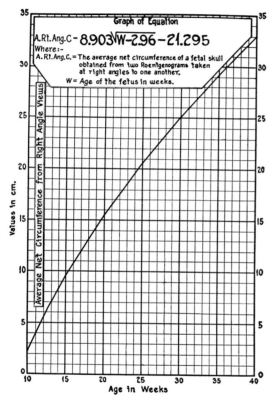

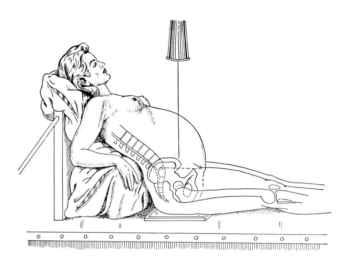

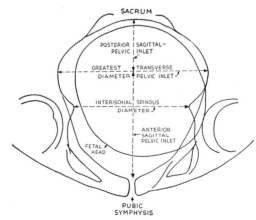

FIGURE 13-11 Graph for calculating fetal age from fetal head circumference. The fetal head circumference is obtained by measuring the average fetal diameter in both the anteroposterior and lateral views, averaging all four values, corrected for magnification. The fetal head circumference may be obtained by direct reference to the nomogram in Figure 13–14 or by multiplying the average diameter by 3.14.

FIGURE 13-12 Tracing of radiograph routinely employed in pelvicephalometry. Special view of pelvic inlet, showing positioning of patient (note the pelvic inlet is parallel to the table top) and tracing of radiograph so obtained.

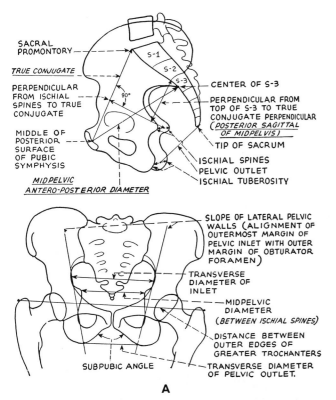

A

FIGURE 13–13 *A*. Diagrams illustrating the various measurements obtained from routine anteroposterior and lateral teleroentgenograms of the pelvis for pelvic measurement. *B*. Format of reporting pelvic measurements. (All measurements are recorded after correction for magnification.)

Format for Reporting Cephalopelvic Measurements

Inlet		Average Normal (cm.)	Volume
(1) A-P		10.5–11.5	
(2) Transverse		11.5–13.5	
Average of A-P and Transverse			*
Midpelvis			*Volumes*
(1) A-P		11.0–12.0	
(2) Post. Sag. Index		Greater than 5.0	
(3) 2 x P.S.I.		Greater than 10.0	
(4) Interischial spinous		10.0–11.0	
Average (1) + (4)			*
Average (3) + (4)			*
Outlet			
Intertub.		9.5–10.5	
Fetal Head		*Average Normal*	*Volumes*
A-P view (a) Long			
(b) + to (a)			
Lat. view (c) Long			
(b) + to (c)			
Ave. a, b, c, d.		10.0–11.0	
Relation of Fetal Head Volume to:		*Head Greater by:*	*Pelvis Greater by:*
	Pelvic inlet	cc.	cc.
	Midpelvis	cc.	cc.

B

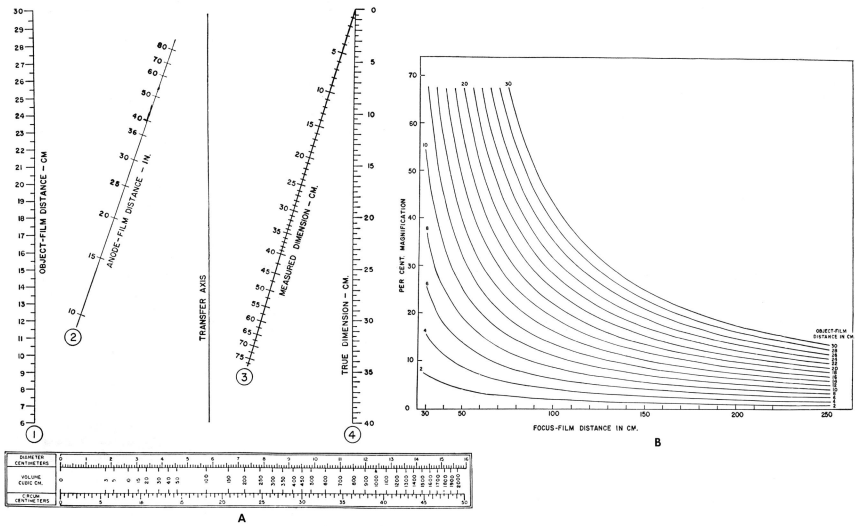

FIGURE 13–14 *A*. Nomograms for correction of magnification and for conversion of diameters to volumes. With a straight edge, a line is drawn from the object-film distance *(1)* of a certain dimension through the anode-film distance *(2)* used when the film was taken to the transfer axis. From this point on the transfer axis, a line is drawn through the dimension as measured on the film *(3)* which intersects *(4)* at the true, corrected dimension. With the table at the bottom of the nomogram a circumference or a diameter measurement in centimeters can be transposed directly to volume of a similar sphere in terms of cubic centimeters. (After Halmquest, from Golden, R.: Diagnostic Roentgenology. Baltimore, The Williams & Wilkins Co., 1963–1969.) *B*. Graph demonstrating the per cent magnification readily obtained when one knows the focus-film distance in centimeters and the object-film distance in centimeters. (Courtesy T. H. Oddie, D.Sc.)

Figure continued on opposite page

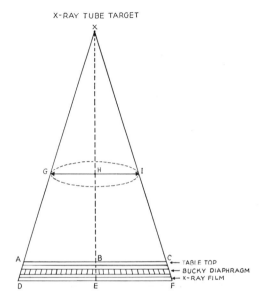

X-RAY TUBE TARGET

XE = TARGET-TO-FILM, DISTANCE (KNOWN)
BE = TABLE TOP-TO-FILM, DISTANCE (KNOWN)
GH = 1/2 THE DIMENSION TO BE MEASURED
DE = THE PROJECTION OF GH ON THE FILM
AND HENCE THE MEASUREMENT OBTAIN-
ED FROM THE FILM (KNOWN)
HB = THE DISTANCE OF DIMENSION GH FROM
THE TABLE TOP (KNOWN FROM FILM IN
OPPOSITE VIEW AFTER CORRECTED FOR
MAGNIFICATION)

C

FIGURE 13-14 *Continued.* *C.* Triangulation method of determining radiographic magnification (see text).

Study of Pelvic Architecture (Fig. 13-15)

PELVIC INLET. In addition to the anteroposterior and lateral projections of the abdomen and pelvis, it may be routine in this radiographic study to obtain a special view of the pelvic inlet as illustrated in Figure 13-12. With this special view, the pelvic inlet can be described as falling into one or another of at least four major pelvic types. There are, of course, many subtypes in these groups but at least these four major types must be understood (Fig. 13-8). Delivery of the fetus is most readily accomplished with the gynecoid pelvis; difficulty is encountered with increasing frequency in the android, platypelloid, and anthropoid types.

If the posterior sagittal portion of the pelvic inlet is diminished, an occiput posterior presentation is favored.

THE SACRUM. Following analysis of the pelvic inlet, the prominence of the sacral promontory and the curvature of the sacrum are studied for architecture (Figs. 13-13 and 13-15). The capacity of the posterior pelvic inlet is related to the width of the sacrosciatic notch and the configuration of its apex. Also the inclination of the sacrum directly affects the capacity of the birth canal, since a forward tilt offers a barrier to normal delivery. The female sacrum is wide and short compared with that of the male. Normally, also, the sacrum is concave anteriorly; when this curvature is absent because of any developmental aberration, the midpelvis is diminished and the progress of labor is impeded.

SIZE OF THE SACROSCIATIC NOTCH. The capacity of the posterior pelvic inlet is related to the width of the sacrosciatic notch and configuration of its apex. The male pelvis shows a long narrow notch with a high rounded apex and the female a wide notch with a blunt apex.

PROMINENCE OF THE COCCYX A prominent coccyx interferes with the passage of the fetus through the birth canal.

PROMINENCE OF THE ISCHIAL SPINES. Ischial spines are classified as sharp, average, or anthropoid. Sharp spines are definitely a male characteristic and may be associated with convergent side walls of the pelvis. Gynecoid spines are blunt and shallow.

SLOPE OF PELVIC WALLS. The slope of the pelvic wall is readily obtained by drawing a tangent along the outer aspect of the obturator foramen connecting with the outermost margin of the transverse diameter of the pelvic inlet. For maximum facility of delivery, the lines so drawn should be parallel. Convergent lines indicate a diminution in either midpelvis or pelvic outlet which may cause some difficulty in delivery.

SUBPUBIC ANGLE. The pubic rami may be delicate, average, or heavy, and the pubic angle may be wide or curved as in the female or narrow and straight as in the male. The capacity of the pelvic outlet to a great extent is regulated by the subpubic angle and the pubic rami.

DIASTASIS OF THE PUBIC SYMPHYSIS. In experimental animals there is a considerable diastasis of the pubic symphysis and resorption of bone along both sides of the pubic symphysis near term. This is an endocrine phenomenon. In the human such resorption of bone or actual diastasis does not ordinarily occur, but a relaxation of the ligaments across the pubic symphysis does occur, and occasionally diastasis persists following parturition. Such diastasis may facilitate delivery.

EXTENT OF ACETABULAR BULGE. Occasionally in association with nutritional deficiencies or hereditary disorders of the bony pelvis, there is a bulging inward of the acetabulum, producing the so-called Otto pelvis or arthrokatadysis. Such abnormality may impede the passage of the fetus through the midpelvis.

METHOD OF REPORTING. In reporting, one section is devoted entirely to the various measurements; these are given in table form (Fig. 13–13 B). The theoretical fetal skull diameter, perimeter, and volume are also indicated relative to the dimensions of the pelvic inlet and midpelvis.

The second portion of the report should refer to pelvic architecture and details concerning fetus, placenta, and amniotic sac.

METHOD FOR CORRECTION OF MAGNIFICATION. The degree of magnification will vary in accordance with the distance between the x-ray tube target and the film, and the distance between the diameter (or distance) to be measured and the film. If the dimension in question is parallel with the film surface, distortion is eliminated. If the target-to-film distance is known and also the object-to-film distance, it is pos-sible to calculate accurately the true measurement of the part. This may be accomplished by graphs or nomograms (Fig. 13–14) (Ball, Snow),* stereoscopic films (Caldwell and Moloy),* metal notched rules placed next to the part being radiographed (Colcher-Sussman),* or perforated metal plates superimposed on the radiograph (Thoms).*

In those methods that employ calculation, graphs, or nomograms to determine the degree of magnification, the basic procedure is as follows:

1. The desired dimension is measured on the one radiograph, whether it be the anteroposterior or lateral view.

2. The distance that this dimension is placed from the film is determined from the other radiograph. Thus, to determine this object-to-film distance for dimensions measured on the anteroposterior view, the lateral radiograph is employed and vice versa.

3. There will, however, be an error of magnification on this second radiograph also, which must be corrected before it can be applied as the object-to-table-top distance.

4. In order to obtain object-to-film distance, the object-to-table-top distance is first calculated, and to this figure is added the known table-top-to-film distance (usually 5 cm.).

5. Only those dimensions in the central ray can be measured, unless the teleroentgenographic method is employed where beam divergence is negligible.

6. The following triangulation laws are applied (Fig. 13–14 C):

$$\frac{GH \text{ (unknown)}}{DE \text{ (known)}} \quad \frac{XH}{XE} = \frac{XE - (HB + BE) \text{ (known)}}{XE \text{ (known)}}$$

From this equation, it is obvious that all factors are known except GH and hence, simple algebraic solution is possible. Snow's special calculator or Ball's nomograms allow this algebraic solution to be obtained directly.

---

*Additional references may be obtained in Meschan, I.: An Atlas of Anatomy Basic to Radiology. Philadelphia, W. B. Saunders Co., 1975, Chapter 17.

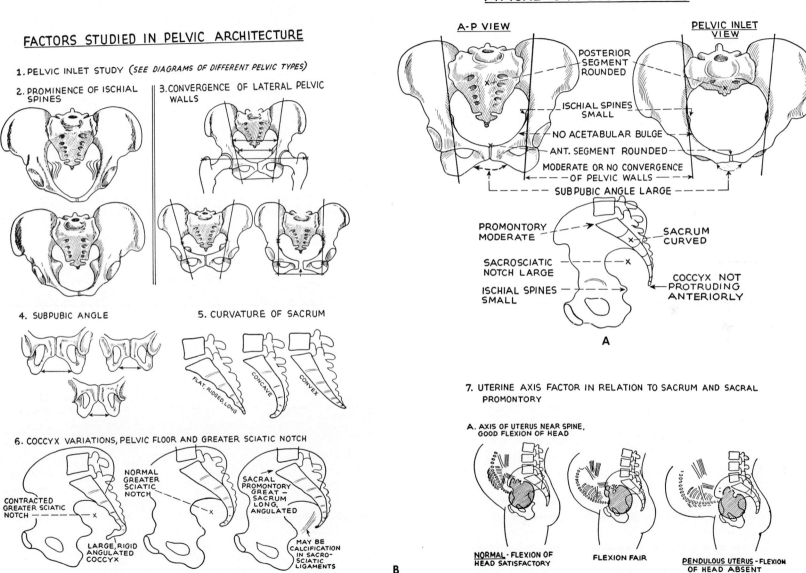

FACTORS STUDIED IN PELVIC ARCHITECTURE

1. PELVIC INLET STUDY *(SEE DIAGRAMS OF DIFFERENT PELVIC TYPES)*

2. PROMINENCE OF ISCHIAL SPINES

3. CONVERGENCE OF LATERAL PELVIC WALLS

4. SUBPUBIC ANGLE

5. CURVATURE OF SACRUM

FLAT, RIDGED LONG   CONCAVE   CONVEX

6. COCCYX VARIATIONS, PELVIC FLOOR AND GREATER SCIATIC NOTCH

CONTRACTED GREATER SCIATIC NOTCH —— x

NORMAL GREATER SCIATIC NOTCH

SACRAL PROMONTORY GREAT - SACRUM LONG, ANGULATED

LARGE, RIGID ANGULATED COCCYX

MAY BE CALCIFICATION IN SACRO-SCIATIC LIGAMENTS

B

TYPICAL GYNECOID PELVIS

A-P VIEW

PELVIC INLET VIEW

POSTERIOR SEGMENT ROUNDED

ISCHIAL SPINES SMALL

NO ACETABULAR BULGE

ANT. SEGMENT ROUNDED

MODERATE OR NO CONVERGENCE OF PELVIC WALLS

SUBPUBIC ANGLE LARGE

PROMONTORY MODERATE

SACRUM CURVED

SACROSCIATIC NOTCH LARGE —— x

ISCHIAL SPINES SMALL

COCCYX NOT PROTRUDING ANTERIORLY

A

7. UTERINE AXIS FACTOR IN RELATION TO SACRUM AND SACRAL PROMONTORY

A. AXIS OF UTERUS NEAR SPINE, GOOD FLEXION OF HEAD

NORMAL - FLEXION OF HEAD SATISFACTORY

FLEXION FAIR

PENDULOUS UTERUS - FLEXION OF HEAD ABSENT

FIGURE 13–15 *A* and *B*. Factors studied in pelvic architecture; diagrammatic description of a typical gynecoid pelvis.

Study of the Nonpregnant Female—
Gynecologic Radiology

X-ray Appearance of Intrauterine Contraceptive Devices.* Most intrauterine contraceptive devices are made of radiopaque materials. Commonly employed devices are illustrated in Figure 13–16. In rare cases pregnancy has occurred with the device *in situ*. Few obstetric difficulties caused by the intrauterine devices have been reported.

X-ray evidence of the intrauterine contraceptive device in the pelvic area is no definite proof that it is within the uterine cavity. In the nonpregnant woman, the definite answer may be supplied by a hysterogram. In pregnancy, the presence or absence of the device should not be determined until the early part of the third trimester to avoid fetal exposure to radiation.

Perforation of the uterus occurs rarely. According to Shimkin et al.,† uterine perforation may occur in about 1 out of 2500 insertions of a coil or loop and in 1 out of 150 insertions of a bow. Perforation occurs especially at the time of insertion or occasionally at attempted blind removal. It may be partial or complete. Perforation at insertion is often asymptomatic and unrecognized.

Hysterosalpingography. The main uses of this procedure are: (1) study of sterility problems; (2) investigation of uterine bleeding; (3) re-establishment of tubal patency; (4) visualization of abnormalities of the uterine cavity or oviducts; and (5) visualization of sinus tracts communicating with the female genital tract.

Technique of examination. As with all contrast procedures, it is always advisable to obtain a preliminary scout film prior to the introduction of the contrast medium (Fig. 13–17). Areas of calcification and soft tissue masses can thereby be delineated prior to the introduction of the special medium. The lithotomy position over an x-ray Bucky table, preferably equipped with image amplification and closed circuit television fluoroscopy, is employed.

A cannula, preferably radiolucent, is inserted into the uterine cervical canal after visualization of the cervix through an appropriate

---

*Lehfeldt, H.: X-ray appearance of intrauterine contraceptive devices. Fertil. Steril., *16*:502–507, 1965.

†Shimkin, P. M., et al.: Radiologic aspects of perforated intrauterine contraceptive devices. Radiology, *92*:353–358, 1969.

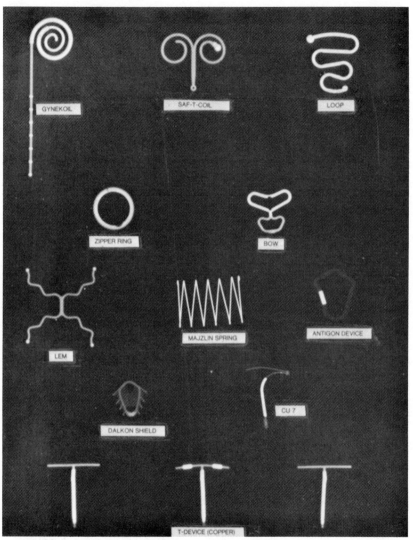

FIGURE 13–16 Radiographic appearances of the ten most frequently encountered intrauterine contraceptive devices. Minor variations in size and form exist, including substitution of thread for beaded tail on Gynekoil. (From Seymour, E. Q., and Williamson, H. O.: A review of commonly used intrauterine contraceptive devices. Radiology, *115*:359–360, 1975.)

speculum. It is best that the cannula be filled with contrast material so that all air bubbles are extracted prior to the insertion into the uterine cervical canal. The introduction of air bubbles may cause confusion in interpretation.

Under fluoroscopic control, while viewing the injection on a television monitor, a fractional injection of an appropriate contrast medium is begun (for example, Sinografin). A spot film may be obtained after each 2 cc. injection if so desired and a total of 6 to 10 cc. is employed. The entire study may be done with video tape recording. The examination can cease after the investigator is satisfied that the entire genital tract has been visualized maximally.

If Salpix is employed, serial films may be obtained at 20 minutes, 60 minutes, 2 hours, and 3 hours (Fig. 13–17 B). Ordinarily, by 3 hours, the soluble absorbable medium has been resorbed and may be found in the urinary bladder. It is important at this time to note whether or not there is any residual dye in loculated areas within the pelvis such as may occur with hydrosalpinx.

HYSTEROSALPINGOGRAPHY WITH OPAQUE OILY SUBSTANCES.* Hysterosalpingography with opaque oily substances is preferred by some because of the denser image produced and because this method permits a 24 hour follow-up study which water soluble substances cannot provide.

The technique is fundamentally the same; care must be exercised, however, to remove the speculum prior to injection so as not to obscure the cervical canal and internal os. The injection is made under image amplifier fluoroscopic control so that venous intravasation may be seen immediately.

Although practically all patients are examined for sterility or habitual abortion, many abnormalities may be visualized. These are summarized and illustrated in *Analysis of Roentgen Signs.*

CONTRAINDICATIONS TO THE PROCEDURE ARE AS FOLLOWS:

1. Uterine bleeding.
2. Pelvic inflammation.
3. Pregnancy. Abortions have been reported.

---

*Fullenlove, T. M.: Experience with over 2000 utero salpingographies. Am. J. Roentgenol., *106*:463–471, 1969.

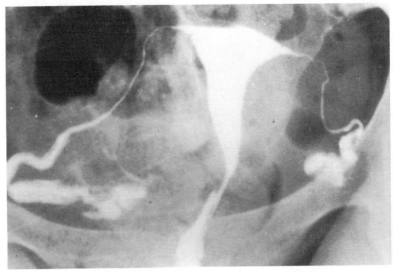

A

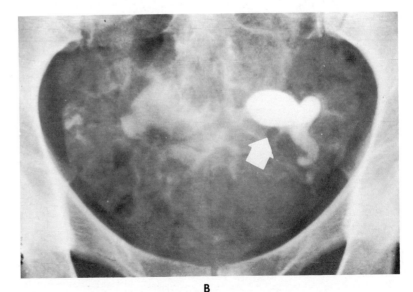

B

FIGURE 13–17 *A.* Normal hysterosalpingogram using water-soluble media. *B.* Appearance of hydrosalpinx on the 30-minute retention film taken afterward.

Gynecography (Pneumoperitoneum of the Pelvis) (Fig. 13–18). This technique allows visualization of the uterine fundus, ovaries, oviducts, and broad ligaments.*

TECHNIQUE. 1000 to 2000 cc. of a gaseous medium (air, carbon dioxide, nitrous oxide) are slowly introduced under pressure not exceeding 12 cm. of water. Films are taken in the position shown in Figure 13–18 *A*.

Anteroposterior and lateral projections are employed. A normal appearance is shown.

*Granjon, A.: La gynécographie. Presse Méd., *16*:1765–1766, 1953.

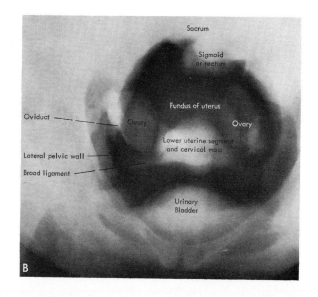

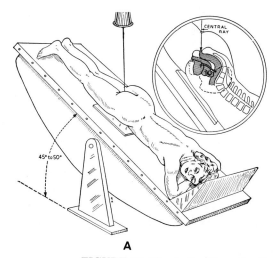

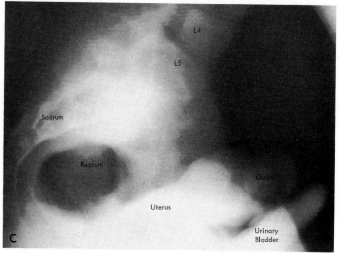

FIGURE 13–18 *A.* Position of patient (after instillation of gas) for radiography. Pneumoperitoneum of the female pelvis in posteroanterior *(B)* and lateral *(C)* projections. This patient was a 29-year-old female with a Stein-Leventhal syndrome proved by surgery, but her ovaries are considered normal in size for a young woman. (Courtesy of Dr. Wilma C. Diner, Department of Radiology, University of Arkansas Medical Center, Little Rock, Arkansas.)

Angiography of the Pelvis. Percutaneous, transfemoral aortography by the Seldinger technique has permitted catheterization of major branches of the iliac arteries. The injections may be made in the aorta above the bifurcation of the iliac arteries or in selective branches.

The techniques of pelvic angiography and pneumoperitoneum have also been combined.* Lymphangiography has also been used as an adjunct to gynecologic roentgenology.† This has been discussed and illustrated in prior chapters.

TECHNIQUE. Reference is made to prior chapters for more detailed technical description. Using mild sedation, sterile technique, and local anesthesia a Seldinger needle is inserted into the femoral artery approximately 2 inches below the inguinal ligament. The needle is usually inserted through both walls of the artery. After the stylet in the needle is withdrawn, the cannula is carefully withdrawn through the posterior wall into the lumen of the femoral artery, when pulsating bleeding is encountered. The stylet is immediately inserted partially and the cannula threaded up the femoral artery a short distance. A long, specially coiled spring guide is then introduced through the cannula and advanced within the arterial lumen under fluoroscopic control. The spring guide must be introduced far enough so that when the cannula is withdrawn over it, it will remain in place. The cannula is then removed entirely and a length of appropriate catheter tubing is pushed over and along the guide into the femoral artery. Fluoroscopy is always employed during manipulation of the guide and tubing. The tip of the catheter is usually localized in the upper abdominal aorta for abdominal aortography and renal arteriography, or at the aortic bifurcation for pelvic arteriography.

The guide is then withdrawn and a few milliliters of heparin-saline solution (10 units of heparin per milliliter of normal saline solution) is injected through the tubing to prevent clotting.

---

*Rådberg, C., and Wickbom, I.: Pelvic angiography and pneumoperitoneum. Acta Radiol. (Diag.), 6:133–144, 1967.

†Howett, M.: Lymphangiography as an adjunct to gynecologic roentgenology. Sem. Roentgenol., 4:289–296, 1969.

During the injection for pelvic arteriography, blood pressure cuffs may be employed as tourniquets about both thighs to prevent the radiopaque agent, such as the diatrizoates, from running off into the leg arteries. The usual dose of contrast agent of 60 per cent methylglucamine or 89 per cent methalamate is 20 to 25 cc., depending upon the location of the catheter and the size of the vessel being injected. This material is injected rapidly and a series of films is obtained, usually two or three per second for the first 3 seconds, and 1 per second thereafter for 7 or 8 seconds.

A mechanical pressure injector is desirable to allow the rapid injection of large volumes of the agent. It is desirable usually to complete the injection within 1 second.

The catheter is removed following the procedure and hemostasis is obtained by constant pressure, followed thereafter by a pressure dressing to be removed in 2 to 4 hours. The patient should be kept under observation for a sufficiently long period to allow detection of recurrence of bleeding at the cannulation site.

SIDE EFFECTS NOTED BY PATIENTS. Usually the injection of the contrast agent produces a sensation of heat in the area of distribution, and occasionally a sudden brief sharp or burning pain in the lower back may be encountered. Usually such pain persists for 10 to 15 seconds only. Care must be exercised that dissection of the artery has not occurred subintimally. Varying degrees of nausea may occur immediately after the injection in occasional patients, but vomiting rarely occurs and the nausea disappears spontaneously. During the week following the procedure, tenderness and ecchymosis are observed at the needle puncture site in the groin, but this may be minimized by prevention of hematoma formation during the procedure and an appropriate pressure dressing thereafter.

Repeated injections may be carried out with adequate time for excretion of the contrast agent in those patients who have normal renal function. Ordinarily, 120 ml. of the contrast agent can be tolerated in the course of 1 hour of such study in such patients. In the presence of disturbed or abnormal renal function, lesser volumes of contrast agent are usually utilized.

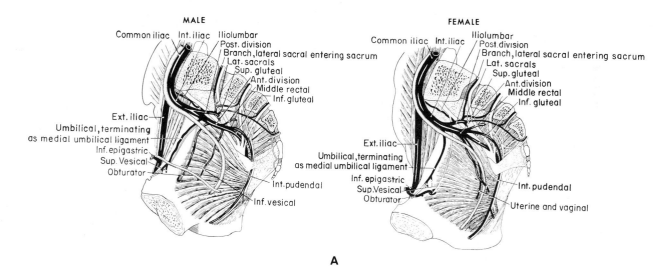

A

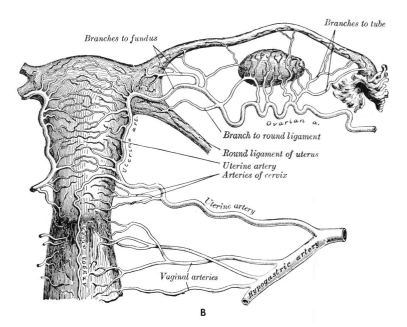

B

FIGURE 13–19 *A.* The arteries of the pelvic cavity in the male and female. (Modified from Roger C. Crafts, A Textbook of Human Anatomy, © 1966. The Ronald Press Company, New York. Modified and redrawn after Jamieson.) *B.* The arteries of the internal organs of generation of the female, seen from behind (after Hyrt). (From Goss, C. M. (ed.): Gray's Anatomy of the Human Body, 29th ed. Philadelphia, Lea & Febiger, 1973.)

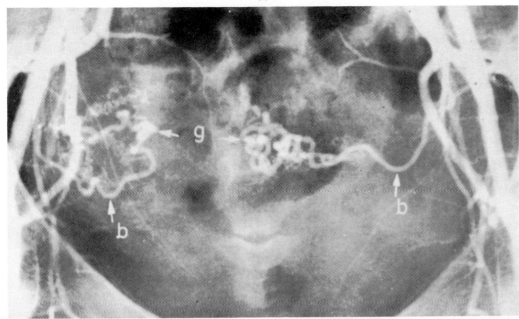

A

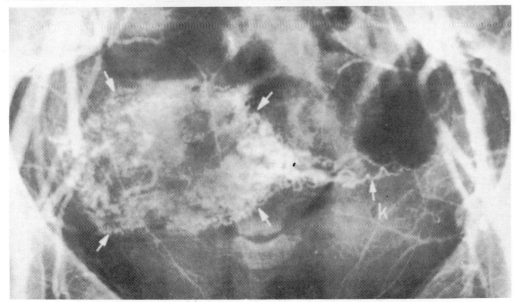

B

FIGURE 13–20 Normal arteriogram. Axial projection of the uterus. *A*. Film taken immediately after the injection of opaque medium. The uterine arteries in the parametrium *(b)* and along the lateral margin of the uterus (g) are seen. A few tortuous intramural arteries within the right half of the uterus begin to opacify. *B*, Film taken two seconds after film *A*. The main trunk of the uterine artery is now faintly outlined. Numerous small, tortuous intramural arteries are visible within the uterus (arrows). The left adnexal branch *(k)* follows a tortuous course. (From Abrams, H. L.: Angiography, 2nd ed., Vol. 2. Boston, Little, Brown & Company, 1971.)

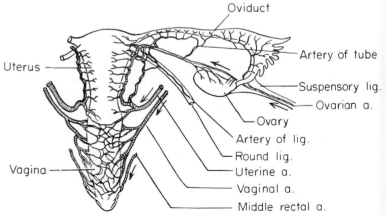

FIGURE 13–21 Diagram of arteries of the female genitalia.

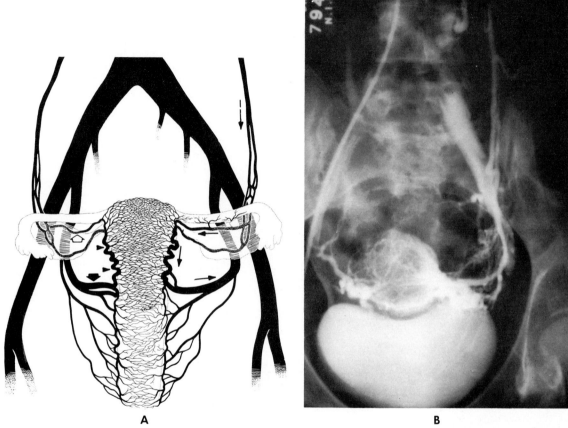

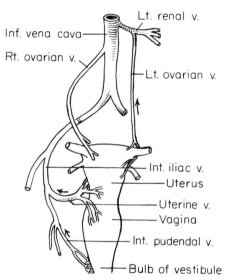

FIGURE 13–23 Veins of the female pelvis depicted diagrammatically.

FIGURE 13–22 *A*. Diagrammatic sketch of the major visceral veins of the pelvis. The right ovarian pedicle (clear arrow), right uterine plexus (arrowheads), and right uterine pedicle or vein (solid arrow) are shown on the left. The direction of flow during retrograde ovarian venography, shown on the right, is down the ovarian vein, medially via the ovarian pedicle to the uterine plexus, down the uterine, and laterally in the uterine pedicle to the internal iliac vein (arrows). This route is invariably demonstrated with satisfactory retrograde injection; filling of the uterine myometrial plexus is less constant.

B. Retrograde left ovarian venogram obtained without bladder distension or angulation of the radiographic tube. The uterus is projected axially above the bladder. (From Doppman, J. L., and Chretien, P.: Radiology, *98*:406, 1971.)

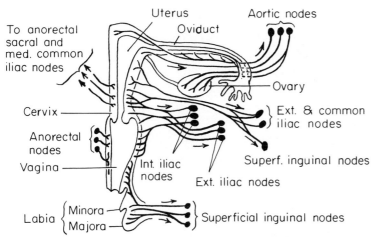

FIGURE 13–24 Lymph vessels of the female genitalia shown diagrammatically.

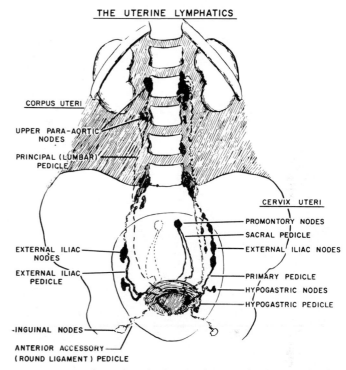

FIGURE 13–25 Diagrammatic sketch of the uterine lymphatic circulation. The solid lymph nodes and pedicles represent the visualized primary drainage areas, the shaded lymph nodes are secondary drainage areas, and the open lymph nodes are nonopacified lymph nodes in our case. (From Hipona, F. A., and Ditchek, T.: Am. J. Roentgenol., *98*:236–238, 1966.)

It is recommended that the x-ray tube be angled 35 degrees cranially with distention of the urinary bladder so as to prevent superimposition of the ovarian pedicle, uterine plexus, and uterine pedicle. Distention of the urinary bladder with gas is to be preferred. One film every second for 15 seconds is adequate.

Combined Pelvic Angiography and Pneumoperitoneum in Gynecologic Diagnosis. These two methods are often complementary. The vascular structure of the pelvis combined with the morphological delineation of detail by pneumoperitoneum makes a valuable contribution to the diagnostic armamentarium.*

---

*Rådberg, C., and Wickbom, I.: Pelvic angiography and pneumoperitoneum. Acta Radiol. (Diag.), 6:133–144, 1967.

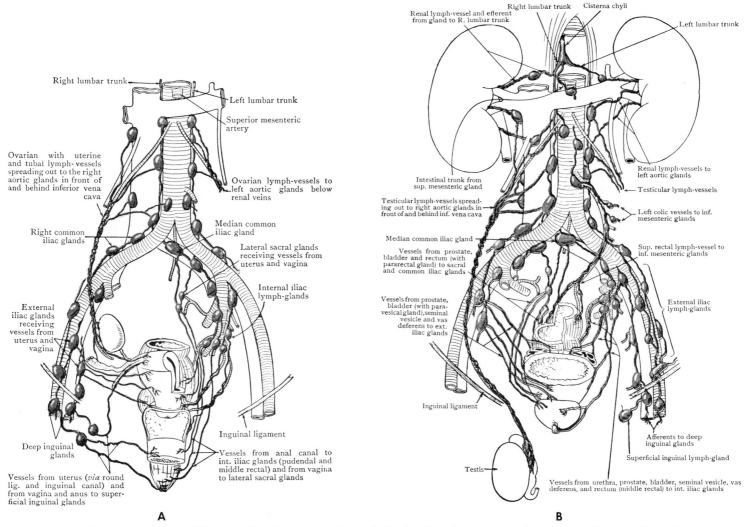

Right lumbar trunk

Left lumbar trunk

Superior mesenteric artery

Ovarian with uterine and tubal lymph- vessels spreading out to the right aortic glands in front of and behind inferior vena cava

Ovarian lymph-vessels to left aortic glands below renal veins

Median common iliac gland

Right common iliac glands

Lateral sacral glands receiving vessels from uterus and vagina

Internal iliac lymph-glands

External iliac glands receiving vessels from uterus and vagina

Deep inguinal glands

Inguinal ligament

Vessels from anal canal to int. iliac glands (pudendal and middle rectal) and from vagina to lateral sacral glands

Vessels from uterus (via round lig. and inguinal canal) and from vagina and anus to superficial inguinal glands

A

Right lumbar trunk   Cisterna chyli

Renal lymph-vessel and efferent from gland to R. lumbar trunk

Left lumbar trunk

Intestinal trunk from sup. mesenteric gland

Renal lymph-vessels to left aortic glands

Testicular lymph-vessels spreading out to right aortic glands in front of and behind inf. vena cava

Testicular lymph-vessels

Left colic vessels to inf. mesenteric glands

Median common iliac gland

Sup. rectal lymph-vessel to inf. mesenteric glands

Vessels from prostate, bladder and rectum (with pararectal gland) to sacral and common iliac glands

Vessels from prostate, bladder (with para-vesical gland), seminal vesicle and vas deferens to ext. iliac glands

External iliac lymph-glands

Inguinal ligament

Afferents to deep inguinal glands

Testis

Superficial inguinal lymph-gland

Vessels from urethra, prostate, bladder, seminal vesicle, vas deferens, and rectum (middle rectal) to int. iliac glands

B

FIGURE 13–26 *A*. Diagram of lymph vessels and lymph glands of female pelvis and abdomen. *B*. Diagram of lymph vessels and lymph glands of male pelvis and abdomen. (From Cunningham's Manual of Practical Anatomy, 11th ed. London, Oxford University Press, 1949.)

Study of the Pregnant Woman with Respect to the Fetus

Introduction. Protection from radiation and potential radiation hazards take on greater significance in this field, since there are at least two or more lives involved (mother and fetuses) and not just that of the patient. The hazards of radiation must be carefully weighed against the benefits to be achieved.

Determination of a Fetal Skeleton in Utero. The viable fetus should not be exposed to irradiation during the first trimester of pregnancy. Hormonal tests are far more sensitive in any case for the detection of early pregnancy, since ossification of the fetal skeleton does not occur prior to the third month of gestation, and radiographically detectable fetal skeletal parts are difficult to find prior to the thirteenth or fourteenth week.

The indications for seeking fetal skeletal parts are (1) an enlarging uterus without other evidence of pregnancy; (2) an enlarging tumor mass of the pelvis that could conceivably be teratomatous or represent an extra-uterine pregnancy; (3) a previously suspected gravid uterus when the clinical situation has changed and pregnancy tests have ceased to be positive; and (4) an abnormal fetus that is strongly suggested by clinical appearances (hydrocephalus; anencephaly).

The fetal parts that lend themselves most readily to early detection are the segmental structures such as those of the spine and ribs; occasionally the extremities and head may be seen in faint outline.

The oblique views of the pelvis are often more helpful than straight anteroposterior views, since the fetal ossified parts may be projected over the sacrum and lost to view.

Determination of Multiple Fetuses. Study for multiple fetuses is not undertaken prior to the later stages of pregnancy, preferably late in the last trimester when radiation hazard to the fetus is minimal. Multiple fetuses can be ascertained, however, after approximately the fourteenth week when fetal ossification may be manifest radiographically. A differentiation of multiple fetuses is particularly useful in patients who have enlarged uteri because of pendulous abdomens, marked lordosis of the lumbar spine, or a tendency to polyhydramnios. The physician may not assume that the 14-week size uterus will necessarily reveal the skeletons of developing twins. The fetal skeletons may not be determinable at this early period, especially with twins.

Fetal Normality. Fetal normality is best studied late in the last trimester. In evaluating the fetal skeleton in utero, it is important to bear in mind the problems related to magnification and distortion. Before diagnosing an abnormal fetus, one must be certain of the finding by means of examinations in various projections and serial studies.

A thin black line surrounding the fetus on the radiograph is called the normal "fetal fat line." This is best developed after the eighth month when the deposition of subcutaneous fat occurs most rapidly. When the fetal fat line is thicker than normal, postmaturity or erythroblastosis of the fetus may be suspected.

Evidence of trauma to the fetus may also be detected on occasion in utero.

Fetal Age and Development. Fetal age determination should rarely be required prior to the third trimester of pregnancy. There are many different bases upon which fetal age can be estimated, but probably the most reliable are estimation of actual fetal length and determination of average fetal head diameter.

Determination of average fetal head diameter can be accurate. There are several tables and graphs available for computing fetal age from roentgen measurements of the fetal skull, based on the anthropometric studies of Scammon and Calkins, Hodges, and others.* These graphs indicate the fetal age in accordance with occipital-frontal diameter in centimeters, biparietal skull diameter, and average net circumference of the fetal skull obtained from two roentgenograms taken at right angles to one another (Fig. 13–11). The average diameter of the fetal skull is obtained by averaging the long and short perpendicular diameters (corrected for magnification) from anteroposterior and lateral teleroentgenograms of the fetal skull (average of two diameters for each view). (Sonics may be used for this purpose.)

---

*References may be obtained in Meschan, I.: An Atlas of Anatomy Basic to Radiology. Philadelphia, W. B. Saunders Co., 1975, Chapter 17.

Prediction of Fetal Maturity. The following criteria are perhaps most important.

1. An ossification center is present in the distal end of the femur in 90 per cent of term fetuses.

2. Proximal tibial epiphyseal ossification is noted at term in 70 to 80 per cent of the newborn.

3. Less practical standards for ossification are (a) ossification of the hyoid bone should be complete; (b) ossification of the central parts of the vertebrae should appear; and (c) the first segments of the coccyx, the metacarpals, and the phalanges may be visualized.

With regard to reliability of some of these criteria, Schreiber et al.* came to the following conclusions:

1. Visualization of the fetal distal femoral ossification centers indicated a mature fetus by several criteria in 92 to 98 per cent of cases, with an average of 96 per cent for all criteria.

2. Approximately one fetus in twenty with visualized distal femoral ossification centers was not mature.

3. Visualization of both the distal femoral and proximal tibial epiphyseal centers on antepartum abdominal films was a highly reliable indicator of fetal maturity. When these centers were present the fetus was mature in 95 to 100 per cent of cases with an average of 98 per cent for all criteria.

4. Presence of ossification centers for the distal femoral epiphyses on postpartum knee films was associated with a mature fetus in 93 per cent of cases. However, 58 per cent of the newborn with absent femoral epiphyseal centers were mature by the same criteria and 61 per cent were mature by clinical estimation.

Therefore, failure to visualize these centers on postpartum knee films was not ipso facto evidence of prematurity in their series. Failure to visualize the distal femoral epiphyseal ossification centers on the antepartum films was also a poor indicator of prematurity because of superimposition of structures and fetal movement during the radiographic exposure.

In a second study (1963)† distal femoral epiphyseal ossification centers were demonstrated on abdominal films in 80 per cent of the cases in which they were visualized subsequently on postpartum films of the knees of the newborn. False positive demonstration of distal femoral epiphyses was obtained in 1.7 per cent of cases.

The determination of fetal maturity by whatever means is often an important decision, since very often it in turn will decide whether or not elective induction of labor or repeat cesarean section may be indicated.

In the unpublished data from the Vanderbilt Fetal Age Study, antepartum radiographic visualization of the fetal ossification centers about the knees was a better indicator of fetal maturity than estimated gestational age, uterine size, and other physical findings.

Fetal maturity may in part be estimated from measurements of the fetal skull and determination of fetal age.

Brosens et al.‡ reported a cytologic test for fetal maturity in combination with a new radiologic method for estimation. They used a lipid contrast medium for intrauterine fetal visualization, which is accomplished by amniocentesis after ultrasonic localization of the placenta. A few milliliters of the amniotic fluid are aspirated and 6 ml. of Ethiodan are injected. An x-ray film is taken 8 to 24 hours later. After 6 to 8 hours Ethiodan outlines the fetal skin clearly through absorption on the vernix. The cytologic method involves counting lipid positive cells in amniotic fluid, using 0.1 per cent aqueous Nile-blue sulfate stain. At birth, maturity was estimated by the pediatrician's using neurological parameters. No complications resulted from the injections. The histologic study of the lungs in live born infants who died soon after delivery showed no abnormalities attributable to Ethiodan inhalation.

A fetal lumbar vertebral length of 52 mm. or more indicated that 95 per cent of the group weighed over 2500 grams, with an actual total length of 49 cm. or more.

---

*Schreiber, M. H., et al.: Reliability of visualization of distal femoral epiphyses as a measure of maturity. Am. J. Obstet. Gynecol., *83*:1249–1250, 1962.

†Schreiber, M. H., et al.: Epiphyseal ossification center visualization: Its value in prediction of fetal maturity. J.A.M.A., *184*:504–507, 1963.

‡Brosens, I., et al.: Prediction of fetal maturity with combined cytologic and radiologic method. J. Obstet. Gynecol. Br. Comm., *76*:20–26, 1969.

Determination of Fetal Viability, Death, or Other Fetal Abnormalities. This is considered outside the scope of this text and the student is referred to *Analysis of Roentgen Signs*.

Presentation of Fetus (Fig. 13–27). The position of the fetal head, small parts, and back is readily determined by consideration of the anteroposterior and lateral radiographs.

A "military" position of the head precludes engagement unless the head is very small and the pelvis is very large. This hyperextended position is more common with cephalopelvic disporportion or other factors that interfere with engagement, such as a distended bladder, pelvic mass, placenta previa, polyhydramnios, or a pendulous uterus. Atypical fetal presentations that can be recognized radiographically are face and brow presentation, transverse, shoulder or arm, breech, footling, or knee.

Roentgenographic pelvic measurements and fetal head mensuration play an important part in management decisions.

When the head is not engaged in a prima gravida, some possibilities to be considered are: obstructing masses in the pelvis such as ovarian cyst or fibroids; placenta previa centralis; a short umbilical cord, or more often a cord twisted around the fetus; fetal malformation such as hydrocephalus and cystic hygroma of the neck; or a pendulous uterus impairing the direction of uterine force.

Study of the Pregnant Woman for Uterine Detail Outside the Fetus

Placenta (Fig. 13–28). Various methods for study of the placenta radiologically are:

1. Routine anteroposterior and lateral projections of the abdomen, inclusive of the entire uterus.

2. A special lateral film employing a wedge filter when the placenta is anteriorly situated in the uterine fundus. (A "wedge filter" is an x-ray filter and medium interposed between the x-ray tube and the patient which will diminish the radiation over the patient's thinner parts so that this area on the radiograph will have equal clarity with the x-ray image of the thicker anatomic portions. This is particularly useful on the lateral view.) The placenta is situated on either the anterior or posterior sur-

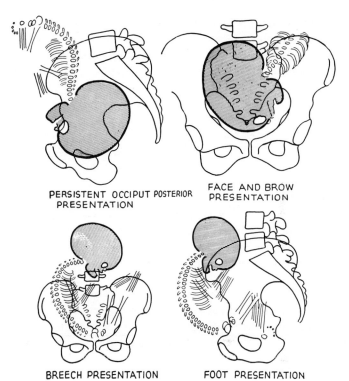

PERSISTENT OCCIPUT POSTERIOR PRESENTATION

FACE AND BROW PRESENTATION

BREECH PRESENTATION

FOOT PRESENTATION

FIGURE 13–27 Diagrams illustrating various types of atypical presentation as they may be seen radiographically.

face of the uterine fundus in most instances and can usually be differentiated as a thick, crescentic, platelike structure with a central thickness of 6 to 8 cm. tapering to each side, and a diameter of approximately 25 cm. Contraction and blood loss after delivery diminish the size of the placenta postnatally. The fetus faces the placenta in about three-quarters of the cases. Occasionally, calcification can be identified within the placenta.

3. Radioisotopic techniques or ultrasound gray scale and B scans (outside the scope of this text) may be utilized for scanning the placenta.

4. Angiographic methods are seldom used in view of the radiation exposure required, but in rare instances they may also be employed.

Amniography

TECHNIQUE. The maternal urinary bladder is emptied and the placenta localized, either radiographically or by image amplifier fluoroscopy. The maternal abdominal wall is punctured at a distance from the placenta so that entrance is made into the amniotic sac. Generally the dosage is 1.5 cc. of Renografin-60 per week of gestation, up to a total of 50 cc.*

Anteroposterior and lateral films of the abdomen are obtained as early as 30 minutes following injection, or as late as 2 to 3 hours afterward.

Hazards, apart from x-ray radiation, may be (1) premature labor may be induced; and (2) in a series of 50 consecutive patients studied in this way for painless vaginal bleeding, the morbidity noted included needle marks in three infants, one of them infected, and postpartum maternal morbidity involving six patients.* (Sonics may be used as a preferable modality, where feasible.)

PURPOSES OF PROCEDURE

1. It provides a positive contrast outline of all structures within or impinging upon the amniotic sac. Thus the method may be used to detect placenta previa.

2. Fetal death can be distinguished with reasonable certainty. In films taken after 2 hours, some of the contrast agent should be detected in the fetal stomach or intestine. In a dead fetus, no swallowing will have occurred.

*Blumberg, M. L., et al.: Placental localization by amniography. Am. J. Roentgenol., *100*:688–697, 1967.

FIGURE 13–28 Radiographic appearance of normal placental implantation compared with appearances of abnormal implantations. The placenta previa is shown in good contrast by means of air distention of both the bladder and the rectum.

ROENTGEN STUDY OF THE PLACENTA

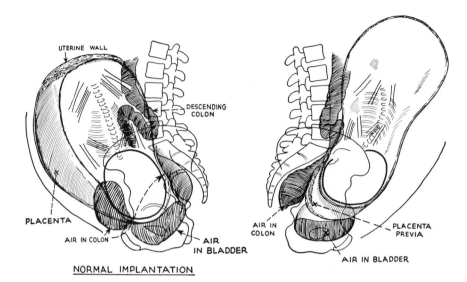

NORMAL IMPLANTATION

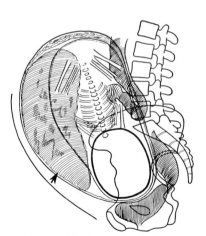

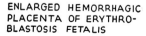
ENLARGED HEMORRHAGIC PLACENTA OF ERYTHRO-BLASTOSIS FETALIS

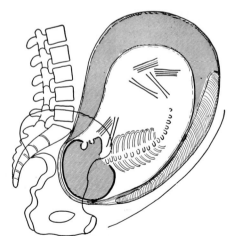

POLYHYDRAMNIOS

3. It can be a guide to fetography and intrauterine fetal transfusion.

4. It assists in diagnosis of uterine or fetal abnormalities.

5. Premature membrane rupture may be diagnosed by leakage of the contrast medium into the vagina.

6. Extrauterine pregnancy can be demonstrated.

7. Removal of the amniotic fluid under fluoroscopic guidance prior to delivery has also been very helpful in determining the onset of deterioration from erythroblastosis fetalis in the fetus.

After 29 weeks of gestation, the prognosis of impending fetal death on the basis of the rise of optical density of the amniotic fluid seems to be quite accurate. Prior to this time the significance of a given rise of optical density of the amniotic fluid is less certain. This has afforded an effective means of selection of fetuses for preterm delivery and post-delivery exchange transfusions (Queenan et al.; Liggans).*

AMNIOGRAPHY AS A GUIDE TO FETOGRAPHY AND INTRAUTERINE FETAL TRANSFUSIONS. During amniography, the fetus swallows the radiopaque medium when it is present in amniotic fluid, and this results in delineation of the fetal gastrointestinal tract.

In 1963 Liley* demonstrated that he could pass a needle through the maternal abdominal wall, the uterine wall, and the abdominal wall of the fetus to instill Rh negative blood into the peritoneal cavity of the fetus. Blood so instilled was absorbed in the fetal peripheral circulation. Others who have repeated this technique have also reported success with it (Queenan et al.; Bowman and Friesen; Duggin and Taylor).*

Image intensifier fluoroscopy is of course essential for such a procedure. It is apparently not unusual to make three or four attempts to enter the peritoneal cavity of a fetus 25 to 26 weeks of age before a successful intraperitoneal approach is achieved.

TECHNIQUE FOR THE TRANSUTERINE INFUSION OF RED CELLS INTO THE FETUS IN ERYTHROBLASTOSIS FETALIS (Ferris et al.).* An 8 inch No. 16 Touhy needle is introduced into the amniotic sac at a point approximating the anterior abdominal wall of the fetus (Fig. 13–29). The needle is thereafter inserted into the peritoneal cavity of the fetus.

Five cc. of methylglucamine diatrizoate are injected to check the needle position. If the end of the needle is free, the opaque medium will outline the diaphragm of the fetus in a crescent shape that can usually be recognized fluoroscopically. Also, contrasted bowel loops of the fetus may be seen. Once the needle is definitely free, 50 to 100 cc. of packed red cells are injected into the peritoneal cavity of the fetus. In their phantom studies Ferris et al.* showed that the radiation to the the fetus was 228 milliroentgens.

USE OF CARBON DIXOIDE AS A CONTRAST AGENT FOR LOCALIZATION (Hanafee and Bashore).* An injection of 2 to 5 cc. of carbon dioxide is made under fluoroscopic control. If the needle-catheter system is correctly placed, all the signs of free intraperitoneal air in the newborn are evident. If the needle is outside the fetus, gas will be spread over a wide arc.

A catheter replaces the needle after the correct position is ascertained, and the blood is allowed to drip in during the next 30 to 60 minutes.

Excessive quantities of carbon dioxide should not be employed since gas may stimulate the fetus to excessive position change.

A grid to aid in film localization of the needle in intrauterine transfusion has been recommended by Wade.*

PRENATAL SEX DETERMINATION. Fort and Riggs* were able to outline the fetal labia in a fetus at 22 weeks of gestation during intrauterine fetal transfusion. Likewise, they were able to visualize a fetal testis in a male fetus. Thus, prenatal sex determination was possible.

Genitography in Intersexual States (Shopfner)

The components of sexual differentiation consist of chromosomal, gonadal, internal genital anatomy, external genital anatomy, hormonal aspects, environmental rearing, and sexual orientation or gender. The

*References may be obtained in Meschan, I.: An Atlas of Anatomy Basic to Radiology. Philadelphia, W. B. Saunders Co., 1973, Chapter 17.

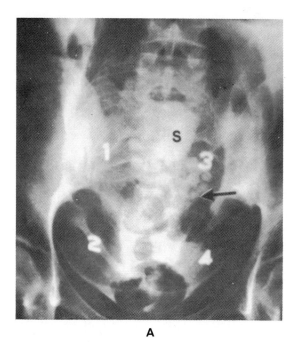

A

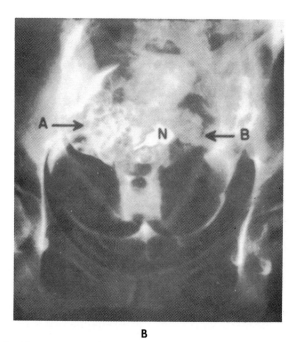

B

FIGURE 13-29 *A*. Complete breech presentation. Radiopaque material may be seen in the fetal stomach (S) and small intestine (arrow). Localizing lead markers surround fetal peritoneal cavity. *B*. Touhy needle (N) in fetal peritoneal cavity. Radiopaque material demonstrated outside fetal small intestine (A) and in small intestine (B). (From Queenan, J. T.: J.A.M.A., *191*:944, 1965.)

last two elements are largely governed by internal and external genital anatomy; in the case of the male, hormonal activity is required as well.

The clinical studies which are of assistance in the determination of these sexual components are sex chromatin pattern, a study of the external genital anatomy, a knowledge of the internal genital anatomy, urinary hormonal excretion, and the nature of the gonads as determined by biopsy.

Genitography is the simplest and best procedure for providing information regarding the internal genital anatomy, particularly prior to the time when knowledge of the nature of the gonads is not essential. Apparently, genitography can provide anatomic information not afforded by other means.

The technique of genitography requires the filling of all genital cavities with opaque media. Two methods may be employed: a flushing technique, or a multiple catheter technique. The examination should be performed under fluoroscopy for proper control. The multiple catheter technique is employed when the flushing technique fails, since in placing a catheter into one cavity, one may miss other passages. The relationship of the urinary bladder may be simultaneously determined by excretory urography. It is suggested that the opaque medium employed be aqueous at first try; if success is not obtained, an oily medium may thereafter be employed.

For further detail in regard to this important subject, the reader is referred to Shopfner's comprehensive monograph.*

---

*Shopfner, C. E.: Genitography in intersexual states. Radiology, *82*:664-674, 1964.

14

THE UPPER
ALIMENTARY TRACT

PRINCIPLES INVOLVED IN STUDY OF THE ALIMENTARY TRACT

The walls of the alimentary tract are intermediate in radiographic density, and hence require some type of contrast material for detection by means of x-rays. Normally, there is a variable amount of gas in the stomach and colon that permits a relatively gross and inadequate visualization of these structures. In the normal adult, gas in the small intestine is considered abnormal and the introduction of contrast material into the small intestine is therefore essential.

Although negative contrast may be employed in the visualization of the gastrointestinal tract, it is usually supplementary to the more significant positive contrast with radiopaque media.

Since the physiology and function of the gastrointestinal tract are readily altered by so many factors such as hypotonicity or hypertonicity, alkalinity, acidity, proteins, fats, carbohydrates, amino acids, and any slight mechanical irritation, it is essential for any opaque contrast medium to be physiologically inert.

The most commonly used medium thus employed in present-day radiography of the gastrointestinal tract is barium sulfate in water suspension. In certain patients, in whom obstruction by barium mixtures may occur, organic soluble iodides are utilized by intubation techniques. In infants or other patients in whom aspiration is a potential danger, small quantities of iodized oil are helpful, at least until it is certain that aspiration is not taking place. Iodized oil is a poor contrast agent beyond the esophagus because it distorts the normal physiologic pattern.

On certain occasions, it is advantageous to use so-called double contrast in which gas is introduced after administering the barium suspension. The gas and barium suspension are thus mixed and are helpful in outlining polyps and small tumors. The gas employed may be air, carbon dioxide, or a mixture of both, as when ginger ale, carbonated water, Seidlitz powder, or "sparklers," manufactured for this purpose are introduced into the stomach.

The usual radiologic methods include: (1) fluoroscopy, (2) spot-film radiography, (3) routine radiography in certain positions; any or all of the usual erect, recumbent, supine, prone, lateral or oblique positions are employed; and (4) computerized tomography.

Other methods of radiologic study of the upper alimentary tract include *hypotonic duodenography, angiography,* and *endoscopic pancreatocholangiography,* as well as other pararadiologic procedures not included in this text, such as ultrasonography and radioisotopic scanning procedures.

Parietography—the demonstration of the walls of the gastrointestinal tract by filling the peritoneal cavity and the lumen of the studied organ simultaneously with air or gas—is a further refinement of the air contrast technique. This may be especially helpful when combined with tomography.

In many of these methods, *pharmacoradiography,* or the injection of drugs in order to influence the radiologic examination, may be employed.

There are two major principles involved in the radiologic anatomy of the gastrointestinal tract:

1. We are examining a dynamic, moving, functioning system of organs. They are not static. Their structure must at all times be considered along with their function, and the two aspects are inseparable.

2. When the lumen of a hollow organ is filled with contrast substance, we can visualize the inner lining with accuracy, but the wall of the organ outside the innermost lining can be studied only indirectly as it affects the lumen or the mucosa. It is conceivable that considerable abnormality may exist outside the lumen within the wall of the organ, which may not be reflected in the mucosal pattern.

(Parietography, does, however, permit visualization of the outer walls of the gastrointestinal tract simultaneously with the lumen of the studied organ, particularly when combined with tomography.)

THE MOUTH AND OROPHARYNX

The mouth and oropharynx are so readily examined by direct inspection and palpation that it is not usual to employ the radiograph except for demonstration of hidden structures.

In a direct lateral view (Fig. 14–1), the air within the mouth and pharynx permits a contrast visualization of the tongue surface, the hard and soft palate, and the nasopharynx and oropharynx.

Special views of the salivary glands may be obtained after the injection of iodized water soluble contrast agents into the ducts. Soft tissue studies of the floor of the mouth or the cheek are also feasible.

Brief mention of the radiography of the teeth has already been made (see Chapter 7), and will not be further discussed in this text.

Soft Tissue Study of the Mouth and Pharynx by Lateral Projection. This projection is identical with that employed for a lateral view of the cervical spine, except that technical factors are varied slightly to emphasize the soft tissues rather than the skeletal structure (see Chapter 8).

The structures demonstrated in profile are the following: the tongue and floor of the mouth, the hard and soft palate and uvula, the vallecula at the base of the tongue and the pyriform sinuses on either side, the nasopharynx above the palate with turbinates and eustachian orifice, the lymphoid structures in the nasopharynx, and the epiglottis.

The width of the soft tissues projected under the sphenoid is considerably narrower in the adult than in the child, owing to the markedly enlarged lymphoid apparatus in the child after 3 to 6 months of age. This view affords a ready means of investigating these lymphoid and adenoid structures.

The width of the retro-oropharyngeal soft tissues in the child is also considerably greater than it is in the adult when these structures are compared with the retrolaryngeal soft tissues between the larynx and the cervical spine. Thus in the newborn and infant, the ratio of the retro-oropharyngeal soft tissues to the retrolaryngeal soft tissues is approximately 1 to 1, while in the adult it is usually in the order of 1 to 3. These measurements are of value in the detection of space-occupying lesions such as inflammations and tumors in these locations, which by direct inspection are difficult to evaluate because they may be posterior to the visible mucosa, or because the patient may be unable to open his mouth.

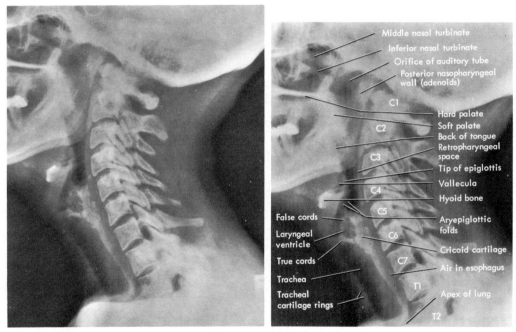

FIGURE 14-1 Lateral soft tissue film of the neck with labeled radiograph.

Soft Tissue Radiography of the Floor of the Mouth with the Aid of the Occlusal Type Dental Film

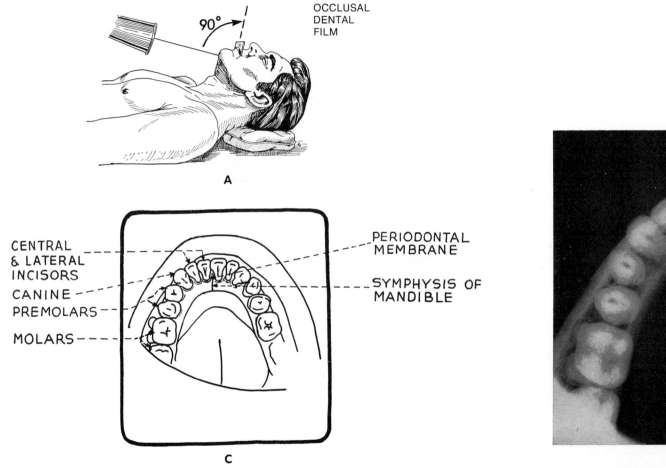

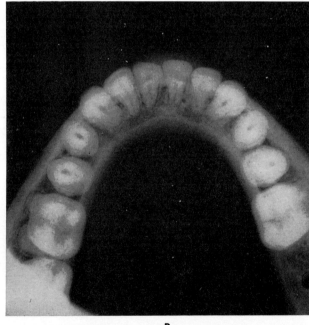

FIGURE 14–2 Occlusal type dental film of floor of mouth. *A*. Position of patient. *B*. Labeled tracing of radiograph. *C*. Radiograph obtained.

Radiography of the Hard Palate

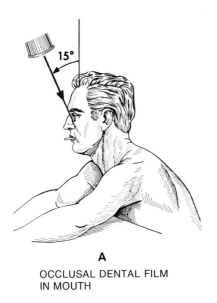

A

OCCLUSAL DENTAL FILM
IN MOUTH

MIDLINE SUTURE
AND TRANSVERSE
PALATINE SUTURE
MAY BE IDENTIFIED

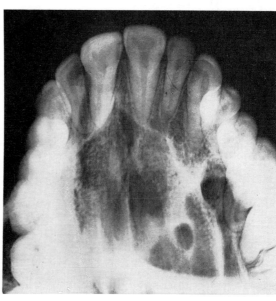

B

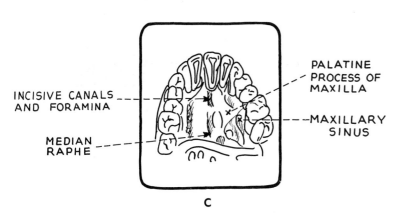

INCISIVE CANALS
AND FORAMINA

MEDIAN
RAPHE

PALATINE
PROCESS OF
MAXILLA

MAXILLARY
SINUS

C

FIGURE 14–3 Method of radiography of hard palate with occlusal type dental film. *A*. Position of patient. *B*. Radiograph. *C*. Labeled tracing of *B*.

THE SALIVARY GLANDS

Radiographic Technique of Examination. The salivary glands may be examined by means of plain radiographs, or after the injection of contrast media into the salivary duct. Plain radiographs are of value only when a calculus is suspected. In other instances, contrast studies are necessary.

With regard to *plain radiographs,* the following studies may be performed:

1. For parotid calculi, a lateral view (in stereoscopic projection preferably) is taken, centering over the gland, with the neck extended and the mouth open.

2. For submaxillary and sublingual calculi, a stereoscopic lateral view is obtained with the mouth closed, and usually it is best to incline the x-ray tube slightly cephalad to prevent superimposition of the two rami of the mandible. Also a view of the floor of the mouth is obtained with the aid of an occlusal type dental film as previously described.

Sialograms are defined as the radiographic demonstration of the salivary ducts and alveoli by the injection of contrast media. The technique is as follows:*†

The duct may be dilated with olive-tipped lacrimal probes. A sterile polyethylene catheter is thereafter inserted with a wire stylus for rigidity for a distance of 3 to 4 cm.

The contrast medium usually employed is a diatrizoate such as Hypaque or Renografin. It may be injected directly or by means of a glass reservoir positioned 70 cm. above the patient's head. If direct injection is employed, the injection is continued until definite pain is experienced by the patient. In the second technique,† underfilling seldom occurs because the film is taken while the contrast medium is still flowing and the pressure is therefore maintained. Moreover, overfilling rarely occurs because of the almost constant pressure. Usually 1 to 2 cc. of the contrast agent is adequate.

Films are obtained in the anteroposterior, lateral, or lateral-oblique positions at the completion of the filling phase. The polyethylene cath-

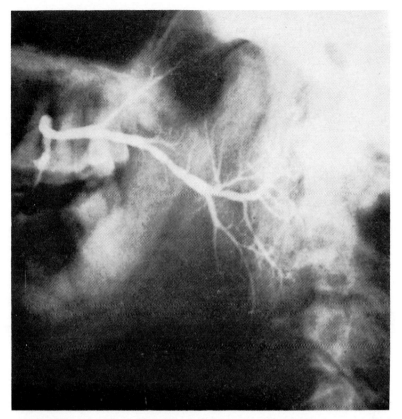

FIGURE 14–4 Normal sialogram of the parotid gland. (Courtesy of Dr. L. B. Morettin, Galveston, Texas.)

eter may be plugged while the films are checked for adequacy. These films are then followed by a secretory film taken 5 minutes after the completion of the filling phase. To insure rapid expulsion of the contrast medium, salivary flow is stimulated by a few drops of lemon juice or by sucking on a lemon for 1 minute, after which the patient rinses his mouth. Normally, the gland should be empty within 5 minutes, although a faint "acinar" cloud may persist for up to 24 hours.

The emptying phase is considered as important as the "filling phase" described.

---

*Chisholm, D. M., et al.: Hydrostatic sialography as an index of salivary gland disease in Sjögren's syndrome. Acta Radiol. (Diag.), *11*:577–585, 1971.

†Park, W. M., and Mason, D. K.: Hydrostatic sialography. Radiology, *86*:116, 1966.

ROENTGENOLOGIC CONSIDERATIONS OF THE HYOID APPARATUS

Basic Anatomy.* The hyoid bone is suspended in the anterior portion of the neck above the larynx, beneath the mandible, and anterior to the epiglottis. It is connected inferiorly by broad membranous bands to the thyroid cartilages of the larynx, and by other broad ligamentous sheaths to the epiglottis. It is suspended from the styloid processes by two ligaments, the stylohyoid ligaments, which may be variably ossified. The stylohyoid ligaments attach to the lesser horns of the hyoid bone, which consists of a body and two pairs of processes, the greater and lesser horns.

There is a synovial articulation between the lesser and greater horns of the hyoid bone, and a synchondrosis of the greater horn with the body of the hyoid bone. The synovial articulations are subject to all diseases of synovia, such as rheumatoid arthritis.

Roentgen Appearance. In the lateral view (Fig. 14–5), the body of the hyoid bone is parallel to the body of the mandible and to the thyroid cartilages.

The stylohyoid ligaments extending from the free tips of the styloid process to the lesser horns vary considerably in degree of ossification as well as in length and width.

The paired lesser horns of the hyoid are small and conical and are united to the body of the hyoid by fibrous tissue and occasionally a synovial joint. As pointed out previously, the lesser horns articulate with the greater horns by means of a synovial joint.

The posterior surface of the hyoid is parallel to the epiglottis and is separated from it by the hyothyroid membrane and loose areolar tissue. Several bursae may be interposed between the membrane and the bone in these regions.

The recognition of hyoid fractures as well as anomalies of this bone require a good appreciation of the normal roentgen anatomy.*

_____

*Porrath, S.: Roentgenologic considerations of the hyoid apparatus. Am. J. Roentgenol., _105_:63–73, 1969.

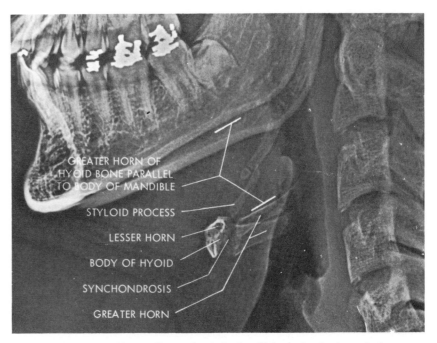

FIGURE 14–5 Xeroradiograph of the hyoid bone in the lateral view.

THE ESOPHAGUS

Gross Anatomy and Relationships of the Esophagus. The esophagus extends from the pharynx at the inferior border of the cricoid cartilage to the cardiac orifice of the stomach opposite the eleventh thoracic vertebra. Its course is in the midline anterior to the vertebral column, but it deviates to the left at the base of the neck for a short distance. At about the level of the seventh thoracic vertebra it passes slowly to the left and anteriorly to reach the esophageal orifice of the diaphragm, and it maintains this direction until it reaches the stomach.

Its length varies between 25 and 30 cm., and its breadth between 12 mm. and 30 or more mm. in its distended state.

In cross section it usually appears as a flattened tube, or a tube with a stellate lumen.

There are certain anatomic relationships of the esophagus (Fig. 14–7) which are of definite importance:

In the neck it is loosely connected by areolar tissue with the posterior aspect of the trachea. It is possible, however, for an abnormal structure such as aberrant thyroid tissue to lie between the trachea and esophagus, and hence it is important to obtain a lateral visualization of the base of the neck with barium in the esophagus when studying the thyroid gland.

In the thorax, the trachea lies anterior to the esophagus as far as the fifth thoracic vertebra near which the trachea bifurcates.

The *arch of the aorta,* passing back to reach the vertebral column, crosses to the left side of the esophagus, causing a *slight deviation of the esophagus to the right.*

The *thoracic aorta* lies first to the left of the esophagus, then posterior to it, and finally, both posterior and to the right of it.

Immediately *below the level of the bifurcation of the trachea,* the esophagus is *crossed by the left bronchus,* and in the rest of its thoracic course it *lies close to the posterior surface of the pericardium.*

In this location it is situated in the posterior mediastinum, and is *separated from the vertebral column by the azygos vein, thoracic duct, and lower thoracic aorta.* It is in *close proximity with the left atrium,* and any enlargement of the latter structure is reflected in displacement of the esophagus posteriorly and to the right (Fig. 14–6).

The two *vagus nerves* descend to the esophagus after forming the anterior and posterior pulmonary plexuses, and unite with the sympathetic branches to form the anterior and posterior esophageal plexuses. The left vagus then winds anteriorly and the right posteriorly, and the two vagi descend in the esophageal sheath through the diaphragm to reach the stomach.

The esophagus is connected with the *esophageal orifice of the diaphragm* by strong fibrous tissue throughout its circumference.

The *abdominal portion of the esophagus* is approximately 1 to 3 cm. in length and runs in the esophageal groove on the posterior surface of the liver.

The esophagus is a tubular structure for the most part, except that its lower end, when relaxed, may form a sac, which is a combination of what has been called the *ampulla* and the *vestibule,* depending upon whether it is above or below the diaphragm. Friedland,* after a very extensive historical review, prefers the term *vestibule.* He has called the junction of the tubular area and saccular portion the *tubulo-vestibular junction (ring "A"* of Wolf et al.).

There are two *sling fibers* of inner muscle of the stomach that are shaped like an inverted "U," arching around the true esophago-gastric junction. The arms of these fibers lie anteriorly and posteriorly and parallel the lesser curvature of the stomach. Their junction with the esophagus is the true *esophago-gastric junction or ring "B"* of Wolf et al.

At rest and during quiet normal breathing, the vestibule is divided into the supradiaphragmatic portion called the ampulla and a subdiaphragmatic segment called by some the vestibule or the cardiac antrum. In normal adults a small amount of sliding of the vestibule through the esophageal hiatus may occur with swallowing or stress, but insignificant esophageal reflux is noted. This sliding does not occur in infants because of the more effective structure of the phrenico-esophageal membrane, and no stomach should protrude into the thorax.

With the formation of a hiatal hernia of the stomach, the elastic fibers of the phrenico-esophageal membrane are stretched (or there may be no elastic tissue) and the esophago-gastric junction is displaced above the esophageal hiatus (Fig. 14–11).

---

*Friedland, G. W.: A Historical Review of Lower Esophageal Anatomy: 430 B.C.–1977 (personal communication, being submitted for publication).

The diaphragm and its ligamentous esophageal attachments (phrenicoesophageal membrane) at the esophageal hiatus produce a valve-like action also called a constrictor cardiae.

Normal Points of Narrowness in the Esophagus. There are four definite constrictions in the normal esophagus (Fig. 14–6): one at its cricoid beginning, a second at the level of the aortic knob, a third opposite the crossing of the left bronchus, and the fourth at the place where it passes through the diaphragm. The lumen at the site of the upper constrictions is smaller than the fourth, and ordinarily, when a foreign body fails to pass down the esophagus, the site of obstruction occurs at one of the upper points of narrowness.

ESOPHAGEAL LIP. The esophageal lip is an indentation on the posterior aspect of the esophagus at its junction with the hypopharynx. It is postulated that this is caused by the cricopharyngeal muscle. Differential diagnosis of this formation from a foreign body or other abnormality may cause some problems. It is probable that the esophageal lip is not associated with dysphagia and is of no definite pathologic significance.*

The Normal Rugal Pattern of the Esophagus. The mucous coat of the esophagus is very loosely connected with the muscular coat by the areolar tissue of the submucous layer. When the esophagus is empty, the mucous coat is thrown into a series of longitudinal folds (Fig. 14–8); otherwise it is very smooth in contrast with the mammillated gastric mucous membrane.

The longitudinal folds of the empty or partially empty esophagus impart to the radiographic picture the typical rugal pattern attributed to this organ. These consist of parallel lines throughout the esophagus which become more closely approximated as the distal funnel end of the esophagus is reached just above the cardia (Fig. 14–8B).

Abnormalities in the esophageal wall are reflected to a great extent in alteration of this normal rugal pattern, either by the appearance of abnormal folds or by the lack of folds.

<hr>

*Siebert, T. L., et al.: Variations in the roentgen appearance of the "esophageal lip." Am. J. Roentgenol., *81*:570–575, 1959.

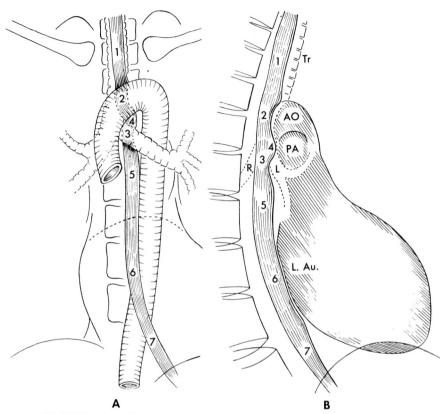

A　　　**B**

FIGURE 14–6 Segments of the esophagus. *A*. The segments of the thoracic esophagus (anteroposterior view): (1) paratracheal segment, (2) aortic segment, (3) bronchial segment, (4) interaorticobronchial triangle, (5) interbronchial segment, (6) retrocardiac segment, (7) epiphrenic segment.

B. The segments of the esophagus (right anterior oblique view). Shown are: trachea (Tr), right (R) and left (L) main bronchi, pulmonary artery (PA), left auricle (L. Au), and the different segments of the paratracheal (1), aortic (2), bronchial (3), interaorticobronchial (4), interbronchial (5), retrocardiac (6), and epiphrenic (7) esophagus. (From Brombart, M.: Roentgenology of the esophagus. *In* Margulis, A. R., and Burhenne, H. J., (eds.): Alimentary Tract Roentgenology, 2nd ed. St. Louis, C. V. Mosby Co., 1973.)

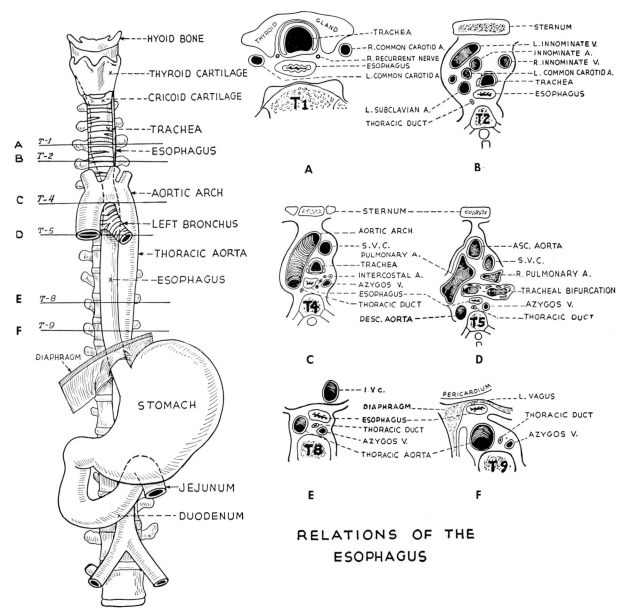

FIGURE 14–7 Relationship of esophagus to contiguous structures at various levels.

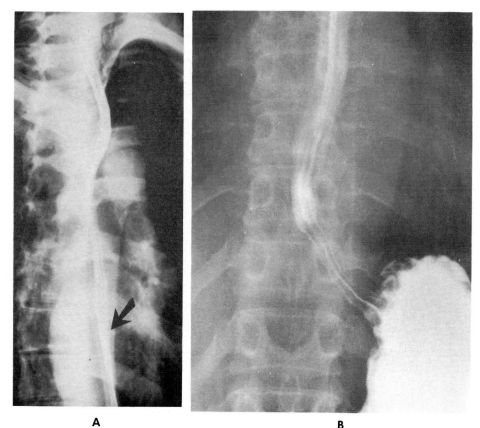

A   **B**

FIGURE 14–8 Rugal pattern of the esophagus. *A*. Upper. *B*. Lower.

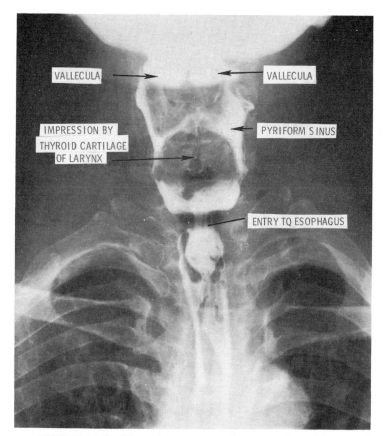

FIGURE 14–9 Normal anteroposterior projection of laryngeal and pharyngeal esophagus with barium: anatomic parts labeled.

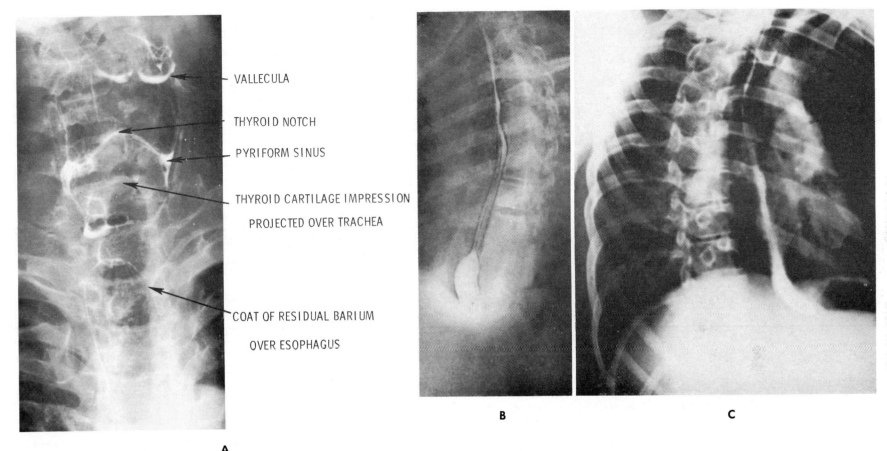

— VALLECULA

THYROID NOTCH

— PYRIFORM SINUS

— THYROID CARTILAGE IMPRESSION
PROJECTED OVER TRACHEA

COAT OF RESIDUAL BARIUM

OVER ESOPHAGUS

A

B

C

FIGURE 14–10 *A*. Pharyngeal region and upper esophagus coated with a thin coat of barium. *B*. and *C*. Radiograph of esophagus in both obliques, with *B* demonstrating the esophageal phrenic ampulla (intensified) and *C* showing the rugal pattern of the esophagus. The ampulla is most likely the supradiaphragmatic portion of the saccular dilatation of the lower esophagus during restful breathing.

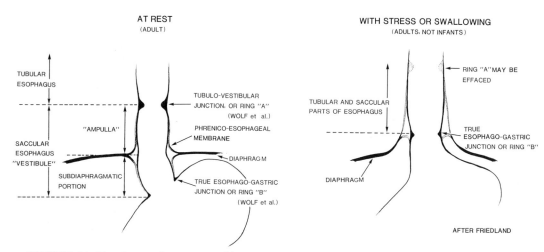

FIGURE 14-11 Anatomic concept of lower esophagus. (After Friedland.)

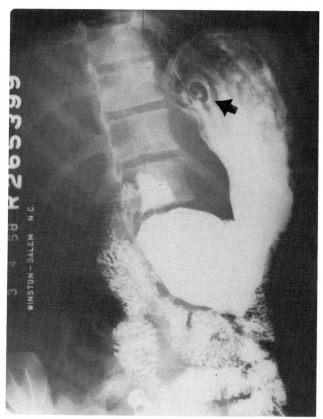

FIGURE 14-12 "Epithelial ring" at the cardioesophageal junction most likely formed by the "sling fibers" of the stomach.

The submerged segment functions most effectively when a portion of the esophagus lies beneath the diaphragm (esophageal vestibule), where the diaphragmatic contraction assists in establishing a high pressure zone to prevent reflux from the stomach to the esophagus. It is when the fundus slides above the diaphragm through a patulous hiatus to create a hiatal hernia that the function of this segment is most vulnerable and the barrier furnished by it to regurgitation and reflux may be inadequate to protect the lower esophagus from the refluxing digestive enzymes of the stomach.

The junction of the vestibule and fundus of the stomach is often demarcated by an epithelial ring which can be identified radiographically ("sling fibers") (Fig. 14-12).

With a hiatal hernia, a ring is often identified between the esophagus and herniated portion of stomach; it is called a "Schatzki ring" or a "Templeton ring." This is in fact a B ring. It is probably of clinical significance when its transverse measurement is less than 13 mm. (Fig. 14-13) and when there is an associated reflux to the level of the tracheal bifurcation.

The constrictor cardiae is at the gastroesophageal junction and ordinarily is located beneath the diaphragm at the junction of the esophageal and gastric mucosa. There is an abrupt change from the squamous epithelium of the esophagus to the columnar epithelium of the stomach at this site. At times, this epithelial line appears as an epithelial ring (Fig. 14-12) as previously illustrated.

FIGURE 14–13 *A*. Summary diagram illustrating herniations of the stomach through the diaphragm. *B*. Radiograph demonstrating Schatzki's ring.

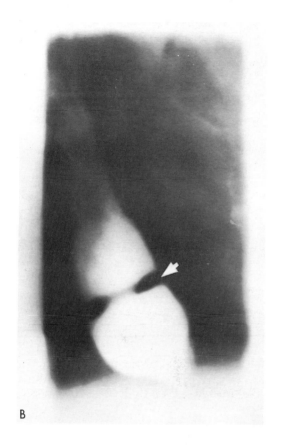

B

HERNIATIONS

SHORT ESOPHAGUS TYPE: CONGENITAL (RARE); POST-ESOPHAGITIS; SCLERODERMA

CONSTRICTION CONSTANT

GASTRIC FUNDAL RUGAL PATTERN

PERITONEUM

SECOND CONSTRICTION

PARA-ESOPHAGEAL HERNIA

PERITONEUM

FOR DEMONSTRATION OF THIS PORTION OF ESOPHAGUS, OBLIQUE VIEWS IMPORTANT TO SHOW FULL LENGTH OF ESOPHAGUS

PRONE POSITION WITH INCREASED INTRA-ABDOMINAL PRESSURE BEST FOR DEMONSTRATION

REDUNDANT ESOPHAGUS TO INDICATE IT IS NOT CON-GENITALLY SHORTENED

REMAINS CONSTANT AND CONTAINS FUNDAL RUGAL PATTERN - THUS DISTINGUISHED FROM ESOPHAGEAL AMPULLA

(SLIDING HERNIA: ESOPHAGUS "CURLED" AND NOT CONGENITALLY SHORTENED)

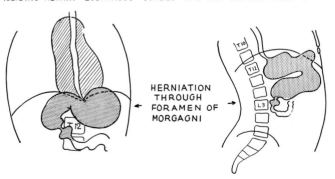

HERNIATION THROUGH FORAMEN OF MORGAGNI

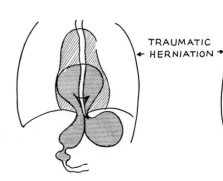

TRAUMATIC HERNIATION

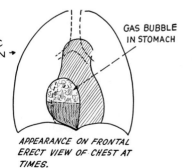

GAS BUBBLE IN STOMACH

APPEARANCE ON FRONTAL ERECT VIEW OF CHEST AT TIMES.

A

Blood Supply of the Esophagus

VENOUS DRAINAGE OF THE LOWER ESOPHAGUS AND ITS IMPOR-
TANCE. The veins of the esophagus form a plexus exteriorly (Fig.
14–15). The venous drainage of the lower esophagus passes to the
coronary vein of the stomach, and the latter vein empties into the portal
vein. Higher up, the veins of the esophagus empty into the azygos system and thyroid veins.

Thus, the esophagus forms a communicating link between the
portal circulation on the one hand and the systemic veins on the other,
since the azygos vein empties into the superior vena cava.

Obstruction of the portal vein from any cause may, in turn, cause
considerable distention of the lower esophageal veins and other tributaries of the coronary vein of the stomach. These irregular distentions
are spoken of as "varices," and have the appearance and the same
physiologic significance as hemorrhoids in the case of the anal canal
(Fig. 14–16). These veins may rupture and cause considerable em-
barrassment from bleeding. They produce a marked irregularity of the
rugal pattern of the lower esophagus, especially when the venous pressure is increased as in the case of forced expiration. Indeed, the relative
disappearance of the irregularity in deep inspiration, and reappearance
with forced expiration is pathognomonic of esophageal varices.

ARTERIAL SUPPLY OF THE ESOPHAGUS. The arterial supply of the
esophagus is derived from esophageal branches of the aorta (Fig. 14–14),
bronchial arteries, the inferior phrenic artery, and left gastric arteries.
Veins accompany these arteries, which usually number three at the
most. At times, esophageal branches are received from the bronchial
arteries. Ascending branches of esophageal arteries from an abnormal
level are also shown.

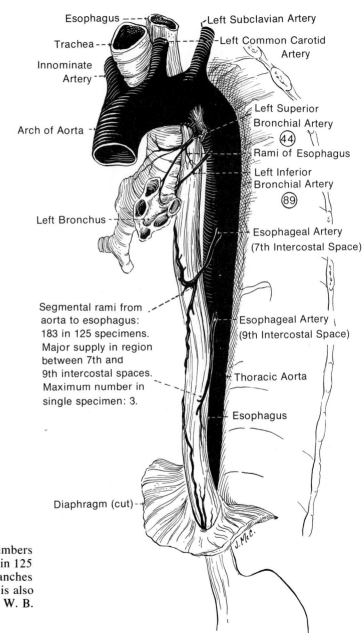

FIGURE 14–14 Thoracic sources of esophageal arteries, diagrammatic. The encircled numbers
represent the frequency with which esophageal rami arose from the particular bronchial artery in 125
dissections. Ascending branches of esophageal arteries from abdominal level and descending branches
of the segmental esophageal arteries of thoracic level are also shown. The innominate artery is also
called the brachiocephalic. (From Anson, B. J.: An Atlas of Human Anatomy. Philadelphia, W. B.
Saunders Co., 1963.)

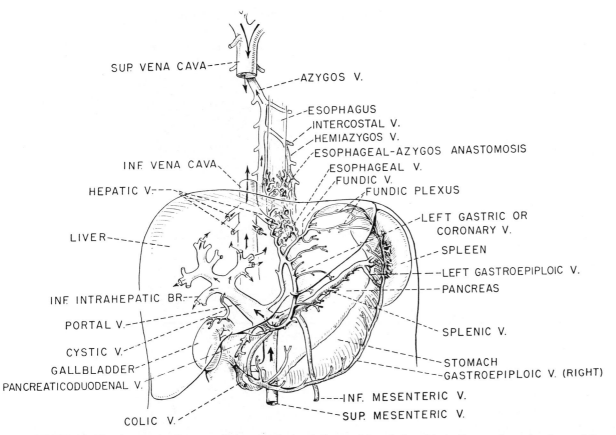

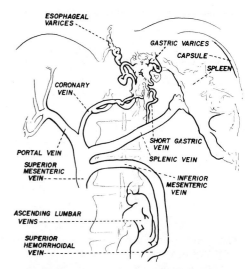

FIGURE 14–15 Anatomic diagram of the portal circulation and its relationship to the esophageal veins and the azygos venous system.

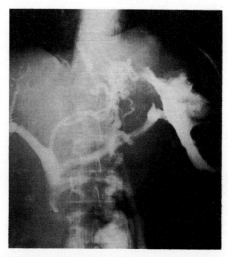

FIGURE 14–16 Roentgenogram at 12 seconds demonstrates coronary vein, gastric, and esophageal varices. The anastomosis between the inferior mesenteric vein and superior hemorrhoid plexus is demonstrated. The latter is also seen to drain into the vertebral venous plexus. Tracing is above. (From Evans, J. A., and O'Sullivan, W. D.: Am. J. Roentgenol. *77,* 1957.)

Technique of Examination of the Esophagus

Fluoroscopy. The proper examination of the esophagus involves a combination of fluoroscopy and radiography, with spot film radiography in selected areas. We now consider cinefluoroscopy and radiography to be an essential part of this examination with respect to the swallowing function.

The sequence is as follows: (1) survey fluoroscopy of chest; (2) survey fluoroscopy of abdomen; (3) the swallowing of a single mouthful of thin barium is studied in frontal and oblique perspective; (4) for mucosal detail, the swallowing of thick barium paste is thereafter viewed in frontal and oblique perspectives; (5) the patient is then placed in the supine position and the study is repeated. When the patient is in the left posterior oblique or prone on a bolus, regurgitation is assayed by gravity and positive pressure (Valsalva maneuver). The water test is done in this position also.

The Trendelenburg position is utilized when a hiatal hernia is suspected.

The prone position for demonstration of a hiatal hernia with the patient straining is particularly useful and is repeated with both thick and thin barium with the patient in the right anterior oblique position. Spot films are obtained in at least two separate sequences.

Films Obtained. (1) Anteroposterior film study of the esophagus, including neck to diaphragm (Figs. 14–17 and 14–18). (2) Right anterior oblique projection (Fig. 14–19). (3) Left anterior oblique projection (Fig. 14–20). (4) A lateral view of the neck with barium in the esophagus (Fig. 14–17 *B*).

Routine Film Studies of the Esophagus

Anteroposterior Film Study of the Neck (Fig. 14–17 *A*)

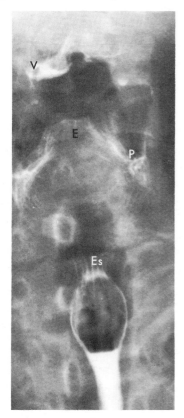

A

FIGURE 14–17 Upper esophagus and hypopharynx. *A*. Anteroposterior projection.

Figure continued on the opposite page.

Lateral Projection of the Upper Esophagus (Fig. 14–17 *B*). The upper esophagus is immediately posterior to the trachea and separated from it by a thin fascial plane.

The Anteroposterior Film Study Below the Neck (Fig. 14–18)

THICK BARIUM PASTE MAY BE PREFERABLE, SINCE IT REMAINS LONGER IN THE ESOPHAGUS FOR FILMING PURPOSES

THE CENTRAL RAY IS CENTERED OVER THE UPPER PORTION OF THE XYPHOID PROCESS

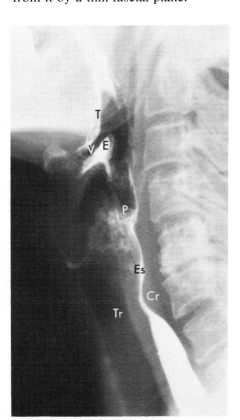

B

FIGURE 14–17 *Continued.* *B*. Lateral projection. (V) Vallecula. (E) Epiglottis. (P) Pyriform sinuses. (Es) Esophagus (T) Tongue. (Cr) Cricopharyngeus muscle indentation on esophagus. (Tr) Trachea.

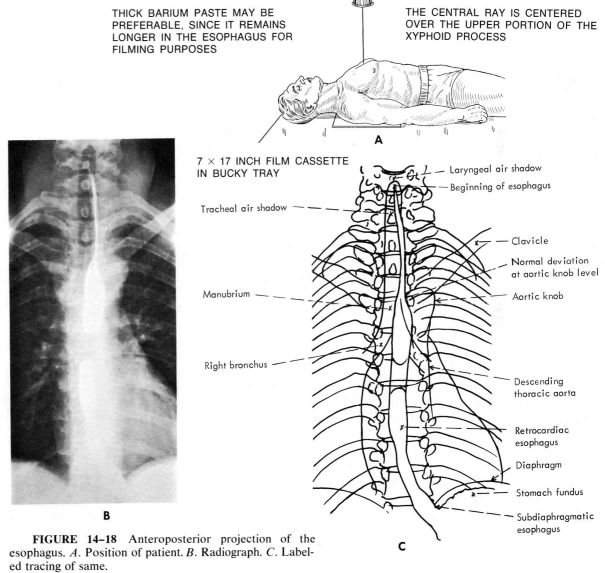

A

7 × 17 INCH FILM CASSETTE IN BUCKY TRAY

— Laryngeal air shadow
— Beginning of esophagus
Tracheal air shadow —
— Clavicle
— Normal deviation at aortic knob level
Manubrium —
— Aortic knob
Right bronchus —
— Descending thoracic aorta
— Retrocardiac esophagus
— Diaphragm
— Stomach fundus
— Subdiaphragmatic esophagus

B

C

FIGURE 14–18 Anteroposterior projection of the esophagus. *A*. Position of patient. *B*. Radiograph. *C*. Labeled tracing of same.

Right Posteroanterior Oblique Projection (Fig. 14–19)

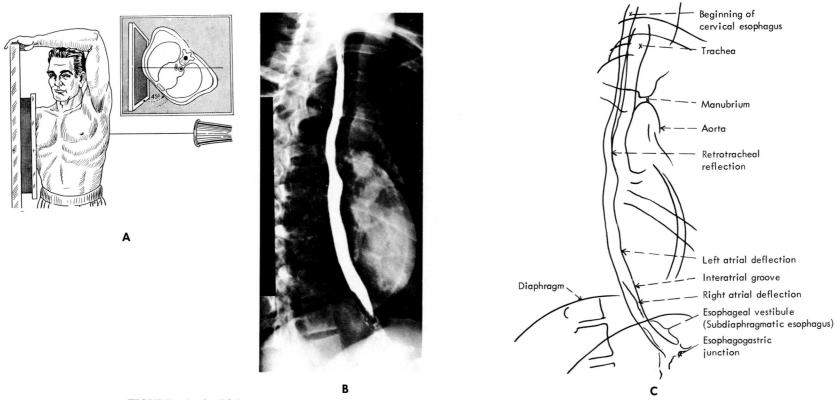

A

B

C

Beginning of
cervical esophagus

Trachea

Manubrium

Aorta

Retrotracheal
reflection

Left atrial deflection

Interatrial groove

Right atrial deflection

Esophageal vestibule
(Subdiaphragmatic esophagus)

Esophagogastric
junction

Diaphragm

FIGURE 14–19 Right posteroanterior oblique projection of esophagus. *A.* Position of patient. *B.* Radiograph *C.* Labeled tracing. (This same projection is frequently taken in the recumbent position as well.)

Iodized Oil Study. Iodized oil is possibly somewhat less irritating when inhaled into the trachea or bronchial tree than is the barium sulfate suspension. On the other hand, it is more expensive and somewhat more irritating to gastric mucosa.

When a patient gives a history of extreme difficulty in swallowing, followed by considerable coughing, it usually indicates that he inhales the swallowed bolus, at least in part. In such instances, an iodized oil such as Dionosil (oily) may be injected by syringe onto the back of the tongue and swallowed. The barium sulfate suspension may be used thereafter if inhalation of the Dionosil has not occurred.

This is particularly true in cases of pharyngeal palsies, pseudo-pharyngeal palsies, and such congenital anomalies as esophageal atresias, where there is usually a communication between the esophagus and the trachea or bronchial tree. Barium sulfate suspension may be used initially, however, if desired, since it has been tolerated as a bronchographic agent also.

Left Posteroanterior Oblique Projection (Fig. 14–20)

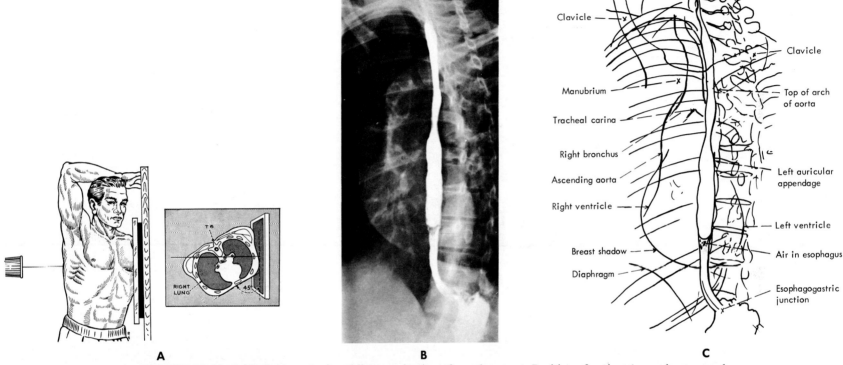

A   B   C

FIGURE 14–20 Left posteroanterior oblique projection of esophagus. *A*. Position of patient (recumbent may also be used). *B*. Radiograph (intensified). *C*. Labeled tracing.

Special Procedure for Suspected Swallowing of Foreign Body. (1) Lateral films of the neck and chest without contrast media. (2) Lateral film of the neck during deglutition, so that the calcified, cartilaginous structures will be elevated, bringing into clear relief any postcricoid foreign body. (3) Routine fluoroscopy of the esophagus as outlined above.

It has been recommended by some that the swallowing of a small cotton ball soaked with barium or a barium-filled gelatin capsule be employed. If this is done, interpretation must be carried forward with great caution since either of these may be delayed in transit and false conclusions drawn.

A plain survey film of the abdomen prior to the introduction of barium is advisable, as is an AP or PA film of the chest to determine whether or not the suspected foreign body has been aspirated into the chest or swallowed into the gastrointestinal tract below the level of the esophagus.

THE STOMACH AND DUODENUM

Subdivisions of the Stomach. The stomach is arbitrarily divided into three parts: the fundus, the body, and the pyloric portion (Fig. 14–21).

The fundus is that portion of the stomach that lies above a horizontal plane through the junction of the stomach and esophagus (this latter being called the "cardiac orifice" or "cardia"), and the pyloric portion is that part that falls between the incisura angularis and the pylorus. The body is represented by the intervening portion.

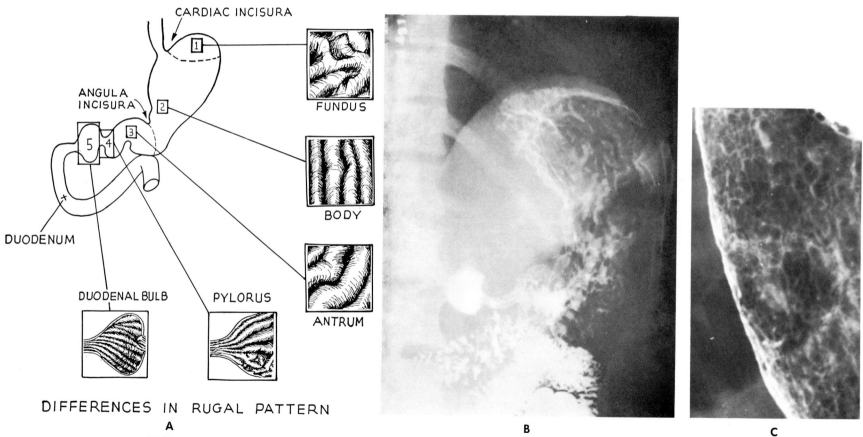

DIFFERENCES IN RUGAL PATTERN

A

B

C

FIGURE 14–21 Stomach. *A.* Subdivisions and rugal pattern. *B.* Radiograph showing rugal pattern. (The distal portion of the pyloric antrum is in a contracted state and its rugal pattern merges imperceptibly with the pattern of the pyloric canal.) *C.* Areae gastricae as shown by high-density double contrast barium-air technique of the stomach. These are the mammillated parts of the stomach as seen grossly when the stomach is opened.

The right wall of the cardia merges into the lesser curvature of the stomach, while the left wall is deeply notched by the cardiac incisura.

A pyloric constriction marks the junction between the stomach and duodenum. The pyloric sphincter is sharply demarcated from the duodenum, but blends imperceptibly with the thickened masculature of the pyloric antrum. The pyloric canal traverses the pyloric sphincter and is approximately 5 mm. in length. The gastric mucous membrane is continued into the duodenum without any alteration visible to the naked eye.

The greater curvature corresponds in its greater part with the attachment of the gastrosplenic and gastrocolic ligaments.

Stomach Contour Variations in Accordance with Body Build (Fig. 14–22). Gastric tone and contour normally follow the habitus of the individual closely. In the individual who is short and stocky, the stomach is usually high in position and "steerhorn" in shape, its lumen being largest above and tapering toward the pylorus. It extends more quickly toward the right. At times, it is even horizontal in position. The incisura angularis is difficult to identify, and occasionally the pylorus is the lowermost part of the stomach.

In the sthenic individual, the eutonic stomach is J-shaped, and the body of the stomach tends to be vertical in the frontal projection and uniform in size. The lowermost part of the stomach in the erect position tends to be at the level of the iliac crests.

In asthenic individuals, the stomach tends to be hypotonic, and shaped rather like a fishhook. The greater curvature tends to sag down into the pelvis, with the greatest diameter between the incisura angularis and the adjoining greater curvature.

Each of the stomach types may occur in individuals of any body build, but in general the hypotonic stomach tends to occur more frequently in underweight individuals, whereas the steerhorn type tends to occur more frequently in the overweight. Indeed, according to a study which we have conducted, when the hypotonic stomach occurs in an overweight individual, it is almost invariably symptomatic. Likewise, a cascade stomach tends to be symptomatic in an overweight person, whereas in normal or underweight individuals the cascade stomach is relatively asymptomatic. The symptoms are vague abdominal distress, sometimes suggestive of peptic ulcer.

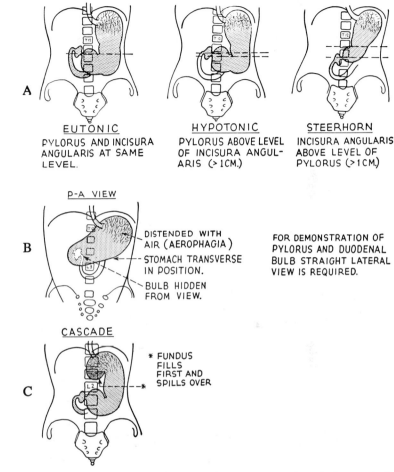

FIGURE 14–22 Variations in stomach contour. *A.* In relation to body build and general stomach type. *B.* The infantile stomach. *C.* The cascade stomach.

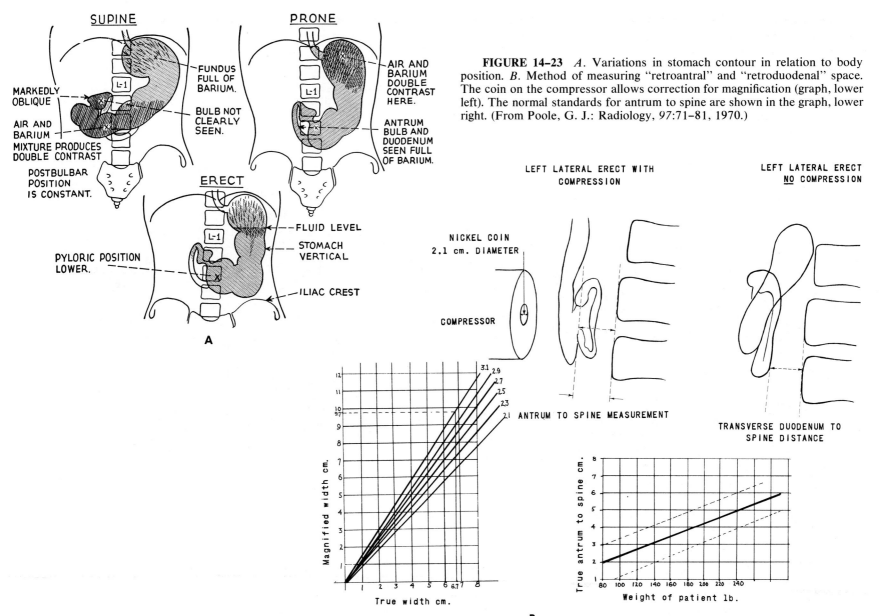

SUPINE

MARKEDLY OBLIQUE

AIR AND BARIUM MIXTURE PRODUCES DOUBLE CONTRAST

POSTBULBAR POSITION IS CONSTANT.

FUNDUS FULL OF BARIUM.

BULB NOT CLEARLY SEEN.

PRONE

AIR AND BARIUM DOUBLE CONTRAST HERE.

ANTRUM BULB AND DUODENUM SEEN FULL OF BARIUM.

ERECT

FLUID LEVEL

STOMACH VERTICAL

PYLORIC POSITION LOWER.

ILIAC CREST

A

FIGURE 14–23 *A*. Variations in stomach contour in relation to body position. *B*. Method of measuring "retroantral" and "retroduodenal" space. The coin on the compressor allows correction for magnification (graph, lower left). The normal standards for antrum to spine are shown in the graph, lower right. (From Poole, G. J.: Radiology, *97*:71–81, 1970.)

LEFT LATERAL ERECT WITH COMPRESSION

LEFT LATERAL ERECT NO COMPRESSION

NICKEL COIN 2.1 cm. DIAMETER

COMPRESSOR

ANTRUM TO SPINE MEASUREMENT

TRANSVERSE DUODENUM TO SPINE DISTANCE

Magnified width cm.

True width cm.

True antrum to spine cm.

Weight of patient lb.

B

The Duodenum. The duodenum is ordinarily examined simultaneously with the stomach, and it is discussed separately here for the sake of convenience only. The first part of the duodenum—the duodenal bulb—is integrated both structurally and functionally with the pyloric antrum. The structure of the remainder of the duodenum resembles that of the small intestine.

The duodenum differs from the rest of the small intestine in several important respects:

1. It has no mesentery, and is fixed to the posterior abdominal wall for the most part.

2. The ducts of the liver, gallbladder, and pancreas open into it (at the duodenal papilla, or ampulla of Vater) in the descending part of the duodenum.

3. The duodenum contains some distinctive glands of its own, the duodenal glands of Brunner, which abnormally may be hypertrophied.

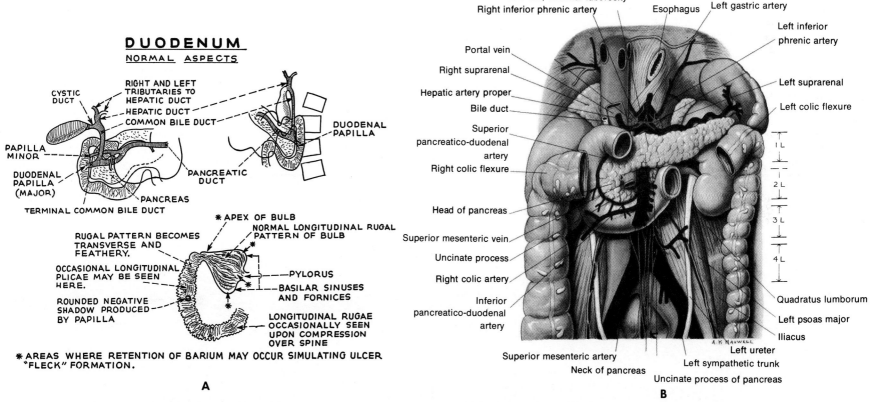

FIGURE 14–24 *A.* Normal relationships of the bile ducts to the duodenum, and the narrow mucosal patterns of the duodenum proper. *B.* A dissection to show the duodenum and pancreas. The right and left hepatic veins have been cut away at their points of entry into the inferior vena cava. The superior hypogastric plexus is shown in front of the sacral promontory and the sympathetic nerves which form it are seen descending across the bifurcation of the aorta, the left common iliac vein and the body of the fifth lumbar vertebra. (In this specimen the left renal artery is situated anterior to the left renal vein at the hilus of the kidney.)

4. It is the shortest, widest, and most fixed portion of the small intestine.

SUBDIVISIONS. The duodenum is variably described as consisting of three or four parts (Fig. 14–24):

1. The superior portion, or duodenal bulb, which runs superiorly backward and to the right, is in direct continuity with the pylorus of the stomach. This portion has a mesentery of its own for a short distance.

2. The descending portion, which begins at the neck of the gallbladder, runs down on the posterior abdominal wall and usually ends approximately opposite the upper border of the fourth lumbar vertebra on the right of the vertebral column.

3. The inferior part is variably described as having one or two separate parts. It consists of a transverse portion, which crosses to the left of the midline, across the vena cava, aorta, and vertebral column; and an ascending portion, which ascends on the left of the vertebral column to the inferior surface of the pancreas. There it bends abruptly forward, forming the duodenojejunal flexure.

The duodenum is in the form of a U, with the superior portion more anterior than the descending part, the transverse portion coming directly forward and to the left, and the ascending portion in the same plane as the superior portion but to the left of the midline.

The rugal pattern of the bulb more closely resembles that of the pyloric antrum than the remainder of the duodenum, tending to be rather parallel, or parallel in spiral fashion from the base to apex. The contraction pattern and motor physiology of the bulb form a transition between that of the antrum and the distal duodenum.

Radiologically, a "fleck" (from the German meaning "spot") is a loculation of barium of any size from a few millimeters to 2 or more centimeters which strongly suggests a break in the normal mucosal structure and ulceration. In view of the great frequency of ulceration in this area, the detection of a fleck in this location is of extreme importance.

There are certain locations in the duodenal bulb, however, where fleck formation may be a normal variant, and these must be differentiated from the pathologic variety: (1) when the pylorus closes, there may be a dimple of mucosa at the base of the bulb in which the barium may accumulate, giving rise to the appearance of a fleck (Fig. 14–25); (2) the outer periphery of the base of the bulb occasionally acts as a groove, or sinus, in which barium may accumulate, and when seen in profile, gives the appearance of fleck formation at the base of the bulb; (3) the concentration of rugae at the apex of the bulb may simulate fleck formation on occasion also; (4) flecks of an inconstant variety may be simulated by peristaltic waves passing over the duodenal bulb.

The anatomic relationships of the bulb which are important are as follows: the duodenal bulb forms the inferior boundary of the foramen epiploicum (foramen of Winslow), and hence a pathologic penetration of the bulb finds ready access into the lesser omental bursa (Fig. 14–28). The hepatic artery is also in contact for a short distance with the superior margin of the bulb. Below, the bulb rests on the head and neck of the pancreas. There are several large blood vessels which come into close contact with this area (Fig. 14–28), and are of considerable importance from the standpoint of possible erosion of an ulcer. On the left side lie the portal vein, gastroduodenal artery (and bile duct); close to the posterior aspect is the right side of the inferior vena cava; and adjoining the inferior margin are the superior pancreaticoduodenal and the right gastroepiploic vessels.

The common bile duct may occasionally indent the bulb, giving rise to an apparent deformity, and the gallbladder lies in close apposition with the superior and right margins of the first part of the duodenum, occasionally producing an indentation of the duodenum.

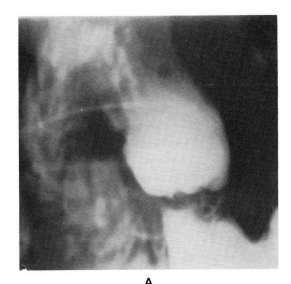
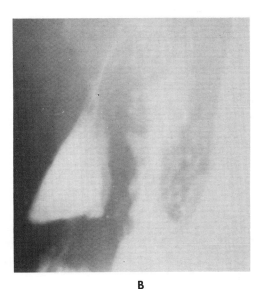
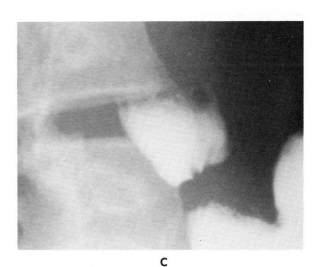

A   B   C

FIGURE 14–25 Spot film radiographs of the duodenal bulb in the right posteroanterior (*A*) and left posteroanterior oblique (*B*) projections. *C*. There is a "dimple" at the base of the duodenal bulb when the pylorus closes normally. The dimple simulates an ulcer niche.

The second, or descending part of the duodenum. Description of villi and plicae circulares. This part of the duodenum is retro-peritoneal in position with the root of the transverse mesocolon, crossing it at its middle. The head of the pancreas is in contact with its left margin (Fig. 14–29) and occasionally overlaps it both anteriorly and posteriorly, and along this margin run the branches of the pancreati-coduodenal arteries. The bile duct, after descending behind the duodenal bulb, passes between the head of the pancreas and this part of the duodenum, where it joins with the pancreatic duct. The two together pierce the duodenal wall obliquely, and open by a common orifice on its inner aspect at the apex of the duodenal papilla (ampulla of Vater) medially (Fig. 14–31).

The mucous membrane of this part of the duodenum, as well as all parts of the small intestine, presents a soft, velvety internal surface which is caused by the presence of the minute mucosal processes known as villi. These begin at the edge of the pyloric valve where they are quite broad, but they become narrower as they proceed down the small intestine. The only place they are not found is immediately over the solitary lymph nodules. These villi play an important part in the absorption function of the small intestine (Figs. 14–24 and 14–26).

The mucous membrane of the small intestine is thrown into numerous folds which may to a great extent disappear upon distention, but there are permanent folds known as the plicae circulares (Fig. 14–30) or valvulae conniventes. They are crescentic folds running around the small intestine in circular fashion. They may bifurcate, and they usually project about 8 mm. into the lumen of the small intestine. *They begin in the second part of the duodenum,* and gradually become more prominent, so that in the region of the duodenal papilla, they are very distinct and remain prominent in the rest of the duodenum. The combination of the plicae circulares and the villi imparts a feathery pattern to the duodenum and jejunum when viewed radiographically in the absence of distention, and this is the typical rugal pattern not only of the duodenum but also of the jejunum. The absence of plicae circulares in the duodenal bulb accounts for its closer resemblance radiographically to the pyloric antrum.

The horizontal portion of the inferior part of the duodenum (third part). This part is somewhat concave upward, is retroperitoneal, and is crossed by the superior mesenteric vessels and the root of the mesentery near the midline. It crosses the inferior vena cava, and is closely applied to the inferior aspect of the head of the pancreas.

The ascending portion of the inferior part of the duodenum (fourth part). This part lies on the aorta, the left renal vein, and occasionally also the left renal artery (Fig. 14–33). As previously indicated, it extends obliquely anteriorly and to the left, and its left side lies in contact with some coils of small intestine. In addition to being clothed by peritoneum anteriorly (as is the case of the second and third parts), it is also covered by peritoneum on its left side.

The duodenojejunal flexure is fixed by the musculus suspensorius (suspensory ligament) of Treitz, opposite the left side of the first or second lumbar vertebrae. This latter suspensory muscle blends with the muscular coat of the duodenum, passes upward behind the pancreas to blend partially with the celiac artery, and then is attached to the right crus of the diaphragm.

In the neighborhood of the ascending part of the duodenum, three peritoneal fossae may frequently be present (Fig. 14–36). Two of these, the superior and inferior duodenal fossae, are formed by slips of fibrous tissue covered by peritoneum extending from the left side of the duodenum to the peritoneal surface adjoining it, and form very small pouches directed caudad and cephalad, respectively. The third, however, which is called the paraduodenal fossa, is produced by a fold of peritoneum formed by the inferior mesenteric vein as it courses along the left lateral side of the ascending part of the duodenum. The inferior mesenteric vein is accompanied in part of its course by the left colic artery. This fossa is capable of forming a hernial sac, and therefore may be of some clinical significance.

Importance of a study of the duodenal contour. The duodenum is in a fixed position for the most part, and hence variations from its normal position become significant in the detection of space-occupying lesions in adjoining structures, such as the pancreas, lesser omental bursa, colon, gallbladder, and biliary ducts.

There is, however, a considerable variation in different individuals in the normal contour of the duodenum. To a great extent, this is correlated with body habitus. Thus in pyknic individuals with high steer-horn stomachs, the duodenal loop appears widened; and in asthenic individuals, portions of the duodenal loop will appear to be very close to one another, and sometimes overlapping. Occasionally, there is a redundancy of the first part of the duodenum (Fig. 14–35) with a greater segment peritonealized than is ordinarily seen. In some individuals, the second part of the duodenum may be virtually lacking, and it would appear that the superior part of the duodenum connects almost directly with the horizontal part of the inferior portion of the duodenum.

These normal variations and anomalies must be constantly borne in mind when radiography of the duodenum is attempted.

Variations in the appearance of the duodenal bulb (Fig. 14–34).

The duodenum distal to the duodenal bulb. The second, third, and fourth portions of the duodenum have the normal feathery mucosal pattern already described. They appear as a single loop, with peristaltic waves carrying the barium around this loop.

Occasionally the duodenal papilla in the middle of the descending part of the duodenum will fill with barium or produce a small filling defect in the contour of the duodenum. This must not be interpreted as abnormal.

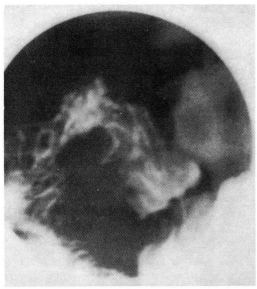

FIGURE 14–26 Mucosal pattern of the duodenal bulb and the change in pattern which occurs at the beginning of the second part of the duodenum.

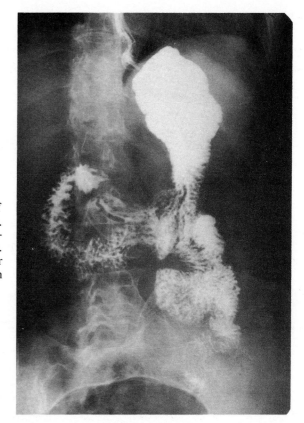

FIGURE 14–27 Anteroposterior projection of stomach in slight left posterior oblique position. Note the excellent double contrast of the distal stomach while the fundus is completely filled with barium. Note also the changes in mucosal pattern which occur more distally in the bulb and duodenum as well as in the jejunum.

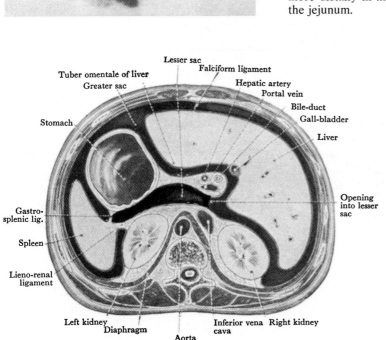

FIGURE 14–28 Transverse section of abdomen to show the arrangement of peritoneum at the level of the opening into lesser sac. (From Brash, J. C. (ed.): Cunningham's Manual of Practical Anatomy, 12th ed., Vol. 2. London, Oxford University Press, 1958.)

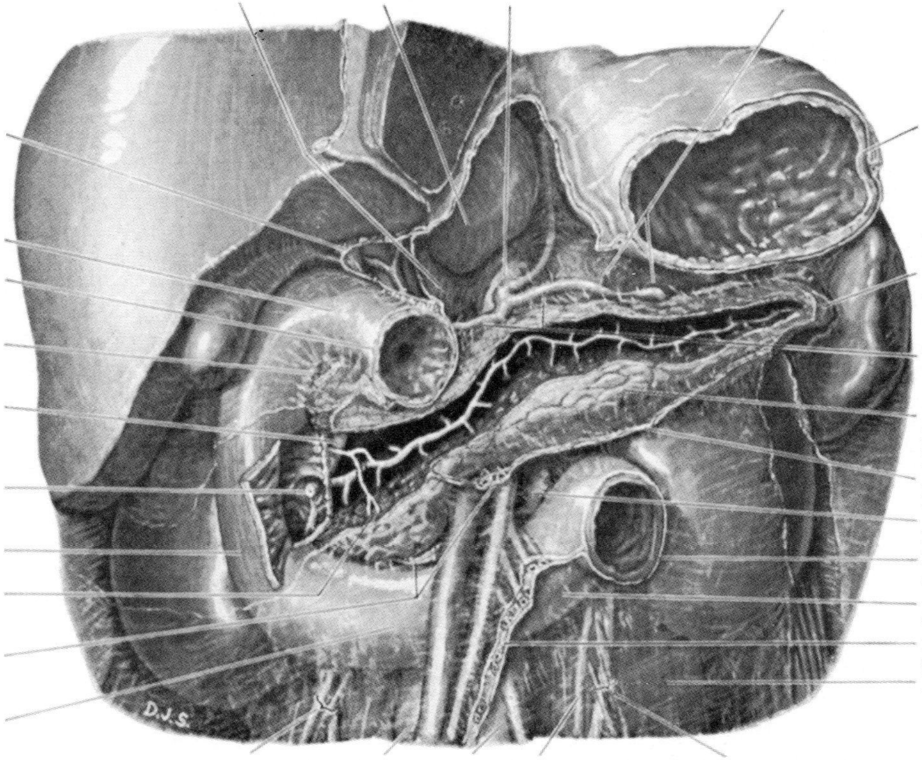

Inf. vena cava

Caudate lobe of liver

Aorta between crura of diaphragm

Left suprarenal gland and kidney

Lesser omentum with bile duct, hepatic a. and portal vein

1st part of duodenum

Pylorus over neck of pancreas

Sup. pancreatico-duodenal vessels

Bile duct
Exit of bile and main pancreatic ducts on duodenal papilla

2nd part of duodenum

Accessory pancreatic duct enters duodenum above main duct

Inf. pancreatico-duodenal and mid. colic vessels

3rd part of duodenum

Upper part of stomach pulled aside

Tail of pancreas at hilum of spleen

Hepatic and splenic brs. of coeliac a.

Body of pancreas, covered by lesser sac

Transverse mesocolon

Uncinate process

Beginning of jejunum

4th part of duodenum

Mesentery, cut

Psoas

Rt. testicular vessels crossing ureter

Inf. vena cava

Aorta

Inf. mesenteric vein

Left testicular vessels crossing ureter

FIGURE 14–29 Dissection of duodenum and pancreas. Transverse colon and part of stomach removed. (Reprinted by permission of Faber and Faber, Ltd.; from Lockhart, Hamilton, and Fyfer: Anatomy of the Human Body. London, Faber and Faber; distributed by J. B. Lippincott Co., Philadelphia.)

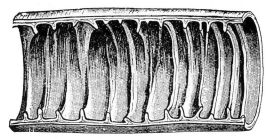

FIGURE 14–30 Anatomic presentation of the plicae circulares of the small intestine (jejunum). (From Cunningham's Textbook of Anatomy, 6th ed. London, Oxford University Press, 1931.)

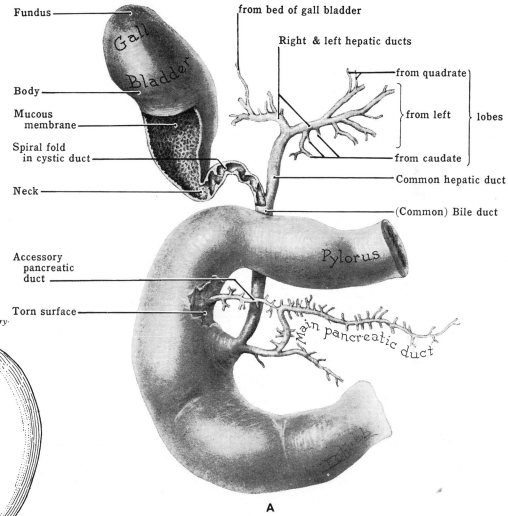

FIGURE 14–31 *A.* Extrahepatic bile passages and the pancreatic ducts. (Reproduced by permission from J. C. B. Grant: An Atlas of Anatomy, 5th ed. Baltimore, The Williams & Wilkins Co., 1962. © 1962 The Williams & Wilkins Co., Baltimore.) *B.* Posterior aspect of the pancreas and duodenum from behind. (From Warwick, R., and Williams, P. L. (eds.): Gray's Anatomy, 35th British ed. Longman, London [for Churchill Livingstone], 1973.)

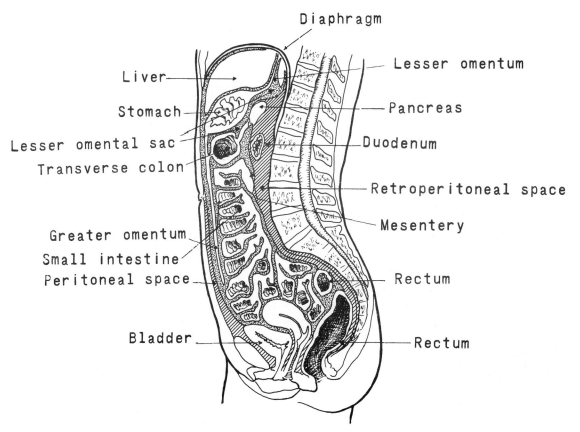

FIGURE 14–32 Sagittal section diagram of the abdomen, demonstrating the retrogastric space and the ligamentous attachments of the transverse mesocolon as well as the small bowel mesentery. Potential spaces around these mesenteries as well as those in the lesser omental bursa are indicated. (After Pernkopf, E.: Atlas of Topographical and Applied Human Anatomy. Philadelphia, W. B. Saunders Co., 1964.)

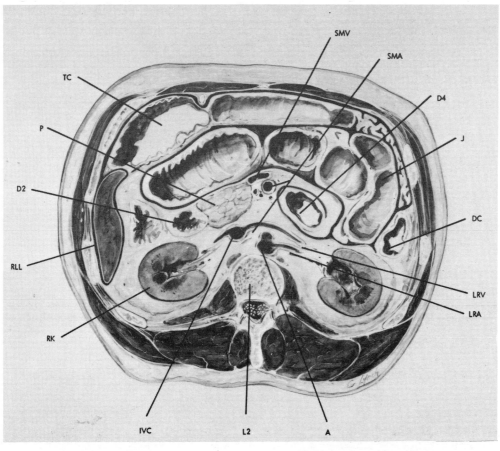

TC	=	TRANSVERSE COLON	SMV	=	SUPERIOR MESENTERIC VEIN
P	=	HEAD OF PANCREAS	SMA	=	SUPERIOR MESENTERIC ARTERY (MORE DISTAL)
D2	=	2nd PORTION OF DUODENUM	OSMA	=	ORIGIN OF SUPERIOR MESENTERIC ARTERY
RLL	=	RT. LOBE OF LIVER	D 4	=	4th PORTION OF DUODENUM
RK	=	RT. KIDNEY	J	=	JEJUNUM
IVC	=	INFERIOR VENA CAVA	DC	=	DESCENDING COLON
L2	=	L2 LEVEL	LRV	=	LT. RENAL VEIN
A	=	AORTA	LRA	=	LT. RENAL ARTERY

FIGURE 14–33 Transverse section through abdomen at the level of the second lumbar vertebra. Section through the hepatorenal space (compartment for liver, colon, duodenum, and kidneys) and retrogastric space (lesser omental bursa) of peritoneal cavity.

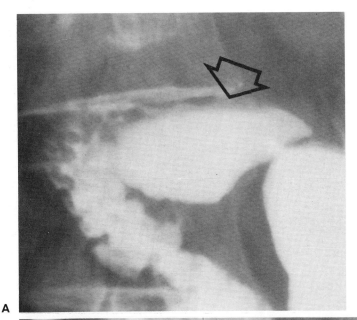

A

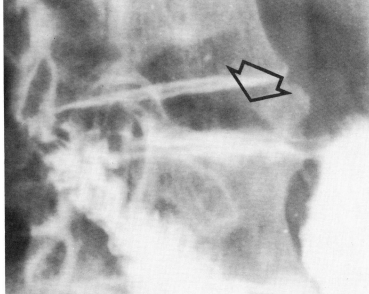

B

FIGURE 14-34 *A* and *B*. Normal duodenal bulb in two stages of contraction. *B* simulates an elongated pyloric canal.

DUODENAL ANOMALIES

DEFECTIVE ATTACHMENT OF DUODENAL MESENTERY

MOBILE DUODENUM

DUODENUM APPEARS INVERTED

DUODENUM HAS NORMAL APPEARANCE

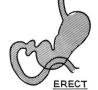

RECUMBENT

ERECT

NONROTATION OF DUODENUM

LOWER DUODENUM CURVES TO RIGHT INSTEAD OF LEFT AND JOINS JEJUNUM IN RIGHT UPPER QUADRANT *(USUALLY NONROTATION OF JEJUNUM ALSO.)*

NOT INVOLVED *(ARISES FROM FOREGUT)*

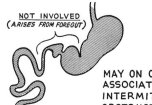

MAY ON OCCASION BE ASSOCIATED WITH INTERMITTENT OBSTRUCTION.

REDUNDANCY – FIRST PART

REDUNDANCY- 3rd PART

INVERTED DUODENUM

MAY PREDISPOSE TO PANCREATITIS DUE TO TWIST OF BILE DUCT AND REFLUX INTO PANCREAS.

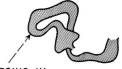

INVERSION BEGINS IN 2nd PART USUALLY.

FIGURE 14-35 Duodenal anomalies.

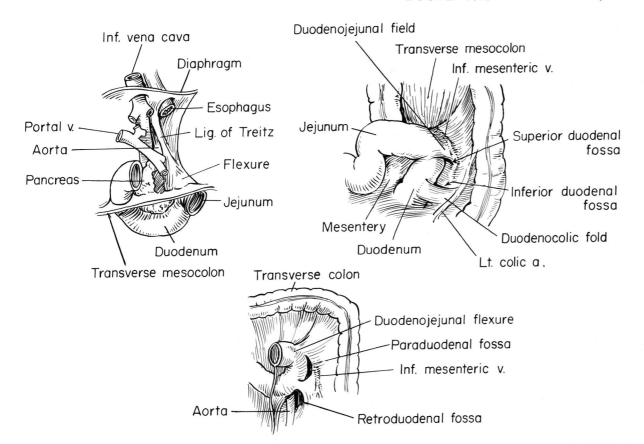

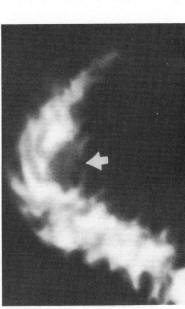

FIGURE 14-37 Occasional normal appearance of the major papilla indenting the second part of the duodenum.

FIGURE 14-36 Line drawing indicating the structures involved at the duodenojejunal flexure and the duodenal fossae and folds. Note the superior duodenal fossa, the inferior duodenal fossa, and the paraduodenal fossa as well as the relationship to the duodenojejunal flexure.

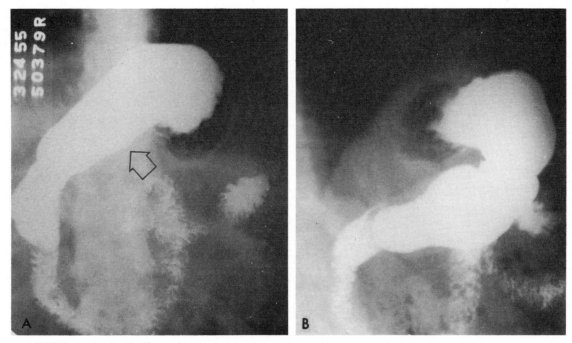

FIGURE 14–38 Radiographs demonstrating an intermittent type of organoaxial rotation of the stomach. In *A* the inferior margin of the stomach is concave and the stomach is situated high under the diaphragm. In *B* the stomach is in a relatively normal position. This type of rotation has also been referred to as "incomplete volvulus."

The Rugal Pattern of Each Subdivision of the Stomach (Fig. 14–21). When the stomach is wholly or partially empty, the muscular layers contract and throw the mucosa into numerous folds or rugae which project into the interior of the stomach. The rugae of the fundus tend to be arranged in a mosaic, which gradually becomes more regular in the body of the stomach. The mosaic appearance is more marked along the greater curvature and this pattern gradually diminishes toward the pylorus.

The rugae tend to remain parallel in a narrow segment on the lesser curvature of the stomach throughout the entire length of the stomach from the cardia to the pylorus. These longitudinal rugae form the "mag-enstrasse," which seems to constitute a channel for the usual descent of the food, although not invariably so.

The rugae in the pylorus are thin parallel folds. These parallel folds continue into the duodenal cap or bulb, where they either remain parallel or spiral toward the apex of the duodenal bulb.

Between the rugae, there are minute depressions caused by the openings of the small gastric glands, and minute ridges around them, giving the stomach mucosa the so-called mammillated appearance. These minute mammillae are recognizable radiographically as the "areae gastricae."

The rugal pattern of the stomach must not be thought of as com-

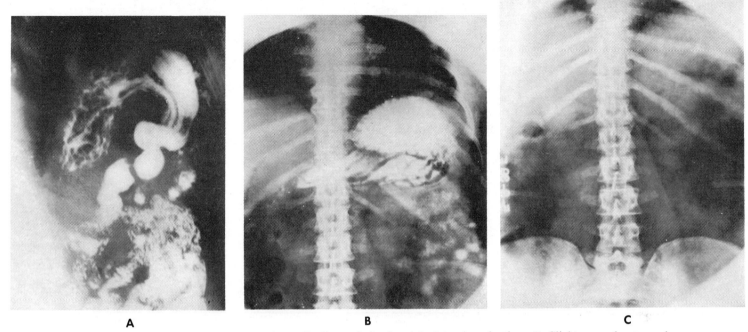

FIGURE 14–39 "Cascade" stomach. *A*. Radiograph in the right lateral projection. *B*. Slight cascade stomach in anteroposterior projection. *C*. Same as *B* without the barium, showing how the fundus of such a stomach may simulate a mass in the left upper quadrant. (*B* and *C* courtesy of Drs. H. L. Friedell and C. C. Dundon, University Hospitals, Cleveland, Ohio.)

pletely static—it can vary in the same individual under different physiologic conditions. Thus, it will vary in accordance with the degree of vascularity of the mucosa and submucosa and also with the degree of distention of the stomach. Cold tends to make the rugae smaller and more numerous, and certain chemicals such as pilocarpine and physostigmine have the same effect, whereas atropine has the opposite effect.

However, the rugal pattern will change in certain pathologic states such as inflammation, ulceration, and neoplastic infiltration, as well as from extrinsic pressure, and the rugae thus become one of the most accurate indices which the radiologic examination of the stomach furnishes. Examination for rugal pattern constitutes one of the most important aspects of the gastrointestinal examination, if not the most important.

"The Areae Gastricae" (Fig. 14–21). The mammillated appearance of the gross specimen of the stomach and its corresponding radiograph are sometimes aggravated in gastritis. (See also Fig. 14–44*B*.)

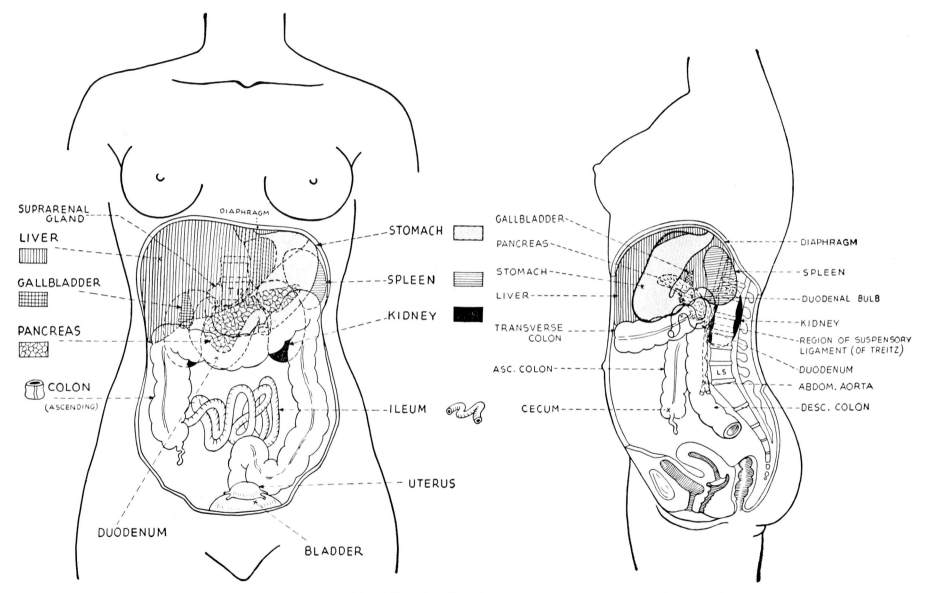

FIGURE 14–40 Important anatomic relationships of the stomach. *A*. Anteroposterior view. *B*. Lateral view (right recumbent).

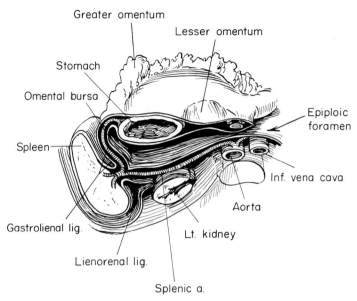

FIGURE 14–41 Cross section showing relation of stomach, spleen, and adjoining structures to lesser omental bursa and epiploic foramen.

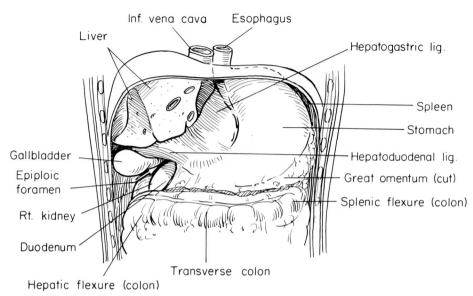

FIGURE 14–42 Stomach in situ, with hepatic ligaments, greater omentum cut.

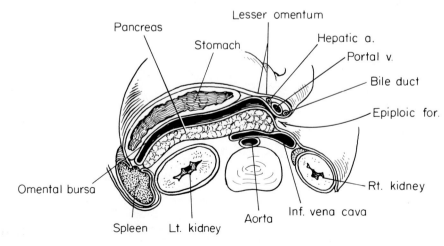

FIGURE 14–43 Transverse section showing relationship of pancreas and stomach to lesser omental sac.

Physiologic Considerations Concerning the Stomach

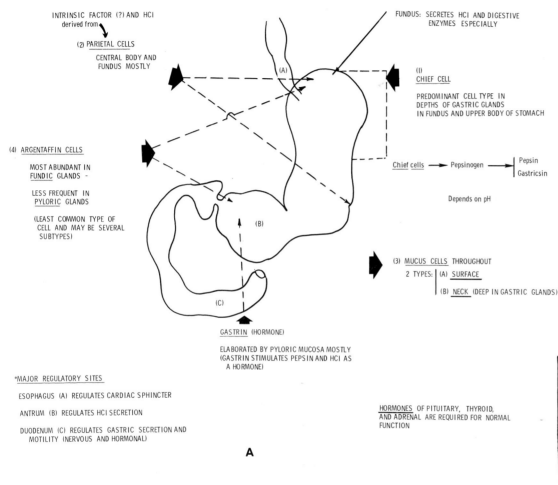

INTRINSIC FACTOR (?) AND HCl
derived from

(2) PARIETAL CELLS

CENTRAL BODY AND
FUNDUS MOSTLY

FUNDUS: SECRETES HCl AND DIGESTIVE
ENZYMES ESPECIALLY

(A)

(I)
CHIEF CELL

PREDOMINANT CELL TYPE IN
DEPTHS OF GASTRIC GLANDS
IN FUNDUS AND UPPER BODY OF STOMACH

(4) ARGENTAFFIN CELLS

MOST ABUNDANT IN
FUNDIC GLANDS -

LESS FREQUENT IN
PYLORIC GLANDS

(LEAST COMMON TYPE OF
CELL AND MAY BE SEVERAL
SUBTYPES)

Chief cells → Pepsinogen → | Pepsin
| Gastricsin

Depends on pH

(B)

(3) MUCUS CELLS THROUGHOUT

2 TYPES: | (A) SURFACE
| (B) NECK (DEEP IN GASTRIC GLANDS)

(C)

GASTRIN (HORMONE)

ELABORATED BY PYLORIC MUCOSA MOSTLY
(GASTRIN STIMULATES PEPSIN AND HCl AS
A HORMONE)

*MAJOR REGULATORY SITES

ESOPHAGUS (A) REGULATES CARDIAC SPHINCTER

ANTRUM (B) REGULATES HCl SECRETION

DUODENUM (C) REGULATES GASTRIC SECRETION AND
MOTILITY (NERVOUS AND HORMONAL)

HORMONES OF PITUITARY, THYROID,
AND ADRENAL ARE REQUIRED FOR NORMAL
FUNCTION

A

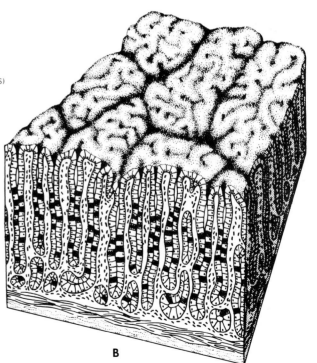

B

FIGURE 14–44 *A.* The sites of origin of the gastric glandular secretions. *B.* Diagram of mucosal islands interlaced by furrows or sulci that make up the radiographic appearance of areae gastricae. (Courtesy of Drs. Gerald Dodd and Harvey Goldstein, M.D. Anderson Hospital and Tumor Institute, Houston, Texas.)

Physiologic Considerations Concerning the Stomach

Gastric and Duodenal Evacuation, Tone and Peristalsis. Usually from two to five simultaneous peristaltic waves are observed in the stomach, with the greatest activity occurring in the distal half. The stomach will empty its contents when the pressure in the stomach exceeds the pressure in the duodenum; regurgitation from the duodenum will occur when there is a reversal of this pressure relationship. The pyloric antrum, pylorus, and duodenal bulb tend to act as a single unit in response to various food stimuli.

After the introduction of barium into the stomach, emptying begins almost immediately, and the main bulk of the barium meal will have left the stomach in 1 to 2 hours, with no residual trace after 3 hours. Hyperacidity in the stomach will permit the retention of a coating of barium on the gastric mucosa that in itself is not an indication of abnormality. Six-hour retention to any significant degree is pathologic, and it is customary to obtain a film 3 to 6 hours later for this purpose. On the other hand, retention in infants may be normal up to 8 hours after a barium meal, but anything beyond 8 hours may be interpreted as pathologic.

The main function of the pyloric sphincter normally is to prevent regurgitation from the duodenum into the stomach.*

"In brief, it is the purpose of the stomach to accept almost anything that is presented to it in almost any volume, by bringing this material to body temperature and proper isotonicity and dilution (fats, condiments, etc.) to make it acceptable to the relatively 'intolerant' duodenum and then deliver it to the duodenum at a moderate rate."†

In the presence of gastric retention it must not be assumed that the obstruction is necessarily pyloric in origin. At times, inadequacy of the evacuation mechanism may result from a hypotonicity of the stomach from some undetermined cause (that is, vagotomy). It would be folly to treat such dysfunction with atropine-like drugs (Fig. 14–45).

---

*Quigley, J. P., and Meschan, I.: The gastric evacuation of fat with special reference to pyloric sphincter activity. Gastroenterology, 4:272–275, 1937.

†Quigley, J. P., and Louckes, H. S.: Am. J. Dig. Dis., 7:672–676, 1962.

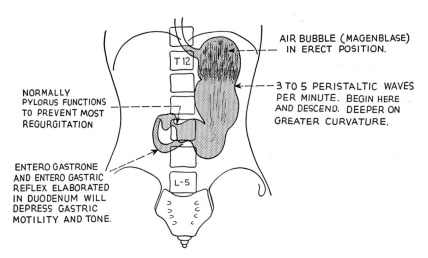

AIR BUBBLE (MAGENBLASE) IN ERECT POSITION.

T 12

NORMALLY PYLORUS FUNCTIONS TO PREVENT MOST REGURGITATION

3 TO 5 PERISTALTIC WAVES PER MINUTE. BEGIN HERE AND DESCEND. DEEPER ON GREATER CURVATURE.

ENTERO GASTRONE AND ENTERO GASTRIC REFLEX ELABORATED IN DUODENUM WILL DEPRESS GASTRIC MOTILITY AND TONE.

L-5

FIGURE 14–45 Diagram illustrating résumé of gastric motor physiology.

Gastric Tone. Vagal stimulation increases gastric tone, whereas sympathetic stimulation decreases it. Thus, when a person is frightened or otherwise emotionally disturbed, the stomach tends to be hypotonic. Pathologic processes in the gastrointestinal tract elsewhere or the biliary tract may also cause changes in the stomach.

Factors Influencing Rate of Gastric Evacuation. Of practical importance are the following normal considerations:

The type of meal will alter the rate of gastric evacuation considerably. The presence of any food will depress gastrobulbar peristalsis and prolong the emptying time by about three times. This function is caused by a reflex or hormone (enterogastrone) operating from the duodenum. The presence of alkali such as sodium bicarbonate in the stomach will increase the rate of gastric evacuation. Only isotonicity, with no food substances contained in the meal, will not alter the rate of evacuation.

Cascade Stomach (Fig. 14–39). Occasionally, the posterior portion of the fundus of the stomach will fill first, and the remainder of the stomach will fill by overflow from the fundus. This is called a cascade stomach. It may be related to overdistention of the splenic flexure of the colon or to localized muscular hypertonus. Occasionally it is related to adhesions between the stomach and the diaphragm, but it cannot be properly called a normal variation under these circumstances.

Methods of Roentgenologic Study of the Stomach and Duodenum

Technique of Fluoroscopy and Spot Film Compréssion Radiography (Figs. 14–46, 14–47, 14–48, 14–49). Full Column Barium Study

1. With the patient standing, after the initial survey of the chest and abdomen, the patient is given a cup of barium suspension containing 100 grams of barium sulfate suspended in a glassful (8 oz.) of water.

2. The manner in which the barium enters the stomach is carefully studied. Ordinarily, this first swallow of barium follows along the "magenstrasse" on the lesser curvature of the stomach. In the presence of excessive fluid in the stomach, the barium drops into the fluid like pellets in a glass of water. Spot films of the rugal pattern of the stomach are obtained at this time, particularly in the right anterior oblique projection; compression is used, if necessary.

3. Otherwise, the patient, still in the right anterior oblique, is given additional swallows of barium, and the swallowing function as well as the stomach are studied. The gastroesophageal junction and the action of the constrictor diaphragmae are particularly noted. The patient is in frontal and right anterior oblique projections at this point, and additional spot film studies of the duodenal bulb are obtained in these projections (Fig. 14–46 *E*).

4. The patient then swallows the remainder of the barium, and peristalsis and contour of the stomach and duodenum are studied in all projections. An additional spot film of the stomach or duodenal bulb in the left anterior oblique projection is obtained if necessary (Fig. 14–46).

This provides a profile study of the duodenal bulb on its anterior and posterior aspect as well as the stomach on its lesser and greater curvature.

5. The patient is then turned with his right side toward the table, arms above his head, leaning slightly in the right anterior oblique, and the tilt table is turned into the horizontal so that the patient is lying somewhat prone on his right side.

6. The gastroesophageal junction, peristalsis of the stomach, and the duodenum are then studied in this right lateral relationship. A spot film of the entire duodenal loop is obtained at this juncture (Fig. 14–46 *G*), and, if desired, an additional film of the gastroesophageal junction.

7. The patient is next turned to the prone or the 45-degree oblique position, and peristalsis of the entire stomach and duodenum is carefully studied and spot films obtained as necessary.

8. Next, the patient is turned onto his left side at an obliquity of 45 degrees. Gas in the stomach will then rise to the pyloric antrum, duodenal bulb, and duodenum. One or two spot films of the entire duodenal loop are taken with the double contrast provided by the air enter-

ing the antrum and the duodenum (Fig. 14–53). Additional spot films of the stomach are obtained with this double contrast evaluation. With the patient lying somewhat flatter on his back, the entire fundus is carefully studied since it is now filled with barium (Fig. 14–46 K).

9. In the same position (45 degrees oblique, supine, left side down), the patient is given an additional half cup of barium to swallow. The entire esophagus is then studied and spot films are obtained of the esophagogastric junction with the patient performing the Valsalva maneuver (Fig. 14–46 K). After several swallows of barium, the patient is encouraged to empty the contents of his mouth, and attempt an additional straining maneuver to see whether or not gastroesophageal reflux is obtained in this projection.

10. Further tests for gastroesophageal reflux may be made by turning the patient into the Trendelenburg position at this time and studying regurgitation with a swallow of water. The barium normally will reflux back somewhat into the esophagus, but abnormally a considerable admixture of water with the barium rises from the stomach back into the esophagus.

11. If a hiatal hernia is noted or if esophageal varices are suspected, thick barium is then administered in order to study the rugal pattern of the lower esophagus with and without the Valsalva maneuver. Varices will impart a wormlike pattern to the lower esophageal rugae which is accentuated by the Valsalva maneuver. This accentuation is virtually pathognomonic of esophageal varices in contrast with other irregularities such as esophagitis, which produce a somewhat similar appearance.

This routine of examination of the esophagus, stomach, and duodenum is the one we have followed satisfactorily for a considerable period of time. Other routines in current use may be found in the study reported by Burhenne* of 15 different institutions in the United States and Europe.

Double-Contrast Studies of the Stomach and Duodenum. In recent years, the importance of double-contrast studies of the stomach has been emphasized by some Japanese and other authors who feel that a double-contrast technique enhances the opportunity to demonstrate minute papillary detail, especially in the stomach. The technique for this type of examination varies; generally, however, it involves the following: (1) administration of high-density barium suspensions (HD 200 — Lafayette, Indiana) with or without simethicone (to adsorb bubbles of gas); (2) administration of gas emitters called "sparklers," which contain a mixture resembling Seidlitz powder (citrates and bicarbonates of sodium); (3) rotation of the patient 360 degrees twice in the recumbent position; (4) obtaining films of the stomach and duodenum every 45 degrees through a complete 360-degree rotation of the patient; and (5) obtaining, finally, films in the semi-erect or erect positions for the best ultimate demonstration of each small segment of the stomach and duodenum. By this technique, even the small mammillary mucosal pattern of the stomach related to the *oreae gastricae* (Fig. 14–21) is shown. It is perhaps somewhat more difficult to determine processes such as atrophic gastritis by this means, since the stomach is so distended that mucosal folds are erased (Fig. 14–52).

---

*Burhenne, H. J.: Technique of examination of the stomach and duodenum. *In* Margulis, A. R., and Burhenne, H. J. (eds.): Alimentary Tract Roentgenology. St. Louis, C. V. Mosby Co., 1973.

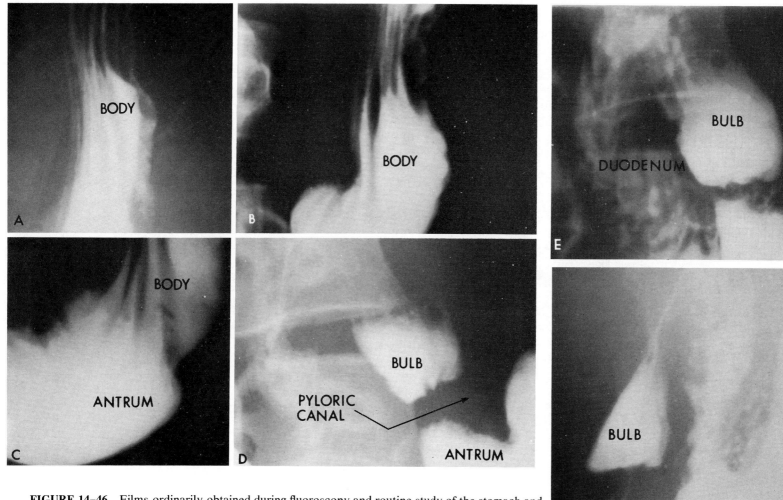

FIGURE 14–46 Films ordinarily obtained during fluoroscopy and routine study of the stomach and duodenum. *A*. Initial spot film of gastric rugae (body of stomach) immediately following the first swallow of barium. *B*. Second spot film showing the rugal pattern of the body and antrum. *C*. Third spot film demonstrates the lower half of the body and antrum of the stomach. *D*. Spot film showing the distal antrum, pyloric canal, and initial filling of the duodenal bulb. *E*. Somewhat later spot film study of the duodenal bulb after the barium has emptied from it into the second part of the duodenum (patient still in the erect position). *F*. Spot film study in the left anterior oblique, demonstrating the full duodenal bulb, especially in relation to its anterior and posterior margins. The apex of the bulb and second part of the duodenum are also well demonstrated.

Figure continued on the following page.

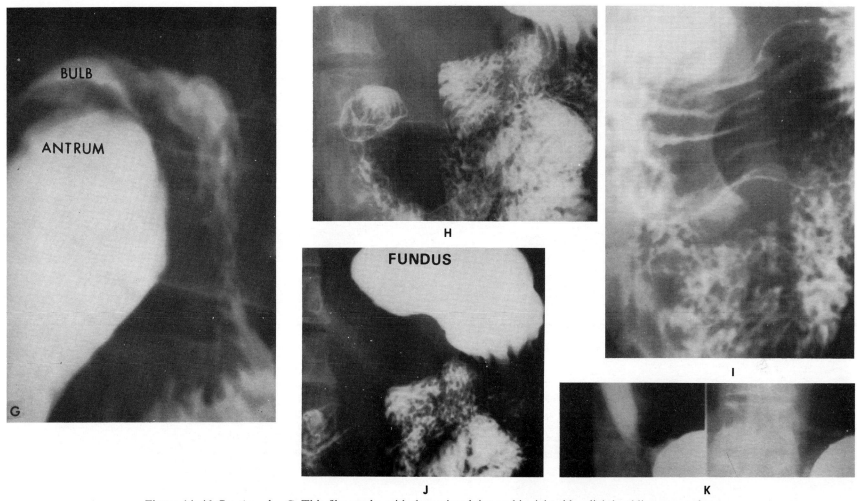

Figure 14–46 *Continued.* *G.* This film study, with the patient lying on his right side, slightly oblique toward prone, demonstrates the relationship of the stomach, the duodenum, and the duodenal bulb. *H.* Patient supine with right side elevated, left side down. The air rises into the duodenal bulb and second part of the duodenum, imparting to these structures a double contrast. A spot film is then obtained. *I.* Patient supine with air occupying the body of the stomach for demonstration of double contrast visualization of the rugae of the body of the stomach. *J.* Patient supine with the barium moving by gravity into the fundus of the stomach. The full contour of the fundus of the stomach is thereby studied. *K.* Patient supine on left side. Additional swallows of barium are given and the esophagus studied both morphologically and physiologically. The patient is asked to strain with the Valsalva maneuver immediately after swallowing and then after the esophagus is emptied. The esophagus is studied for possible gastroesophageal reflux. This may be followed by a "water test" in all cases where hiatal hernia is demonstrated and where esophageal reflux is suspected.

Routine Films Obtained Following Fluoroscopic Study

In addition, the *routine radiographs usually obtained are:* (1) recumbent posteroanterior (prone), straight frontal projection (Fig. 14–47); (2) right anterior oblique prone (Fig. 14–48); (3) right lateral recumbent (Fig. 14–49); (4) posteroanterior full abdominal view in 4 or 6 hours for study of the extent of gastric evacuation (Fig. 14–51).

Posteroanterior Projection. The patient is prone, with median plane of his body centered to the center of the table. The cassette in the Bucky tray is centered to the stomach. The central ray is centered to the midpoint of the film.

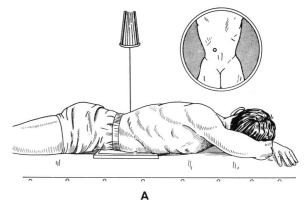

A

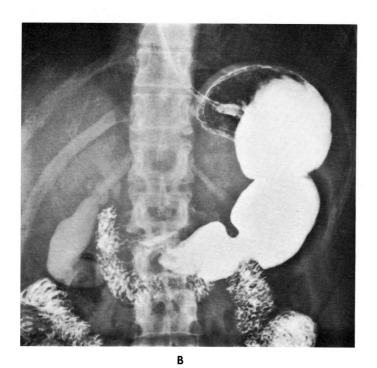

B

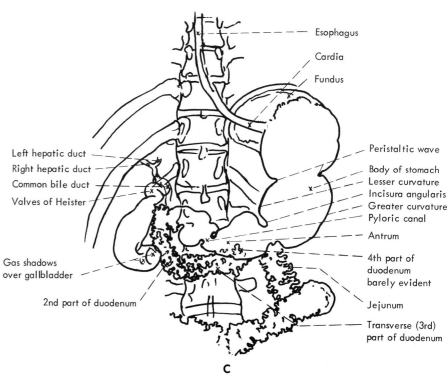

C

FIGURE 14–47 Recumbent posteroanterior projection of stomach and duodenum (an oral cholecystogram was also obtained at this time in the film illustrated). *A.* Position of patient. *B.* Radiograph. *C.* Labeled tracing.

Right Posteroanterior Oblique Prone Projection (Fig. 14–48). The arm is down by the side. The left arm and leg are flexed as shown. The body is rotated approximately 30 degrees, or a second film may be obtained with a 45-degree rotation. The midline of the table falls midway between the spine and forward aspect of the patient's body. The cassette is in the Bucky tray, centered longitudinally to the stomach; the central ray is centered to the midpoint of the film.

Gastric peristalsis is very active when the patient is in this position.

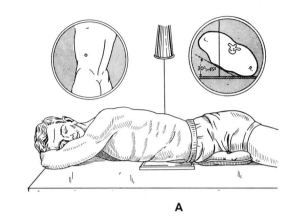

A

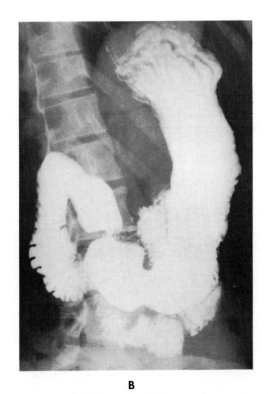

B

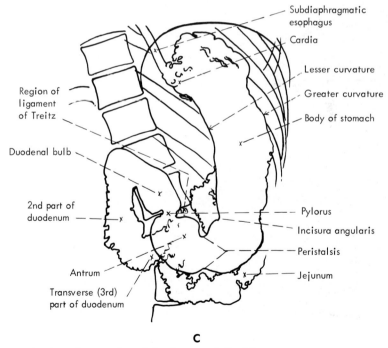

C

FIGURE 14–48   Right posteroanterior oblique prone projection of stomach and duodenum. *A*. Position of patient. *B*. Radiograph. *C*. Labeled tracing.

Right Lateral Recumbent Projection of the Stomach and Duodenum (Fig. 14–49). The knees are flexed. The table is centered to the midaxillary plane of the body. The cassette is in the Bucky tray beneath the stomach and duodenum; the central ray is centered to the midpoint of the film. The stomach, in the recumbent position, swings like a hammock away from the spine.

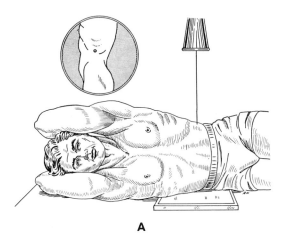

A

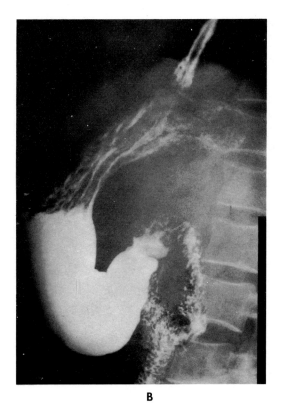

B

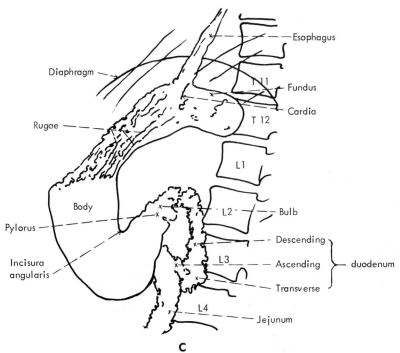

C

FIGURE 14–49   Right lateral recumbent projection of stomach and duodenum. *A.* Position of patient. *B.* Radiograph. *C.* Labeled tracing.

Left Lateral Erect Projection of Stomach and Duodenum (Fig. 14–50).
The left lateral erect view of the stomach and duodenum is most useful
to demonstrate the exact relationship of the stomach to retrogastric
structures. Anatomic detail is obscured, and hence this film study is
obtained when especially indicated by clinical history suggesting
pancreatic or retrogastric disease.

The midaxillary line coincides with the midline of the table. The
film is centered 2 to 4 inches lower than in the recumbent position. The
central ray is centered to the midpoint of the film. In this view the retrogastric and retroduodenal space may be measured if a pressure device
with a coin in view (for correction of magnification) is applied to the
stomach (Poole's method; see text, page 598).

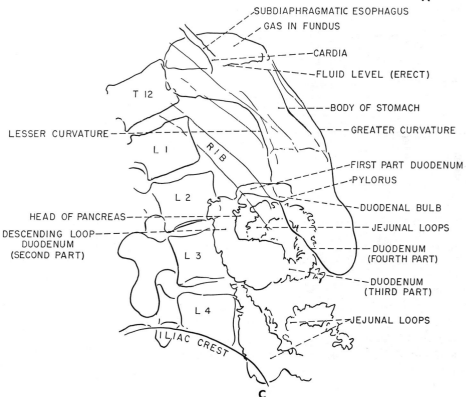

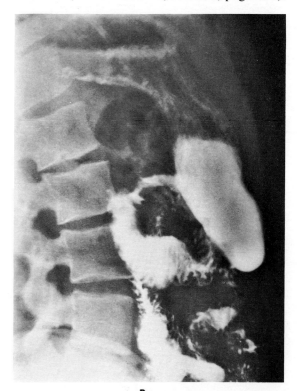

FIGURE 14–50 Left lateral erect projection of stomach. *A*. Position of patient. *B*. Radiograph. *C*.
Labeled tracing of *B*. (Very often this view is combined with the Poole type of compression view with compression of the stomach and duodenum against the spine, as illustrated in Figure 14–23.)

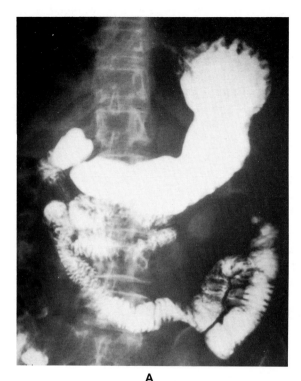

A

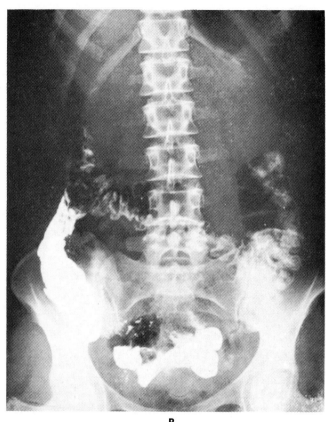

B

FIGURE 14–51 *A.* The full 14 × 17 posteroanterior projection of the stomach and proximal small intestine obtained with routine Bucky technique, immediately following the fluoroscopy. *B.* Six-hour film study of gastric evacuation.

Anteroposterior Projection of Stomach in Slight Left Posterior Oblique (Fig. 14–46 *I*). In this position, the air in the stomach rises and when admixed with the barium furnishes a double contrast visualization of the body, antrum, and bulb, and a completely barium-filled fundus. Filling defects and mucosal disturbances are thereby sometimes intensified in these areas.

Double-Contrast Examination of the Stomach. As previously in-

dicated, there are several useful variations of this method. The one most advantageous to us has been the utilization of high-density barium suspension (200 per cent weight per volume, 3 to 4 ounces in the total mixture). Immediately after ingestion of the barium, the patient is given small carbon dioxide–producing granules in a quantity sufficient to produce about 300 ml. of gas. The granules contain mixtures of sodium bicarbonate, tartaric acid, citric acid, and foam-absorbing agents such as dimethyl polysiloxane (simethicone). The patient is then placed in the left lateral projection, is recumbent, and is rotated 360 degrees twice.

The most useful views thereafter are the following: the anteroposterior supine; the left posterior oblique; the right lateral recumbent, then the table is elevated 45 degrees upright, and an additional right posterior oblique film is obtained. Often, a straight anteroposterior upright film is also obtained.

A view which is sometimes added, especially to emphasize the anterior wall of the stomach, is a steep right anterior oblique view, with the patient in a steep Trendelenburg position.

Some investigators have emphasized the importance of obtaining films in the recumbent position at 45-degree intervals, of rotating the patient through 360 degrees, coupled with the 45-degree upright right posterior oblique, and the Trendelenburg right anterior oblique position.

Spot films of the duodenal bulb and entire duodenal loop are obtained as previously described and required, especially in the supine and erect positions.

Special Studies of the Stomach and Duodenum

Hypotonic Duodenography. Hypotonic duodenography refers to a barium and gas study of the duodenum after the administration of a gas-producing medication or intubation, followed immediately by an atropinelike drug. Double contrast visualization of the duodenum has proved to be of considerable value in studying both intraluminal and extraluminal disorders of this area. Thirty to 60 mg. of Pro-Banthine is administered intramuscularly (or 30 mg. intravenously, adult dose) for this purpose. The barium may be injected by tube also if a duodental tube is used for the introduction of the air. At times, it may be satisfactory to allow air to enter the duodenum from the stomach at the time the antivagal drug is administered. The patient should be in the supine left posterior oblique position. *Pro-Banthine is contraindicated in pa-tients with heart abnormalities or glaucoma. One to five mg. of glucagon may be used instead in nondiabetic patients.*

Some advantages of double contrast in the duodenum and hypotonic duodenography are shown in Figure 14–53.

Duodenal atony occurs about 5 minutes after the intramuscular introduction of 60 mg. of Pro-Banthine and lasts about 20 minutes. The subtle alteration in the pancreaticoduodenal interface has been carefully studied by this method in the normal (Ferrucci et al.).* The method allows: (1) differentiation of duodenal mucosal fold effacement, (2) differentiation of pathologic papillary defects from normal papilla, and (3) straightening of the contour of the duodenum. Lesions of the tail of the pancreas cannot be studied in this way.

Utilization of Water-Soluble Contrast Media for Gastrointestinal Study. Water soluble contrast media have been recommended by some (Rea; Jacobsen et al.),* when barium is contraindicated. This is best administered by gastric tube since it is bitter to taste. A flavoring agent may be added to make it more palatable but this may alter normal physiologic responses.

Sixty cc. of 60 per cent Hypaque or Gastrografin or 50 grams of powdered Hypaque dissolved in 75 cc. of sterile water, to which 10 drops of a wetting agent (Tween-80) have been added, are utilized as the contrast agent.

For examination of the lower gastrointestinal tract, or in dehydrated patients, the use of these water soluble media is probably contraindicated since they are hyperosmotic and cause further water imbalance. They are also probably contraindicated in infants, in whom dehydration by the hyperosmotic medium may be disturbing unless intravenous fluids are administered simultaneously. However, in general, these agents (Hypaque or Gastrografin) may be used whenever barium mixtures can be used, with the proviso that small quantities be employed (Sidaway; Neuhauser).*

---

*References may be obtained in Meschan, I.: An Atlas of Anatomy Basic to Radiology. Philadelphia, W. B. Saunders Co., 1975, Chapter 13.

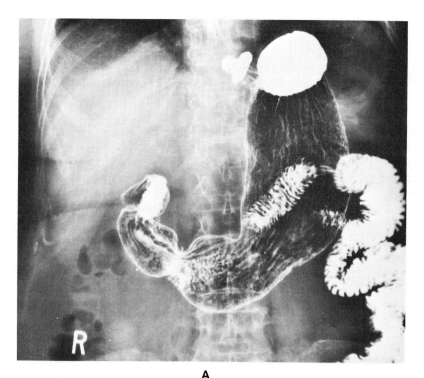

A

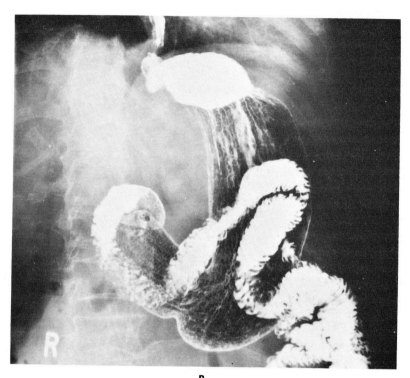

B

FIGURE 14–52 Examples of double-contrast high-density barium–air studies of the stomach. *A.* In the posteroanterior projection. *B.* In the right anterior oblique projection.

Figure continued on opposite page.

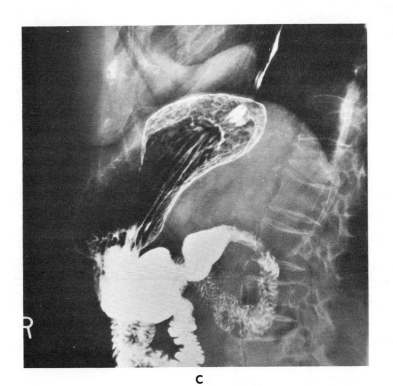

C

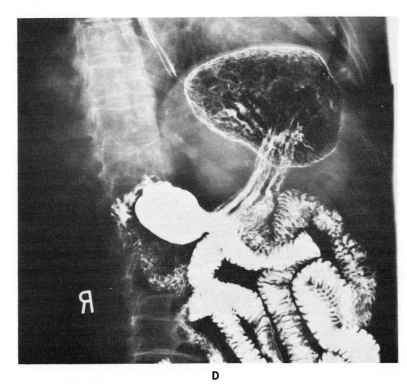

D

FIGURE 14–52 *Continued.* *C.* In the right lateral projection. *D.* Patient supine with left side elevated and right side lower, angulation approximately 30°.

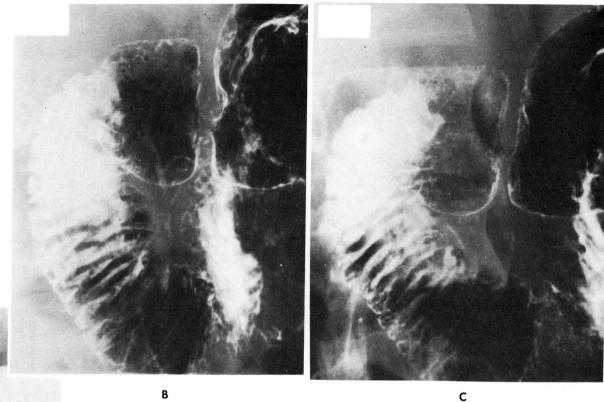

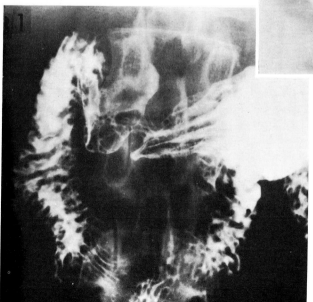

FIGURE 14–53 The difference between the depiction of the duodenum with and without hypotonic duodenography. *A.* Routine filling of the duodenum. *B.* and *C.* The duodenum has been paralyzed by the prior administration of 1 mg. of glucagon intramuscularly and by the introduction in the left posterior oblique position of the patient lying on his back of air from the stomach so that a high-density double-contrast barium-air visualization of the duodenal bulb and duodenum can be obtained.

Emergency Study of the Upper Gastrointestinal Tract for Bleeding. When patients are unable to stand for any reason, we have modified our technique for fluoroscopy as follows:

1. The patient lies obliquely on his right side, prone, facing the examiner. He drinks one or two swallows of barium from a straw.

2. The swallowing function and esophagus are studied as the barium is swallowed and moves into the stomach.

3. The stomach is then studied with small and large quantities of barium, first in this position (right oblique, prone), then with the patient on his left side, and finally rotating the patient onto his back

4. When the patient is supine, he is turned toward his left and lies obliquely on his left side, permitting a double contrast visualization of the antrum and duodenum.

5. Thick barium may be administered, particularly if esophageal varices are suspected. The patient may be asked to carry out, with caution, the Valsalva maneuver.

6. Spot films are taken as necessary throughout the procedure. There is a greater tendency in this examination to make "full spot" films of the entire stomach and duodenum rather than the smaller, more confined views.

7. Routine posteroanterior, right anterior oblique, right lateral, and left posterior oblique projections are obtained. A left lateral decubitus may be obtained if desired.

This procedure is not intended to replace the routine gastrointestinal examination, which is repeated at a suitable interval after cessation of the emergency (Knowles et al.; Hampton).*

Pharmacoradiology in Evaluation of Gastrointestinal Disease. Smooth muscle stimulation by means of pharmacodynamic agents has long been recommended for evaluation of stomach and duodenum (Pancoast; Ritvo; Adler et al.: Bachrach; Rasmussen; Silbiger and Donner).* Such agents as insulin, morphine, Dilaudid, atropine, Prostigmin, pethidine, Pro-Banthine, opium derivatives, Mecholyl, physostigmine, Benzedrine, and Pantopon have found their proponents.

Morphine has been considered by some as the most reliable stimulant of gastric peristalsis. One milligram of morphine is employed. Within 2 to 10 minutes following intravenous administration, there was an increase in peristalsis which lasted 20 to 45 minutes. There was a second phase of prolonged depression of intestinal propulsion and diminution of tone. Neoplastic infiltrates of the gastric wall invariably resulted in disordered peristaltic patterns. Gastric ulcers, the postoperative stomach, and various infiltrating lesions may be studied to good advantage this way. Active intestinal bleeding and hypersensitivity to the drug are considered contraindications.

Parietography. In this examination, the gastric wall is isolated between two layers of air by gastric inflation and pneumoperitoneum. Body section radiography is also employed. This procedure permits definition of wall thickness of the suspected region and defines the extent of a tumor if present. Approximately 800 to 1200 ml. of air are introduced in the peritoneal cavity on the evening prior to the examination. The gas in the stomach is derived from tartaric acid which becomes mixed with a succeeding dose of sodium bicarbonate (250 to 300 ml. of gas estimated). Body section radiographs are obtained at 1 cm. intervals ordinarily, at 11 to 19 cm. from the posterior skin surface (Porcher and Buffard).*

Celiac Angiography for Visualization of the Stomach, Duodenum and Pancreas. See No. 10 in the following section on techniques of examination of the pancreas.

THE PANCREAS

Basic Anatomy. The pancreas is both an endocrine and an exocrine gland, its endocrine function being carried forward by the islets of Langerhans. The two hormones secreted are insulin and glucagon. These hormones help regulate glucose, lipid, and protein metabolism. The acini of the pancreas secrete digestive juices into the duodenum.

The pancreas is arbitrarily divided into four parts: *head, neck, body* and *tail.*

Head. The head of the pancreas lies within the curvature of the duodenum (Fig. 14–24). The prolongation of the left and caudal border of the head of the pancreas is called the "uncinate process." As shown in the posterior view of the pancreas and duodenum, the superior mesenteric artery and vein cross the uncinate process on its right aspect.

---

*References may be obtained in Meschan, I.: An Atlas of Anatomy Basic to Radiology. Philadelphia, W. B. Saunders Co., 1975, Chapter 13.

The posterior surface of the pancreas is without peritoneum and is in contact with the aorta, inferior vena cava, common bile duct, renal veins, and right crus of the diaphragm (Fig. 14–43). The anterior surface is, in its lower part, below the level of the transverse colon, and is covered by the peritoneum and separated from the transverse colon by the transverse mesocolon.

The *neck* of the pancreas is that constricted portion just to the left of the head (Fig. 14–54). Superiorly it adjoins the pylorus. It is proximal to the origin of the portal vein and the gastroduodenal artery.

The *body* of the pancreas is separated anteriorly from the stomach by the omental bursa. The posterior surface of the body of the pancreas is closely related to the aorta, splenic vein, left kidney and its vessels, left suprarenal, the origin of the superior mesenteric artery, and the crura of the diaphragm. The inferior surface of the body is coated by peritoneum and is in close proximity to the duodenojejunal flexure, the coils of the jejunum, and the left flexure of the colon. Along its anterior aspect, the layers of the transverse mesocolon diverge. The superior border of the body of the pancreas is close to the celiac artery, with the hepatic artery to the right and the splenic artery to the left (Fig. 14–54).

The *tail* of the pancreas extends laterally toward the left to the surface of the spleen and is situated in the phrenicolienal ligament.

The exocrine secretions of the pancreas empty into the duodenum through two ductal systems: first, a *major duct* (of Wirsung), which extends the full length of the pancreas toward the right, opening into the descending duodenum at a common orifice with the common bile duct, the *major papilla* (ampulla of Vater). Second, the *minor pancreatic duct* (of Santorini) drains part of the head of the pancreas and enters the duodenum just above the duct of Wirsung by a separate opening in the duodenum.

The arterial blood supply of the pancreas (Fig. 14–54) is derived from *four* main sources: (1) numerous small branches from the *splenic* artery; (2) the retroduodenal branch of the *gastroduodenal* artery; (3) the *superior pancreaticoduodenal* arising from the gastroduodenal artery; and (4) the *inferior pancreaticoduodenal* which arises from the superior mesenteric artery and anastomoses with the superior pancreaticoduodenal in and surrounding the head of the pancreas.

A *dorsal pancreatic artery* may give rise from the celiac artery just distal to the origin of the splenic artery and opposite the point of origin of the left gastric. This supplies the body of the pancreas centrally with branches extending toward the head and tail. This artery, called by some the superior, instead of arising from the celiac trunk may originate from the superior mesenteric artery.

The *superior pancreaticoduodenal* artery may divide into two main segments, one anterior and one posterior, surrounding the head of the pancreas and its uncinate process. The arcade formed around the head of the pancreas also supplies the duodenum on its ventral aspect.

The pancreas also receives branches directly from the *common hepatic artery*.

One of the branches from the splenic artery is often sufficiently large to be identified as a single branch called the *pancreatica magna artery*. It is distributed along the pancreatic duct.

The pancreatic veins drain directly into the portal vein by means of the *splenic and superior mesenteric veins*.

The *lymphatics* terminate in numerous lymph nodes near the root of the superior mesenteric artery, following the course of blood vessels and terminating in the pancreaticolienal, pancreaticoduodenal, and pre-aortic lymph nodes.

Pancreatic Exocrine Secretions. Pancreatic juice contains enzymes for digesting all three major types of food: proteins, carbohydrates, and fat. There are a number of proteolytic enzymes which, as synthesized in the pancreas, are inactive but become active after they are secreted into the intestinal tract by enzymes released from the intestinal mucosa whenever chyme comes in contact with the mucosa. If this were not the case, the pancreatic juice might digest the pancreas itself. There is additionally, however, another substance called trypsin inhibitor stored in the cells of the pancreas which prevents the activation of pancreatic proteolytic enzymes.

Pancreatic secretion, like gastric secretion, is regulated by both nervous and hormonal mechanisms. The most important hormone in this regard is *secretin*. A second hormone is *pancreozymin*. When chyme enters the intestine it causes the release and activation of secretin, which is absorbed into the blood and in turn causes the pancreas to secrete large quantities of fluid containing a high concentration of bicarbonate ion and a low concentration of chloride ion. Hydrochloric acid, particularly in the chyme, is capable of causing a great release of secretin, although almost any type of food will cause at least some release. The secretin response is particularly important in the prevention of too great acidity in the small intestine, since the small intestine cannot withstand the intense digestive properties of gastric juice. Moreover, the tendency toward alkaline environment assists the action of the pancreatic enzymes per se.

Pancreozymin is largely responsible for secretion of the digestive enzymes from the pancreas and is somewhat similar to the effect of vagal stimulation.

Technique of Examination of the Pancreas

1. Plain Films of the Abdomen. Anteroposterior and lateral projections of the abdomen centered over the pancreas (with oblique views taken as necessary) are helpful from the standpoint of revealing (a) pancreatic calcification; (b) an abnormal gas distribution, such as free air in the immediate vicinity of the pancreas or lesser omental bursa; or (c) displacement of adjoining organs such as the stomach, duodenum, kidney, or spleen.

2. Air Contrast Studies of the Stomach and Duodenum. Air contrast may be used in the stomach and duodenum to accentuate the pancreatic region, particularly when calcareous masses are noted therein. Air contrast ordinarily does not obscure the areas of calcification, whereas barium contrast introduced into the stomach and duodenum might do so. Body section radiography may be used in conjunction with the air contrast to enhance its efficiency.

3. Endo- and Perigastric Gas with Selective Celiac Arteriography During the Phase of Maximal Secretion (stimulation by pharmacologic agents).* This combination of an angiographic identification of the pancreas, plus the visualization of the stomach and duodenum by gas intraluminally, permits the identification of the pancreas in conjunction with the gastric mucosa and thickness of the gastric wall.

Selective celiac arteriography in itself is very helpful in identifying certain lesions of the pancreas (Fig. 14–56). However, the interpretation of angiograms of the pancreas offers some difficulty and the efficacy of this technique for identification of carcinoma in the pancreas, for example, is somewhat controversial.

4. Intubation of the Stomach and Duodenum with Opaque Tube. The main purpose of this examination is to delineate the region of the

pancreas for better visualization of any suspicious oblique or negative shadows in this area (Weens and Walker).† A discussion of pancreatic calculi or calcified cysts of the pancreas is outside the scope of this text and the student is referred to special reports of these disorders for further information (Stein et al.; Poppel; Becker et al.).†‡

5. Opaque Meal in Stomach and Duodenum. The close relationship of the pancreas to the stomach and duodenum has already been described. Impressions upon the stomach and alterations of the detailed mucosal pattern of the duodenum may be the only evidence of pancreatic abnormality. Cinefluorography and cineradiography are particularly useful for detailed analysis of areas of pliability or incipient rigidity in the second part of the duodenum (Salik).* Greater variability in appearance, less rigidity and induration, and the absence of fixed corrugations favor a diagnosis of pancreatitis over carcinoma. Hypotonic duodenography is particularly helpful with opaque studies of the stomach and duodenum in revealing minute abnormalities related to the pancreas (Fig. 14–53).

6. Barium Enema (see Chapter 15). The peritoneal reflection of the transverse mesocolon lies in very close proximity to the pancreas; hence, lesions of the pancreas may extend to and involve the colon, especially its transverse portion. The barium enema may corroborate plain films of the abdomen that reveal inordinate shadows in the immediate vicinity of the transverse colon (Salik; Eyler et al.).†

7. Excretory Urogram (see Chapter 12). The tail of the pancreas may lie just anterior to the left kidney and extends to the hilum of the spleen. Abnormal enlargement of the pancreas, especially involving the lesser omental bursa, may displace or distort the left kidney, ureter, or spleen (Marshall et al.).†

8. Cholecystograms and Cholangiograms. Cholecystograms and cholangiograms may at times reveal evidence of an obstructed or a displaced common duct. The maximum diameter of the common duct in chronic pancreatitis, for example, seldom if ever exceeds 25 mm. Obstruction of the common duct due to carcinoma may cause an enlargement of over 30 mm. Unfortunately, intravenous cholangiography fails in about one third of the cases of acute inflammations of the pancreas

---

*Taylor, D. A., et al.: New method of visualizing gastric wall. Further studies. Radiology, 86:711–717, 1966.

---

†References may be obtained in Meschan, I.: An Atlas of Anatomy Basic to Radiology. Philadelphia, W. B. Saunders Co., 1975, Chapter 13.

‡See also Meschan, I.: Analysis of Roentgen Signs in General Radiology. Philadelphia, W. B. Saunders Co., 1973, Chapter 28.

(Schultz).* Conspicuous dilatation of the pancreatic duct and its tributaries coupled with narrowness of the transduodenal portion of the common duct may also indicate inflammations of the pancreas (Sachs and Partington).*

9. Percutaneous Cholangiography. When complete obstruction of the common bile duct occurs at its site of entry into the pancreas, considerable dilatation of the more proximal regions in the biliary tree results. Direct percutaneous injection of a contrast agent through the liver into one of the dilated constituent branches will not only demonstrate severe dilatation, but also the more characteristic appearances of the common bile duct. At the site of obstruction, there may be a jagged, notched appearance and a reversal of the usual convexity of the common bile duct toward the left (Flemma et al.; Evans; Darke and Beal).*

10. Further Comments About Selective Pancreatic Angiography. As indicated earlier, the arterial supply of the pancreas is somewhat variable, with the major supply coming from the splenic, celiac, gastroduodenal, and superior mesenteric arteries. Selective study of the pancreas is probably best accomplished by celiac or superior mesenteric angiograms. Inflation of the stomach in conjunction with this study is helpful (Lunderquist).* Superselective catheterization of the hepatic, splenic, gastroduodenal, dorsal pancreatic, inferior pancreatic, or duodenal arteries has been attempted, and it has been noted that injections must be made at least into both gastroduodenal and splenic arteries for adequate demonstration of the entire pancreas. It is probable that pharmacologic agents will serve to enhance these techniques (Bierman).*

11. Splenoportography. The splenic vein and tail of the pancreas are in close contiguity with one another. Splenic vein occlusion and distortion have been described in association with pancreatic tumors or large masses (pseudocysts) of the pancreas.

12. Retropneumoperitoneum with Body Section Radiography. This method involves a combination of the retroperitoneal insufflation of a gas, gaseous distention of the stomach, and body section radiography in both the sagittal and coronal planes. Simultaneous pneumo-peritoneum, introduction of contrast agent in the stomach, urinary tract, or biliary tree, and other expedients have also been utilized in conjunction with this method. These methods are still in the process of evaluation and it is questionable whether the discomfort and perhaps even the dangers of the procedure are justified when compared with other possible methods that might be employed in identical cases.

13. Direct Pancreatography. This method involves direct insertion of a needle or catheter into the pancreatic duct at surgery. The original method involved transduodenal sphincterotomy and direct injection of a suitable contrast agent (from 2 to 5 ml. of 50 per cent sodium diatrizoate is recommended). This injection is made slowly during a 5-minute period, with the last 2 ml. introduced during the x-ray exposure. The tube may be left in place for drainage. Normal pancreatograms reveal only the main ducts of the pancreas. With acute inflammation the radiopaque solution permeates the acinar tissue, showing not only the smaller ramifications but even some of the parenchymal tissue. Serial pancreatograms will depict resolution of such inflammation.

14. Endoscopic Pancreatocholangiography (peroral pancreaticobiliary ductography). Cannulation of the ampulla of Vater through a fiberoptic duodenoscope may be performed with the aid of x-ray television. The technique of the examination is described as follows: A fiberopticduodenoscope, Model JF-B of the Olympus Company, Tokyo, has been used. This instrument, 10 mm. in diameter and 1250 mm. long, is inserted perorally into the stomach and thereafter into the duodenum. Its tip is equipped with a rigid lens system that can be bent at will 120 degrees up and down, and 90 degrees right and left. It contains lenses and holes for illumination, fixed focus for visualization and photography, a small hole for injecting air and washing fluid, and a larger hole for passing a forceps and cannula. A Teflon cannula 1.7 mm. in external diameter is passed through the duodenoscope into the ampulla of Vater and sodium meglumine diatrizoate is then injected into the cannulated duct system. Usually only 2 to 3 cc. are required. The injection is terminated and left lateral and posteroanterior (sometimes left oblique) roentgenograms are taken. The cannula and scope are withdrawn and several more roentgenograms are taken in various projections, including the right oblique view and erect positions. The speed of disappearance or excretion of the contrast medium into the duodenum is checked on the

---

*References may be obtained in Meschan, I.: An Atlas of Anatomy Basic to Radiology. Philadelphia, W. B. Saunders Co., 1975, Chapter 13.

television screen. If too great a volume of contrast agent is used, a pancreatitis may ensue and this should be avoided. After the procedure an antibiotic is used to prevent acute pancreatitis and infection.

After successful pancreatography the common duct may be visualized with a cannula withdrawn halfway and contrast medium reinjected (Fig. 14–58). The accessory pancreatic duct may be visualized as communicating with the duct of Wirsung. Usually, barium swallow study and hypotonic duodenography are carried out prior to the duodenoscopy. Representative ductograms are shown in Figure 14–58.

Okuda et al.* note that the length of the normal pancreatic duct by this technique is usually 15.8 mm. on the average, and slightly longer in the presence of inflammation. The maximum duct diameter of the head of the normal pancreas is 3.9 mm., but this measurement is considerably larger in the presence of chronic pancreatitis. (There is no indication in this report of magnification in relation to these measurements.) Normally, the ductal system clears in an average of 4 minutes and 6 seconds, but considerably longer retention occurs in abnormal states.

15. Measurement of the Retrogastric and Retroduodenal Spaces: an Index of Pancreatic or Lesser Omental Bursal Involvement. Various methods have been proposed for measurement of the retrogastric space (Poppel et al.; Scheinmel and Mednick; Meschan et al.; Poole).† The normal range of distances in centimeters between the stomach and duodenum and the spine on left lateral roentgenograms of the abdomen according to body habitus has been proposed by a number of investigators. The limits of normal vary considerably according to the gross judgment of body habitus. Such great variations of normal make the validity of measurement difficult to interpret except in the presence of "extrinsic tumor impression on the viscera [which was] . . . the single most important statistical factor in evaluating the presence of a retroperitoneal mass" (Herbert and Margulis).† Poole, in studying this issue, noted that "the only variable measurements in the midline cross-section at the level of the stomach are the thicknesses of the prepancreatic fat, and the width of the pancreatic neck, which is 1 to 1.5 cm. thick normally in the midline. Many other structures, however, are present such as the lesser sac, fat, aortic lymph nodes, and the aorta itself." Poole devised an anterior abdominal wall compression device which contained a nickel coin (measuring 2.1 cm. in diameter) on its flat surface. He used this device to press the midline stomach against the retroperitoneal structures. After the barium was swallowed, the fluoroscopic pressure cone was applied to the midline puddle of barium with sufficient force to splay the mucosal folds and flatten the column of barium. Adequate compression was noted by displacement of the central midbarium column to both sides of the midline. A lateral spot film was taken. The midline antrum-to-spine distance was measured from the posterior pressure defect to the anterior vertebral body. After the antrum-to-spine measurement, the patient was placed in the right lateral decubitus position to allow barium to enter the horizontal duodenum, and then he was brought upright and placed in the posteroanterior position. When the midline duodenum was identified in the posteroanterior projection, the patient was then turned laterally and a spot film taken without pressure (Fig. 14–23). The duodenum-to-spine distance was measured from the posterior aspect of the midline horizontal duodenum to the spine. The measurements obtained from spot films were corrected for magnification by the magnification of the coin marker on the compressor device. A nomogram is provided to correct for such magnification (Fig. 14–23). A direct linear correlation exists between the weight of the normal individual and his true antrum-to-spine measurement. For an average weight of 148 pounds the average corrected antrum-to-spine distance was 3.14 cm. The 95 per cent confidence limits are shown in the accompanying graph. The duodenum-to-spine normal measurement exhibited no relationship to body weight. The mean value was 1.3 cm., with a standard deviation of 5 mm. The upper limit of normal was 2.3 cm. (two standard deviations). This method obviates many of the variables previously noted by compressing the barium-containing midline viscus against the retroperitoneum, thus accurately defining its anterior margin.

Computerized Whole Body Axial Tomography. This technique may prove to be our most valuable method of study. (See special section on Computed Tomography.)

Radioisotope Techniques. These are of only moderate usefulness and are outside the scope of this text.

Ultrasonography. This method is also outside the scope of this text.

---

*Okuda, K., et al.: Endoscopic pancreato-cholangiography. Am. J. Roentgenol., *117*:437–445, 1973.

†References may be obtained in Meschan, I.: An Atlas of Anatomy Basic to Radiology. Philadelphia, W. B. Saunders Co., 1975, Chapter 13.

PANCREAS

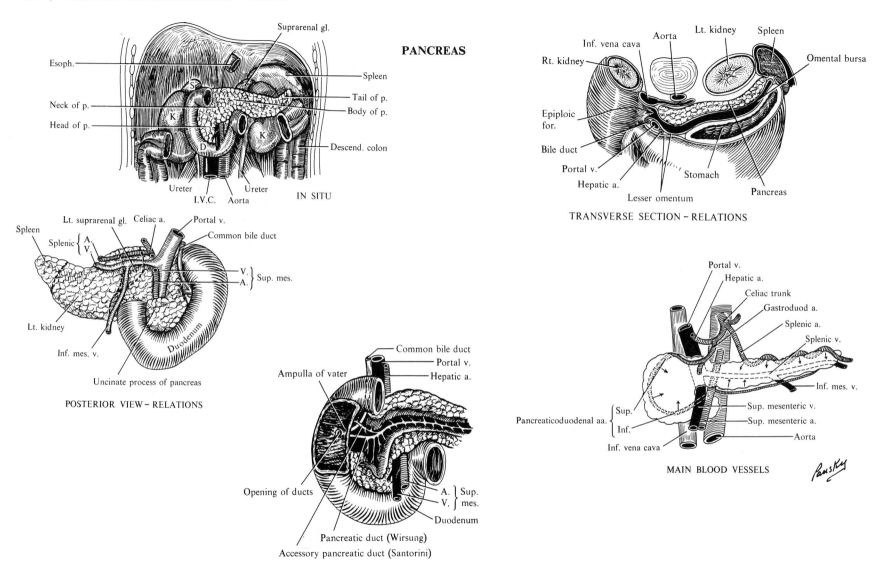

IN SITU

POSTERIOR VIEW – RELATIONS

TRANSVERSE SECTION – RELATIONS

PANCREATIC DUCTS

MAIN BLOOD VESSELS

FIGURE 14–54 Summary of anatomic details of the pancreas: *in situ,* from posterior view, pancreatic ducts, transversely, and main arterial supply and venous drainage. (K) kidney, (D) duodenum, (I.V.C.) inferior vena cava, (a.) artery, (v.) vein, (aa) arcades. (From Pansky, B., and House, E. L.: Review of Gross Anatomy. New York, Macmillan Company, 1964.)

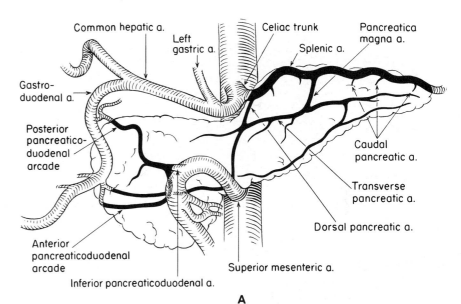

Common hepatic a.

Left gastric a.

Celiac trunk

Pancreatica magna a.

Splenic a.

Gastro-duodenal a.

Posterior pancreatico-duodenal arcade

Caudal pancreatic a.

Transverse pancreatic a.

Dorsal pancreatic a.

Anterior pancreaticoduodenal arcade

Inferior pancreaticoduodenal a.

Superior mesenteric a.

A

FIGURE 14–55. *A.* Line drawing of arterial supply of the pancreas. The pancreatic branches are enlarged for emphasis. In this example, the dorsal pancreatic artery arises from the splenic artery and gives off the transverse pancreatic artery. It receives an anastomotic branch from the anterior pancreaticoduodenal arcade. The relationships of the pancreatic arteries are variable and must be evaluated in each patient. (From Reuter, S. R., and Redman, H. C.: Gastrointestinal Angiography. Philadelphia, W. B. Saunders Co., 1972.) *B.* Regulation of pancreatic secretion. (From Guyton, A. C.: Textbook of Medical Physiology, 4th ed. Philadelphia, W. B. Saunders Co., 1971.)

Acid from stomach releases secretin from wall of duodenum

Common bile duct

Vagal stimulation releases large quantities of enzymes

Secretin absorbed into blood stream

Secretin causes copious output of pancreatic juice weak in enzymes

Pancreozymin is absorbed like secretin and produces large quantities of enzymes

B

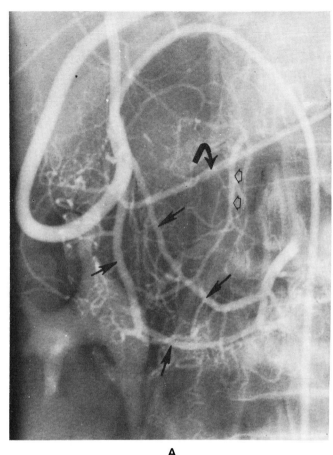

A

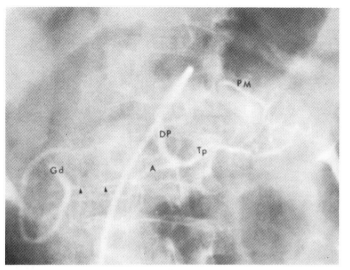

B

FIGURE 14–56 *A.* Normal pancreatic arcades. Direct serial magnification angiography during a gastroduodenal artery injection clearly demonstrates the pancreatic arcades (*straight arrows*), the transverse pancreatic artery (*curved arrow*) and the dorsal pancreatic artery (*open arrow*). (From Baum, S., and Athanasoulis, C. A.: Angiography. *In* Eaton, S. B., and Ferrucci, J. T. (ed.): Radiology of the Pancreas and Duodenum. Philadelphia, W. B. Saunders Co., 1973.) *B.* Selective dorsal pancreatic injection. Catheter passed via celiac artery. (*DP*). Dorsal pancreatic artery, (A and arrowheads), anastomotic branch from dorsal pancreatic artery to pancreaticoduodenal arcade, (*Gd*) gastroduodenal artery, (*Pm*) pancreatic magna, (*Tp*) transverse pancreatic. (From Ruziska, F. F., Jr., and Rossi, P.: Radiol. Clin. North Am., 8:3–28, 1970.)

PANCREAS - BLOOD SUPPLY

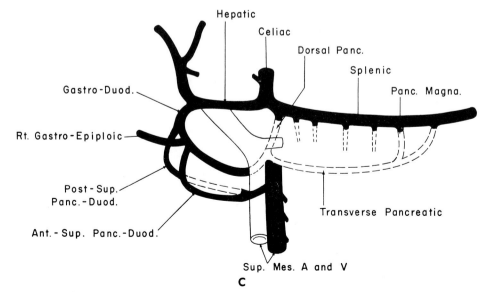

C

FIGURE 14–57 *C. See legend on opposite page*

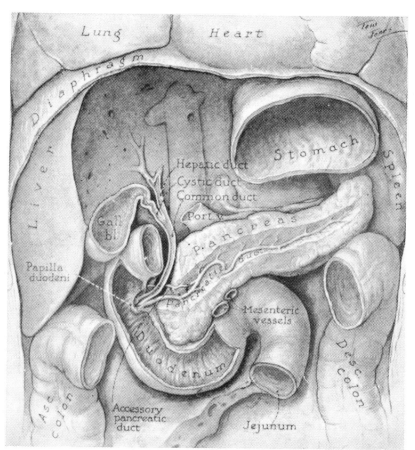

A

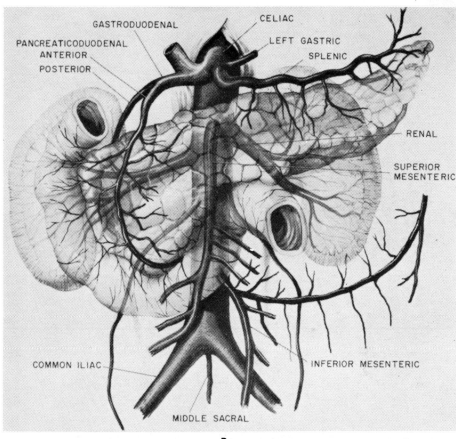

B

FIGURE 14–57 *A.* The gross anatomy of the biliary system. (From Jones, T.: Anatomical Studies. Jackson, Michigan, S. H. Camp and Co., 1943.) *B.* Arterial circulation of the pancreas (isometric diagram). *C.* Pancreatic blood supply in simple diagram to demonstrate the anterior and posterior pancreaticoduodenal arcade in conjunction with the celiac axis and the superior mesenteric arteries and veins. The transverse pancreatic artery is also shown, in its relationship to the splenic artery and the pancreatica magna artery. (*B* and *C* from Bierman, H. R.: Selective Arterial Catheterization. Springfield, Ill., Charles C Thomas, Publisher, 1969. Courtesy of Charles C Thomas, Publisher.)

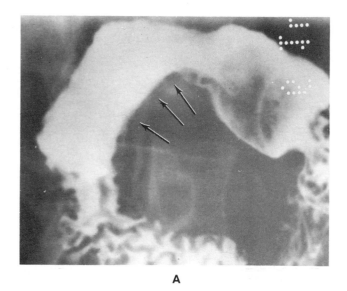

A

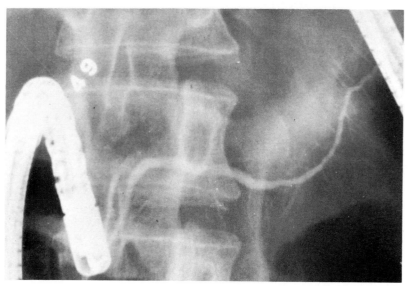

B

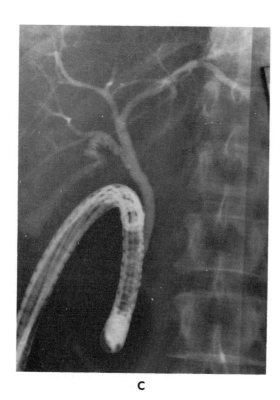

C

FIGURE 14–58 Detection of malignant disease by peroral retrograde pancreaticobiliary ductography. (From Robbins, A. J., et al.: Am. J. Roentgenol., *117*:432–436, 1973.) *A.* Barium studies suggest pressure defect on second part of duodenum. *B.* Main pancreatic duct is normal and other branches are normal as well (patient had chronic pancreatitis). *C.* A normal cholangiogram obtained at this time.

Operation   Roentgen-anatomy   Terminology

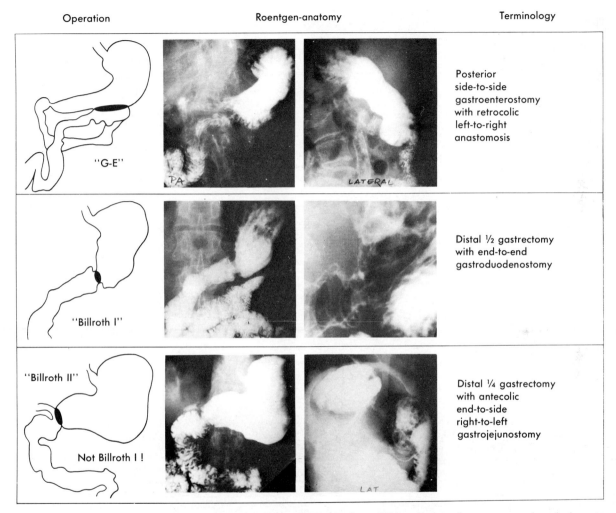

FIGURE 14-59 *A*. Operation, roentgen-anatomy, and terminology. When compared to eponyms, descriptive terminology is clear and widely understood. (From Burhenne, H. J.: Am. J. Roentgenol., *91*:731, 1964.)

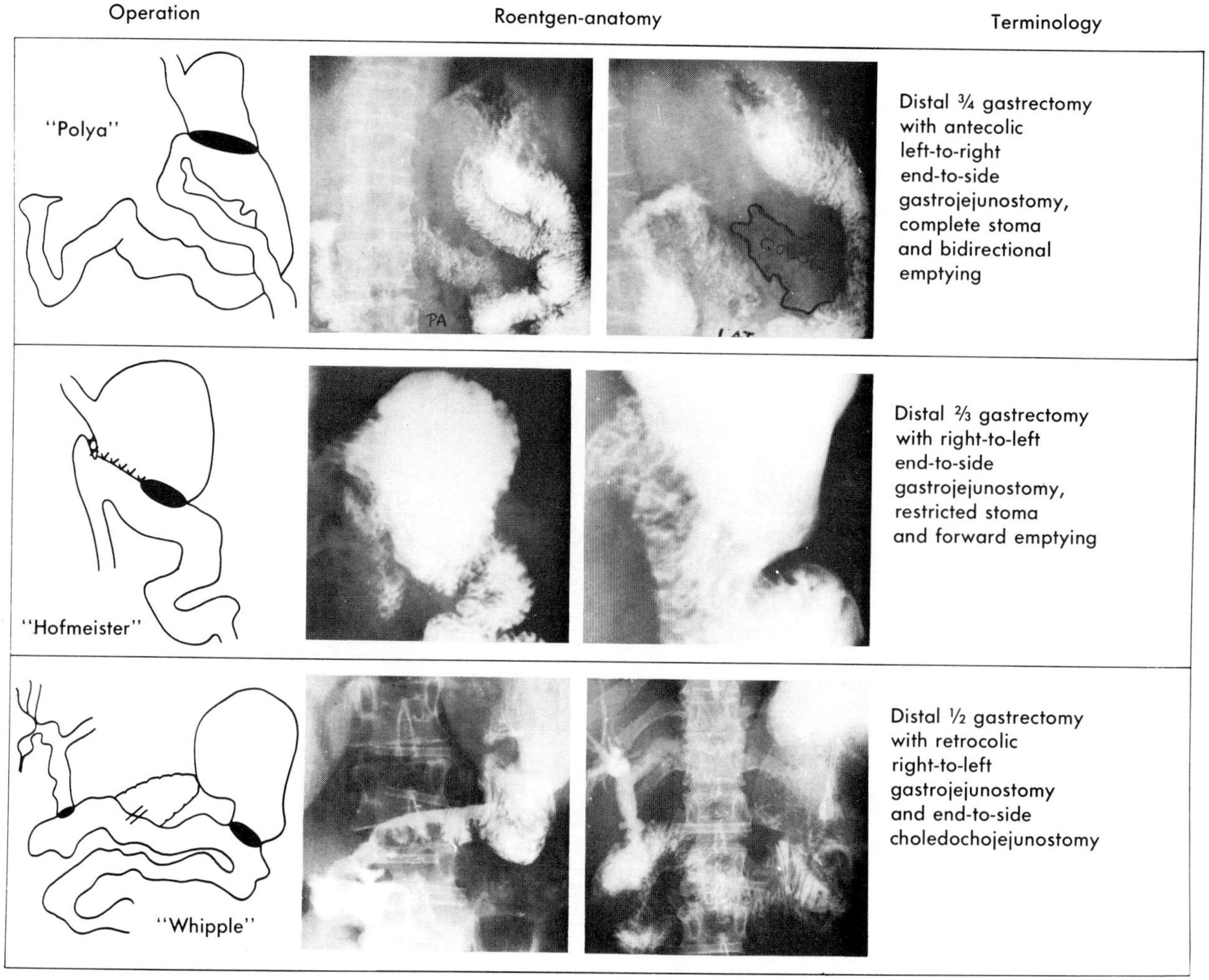

Operation	Roentgen-anatomy	Terminology
"Polya"		Distal ¾ gastrectomy with antecolic left-to-right end-to-side gastrojejunostomy, complete stoma and bidirectional emptying
"Hofmeister"		Distal ⅔ gastrectomy with right-to-left end-to-side gastrojejunostomy, restricted stoma and forward emptying
"Whipple"		Distal ½ gastrectomy with retrocolic right-to-left gastrojejunostomy and end-to-side choledochojejunostomy

FIGURE 14–59 *Continued.* *B.* Descriptive terminology is best suited for all purposes. (From Burhenne, H. J.: Am. J. Roentgenol., *91*:731, 1964.)

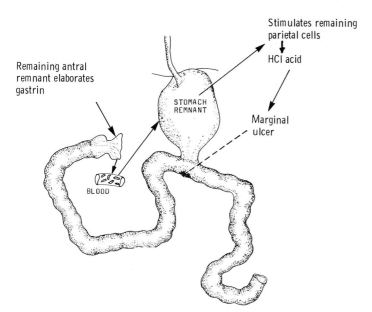

Remaining antral
remnant elaborates
gastrin

Stimulates remaining
parietal cells

HCl acid

STOMACH
REMNANT

Marginal
ulcer

BLOOD

FIGURE 14-60 Antral remnant syndrome.

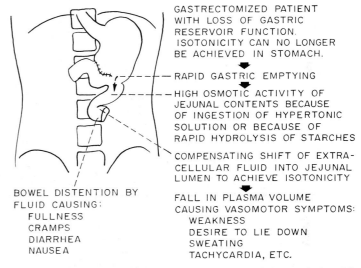

GASTRECTOMIZED PATIENT
WITH LOSS OF GASTRIC
RESERVOIR FUNCTION.
ISOTONICITY CAN NO LONGER
BE ACHIEVED IN STOMACH.

RAPID GASTRIC EMPTYING

HIGH OSMOTIC ACTIVITY OF
JEJUNAL CONTENTS BECAUSE
OF INGESTION OF HYPERTONIC
SOLUTION OR BECAUSE OF
RAPID HYDROLYSIS OF STARCHES

COMPENSATING SHIFT OF EXTRA-
CELLULAR FLUID INTO JEJUNAL
LUMEN TO ACHIEVE ISOTONICITY

BOWEL DISTENTION BY
FLUID CAUSING:
  FULLNESS
  CRAMPS
  DIARRHEA
  NAUSEA

FALL IN PLASMA VOLUME
CAUSING VASOMOTOR SYMPTOMS:
  WEAKNESS
  DESIRE TO LIE DOWN
  SWEATING
  TACHYCARDIA, ETC.

FIGURE 14-61 Diagram illustrating the physiology of the "dumping syndrome." (After Burhenne.)

GASTRIC AND DUODENAL ANGIOGRAPHY

Blood Supply of the Stomach

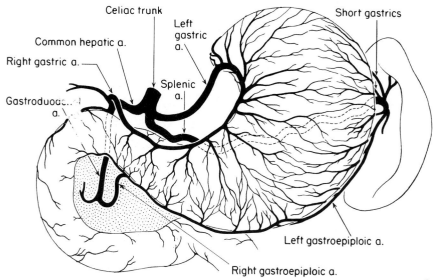

B

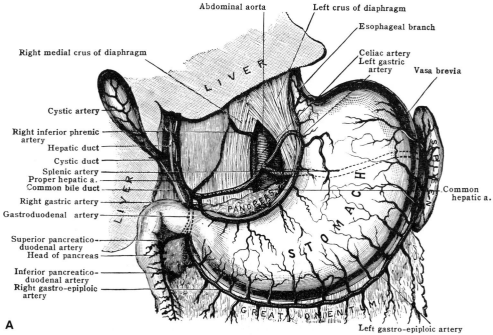

A

FIGURE 14–62 *A.* Celiac artery and its usual main branches. (From Anson, B. J. (ed.): Morris' Human Anatomy, 12th ed. Copyright © 1966 by McGraw-Hill, Inc. Used by permission of McGraw-Hill Book Company.) *B.* Line drawing of arterial supply of the stomach. The arteries to the stomach are enlarged for emphasis. The left gastroepiploic and right gastric arteries are frequently not identified at angiography unless they are serving as a collateral pathway. (From Reuter, S. R., and Redman, H. C.: Gastrointestinal Angiography. Philadelphia, W. B. Saunders Co., 1972.)

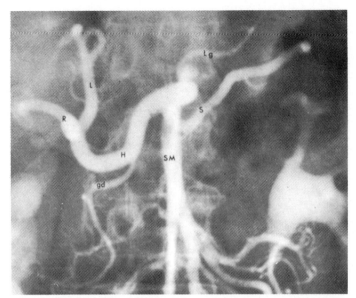

FIGURE 14–63 Simultaneous selective celiac and superior mesenteric artery injections show type I pattern. Anteroposterior view. (*S*) Splenic artery, (*SM*) superior mesenteric. (*gd*) gastroduodenal, (*H*) proper hepatic, (*R*) right hepatic, (*L*) left hepatic, (*Lg*) left gastric. (From Ruzicka, F. F., and Rossi, P.: Radiol. Clin. North Am., *8*:3–29, 1970.)

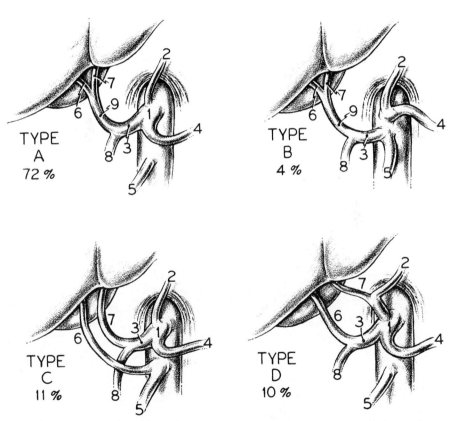

FIGURE 14–64 (*1*) Celiac trunk, (*2*) left gastric artery, (*3*) common hepatic artery, (*4*) splenic artery, (*5*) superior mesenteric artery, (*6*) right hepatic artery, (*7*) left hepatic artery, (*8*) gastroduodenal artery, (*9*) proper hepatic artery. (From Ruzicka, F. F., and Rossi, P.: N.Y. State J. Med., *23*:3032–3033, 1968. Reproduced with permission.)

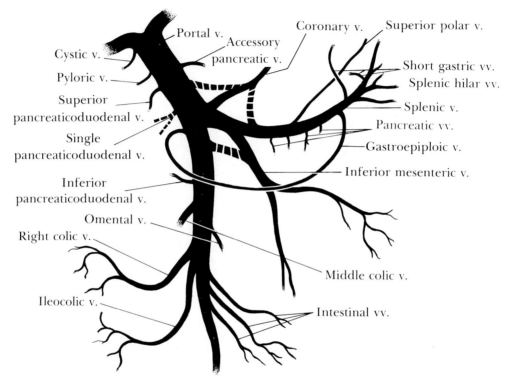

FIGURE 14–65 Portal venous system. Solid line drawing represents the most frequent pattern. Interrupted lines show variations of coronary, inferior mesenteric, and pancreaticoduodenal veins. When the pancreaticoduodenal vein is single, it empties into the right wall of the portal vein just above the confluence of the splenic and superior mesenteric veins. (From Ruzicka, F. F., Jr., and Rossi, P.: Radiol. Clin. North Am., 8:3–29, 1970. Modified from Douglas, B. E., Baggenstoss, A. H., and Hollinshead, W. H.: Surg., Gynecol., Obstet., *91*:562–576, 1950. Reproduced by permission of Surgery, Gynecology, and Obstetrics.)

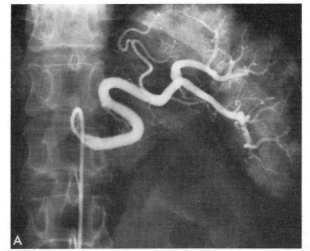

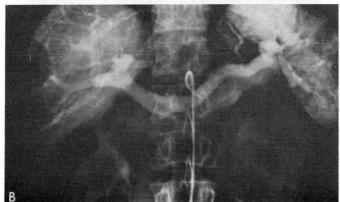

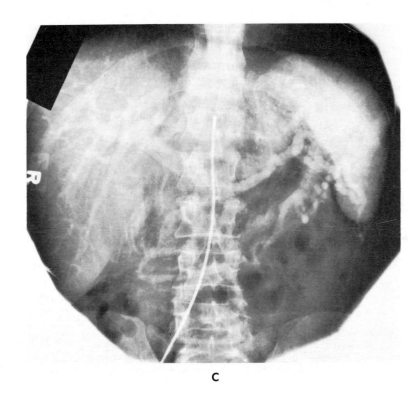

FIGURE 14–66   Normal splenic arteriogram in the evaluation of the pancreatic body and tail.

A. Arterial phase of a selective splenic arteriogram demonstrates the pancreatica magna and short pancreatic arteries supplying the body and tail of the pancreas.

B. During the venous phase of the same injection, the splenic vein and portal vein are optimally visualized. The close association of the splenic vein with the opacified normal pancreatic body and tail is apparent. (From Eaton, S. B. and Ferrucci, J. T., Jr., Radiology of the Pancreas and Duodenum. Philadelphia, W. B. Saunders Co., 1973.)

C. Portal or splenoportal venogram following celiac arteriogram.

REFERENCES

Aoyama, D.: Radiological diagnosis of chronic gastritis. *In* Recent Advances in Gastroenterology. Proceedings of the Third World Congress of Gastroenterology. Tokyo, Nankado Co., 1967, Vol. 1, 209.

Cooke, A. R.: Drugs and peptic ulceration. *In* Sleisenger, M. H., and Fordtran, J. S. (eds.): Gastrointestinal disease. Philadelphia, W. B. Saunders Co., 1973, pp. 642–52.

Frik, W.: Rontgenbefunde am Falten-Und Feinrelief des Magens bei Chronesher Gastritis. Radiologe., *4*:69, 1964.

Frik, W.: Neoplastic diseases of the stomach. *In* Margulis, A. R., and Burhenne, H. J. (eds.): Alimentary Tract Roentgenology. St. Louis, The C. V. Mosby Co., 1973, pp. 662–681.

Gelfand, D. W.: The double-contrast upper gastrointestinal examination in the Japanese style. Am. J. Gastroenterol., *63*:216–20, 1975.

Gelfand, D. W.: The Japanese-style double contrast examination of the stomach. Gastrointest. Radiol., *1*:7–17, 1976.

Goldberg, H. I.: Air barium: contrast radiography of the upper gastrointestinal tract. *In* Margulis, A. R., and Gooding, C. A. (eds.): Diagnostic Radiology. University of California at San Francisco. Extended programs in medical education, 1977.

Goldstein, H. M.: Double-contrast gastrography. Am. J. Dig. Dis., *21*:797–803, 1976.

Hunt, J. H., and Anderson, I. F.: Double contrast upper gastrointestinal studies. Clin. Radiol., *27*:87–97, 1976.

Ichikawa, H.: The Basic Concepts of Double-Contrast Radiography of the Stomach. Tokyo, Fuji Photo Film Co. Ltd., 1973.

Koga, M., Nakata, H., Kiyonari, H., et al.: Minute mucosal patterns in gastric carcinoma. Radiology, *120*:199–202, 1976.

Laufer, I.: The diagnostic accuracy of barium studies of the stomach and duodenum—correlation with endoscopy. Radiology, *115*:569–573, 1975.

Laufer, I.: Assessment of the accuracy of double-contrast gastroduodenal radiology. Gastroenterol., *71*:874–78, 1976.

Laufer, I., Hamilton, J., and Mullen, J. E.: Demonstration of superficial gastric erosions by double-contrast radiography. Gastroenterol., *68*:387–91, 1975.

Miller, R. E.: The air contrast stomach examination: an overview. Radiology, *117*:743–744, 1975.

Poplack, W., Paul, R. E., Goldsmith, M., et al.: Demonstration of erosive gastritis by the double-contrast technique. Radiology, *117*:519, 1975.

Shirakabe, H.: Double Contrast Studies of the Stomach, Stuttgart, Georg Thieme, 1972.

Shirakabe, H., Ichikawa, H., Kumakura, H., Nishizawa, M., Higurashi, K., Hayakawa, H., and Murakami, T.: Atlas of X-ray Diagnosis of Early Gastric Cancer. Tokyo, Igaku Shoin Ltd., 1966.

Shirakabe, H., Ichikawa, H., Kumakura, K., et al.: Atlas of X-ray diagnosis of early gastric cancer. Philadelphia, J. B. Lippincott Co., 1966.

15

SMALL INTESTINE, COLON, AND BILIARY TRACT

THE SMALL INTESTINE

Gross Anatomy

The jejunum and ileum are completely covered with peritoneum and therefore vary considerably in position, except at the two ends where relative fixation occurs. However, the small intestine is usually distributed in the abdomen according to a fairly regular pattern (Fig. 15–1). Thus, the proximal jejunum usually lies in the left half of the abdomen between the level of the pancreas and the intercrestal line. The distal ileum usually lies deep in the pelvis posteriorly, with the terminal ileum arising out of the pelvis to meet the cecum in the right lower quadrant anteriorly. The distal jejunum and proximal ileum are distributed in the right half of the abdomen for the most part.

The root of the mesentery, about 15 cm. long, is attached to the posterior abdominal wall along a line running obliquely from the left side of the body of the L2 vertebra to the right sacroiliac joint, crossing the third part of the duodenum, the aorta, the inferior vena cava. the right gonadal vessels, the right ureter, and the right psoas muscle. It is approximately 20 cm. broad, on the average, tending to become narrower as it reaches the lower end of the ileum. The mesentery contains blood vessels, lymphatics, lymph nodes, and nerves of the small intestine, as well as fat.

The mucous membrane of the small intestine is enormously increased in surface area by the formation of circular folds (valvulae conniventes), upon which are mounted intestinal villi (Figs. 15–2, 15–3, and 15–4). The circular folds give a characteristic coiled-spring appearance to the inner aspect of the small intestine. These folds reach their maximum development in the distal half of the duodenum and proximal part of the jejunum, where they may be as much as 8 mm. in height and extend around two-thirds of the circumference of the bowel, branching in the course of their extension. Thereafter they gradually become smaller and less numerous so that they are virtually absent in the lower ileum (Fig. 15–2). Although they extend through the wall of the bowel and involve the whole thickness of the mucous membrane and a core of submucosa, they do not involve the serosa, unlike the valvulae semilunares of the colon.

The intestinal villi are mounted on these folds and measure less than half a millimeter in height. They begin at the pyloric orifice where they are broad and short, becoming longer and narrower as they approach the ileocecal valve. These villi are actually present on and between the circular folds but never over solitary lymph nodules. In the center of each villus there is a lymph channel—a central lacteal—which joins the submucous lymph plexuses and a vascular capillary network that drains into a vein at the base of the villus.

Major Differences Between Jejunum and Ileum. The main differences between the jejunum and ileum from the radiographic standpoint can be summarized as follows:

1. There is a gradual diminution in diameter as the cecum is approached, and thus the lumen of the ileum is smaller than that of the jejunum. The average diameter of the jejunum measures 3 to 3.5 cm.; that of the ileum, 2.5 cm. or less.

SCHEME OF NORMAL POSITION OF SMALL INTESTINE

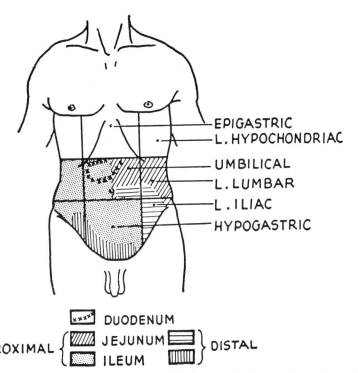

EPIGASTRIC
L. HYPOCHONDRIAC
UMBILICAL
L. LUMBAR
L. ILIAC
HYPOGASTRIC

PROXIMAL { DUODENUM — JEJUNUM — ILEUM } DISTAL

FIGURE 15-1 Approximate distribution of the small intestine within the abdomen.

SCHEMATIC ILLUSTRATION OF DISTENDED BOWEL

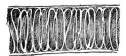

JEJUNUM
(NO INDENTED SEROSA; COILED SPRING APPEARANCE)

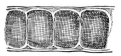

ILEUM
(NO INDENTED SEROSA)

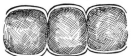

COLON
(NOTE INDENTED SEROSA BY HAUSTRAE)

FIGURE 15-2 Differences in roentgen appearance of distended small and large intestines.

2. The plicae circulares commence in the second part of the duodenum (see the description in the preceding chapter). The maximum number and size of plicae circulares are found in the midjejunum, and they diminish toward the ileum, practically ceasing a little below the middle of this portion. This fact is important because the mucosal pattern of the ileum differs from that of the proximal jejunum by being consider-

ably smoother and less feathery (Fig. 15–3*B*). Barium tends to have a more clumped appearance in the ileum than in the jejunum as a result of this fundamental difference. In the ileocecal region, the rugae tend to be parallel in type, approaching the appearance of the rugae in the pylorus.

3. The aggregate lymphatic nodules, or Peyer's patches, are most numerous in the ileum and considerably fewer in number in the jejunum. They are more prominent in young people and tend to atrophy as age advances. They are not ordinarily distinguishable radiographically and normally do not play a significant role in radiographic diagnosis.

4. In the adult, because the mesentery of the ileum contains considerably more fatty tissue than that of the jejunum, it appears to be considerably thicker than the latter structure.

Motility Study of the Small Intestine. It has been well established that many systemic diseases (such as vitamin deficiency, protein deficiency, certain anemias, allergic states, and so on) are capable of producing considerable changes in the motility pattern of the small intestine, and for that reason, a close study of the normal small intestinal motility is imperative.

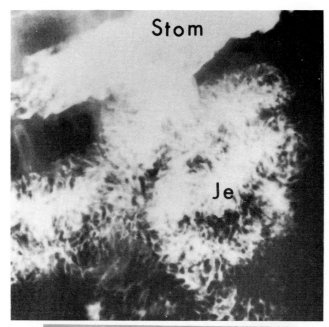

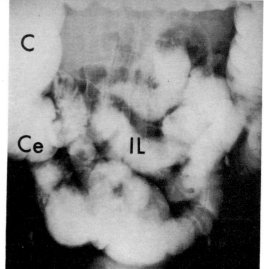

FIGURE 15-3 *A*. Radiograph of jejunal mucosal pattern. *B*. Radiograph of ileal mucosal pattern.

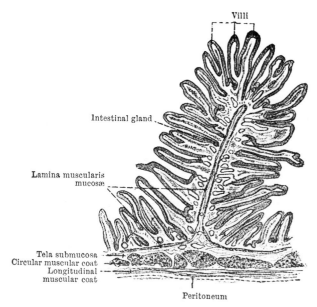

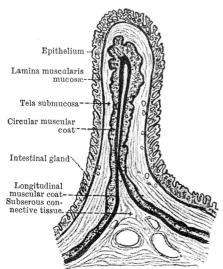

FIGURE 15-4 Diagrammatic presentation of the differences in transverse section between the plicae circulares of the small intestine and plicae semilunares of the large intestine. (From Cunningham's Textbook of Anatomy, 6th ed. London, Oxford University Press, 1931.)

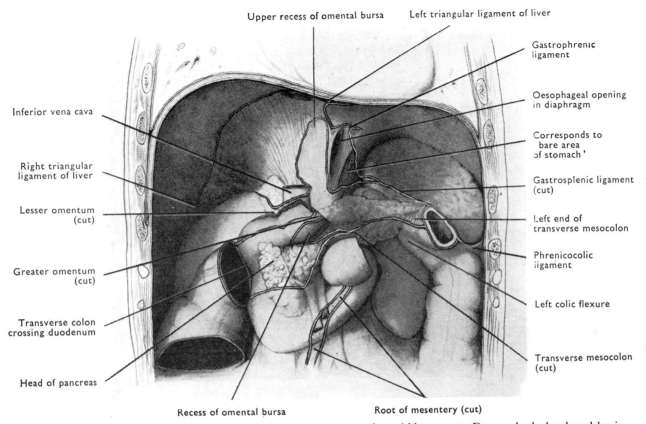

FIGURE 15–5 Peritoneal relations of duodenum, pancreas, spleen, kidneys, etc. From a body hardened by injection of formalin. When the liver, stomach, and intestines were removed the lines of the peritoneal reflections were carefully preserved. (From Cunningham's Textbook of Anatomy, 10th ed. London, Oxford University Press, 1964.)

Special Anatomy of the Ileocecal Valve (Valvula Coli). The terminal ileum projects into the cecum at its termination, producing folds or a papillary protrusion that functions as a sphincter. The serosa of the ileum does not participate in this protrusion and helps to prevent abnormal invagination of the terminal ileum into the ascending colon (called "intussusception"). The filling defect produced by this anatomic structure is readily visualized radiographically (Figs. 15–6 and 15–7).

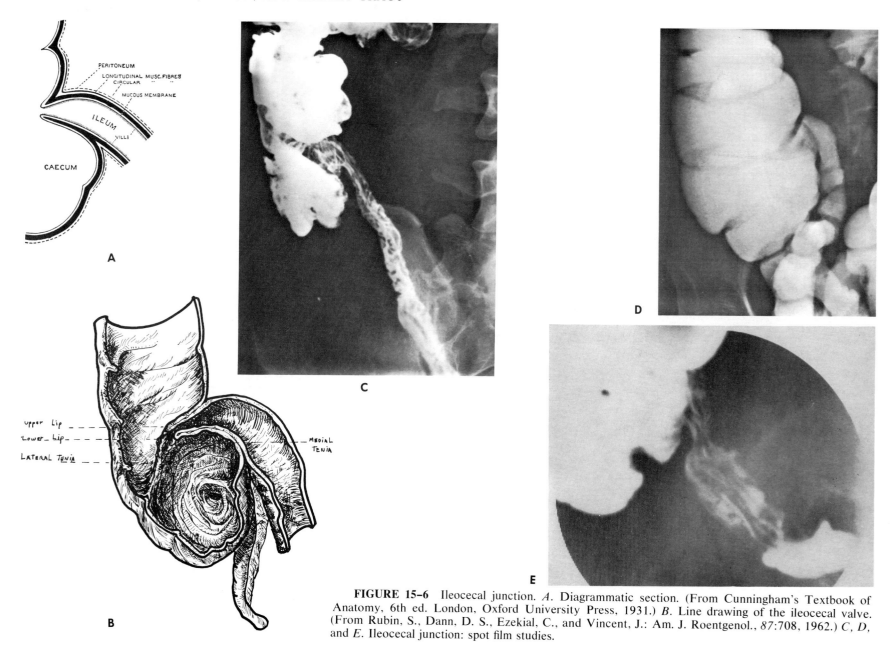

FIGURE 15–6 Ileocecal junction. *A.* Diagrammatic section. (From Cunningham's Textbook of Anatomy, 6th ed. London, Oxford University Press, 1931.) *B.* Line drawing of the ileocecal valve. (From Rubin, S., Dann, D. S., Ezekial, C., and Vincent, J.: Am. J. Roentgenol., *87*:708, 1962.) *C, D,* and *E.* Ileocecal junction: spot film studies.

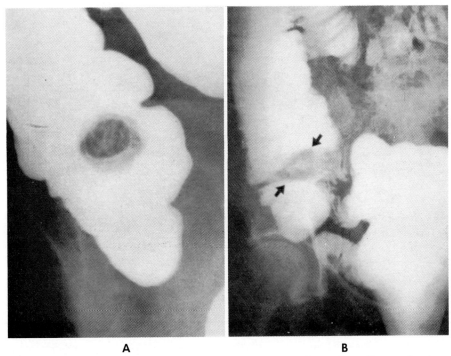

FIGURE 15–7   Difference between prolapse (*A*) and prominent ileocecal valves (*B*). In the former, the central slitlike valve orifice is not filled with barium, whereas in the latter it stands out clearly. This is a posteriorly situated valve. (From Hinkel, C. L.: Am. J. Roentgenol., *68*, 1952.)

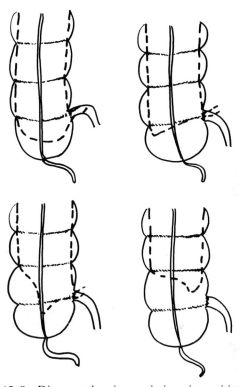

FIGURE 15–8   Diagram showing variations in position of the posterior peritoneal attachment of the cecum.

THE LARGE INTESTINE

Gross Anatomy

The large intestine is approximatly 5 to 5½ feet in length and varies in diameter from 1½ to 3 inches. Commencing at the cecum, it is further subdivided into ascending colon, transverse colon, descending and iliac colon, sigmoid or pelvic colon, and rectum.

The cecum is found in the right lower quadrant of the abdomen ordinarily, but its position is most variable. It is usually situated anteriorly, with only the omentum and abdominal wall lying over it. The terminal ileum joins the cecum usually on its medial or posterior aspect, and the vermiform appendix springs from the cecum on the same side as the ileocecal junction. Variations in the contour and position of the cecum, terminal ileum, and appendix, when on the right side of the abdomen, are shown in Figure 15–9.

The vermiform appendix is part of the cecum. It arises from the point where the three taeniae of the large intestine merge into one uniform coat of longitudinal muscle. It varies considerably in length from 2.5 to 25 cm., averaging 6 to 9 cm.

The transverse colon has a long mesentery, and as a result is subject to wide variation in length and position. It usually hangs down in front of the small intestine, at a considerable distance from the posterior abdominal wall, with only the greater omentum and anterior abdominal wall lying over it. *Along its first few centimeters, however, it is usually firmly attached to the anterior surface of the second part of the duodenum and the head of the pancreas* — a factor of considerable importance when these structures are distended by a space-occupying lesion, since there is in such cases a secondary displacement of this portion of the colon. Toward the left, the mesentery shortens, bringing this segment close to the tail of the pancreas, with the stomach lying anterior and to the right. At the inferior surface of the spleen, it passes into the splenic flexure, which is again retroperitoneal *but at a higher level than the hepatic flexure.*

The posterior surface of the greater omentum adheres to the upper surface of the transverse mesocolon and to the serosal coating on the anterior side of the transverse colon. The omentum droops down from the greater curvature of the stomach, forming a double fold over the middle part of the transverse colon.

The splenic flexure is perhaps the most constant part of the colon, being held in position by the phrenicocolic ligament, which is attached laterally to the diaphragm opposite the ninth to the eleventh rib posteriorly.

The descending and iliac portions of the colon are the narrowest parts. The descending colon first lies in contact with the lateral margin of the left kidney, and then in a comparable position with the ascending colon on the right. The posterior surface is not peritonealized and the descending colon is less mobile ordinarily than the ascending.

The iliac colon lies in the iliac fossa and, like the descending colon, is not peritonealized on its posterior surface.

The pelvic or sigmoid colon has a mesentery of its own, which accounts for the mobility of this portion of the colon, and is somewhat variable in width. It usually lies for the most part in the pelvis minor, but occasionally with marked redundancy it may escape above into the abdominal cavity.

The rectosigmoid junction is usually the narrowest point in the colon, and this narrowness may extend for 1 to 1.5 cm. *This narrowness sometimes is difficult to distinguish from an abnormal constriction*, and the radiologist must be thoroughly familiar with the normal variations of this region. Ordinarily, the rectosigmoid junction is found at the level of the third sacral vertebra. The peritoneal coat continues down from the sigmoid but only over the anterior and lateral rectal walls for about 1 to 2 cm.

The rectum is a true retroperitoneal organ. The peritoneal reflection between the rectum and the bladder in the male, or between the rectum and the uterus in the female forms the *rectovesical* or *rectouterine recess* or *pouch.*

The descending segment of the colon is without a mesentery in 64 per cent of the cases, while 36 per cent do have a mesocolon.*

The relationship of frontal and lateral perspectives of the colon has been very carefully documented by Whalen and Riemenschneider, and is shown in Figure 15–13.†

Rectum and Anal Canal.   The rectum has only a partial covering of peritoneum, and no sacculations; it is very distensible, particularly in its midportion, and this area is therefore called the rectal ampulla. The rectum first follows the hollow of the sacrum and coccyx, and then turns gently forward and finally abruptly downward to join the anal canal. There are three (and sometimes as many as five) crescentic folds, called the plicae transversales (plicae of Houston), which project into the lumen of the rectum. These pass around two-thirds of the rectal circumference and produce indentations on the radiograph of the rectum. They are variable in position and occasionally are poorly developed or virtually absent.

---

*Treves, V. F.: Anatomy of intestinal canal and peritoneum in man. Br. Med. J., *1*:580–583, 1965.

†Whalen, J. P., and Riemenschneider, P. A.: An analysis of the normal anatomic relationships of the colon as applied to roentgenographic observations. Am. J. Roentgenol., *99*:55–61, 1967.

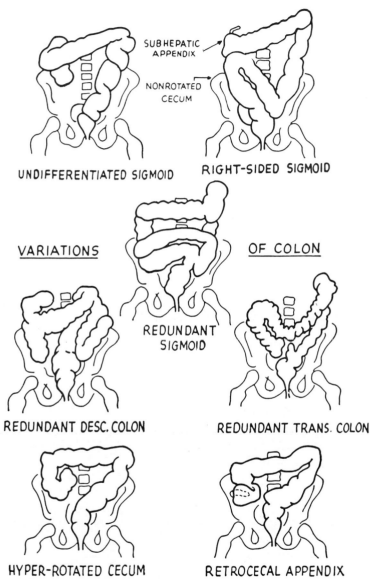

SUBHEPATIC APPENDIX

NONROTATED CECUM

UNDIFFERENTIATED SIGMOID

RIGHT-SIDED SIGMOID

VARIATIONS

OF COLON

REDUNDANT SIGMOID

REDUNDANT DESC. COLON

REDUNDANT TRANS. COLON

HYPER-ROTATED CECUM

RETROCECAL APPENDIX

FIGURE 15–9 Variations in contour and position of the cecum. The redundancy of various parts of the colon is also illustrated.

THE COLON

ANOMALIES OF THE CECUM, ABNORMALITIES OF POSITION

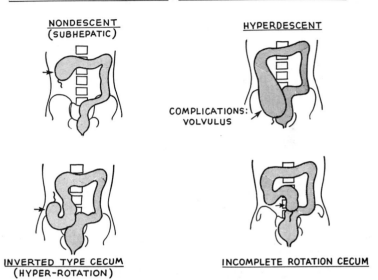

NONDESCENT (SUBHEPATIC)

HYPERDESCENT

COMPLICATIONS: VOLVULUS

INVERTED TYPE CECUM (HYPER-ROTATION)

INCOMPLETE ROTATION CECUM

FIGURE 15–10 Variations of the contour of the ascending colon in particular, demonstrating abnormalities of contour as well as position of the cecum.

Distinguishing Features Between the Large and Small Intestines. Those features which distinguish the large from the small intestine are: (1) the *taeniae coli,* which are longitudinal bands of muscle running along the outer surface of the large intestine and symmetrically placed around its circumference; (2) the *appendices epiploicae,* which are small peritoneal processes projecting from the serous coat of the large intestine; and (3) the *haustral sacculations* of the large intestine (Fig. 15–11).

Special Anatomy of the Vermiform Appendix. The appendix usually arises from the cecum on its medial or posterior aspects, about 2.5 to 4 cm. from the ileocecal valve. It is extremely variable in size and position (Figs. 15–9 and 15–10). There is a "valve" at its orifice in the cecum that probably does not function in life, although occasionally the appendix even with a patent lumen will not fill immediately at the time of a barium enema and will be seen to contain barium 24 or more hours later.

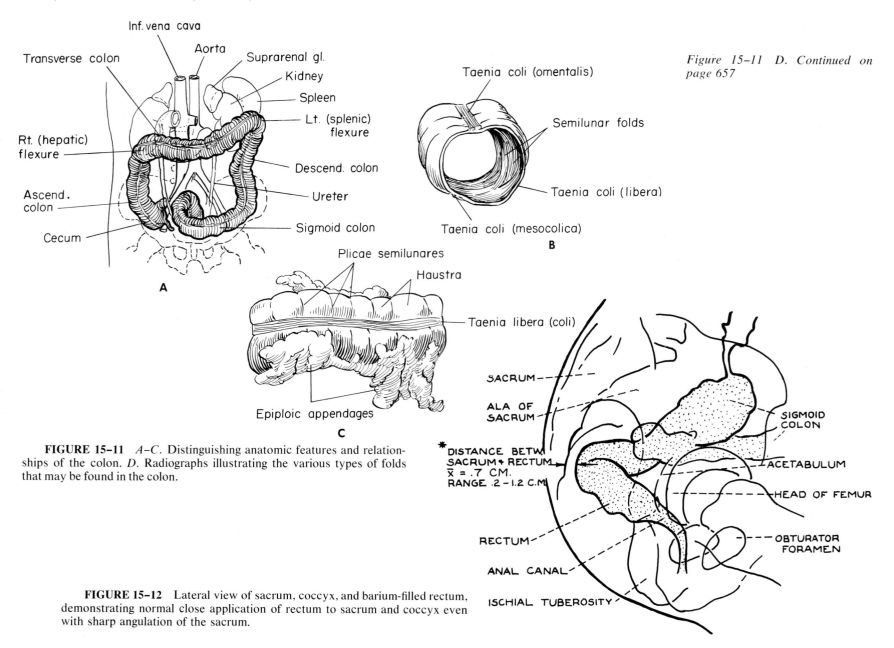

Figure 15–11 D. Continued on page 657

FIGURE 15–11 *A–C.* Distinguishing anatomic features and relationships of the colon. *D.* Radiographs illustrating the various types of folds that may be found in the colon.

FIGURE 15–12 Lateral view of sacrum, coccyx, and barium-filled rectum, demonstrating normal close application of rectum to sacrum and coccyx even with sharp angulation of the sacrum.

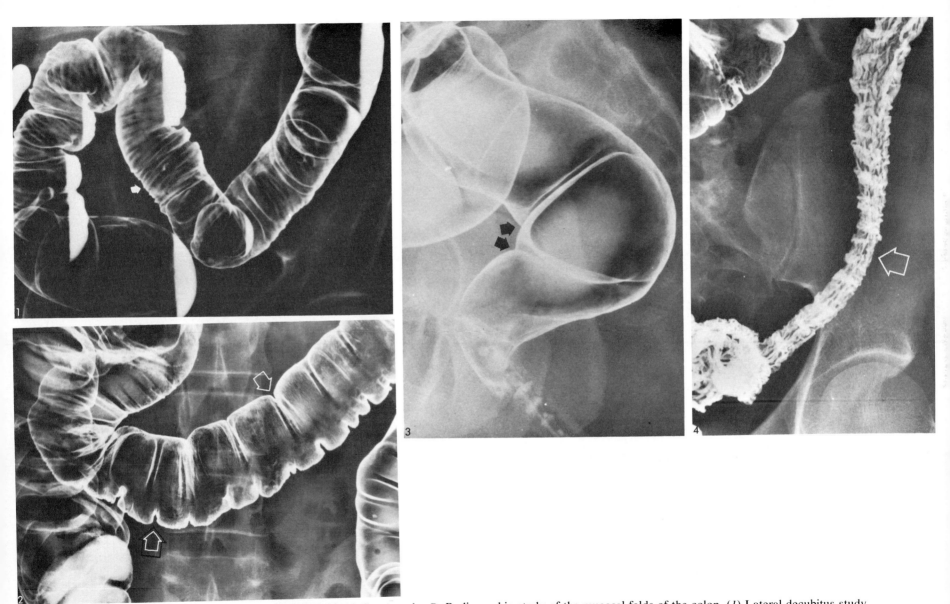

FIGURE 15–11 *Continued.* *D*. Radiographic study of the mucosal folds of the colon. (*1*) Lateral decubitus study of the ascending and transverse colon, showing innominate lines producing a faint serration of the margin of the transverse colon (arrow). (The film is shown in routine rather than decubitus relationship.) (*2*) Haustrations of the colon in a double-contrast study. (*3*) Double-contrast lateral view of rectum showing valves of Houston. (*4*) Mucosal pattern of the descending colon in its contracted state.

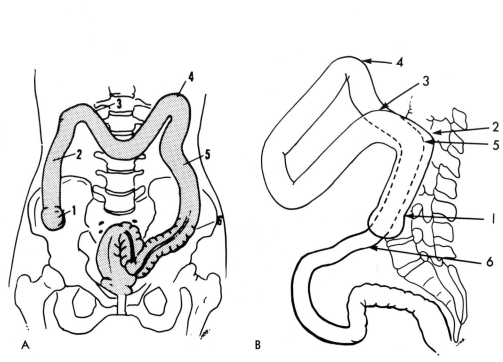

FIGURE 15–13 Diagrammatic drawings of the entire colon in frontal (*A*) and lateral (*B*) views. The known anatomic portions of the colon are labeled from 1 to 6. (*1*) Ileocecal area; (*2*) the most distal portion of the fixed retroperitoneal right colon, the most posterior portion of the right flexure; (*3*) the area of the colon as it passes over the second portion of the duodenum, where the mesentery begins to lengthen; (*4*) the roentgenographic splenic flexure; (*5*) the anatomic splenic flexure; (*6*) that portion of colon which again becomes mesenteric, the beginning of the sigmoid colon. (From Whalen, J. P., and Riemenschneider, P. A.: Am. J. Roentgenol., 99:55–61, 1967.)

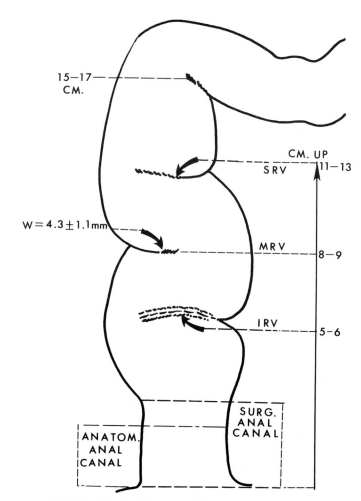

FIGURE 15–14 Diagram illustrating the rectum, the valves of Houston, and the position of the rectosigmoid junction. (W) width, (SRV) superior rectal valve, (MRV) middle rectal valve, (IRV) inferior rectal valve.

TECHNIQUE OF RADIOLOGIC EXAMINATION OF THE SMALL INTESTINE (EXCEPT ANGIOGRAPHY)

Barium Meal. Many different types of barium meals have been tested and many different adjuvant agents have been employed. Generally, nonflocculating barium 85 per cent weight/volume is considered most satisfactory.

Different volumes have been recommended—some have used 8 ounces, others 19 ounces (Schlaeger);* Marshak* has recommended at least 16 ounces and at times 20 ounces.

Our own experience has favored the utilization of 8 ounces initially under fluoroscopic control. During this time the esophagus, stomach, and duodenum are examined, thereafter an additional 8 ounces are administered prior to the routine film studies. At predetermined intervals (30 to 60 minutes) each film is viewed before the next, and spot filming is done as necessary.

Acceleration of the Barium Meal. From time to time different drugs have been advocated to enhance motility and shorten the time of the small bowel examination. Marshak and Lindner* recommend a subcutaneous or intramuscular injection of 0.5 mg. neostigmine. They do not, however, recommend the use of this drug in the elderly or in patients with heart disease, asthma, or mechanical intestinal or urinary tract obstruction. Atropine should be readily available in case a reaction should occur. Sovenyi and Varro* have recommended the addition of 30 grams of sorbitol to a barium meal consisting of 400 cc. of water and 125 to 130 grams of nonflocculent barium for study of the small intestine. The small intestinal transit time is thereby shortened to approximately 40 to 60 minutes, and they claim that there is no apparent interference with accuracy of study.

Goldstein et al.* compared various methods for acceleration of the small intestinal radiographic examination such as 0.5 mg. neostigmine methylsulfate, the right lateral decubitus position except during roentgenography, and the addition of Gastrografin to the barium mixture.

They concluded that adding 10 ml. of Gastrografin to the barium mixture was the most effective method.

Other drugs have also been utilized but may tend to alter the size of the small intestine or its motility—hence, serious doubt is cast on the use of any medication to alter the procedure.

Cold isotonic saline has also been shown to hasten both motility of the small intestine and gastric evacuation (Weintraub and Williams).* After the administration of barium sulfate in examination of the stomach and duodenum, the patient is given a glass of cold isotonic saline to drink. One half hour later he is given another glass of the saline. Under these circumstances the ileocecal region is reached in a half hour or an hour instead of the usual longer interval. In a variance of this basic technique, the second glass of isotonic saline is mixed with approximately 100 grams of barium which may enhance the contrast within the small intestine.

Conventional Small Intestinal Series. It is always desirable to have a film of the abdomen without contrast prior to the introduction of any contrast agent.

The patient is allowed no food or drink following the evening meal on the night before the examination.

A routine examination of the esophagus, stomach, and duodenum is carried out as previously described (Chapter 14). The barium column is watched as it passes into the jejunum. When it appears relatively stationary, it has been our practice to administer another 8 ounces of nonflocculent barium mixture as described above and then to obtain a film of the abdomen. Fifteen to thirty minutes later another film of the abdomen is obtained. This film is inspected, and time intervals are designated for the further examination of the passage of the barium in the small bowel. Usually these intervals are approximately 30 to 60 minutes. When the barium has reached the ileocecal region, the patient is examined fluoroscopically once again and spot-film compression studies of the ileocecal region are obtained.

---

*References may be obtained in Meschan I.: An Atlas of Anatomy Basic to Radiology. Philadelphia, W. B. Saunders Co., 1975, Chapter 13.

If any abnormalities are seen in the course of the small intestinal series, the patient is restudied by fluoroscopy and the area in question is carefully compressed, palpated, and refilmed by spot-film compression techniques.

A representative routine series is shown in Figure 15–15.

If small bowel or large intestinal obstruction is suspected, a routine series of films for investigation of the abdomen without additional contrast is used prior to the small bowel series. These include chest film, supine anteroposterior view of the abdomen, and upright film of the abdomen or a lateral decubitus if the patient is unable to stand (see Chapter 8). If obstruction is suspected in the large intestine, we have preferred to administer a barium enema first to make certain of the site of the obstruction.

An obstruction in the small intestine is not considered a contraindication to examination with oral barium (Frimann-Dahl; Nelson et al.).*

Small Intestinal Enema. Following the passage of a tube into the duodenum, 500 to 1000 cc. of thin barium solution may be given in a continuous stream by gravity. Thereafter, the entire small bowel is studied as this continuous stream of barium passes through it. Schatzki* has indicated that barium reaches the cecum in about 15 minutes under these circumstances.

Modification of Technique with the Postoperative Partially Resected Stomach. The basic modification required for examination of a patient with a partially resected stomach is the study of the small intestine at more frequent intervals, particularly shortly after the administration of the oral barium. Motility through the proximal small intestine is more rapid than normal, but as the barium column reaches the ileum and beyond, motility occurs at normal time intervals.

Intubation Techniques for Study of Small Foci of Involvement. A Miller-Abbott or Cantor tube may be passed and allowed to move down the small intestine until it meets a point of delay or obstruction. The barium mixture is injected through the tube at this point, and the intestine at the site of obstruction is carefully studied without interference of adjoining loops. This technique is particularly useful for studying an area of obstruction, either partial or complete. A length of 6 to 8 feet of tubing is sufficient to extend from the pylorus to the cecum ordinarily. Approximately 3 hours are required for passage. The tube is withdrawn when it has reached the cecum if an obstruction is not present. The instillation of 4 to 8 cc. of liquid metallic mercury into the rubber balloon of the tube facilitates the passage of the tube through the pylorus and increases the rapidity with which the tube passes down the small intestine.

Radiologic Study of the Small Intestine with Water Soluble Iodinated Contrast Media. Various mixtures of water soluble iodide have been utilized for examination of the gastrointestinal tract both orally and rectally.

1. Forty per cent sodium diatrizoate solution (Hypaque) (Shehadi).*
2. Forty per cent sodium diatrizoate with oxyphenisatin.
3. Twenty-five per cent diatrizoate solution plus an equal volume of barium sulfate suspension.
4. Forty per cent sodium diatrizoate or methylglucamine diatrizoate (Gastrografin).
5. Fifty grams of sodium diatrizoate dissolved in 75 cc. of sterile water to which 10 drops of a wetting agent such as Tween-80 have been added, to aid in the coating of the mucosa (Jacobson et al.).* A flavoring agent must be added if this is used orally.

Because of the high tonicity of these water soluble agents, they have not been recommended, especially in children (Neuhauser; Nelson et al.).* The high tonicity of these contrast agents has another result — they are diluted in the small intestine and become less radiopaque in the jejunum and ileum. However, in the colon water is reabsorbed and the contrast improves. The transit time is more rapid than with barium (30 to 90 minutes unless obstruction is encountered).

---

*References may be obtained in Meschan, I.: An atlas of Anatomy Basic to Radiology. Philadelphia, W. B. Saunders Co., 1975, Chapter 13.

Differences in Infants and Children. Small barium feedings of 1 to 3 ounces are utilized for infants and children. The transit time may be long in the very young (Lonnerblad).* Fluroscopy should be limited to the smallest possible field.

In the first weeks and months of life the normal feathery pattern of the small intestine does not appear. Distinct jejunal markings, however, are usually visible after the fifth month. Segmentation persists much longer (Fig. 15–15*D*).

During the first year and until the infant assumes the erect posture, the small intestine lies almost entirely above the pelvis.

Large amounts of gas may be found in the jejunum and ileum during the first two or three years of life.

In general, clumping and segmentation of the barium column are so relatively common in the child (both healthy and sick) that this adult criterion of abnormality cannot be applied (Fig. 15–15*D*). Also, the mucosal contours in the terminal segment of the ileum that are usually longitudinal and linear in the adult may normally have a cobblestone pattern in the child. They are probably caused by the greater abundance in the child of solitary and conglomerate lymph follicles, and are largest in the terminal ilcum during preadolescence and adolescence.

A persistent deficiency of gas in the small intestine of the newborn infant beyond the first day may be a cardinal sign of intestinal obstruction. However, there are other entities which may be responsible for this appearance, such as adrenal insufficiency, dehydration, diarrhea, and other interference with the normal transport mechanisms.

Intestinal Biopsy Techniques (Wood et al.; Tomenius).* In general, these instruments consist of flexible tubes at the lower end of which is a small metal cylinder provided with a circular lateral hole about 2 to 3 mm. in diameter. The capsule contains a circular knife blade. Suction applied with a vacuum pump or a large syringe aspirates a fragment of the mucosa through the opening of the capsule. The knife blade is released, cutting the mucosa fragment, which is then contained within the capsule. In the Crosby capsule the hole is somewhat enlarged, minimizing the occurrence of hemorrhagic artefacts. The capsule is removed as quickly as possible from the gastrointestinal tract, the terminal cylinder is unscrewed, and the mucosal fragments are collected and oriented on a small piece of wet lens paper with the cut surface downward. They are promptly immersed in 10 per cent formalin or a modified Bouin's solution and embedded in paraffin. They are thereafter stained with hematoxylin-eosin or by special staining techniques.

String Test for Bleeding in Upper Gastrointestinal Tract. The original Einhorn string test of 1909 has been modified in two important ways: (1) the application of guaiac stains to the string, and (2) the administration of sodium fluorescein (20 ml., 5 per cent solution) intravenously and the withdrawal of the string 4 minutes thereafter. The string is then examined for fluorescence with a Wood's lamp. The string is a common type with a mercury bag tied to its end. There are small radiopaque gauze markers tied to the string at designated intervals. Approximately the first 40 cm. on the string lie in the esophageal area, 40 to 55 cm. in the gastric area, and beyond 55 to 60 cm. in the duodenal and jejunal areas. The total string length is approximately 150 cm. (Traphagen and Karlan; Smith; Haynes and Pittman).*

According to Smith, the incidence of false negative tests is 1.2 per cent. False positive tests can be attributed to eating of meats, beets, tomatoes, gelatin, cherries (red), or chocolate, or to trauma in passing the string. The string must be withdrawn 4 minutes after the intravenous administration of the fluorescein, since fluorescein would be excreted by the major papilla (of Vater) if the procedure is prolonged.

---

*References may be obtained in Meschan, I.: An Atlas of Anatomy Basic to Radiology. Philadelphia, W. B. Saunders Co., 1975, Chapter 13.

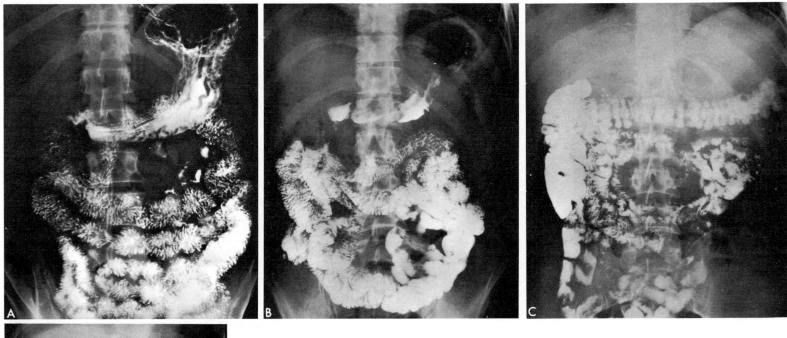

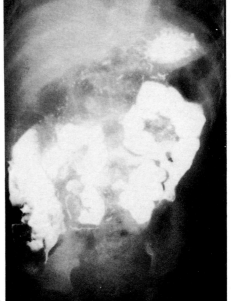

FIGURE 15-15 Illustrations to demonstrate frequent-interval film and fluoroscopy method for examination of small intestine: *A*. At 1 hour following administration of the barium; *B*. at 2 hours; *C*. at 3 hours; *D*. Representative small intestinal pattern of a normal infant on a predominantly milk diet. Note that the clumping and scattering are relatively normal for infants at this stage of development.

TECHNIQUE OF RADIOLOGIC EXAMINATION OF THE COLON (EXCEPT ANGIOGRAPHY)

The methods of examination are: (1) the plain radiograph of the abdomen; (2) the full-column barium enema, under fluoroscopic visualization, and accompanied by spot-film compression radiography, in addition to certain routine film studies; (3) the barium meal, followed through until the colon is visualized, and thereafter at 6 hours, 24 hours, and further intervals if desired; and (4) the barium-air double contrast enema (see Fig. 15–26).

Preliminary Plain Radiograph of the Abdomen. If a film of the abdomen has not been obtained in the course of other studies prior to the barium enema, it is well to obtain a posteroanterior film of the abdomen prior to the introduction of any contrast agent. The routine base line film of the abdomen is not only useful from the standpoint of later evaluation after contrast is introduced, but in itself it may reveal significant abnormality.* Moreover, the appearance of dense inspissated fecal material may indicate the presence of a bowel obstruction. This appearance must also be differentiated at times from extraluminal gas which may produce a somewhat similar appearance.

The Routine Barium Enema

Preparation of the Patient. Thorough cleansing of the colon prior to the barium enema is essential, since any fecal material will obscure the normal anatomy and give rise to false filling defects and mucosal aberrations. This is best accomplished, in our experience, by the following routine:

1. Clear liquid diet for at least 24 hours prior to the examination forcing liquids.

2. One and one-half ounces of X-Prep liquid or its equivalent for

---

*Rosenbaum, H. D., et al.: Routine survey roentgenogram of the abdomen on 500 consecutive patients over 40 years of age. Am. J. Roentgenol., *91*:903–909, 1964.

catharsis, at 6 P.M. on the evening prior to the examination. Two ounces of castor oil may be preferred. As an alternative, a 10-ounce dose of liquid magnesium citrate (U.S.P.) may be administered at 8:00 P.M., followed by 4 Dulcolax tablets (5 mg. bisacodyl each) at 10:00 P.M. If magnesium citrate is used, the *patient must drink about 6 glasses of water additionally before midnight.* A Dulcolax suppository is administered in the morning to clear the watery content in the large intestine.

3. Cleansing enemas prior to the barium enema examination until the returning fluid is clear, unless thorough cleansing of the colon has otherwise been accomplished following the catharsis. A Dulcolax suppository (10 mg.) in the rectum at 7:00 A.M. may be used, or the barium enema may be postponed for 1 to 2 hours to obtain complete evacuation of the cleansing enemas.

Ordinarily, the patient is examined without breakfast, as the breakfast meal will introduce gas in the stomach and occasionally in the colon.

Flocculent-resistant barium sulfate suspension is used (Barotrast or its equivalent) and is made by mixing the compounds in a 1 to 4 or up to 1 to 6 mixture, depending upon preference; 15 per cent barium weight per volume may be obtained commercially already packaged in its antiflocculent form in plastic bags (tubing and bag to be discarded after use), thus preventing reflux contamination.

Barium-Air Double Contrast Enema. The preparation of the patient must be especially carefully done under these circumstances. We have preferred placing the patient on a low residue diet for a period of 2 days, and on 2 successive nights prior to the morning of the examination we have recommended the administration of 1½ ounces of X-Prep liquid. *If 2 ounces of castor oil are used, they should be given on only one occasion, the evening before the examination as in the routine barium enema examination.*

Breakfast is omitted on the morning of the examination and *further cleansing enemas may be given if it is thought necessary.* It has been our usual experience that after 2 such consecutive days of preparation (sometimes 3), the colon is thoroughly cleansed and no further cleansing enemas are necessary.

One-half to 2 mg. of glucagon are administered intramuscularly just prior to the injection of the air.

A colloidal barium mixture of fairly high density (85 per cent weight per volume) is utilized. It may be given in several differing ways: Our preference is to introduce this barium to the mid-ascending colon *with the patient prone*, utilizing gravity tilt of the table and rotation of the patient (with shoulder rests to prevent the patient's sliding when head down). The barium need not be forcibly introduced. The patient is then allowed to go to the toilet to evacuate as much as possible. He then returns to the examination table. Only air is introduced, while the patient is rotated from the prone to the oblique and even supine positions, so long as the mixture is not forced into the terminal ileum. Terminal ileum visualization may obscure the rectum and sigmoid. The tubing and enema tip are of a large bore.

An alternate method is to introduce the barium only to the hepatic flexure, aspirate it into a bag, and then inject the air forcibly thereafter.

In either method, the combination of the barium and air is followed closely throughout the rectum, the sigmoid in all of its flexure, the descending colon, the splenic flexure, the transverse colon, the hepatic flexure, the ascending colon and cecum, and spot films are obtained as each area comes into good view. The patient is rotated, and the tilt-table is elevated or lowered as required.

Routine films (Fig. 15–25) are thereafter obtained in the posteroanterior (prone), both obliques, as well as left and right lateral decubitus projections. A prone view of the rectosigmoid with the tube angled about 30 degrees toward the feet and a lateral view of the rectum and sigmoid to include the sacrum are also obtained. Occasionally, the Chassard-Lapiné view and other oblique views of the rectosigmoid junction may be required.

Although the barium-air double contrast enema was originally thought to be contraindicated in cases of ulcerative colitis, granulomatous colitis, diverticulosis, this is no longer the case; we do, however, prefer the low-pressure technique in these cases.*

---

*Fraser, G. M., and Findlay, J. M.: The double contrast enema in ulcerative and Crohn's colitis. Clin. Radiol., 27:103–112, 1976.

In cases of diverticulitis, some prefer the full column technique first to avoid perforation of the colon.

After all of the films are obtained, the patient may be studied in the supine position for visualization of the terminal ileum, if this is indicated by the history.

We usually allow the patient to wait about 45 minutes after the last cleansing enema to allow the colonic mucosa to dry somewhat, before administering the double-contrast enema.

It is unfortunate that the routine full-column barium enema is so often limited by retained fecal material in the colon, causing small polypoid lesions to be obscured. It is now our preference to perform the double-contrast enema wherever feasible, especially in any patient who is suspected of malignancy or has been bleeding through the rectum.

THE FLUOROSCOPIC-RADIOGRAPHIC EQUIPMENT. The radiographic equipment should be capable of high kilovoltage and high milliamperage with short exposure times. The kilovoltage should be at least 120 Kv. to permit overpenetration of the barium. Photo-timing for spot films is desirable. Image amplifier fluoroscopy is also preferred.

It is our preference to use one hand (left) for manipulation of the exposures and the fluoroscopic screen; the right hand, protected by a heavy lead glove, and kept over the heavy column of barium or outside the direct beam, is used to palpate the patient's abdomen.

ROUTINE FOR FLUOROSCOPY. The routine for fluoroscopy in a single contrast barium enema is as follows:

1. The patient's abdomen and chest are initially surveyed.
2. Following this survey, the examination is carried out as detailed in Figure 15–17. The patient first lies on his left side, at an angle of about 60 degrees to the table. The barium mixture is allowed to flow slowly into the rectum to permit the patient to adjust to the liquid mixture being introduced. It should have been warmed to body temperature prior to introduction.

A spot film of the rectosigmoid junction is obtained when this junction is observed to fill and the barium flow momentarily stops (Fig. 15–16).

The patient is then lowered slightly to a 45-degree angle and a small amount of barium is introduced so that the entire sigmoid and lower descending colon are filled. Once again there is a cessation of the barium flow and a second spot film is obtained to demonstrate the entire sigmoid and junction with the descending colon (Fig. 15–18 *A*).

The patient then is turned on his back, fully supine, and the barium mixture is again allowed to flow until the descending colon to the level of the splenic flexure can be carefully examined.

The patient is then slowly turned to his right side as the barium mixture is allowed to flow around the splenic flexure, and again the flow ceases while a spot film is obtained of the splenic flexure (Fig. 15–18 *B*).

With the patient supine once more the barium is allowed to flow to fill the transverse colon and the beginning of the ascending colon around the hepatic flexure. The patient is then turned on his left side at an angle of approximately 45 degrees so that the hepatic flexure is completely unwound, and another spot film is obtained (Fig. 15–18 *C*).

With the patient once again supine, the barium flow continues until the entire cecum is identified and reflux into the ileum through the ileocecal junction is obtained if possible. The patient is turned so that the ileocecal junction is seen to best advantage without interference from adjoining loops of bowel. A spot film is obtained (Fig. 15–18 *D*).

Usually the patient will experience moderate discomfort once the barium column has passed the hepatic flexure into the ascending colon, and the examination must be carried forward expeditiously at this point. Routine films are immediately obtained after the filling and reflux into the distal ileum.

Each of the films must be carefully inspected before the patient is allowed to leave. A repeat study may be undertaken if any questionable areas are seen during the film review. Air may also be injected at this time if necessary, although the ideal double contrast barium enema is a separate examination.

Routine films following fluoroscopy and spot filming are taken as follows: (1) a high kilovoltage posteroanterior view of the entire colon (Fig. 15–19); and (2) a right or left lateral film of the colon centered at the rectosigmoid (Fig. 15–21). Oblique films are ordered as required. The spot films may be adequate for this purpose.

Special studies of the rectosigmoid, such as the Chassard-Lapiné view of the rectum and sigmoid may be employed to "unravel" a tortuous and redundant sigmoid (Figs. 15–22 and 15–23). An alternate oblique study of the rectosigmoid and sigmoid colon may be obtained as shown in Figure 15–23. Here, the patient lies prone and the central x-ray beam, centered at the level of the anal canal, is directed approximately 35 degrees cephalad. A view very similar to the Chassard-Lapiné view is thereby obtained.

Following colonic evacuation, another posteroanterior prone film of the empty colon is obtained. If the evacuation has not been sufficient, the patient is asked to return after further evacuation for more film studies of the empty colon (Fig. 15–24).

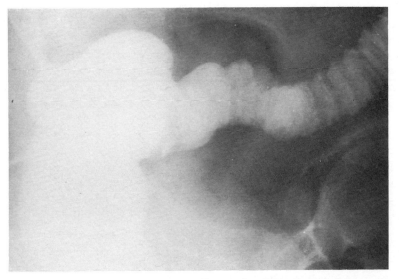

FIGURE 15–16 Example of spot film study obtained during fluoroscopy of the rectosigmoid colon.

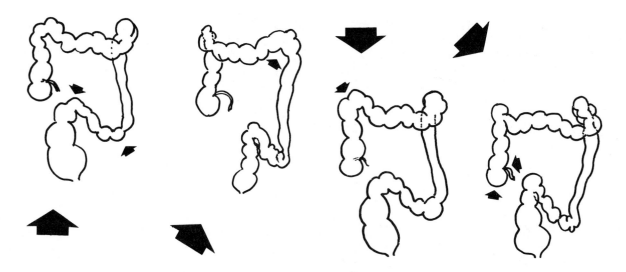

RADIOLOGIC EXAMINATION OF THE COLON (FULL BARIUM COLUMN)

(1)
Patient lying on left
  side
Two spot films, 45° and 60°
Study rectum and sigmoid

(2)
Patient supine
Study descending
  colon

(3)
Patient lying on right
  side
Spot film, 45°
Splenic flexure

(4)
Patient supine
Study transverse colon

(5)
Patient on left side
Spot film, 45°
  oblique hepatic flexure

(6)
Patient supine, then to
  right side
Study ascending colon,
  cecum
Spot ileo-cecal junction
  when visualized at
  maximum

Return for repeat
  fluoroscopy, injection of
  air or repeat injection of
  barium if necessary

FIGURE 15–17 Technique of fluoroscopic examination and spot filming of the colon.

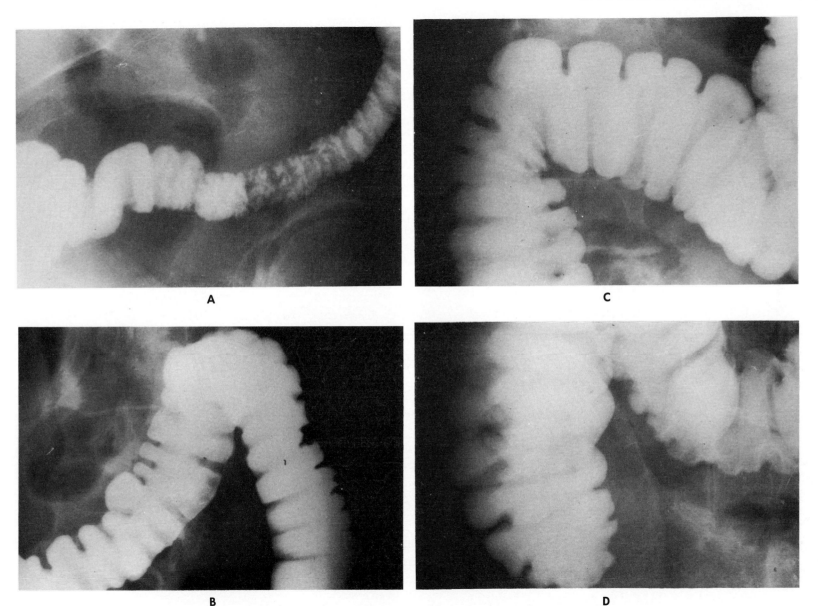

FIGURE 15–18 Spot film studies. *A*. Sigmoid. *B*. Splenic flexure. *C*. Hepatic flexure. *D*. Cecum.

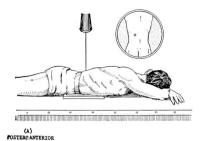

(A)
POSTERO ANTERIOR

A

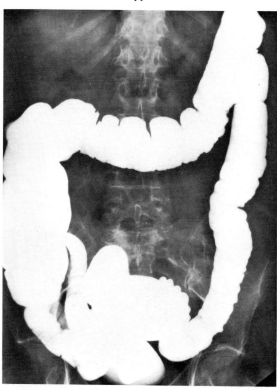

B

POINTS OF PRACTICAL INTEREST ABOUT FIGURE 15–19

1. The exposure should be "high kilovoltage" to permit good penetration of the barium-filled colon. In this way, filling defects may be shown that otherwise could not be demonstrated readily.

2. The central ray is directed through the center of the abdomen about 1 cm. above the iliac crest.

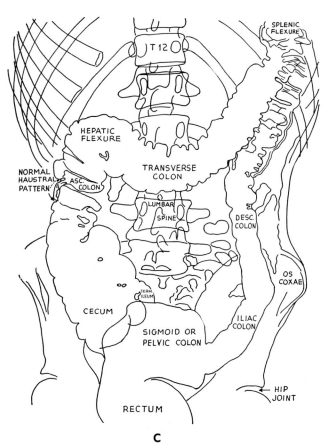

C

FIGURE 15–19 Full-column barium enema. *A*. Position of patient. *B*. Radiograph obtained in posteroanterior projection. *C*. Labeled tracing.

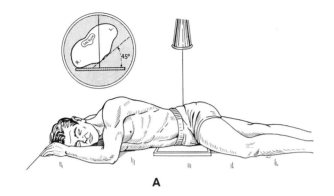

A

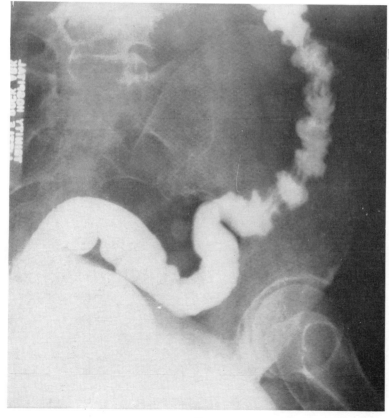

B

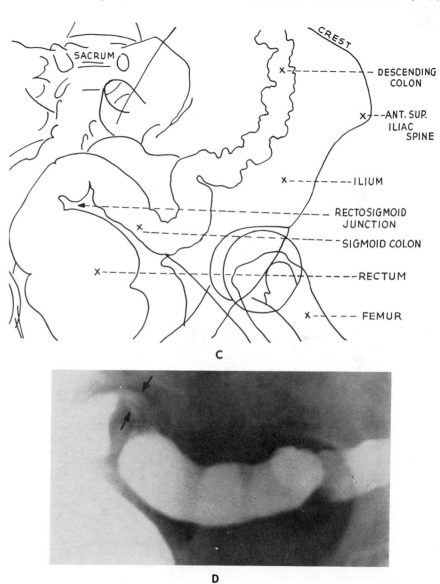

C

D

FIGURE 15–20 Oblique study of pelvic and iliac colon. *A*. Position of patient. *B*. Radiograph obtained. *C*. Labeled tracing. *D*. Film study demonstrating narrowness that may be normal at the rectosigmoid junction.

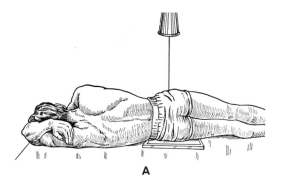

A

POINTS OF PRACTICAL INTEREST ABOUT FIGURES 15–21 AND 15–23

1. Figure 15–22 may be supplemented by a view obtained with the patient prone, and the central ray angled 15 to 30 degrees toward the feet, centering over the anal canal. This position may be more tolerable for the uncomfortable patient than that illustrated in Figure 15–23, and a somewhat similar, distorted view of the rectosigmoid region will be obtained.

If the patient cannot be turned into the prone position, the central ray is angled similarly toward the head, with the patient lying on his back.

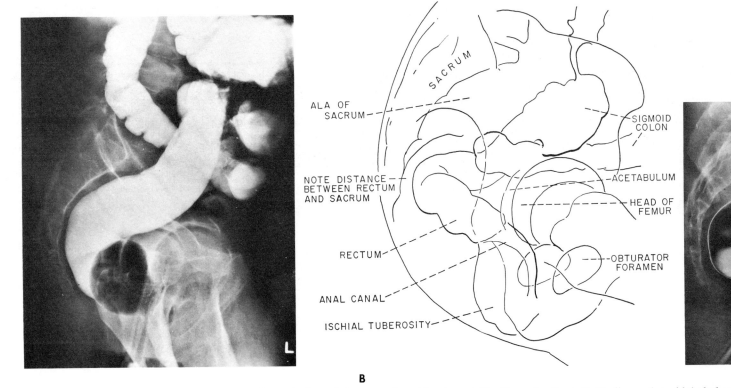

B

ALA OF SACRUM
NOTE DISTANCE BETWEEN RECTUM AND SACRUM
RECTUM
ANAL CANAL
ISCHIAL TUBEROSITY

SACRUM
SIGMOID COLON
ACETABULUM
HEAD OF FEMUR
OBTURATOR FORAMEN

C

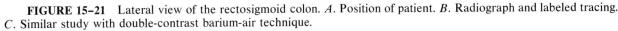

FIGURE 15–21 Lateral view of the rectosigmoid colon. *A.* Position of patient. *B.* Radiograph and labeled tracing. *C.* Similar study with double-contrast barium-air technique.

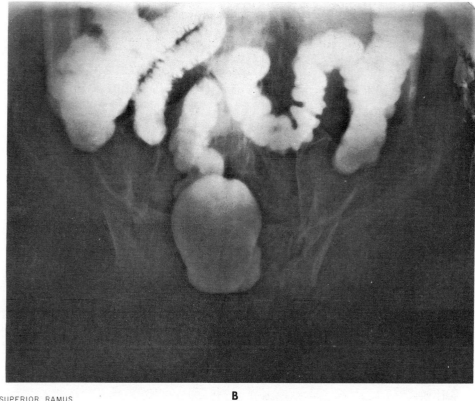

B

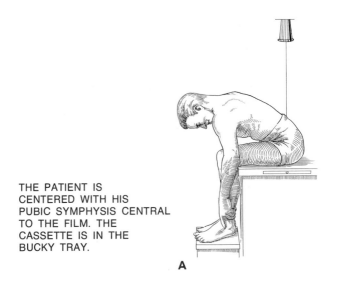

THE PATIENT IS
CENTERED WITH HIS
PUBIC SYMPHYSIS CENTRAL
TO THE FILM. THE
CASSETTE IS IN THE
BUCKY TRAY.

A

FIGURE 15–22 Chassard-Lapiné projection of the rectum and sigmoid colon. The patient is centered with his pubic symphysis central to the film and the cassette in the Bucky tray. *A.* Position of patient. *B.* Radiograph. *C.* Tracing.

SIGMOID
COLON

SUPERIOR RAMUS
OF PUBIS

ILIAC CREST

OBTURATOR
FORAMEN

ILEOPECTINEAL
LINE

HEAD OF FEMUR

HIP JOINT

INFERIOR RAMUS OF PUBIS

ALA OF SACRUM

RECTUM

ISCHIAL TUBEROSITY

SACROILIAC JOINT

COCCYGEAL SEGMENTS

C

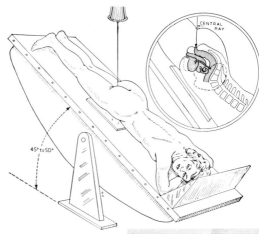

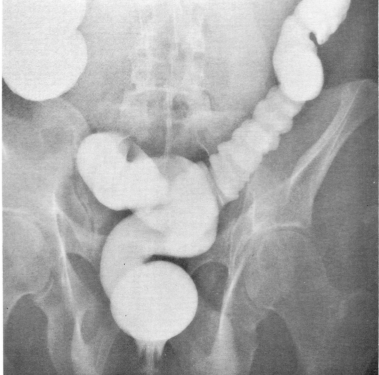

FIGURE 15–23 Distorted view of sigmoid colon. *A*. Position of patient in relation to central x-ray beam. *B*. Radiograph so obtained.

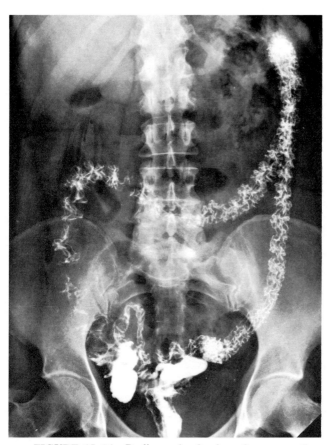

FIGURE 15–24 Radiograph of colon after evacuation of barium.

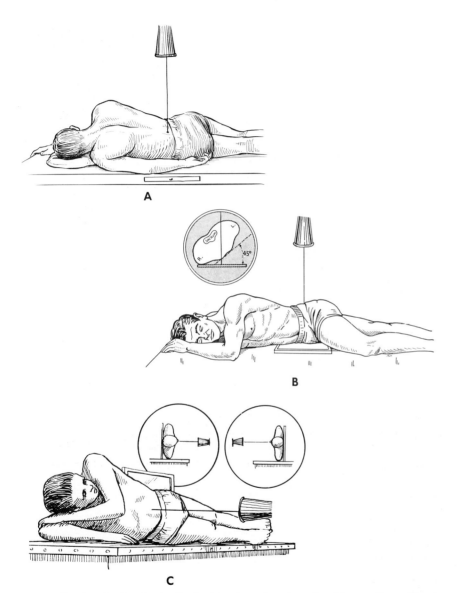

FIGURE 15–25 *A. B. C.* Positioning of patient for film studies with a double-contrast enema. In addition to the two oblique and the two horizontal beam projections shown, straight posteroanterior and left lateral projections are also obtained.

Limitations of the Routine Barium Enema. The barium enema examination should not be considered a substitute for the digital or sigmoidoscopic examination of the rectum. The rectum is often obscured by its voluminous barium content, or by a balloon, if such was employed, and in the postevacuation study the sigmoid and rectal loops may fold over one another in such a way as to mask a lesion. The double-contrast high-density barium and air enema has significantly enhanced the accuracy of diagnosis not only of polypoid lesions of the colon, but also of lesions of the rectum and sigmoid, when it is properly performed.

Redundancy and overlapping of portions of the colon may obscure one of the anatomic parts—hence, a complete examination of all flexures in the fluoroscopic visualization is essential. Occasionally, such complete examination is virtually impossible and careful notation of this inadequacy should be made.

Haustral points of narrowness and the rectosigmoid junction may give the impression of abnormal areas of narrowness unless the examiner is thoroughly conversant with the wide variation in the normal appearance of the colon.

Unless the terminal ileum or appendix has been visualized, it is difficult to be completely certain that the cecum has been seen, and for that reason caution must be exercised in assuming that the colon has been completely filled when the terminal ileum and appendix have not been visualized. Unfortunately, it is sometimes impossible to fill the terminal ileum and appendix, so experience must dictate when the colon has been entirely distended with barium. *The terminal ileum should not be filled in the double-contrast enema, since this may obscure the accuracy of the study of the rectum and sigmoid. To avoid filling the terminal ileum, the patient should be filled and studied in the* prone *position throughout the double-contrast study.*

Fluoroscopy is not as accurate as film studies for revealing minute mucosal changes such as those seen in the earliest aberrations of mucosal structure. It is important to become familiar with the normal appearance of both the full and empty colon in this regard, so that minimal abnormalities may be recognized on film.

When patients are unable to retain the enema and evacuation is forced before complete filling of the colon and cecum, it must not be assumed that an obstructive abnormality of an organic type necessarily exists in the colon. A repeat examination, especially with the aid of a carefully inserted rectal balloon, may be necessary.

The importance of proctosigmoidoscopy is shown by the fact that this adjunctive study may permit observation of: thromboulcerative colitis; ulcerations occurring in amebic, bacillary, and tuberculous colitis; 90 per cent of the organic pathology occurring in the colon; 70 per cent of the nonmalignant tumors; 75 per cent of the malignant tumors originating in the colon; factitial prostatitis and lymphogranuloma venereum; foreign bodies; rectovesical and rectourethral fistulas; and perforation of the rectum or sigmoid by foreign bodies.

Indications for Single- and Double-Contrast Barium Enema

The single-contrast full-column examination has wide usefulness in detecting most abnormalities of the colon, including the right half of the colon, ulcerative disease, and terminal ileal disease in many cases. *It is less efficient than the double-contrast enema in detecting small intraluminal tumors.* It is unfortunate that both examinations cannot be done on the same day. They are best done one or two days apart as indicated by clinical history. In patients with unexplained rectal bleeding (bright red or dark), with a history of polyps, or with polyps found at proctoscopy, the colloidal barium double-contrast enema is performed.

We have also employed a low-residue diet for three successive days, and X-Prep Liquid® (2½ ounces) for three successive nights prior to the examination. This has given us successful preparation and is reasonably well tolerated.

Complications of a Barium Enema

Perforation or rupture of the colon, which may be either *intra- or extraperitoneal.*

Perforation of the colon into the venous system (Rosenberg and Fine; Zatzkin and Irwin).*

Water intoxication, especially in children (Steinbach et al.).*

Colonic intramural barium (Seaman and Bragg).* This complication results from mucosal rupture, which permits the barium to dissect into the colonic wall. The outstanding roentgen feature is a transverse striated pattern that is probably produced by the inner layer of circular muscle fibers.

Examination of the Colon Through a Colostomy. In preparation of and patient, a low residue diet for 24 to 48 hours and thorough cleansing of the colon through the colostomy is ordinarily sufficient.

If a Foley catheter is employed as the enema tip in order to prevent spillage of the barium out of the colostomy, the inflation of the Foley bag must be carried out with great caution after insertion far into the bowel and *under careful fluoroscopic control. Perforation of the bowel may result* (Seaman and Wells).* *Some have urged that a Foley catheter with a long tubular section ahead of the balloon be employed*, the balloon being applied with pressure on the outside of the colostomy to prevent spillage (Margulis).* Various other techniques for preventing spillage have been advocated.

The introduction of the barium and the rolling of the patient from one side to the other is very much the same as previously described for the routine barium enema. Spot films are taken as necessary. Likewise, the routine filming following the enema through the colostomy is very similar, care being exercised once again to obtain the films as quickly as possible after the filling to prevent spillage.

---

*References may be obtained in Meschan, I.: An Atlas of Anatomy Basic to Radiology. Philadelphia, W. B. Saunders Co., 1975, Chapter 14.

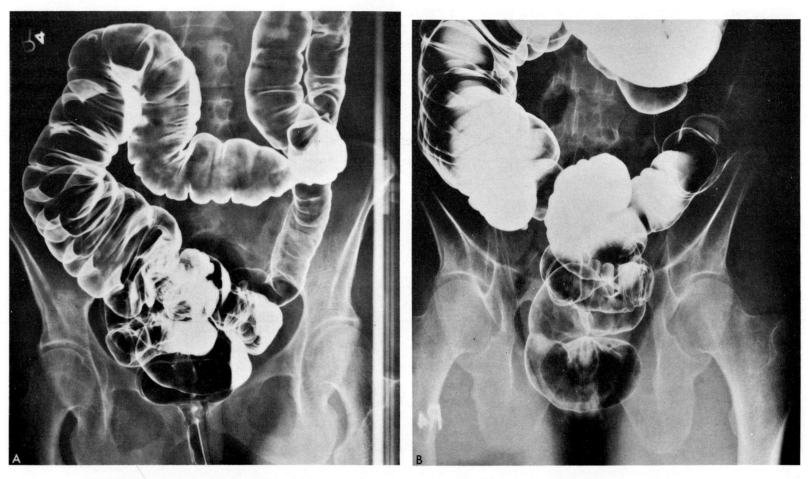

FIGURE 15–26 Sample radiographs of double-contrast high-density barium air enemas: *A*. Routine posteroanterior projection. *B*. Special projection with the patient prone, table tilted with head down for better visualization of double contrast of the rectum and sigmoid.

Figure continued on following page.

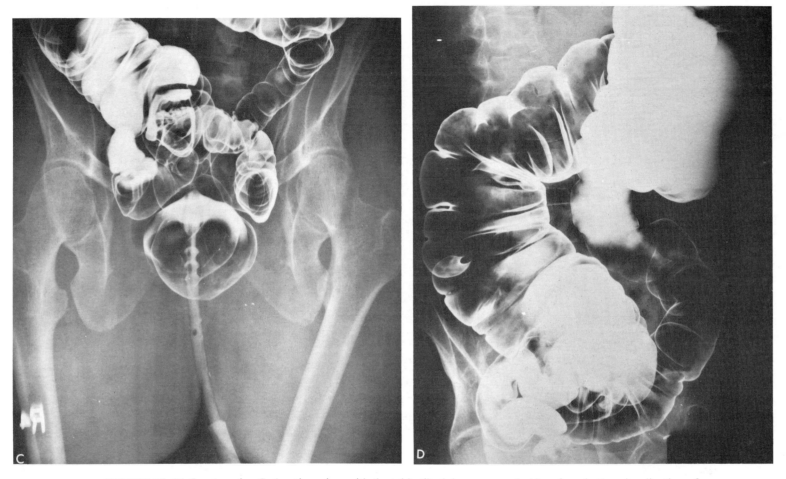

FIGURE 15–26 *Continued.* C. Another view with the table tilted down somewhat less for a better visualization of the sigmoid in double contrast. *D.* Patient supine with left side elevated for best double contrast of both the hepatic flexure and sigmoid.

Figure continued on opposite page.

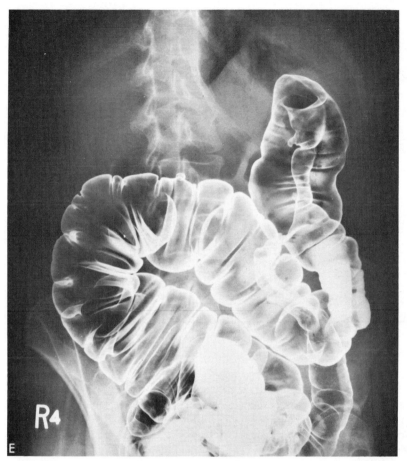

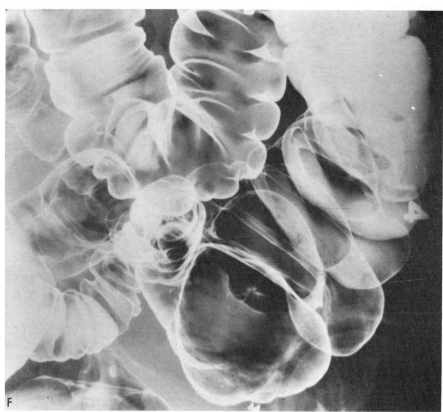

FIGURE 15–26 *Continued.* *E*. Patient supine, left side down, right side up for best double contrast visualization of the hepatic flexure. *F*. Patient prone, table tilted down for best visualization of the cecum.

Figure continued on following page.

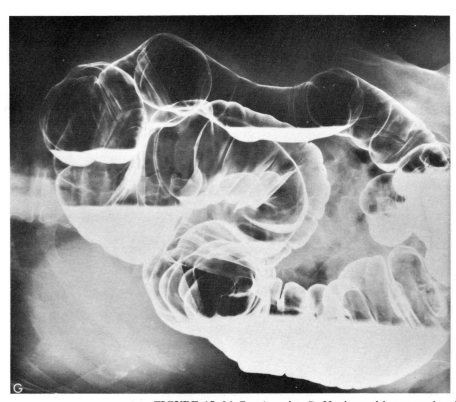
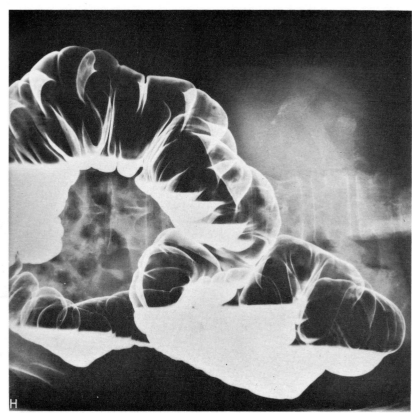

FIGURE 15–26 *Continued.* *G.* Horizontal beam study with patient's left side uppermost for best visualization of the descending colon in particular but also for some double contrast visualization of portions of the transverse colon. *H.* Horizontal beam study with the patient's right side uppermost for best visualization of the right half of the colon in double contrast.

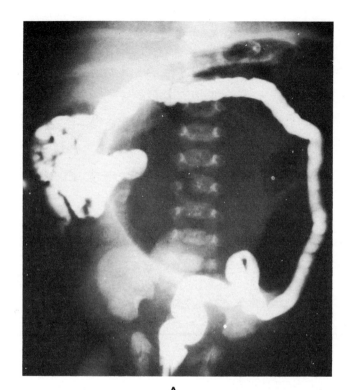

A

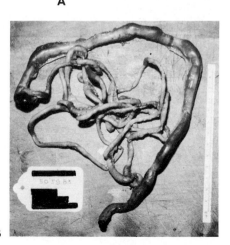

B

FIGURE 15–27 *A*. Barium enema in an "unused colon" in a neonate with a large peritoneal abscess. *B*. Photograph of a neonatal "unused colon." *C*. Barium enema in a neonate with jejunal atresia, but with meconium in the colon.

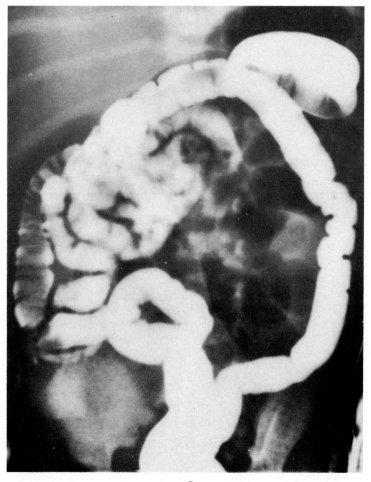

C

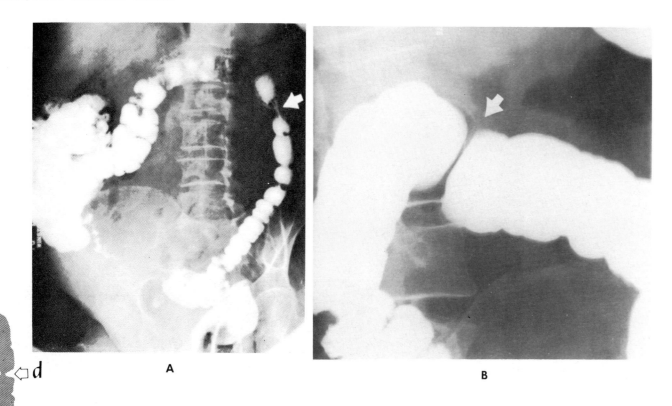

A

B

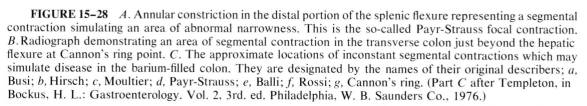

C

FIGURE 15–28 *A.* Annular constriction in the distal portion of the splenic flexure representing a segmental contraction simulating an area of abnormal narrowness. This is the so-called Payr-Strauss focal contraction. *B.* Radiograph demonstrating an area of segmental contraction in the transverse colon just beyond the hepatic flexure at Cannon's ring point. *C.* The approximate locations of inconstant segmental contractions which may simulate disease in the barium-filled colon. They are designated by the names of their original describers; *a,* Busi; *b,* Hirsch; *c,* Moultier; *d,* Payr-Strauss; *e,* Balli; *f,* Rossi; *g,* Cannon's ring. (Part *C* after Templeton, in Bockus, H. L.: Gastroenterology. Vol. 2, 3rd. ed. Philadelphia, W. B. Saunders Co., 1976.)

Figure continued on the opposite page

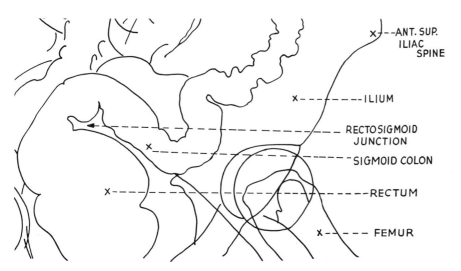

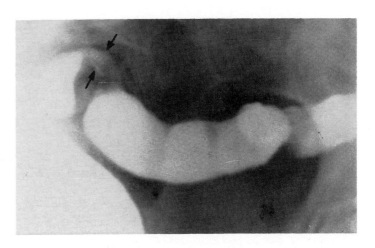

D

FIGURE 15–28 *Continued.* *D.* Oblique study of the rectosigmoid junction demonstrating a frequently encountered normal narrowness. A labeled tracing from another normal patient is shown for comparison.

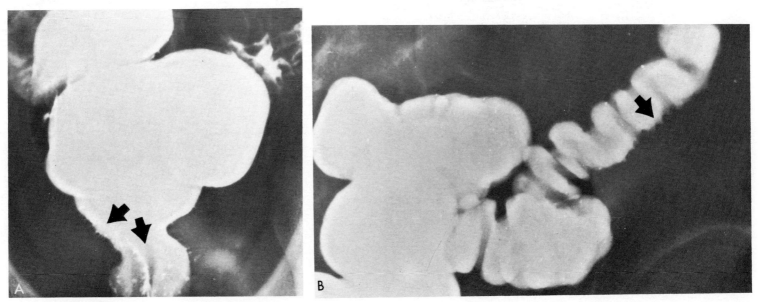

FIGURE 15–29 *A*, Radiograph demonstrating barium sulfate entering small crypts (normal) in the rectum. When perpendicular to the surface, these crypts present a "dotlike" pattern. *B*. Similar granular crypts demonstrated in profile in the region of the sigmoid, simulating diverticulosis.

ANGIOGRAPHY OF THE SMALL AND LARGE INTESTINES

Basic Arterial Anatomy

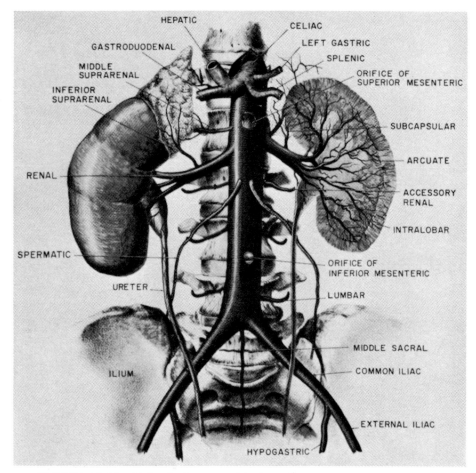

FIGURE 15–30 Abdominal aorta and its branches. (From Bierman, H. C.: Selective Arterial Catheterization. Springfield, Ill., Charles C Thomas, Publisher, 1969. Courtesy of Charles C Thomas, Publisher.)

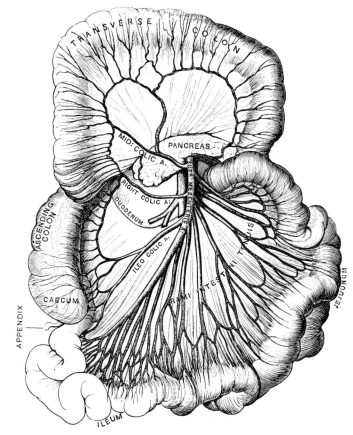

FIGURE 15–31 Superior mesenteric artery and its branches. "Rami intestini tenuis" = jejunal and ileal arteries. (From Brash, J. C., (ed.): Cunninghan's Manual of Practical Anatomy, 12th ed. Vol. 2. London, Oxford University Press, 1958.)

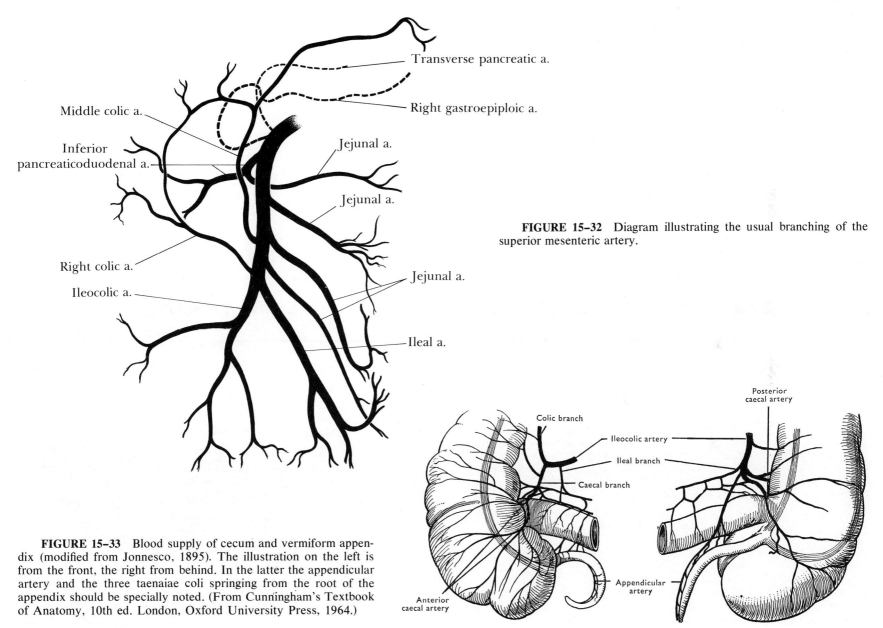

Middle colic a.

Inferior
pancreaticoduodenal a.

Right colic a.

Ileocolic a.

Transverse pancreatic a.

Right gastroepiploic a.

Jejunal a.

Jejunal a.

Jejunal a.

Ileal a.

FIGURE 15–32 Diagram illustrating the usual branching of the superior mesenteric artery.

Colic branch

Ileocolic artery

Ileal branch

Caecal branch

Posterior
caecal artery

Anterior
caecal artery

Appendicular
artery

FIGURE 15–33 Blood supply of cecum and vermiform appendix (modified from Jonnesco, 1895). The illustration on the left is from the front, the right from behind. In the latter the appendicular artery and the three taenaiae coli springing from the root of the appendix should be specially noted. (From Cunningham's Textbook of Anatomy, 10th ed. London, Oxford University Press, 1964.)

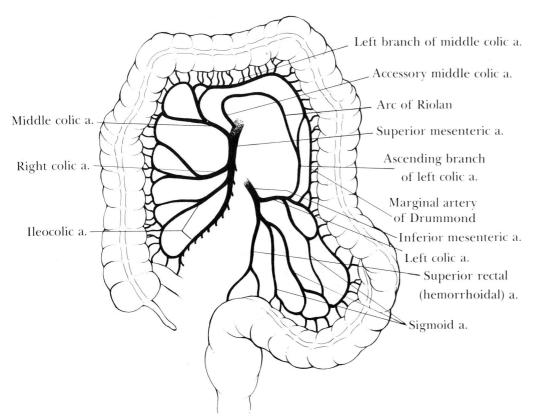

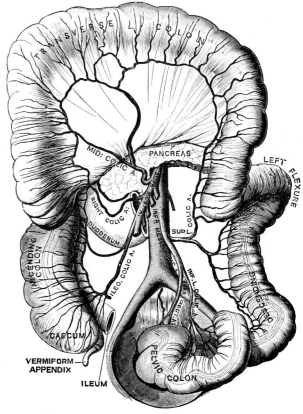

FIGURE 15-34 Superior and inferior mesenteric arterial systems, showing the arc of Riolan and the marginal artery of Drummond. The arc of Riolan is made up of the accessory middle colic artery, the ascending branch of the left colic artery, and an anastomotic branch between the two. The marginal artery of Drummond is shown here as a continuous vessel from sigmoid to cecum. In actuality, it is often interrupted, especially in the right colon. (From Ruzicka, F. F., and Rossi, P.: Radiol. Clin. North Am., 8:3–29, 1970.)

FIGURE 15-35 Superior and inferior mesenteric arteries and their branches. Usually, there is more than one inferior left colic (sigmoid) artery. (From Brash, J. C. (ed.): Cunningham's Manual of Practical Anatomy, 12th ed. Vol. 2. London, Oxford University Press, 1958.)

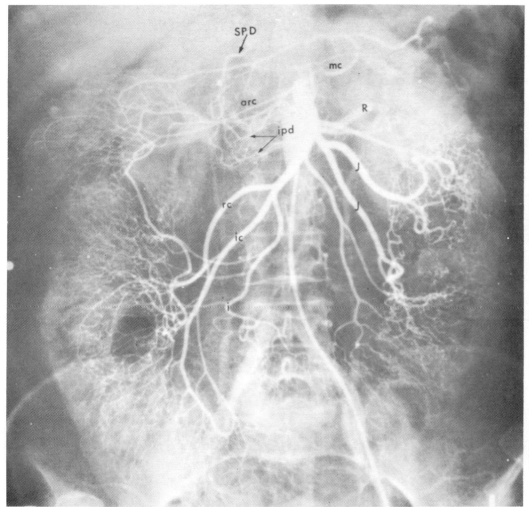

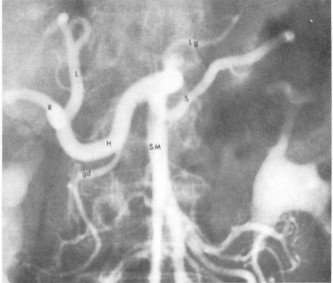

FIGURE 15-37 Simultaneous selective celiac and superior mesenteric artery injections show type I pattern. Anteroposterior projection. (*S*) Splenic artery, (*SM*) superior mesenteric, (*gd*) gastroduodenal. (*H*) proper hepatic. (*R*) right hepatic, (*L*) left hepatic, (*Lg*) left gastric. (From Ruzicka, F. F., Jr., and Rossi, P.: Radiol. Clin. North Am., *8*:3–29, 1970.)

FIGURE 15-36 Superior mesenteric arteriogram. Some reflux of contrast agent into aorta opacifies both renal arteries. Note filling of pancreaticoduodenal arcades and superior pancreaticoduodenal artery from inferior pancreaticoduodenal arteries. (*R*) Renal, (*J*) jejunal artery, (*i*) ileal artery, (*ic*) ileocolic artery, (*rc*) right colic, (*mc*) middle colic, (*arc*) accessory right colic, (*ipd*) inferior pancreaticoduodenal, (*SPD*) superior pancreaticoduodenal artery. (From Ruzicka, F. F., Jr., and Rossi, P.: Radiol. Clin. North Am., *8*:3–29, 1970.)

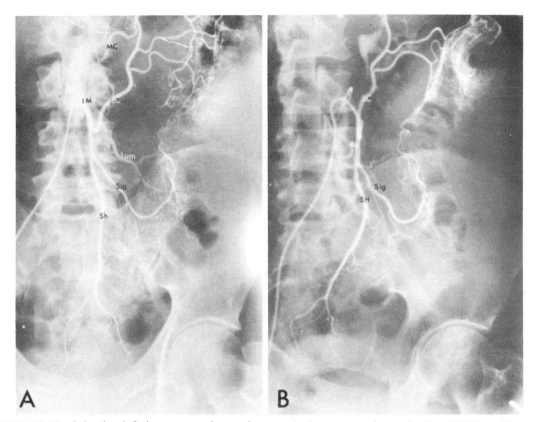

FIGURE 15–38 Selective inferior mesenteric arteriogram. *A.* Anteroposterior projection. Middle colic artery fills via communications (not shown) with left colic branches. A small amount of reflux defines adjacent aorta, and lumbar artery is also opacified because of this reflux. (MC) Middle colic, (LC) left colic, (Lum) lumbar artery, (Sig.) sigmoid, (Sh) superior hemorrhoidal, (IM) inferior mesenteric artery. *B.* Left posterior oblique projection. (From Ruzicka, F. F., Jr., and Rossi, P.: Radiol. Clin. North Am., *8*:3–29, 1970.)

Neonatal Umbilical Catheterization and Angiography

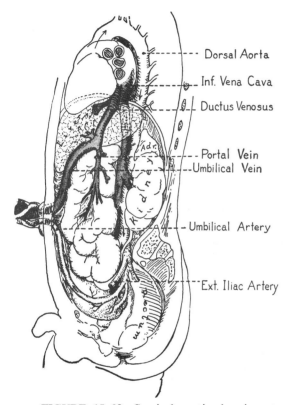

- - - Dorsal Aorta

- - - Inf. Vena Cava

- - - Ductus Venosus

- - - Portal Vein
- - Umbilical Vein

- - - Umbilical Artery

- - - Ext. Iliac Artery

FIGURE 15–39 Semischematic drawings to show the vestiges in the adult of the umbilical vessels of the fetus. (From Cullen, The Umbilicus and Its Diseases, *in* Anson, B. J. (ed.): Morris' Human Anatomy, 12th ed. New York, McGraw-Hill Book Company, 1966. Copyright © 1966 by McGraw-Hill, Inc. Used by permission of Mc-Graw-Hill Book Company.)

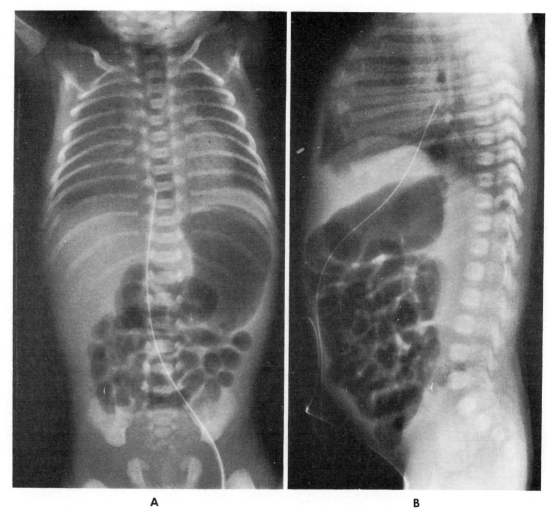

A

B

FIGURE 15–40 *A*. Anteroposterior projection of newborn whose umbilical vein has been catheterized. *B*. Lateral view of infant in *A*.

Figure continued on the following page

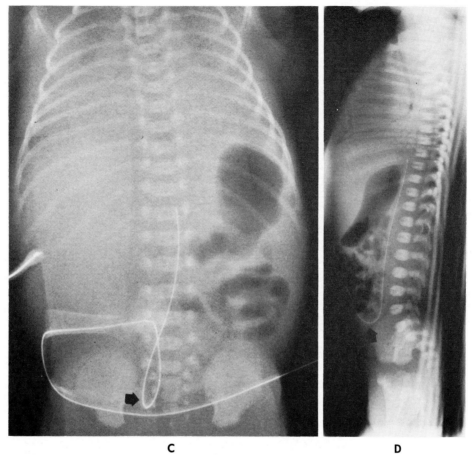

C   **D**

FIGURE 15–40 *Continued.*   *C.* Umbilical catheter in hypogastric artery: Anteroposterior (*C*) and lateral (*D*) projections. The arrow points to the loop that extends into the hypogastric artery, which in frontal prospective establishes the arterial position of the catheter.

Venous Drainage of the Small and Large Intestines

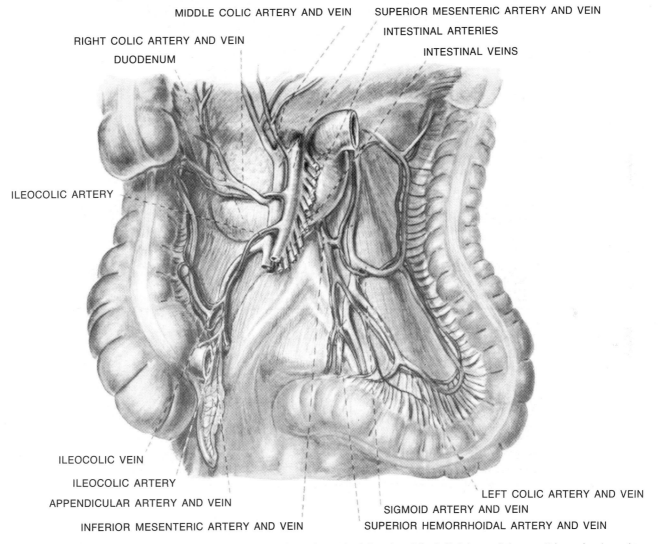

MIDDLE COLIC ARTERY AND VEIN

SUPERIOR MESENTERIC ARTERY AND VEIN

RIGHT COLIC ARTERY AND VEIN

INTESTINAL ARTERIES

DUODENUM

INTESTINAL VEINS

ILEOCOLIC ARTERY

ILEOCOLIC VEIN

ILEOCOLIC ARTERY

LEFT COLIC ARTERY AND VEIN

APPENDICULAR ARTERY AND VEIN

SIGMOID ARTERY AND VEIN

INFERIOR MESENTERIC ARTERY AND VEIN

SUPERIOR HEMORRHOIDAL ARTERY AND VEIN

FIGURE 15–41 Blood supply to the large intestine. The jejunal and ileal divisions of the small intestine have been removed in order to expose the arterial branches of the inferior mesenteric and the corresponding veins of colic drainage. (From Warren: Handbook of Anatomy, Harvard University Press.)

THE BILIARY TRACT

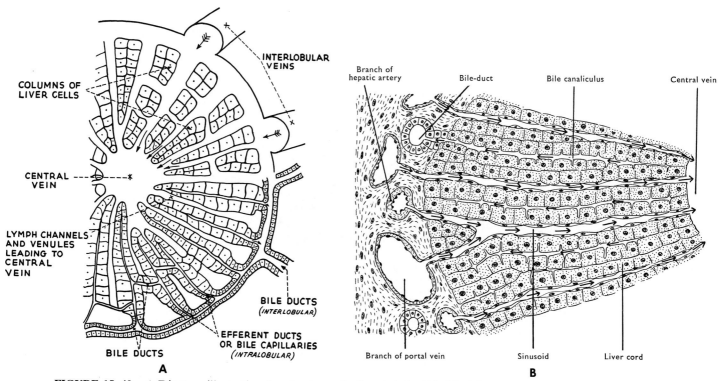

FIGURE 15–42 *A.* Diagram illustrating the structure of a liver lobule. (Modified from Cunningham's Textbook of Anatomy, 10th ed. London, Oxford University Press, 1964.) *B,* The structure of the human liver lobule. (From Cunningham's Textbook of Anatomy, 10th ed. London, Oxford University Press, 1964.)

FIGURE 15-44 Schema of portal system of veins and its connections with systemic veins. It must be remembered that the systemic blood carried by the hepatic artery also enters the capillaries of the liver, and the hepatic veins contain therefore both portal and systemic blood. (Modified from Cunningham's Manual of Practical Anatomy, 11th ed. Vol. 2. London, Oxford University Press, 1949.)

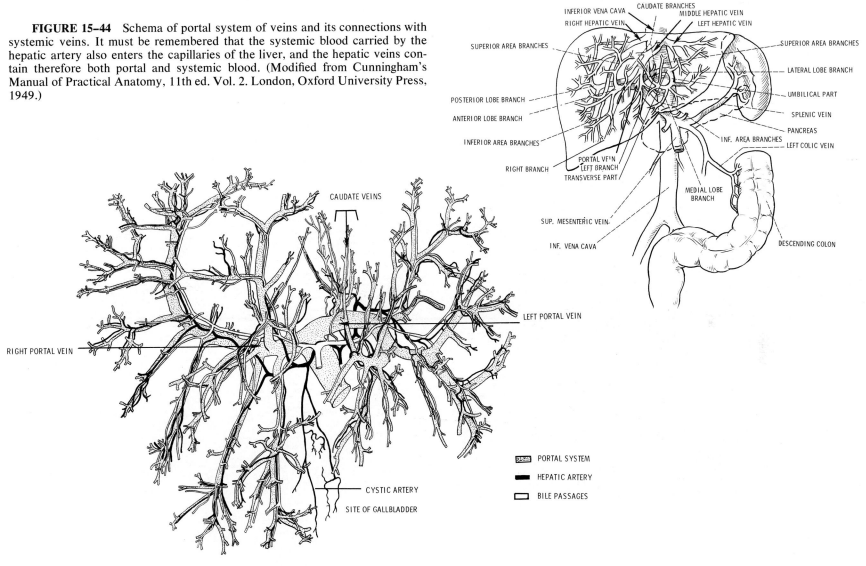

INFERIOR VENA CAVA

CAUDATE BRANCHES

MIDDLE HEPATIC VEIN

RIGHT HEPATIC VEIN

LEFT HEPATIC VEIN

SUPERIOR AREA BRANCHES

SUPERIOR AREA BRANCHES

LATERAL LOBE BRANCH

POSTERIOR LOBE BRANCH

UMBILICAL PART

ANTERIOR LOBE BRANCH

SPLENIC VEIN

PANCREAS

INFERIOR AREA BRANCHES

INF. AREA BRANCHES

LEFT COLIC VEIN

RIGHT BRANCH

PORTAL VEIN

LEFT BRANCH

TRANSVERSE PART

MEDIAL LOBE BRANCH

SUP. MESENTERIC VEIN

DESCENDING COLON

INF. VENA CAVA

CAUDATE VEINS

LEFT PORTAL VEIN

RIGHT PORTAL VEIN

CYSTIC ARTERY

SITE OF GALLBLADDER

PORTAL SYSTEM

HEPATIC ARTERY

BILE PASSAGES

ANTERO-INFERIOR VIEW

FIGURE 15-43 Venous drainage of the liver into the caval system as compared with the portal venous system.

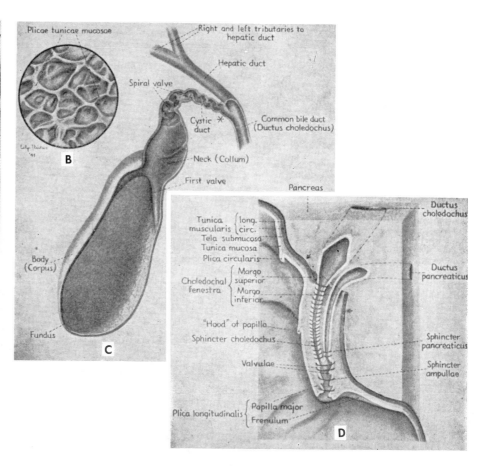

FIGURE 15–45 *A.* The gross anatomy of the biliary system. (From Jones, T.: Anatomical Studies. Jackson, Michigan, S. H. Camp and Co., 1943.) *B.* Gross anatomy of the biliary tract with the interior of the gallbladder (*B*) and the gross outline of the gallbladder and cystic duct (*C*) demonstrated. *D.* Diagram of frontal section through duodenum at the inferior duodenal flexure showing the structure and relations of the papilla major (duodenal papilla). (After Boyden in Surgery. From Jackson, C. M., and Blount, R. F., *in* Jackson, C. M. (ed.): Morris' Human Anatomy. New York, The Blakiston Co.)

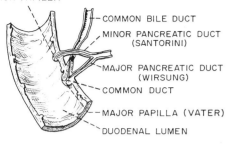

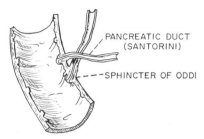

FIGURE 15–46 Anatomic sketch depicting the relationship of the major and minor papillae, the common bile duct, and the pancreatic duct. (After Daves.)

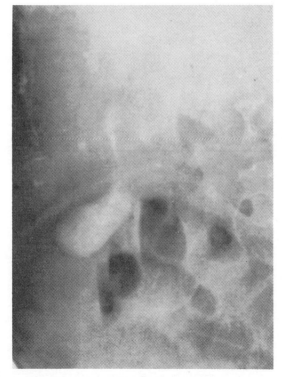

A

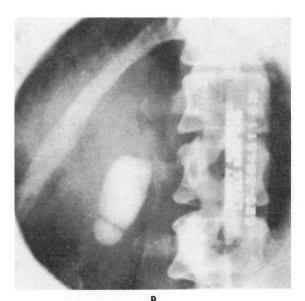

B

FIGURE 15–47 Variations in gallbladder of radiographic significance. *A*. Ptotic gallbladder lying in the iliac fossa. *B*. Mucosal or serosal fold of gallbladder, known as a Phrygian cap.

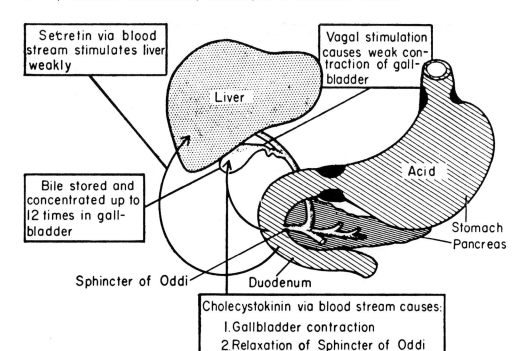

FIGURE 15–48 Mechanisms of liver secretion and gallbladder emptying. (From Guyton, A. C.: Textbook of Medical Physiology. 5th ed. Philadelphia, W. B. Saunders Co., 1976.)

TABLE 15–1. Selection of Patients for Oral Cholangiography and Cholecystography

Test	Values	Probability of Success
Serum bilirubin		
(Mandel)	< 5 mg.%	Worth trying
	> 10 mg.%	Failure
(Shehadi)	< 1 mg.%	Excellent
	< 2 mg.%	Satisfactory
	3 mg.% or	Poor or unlikely
	> 4 mg.%	Not possible
Bromsulphalein (BSP) retention		
(Etess and Strauss)	5–20%	Should not interfere
	> 20–23%	Failure
(Blornstrom and Sandstrom)	> 40%	Failure

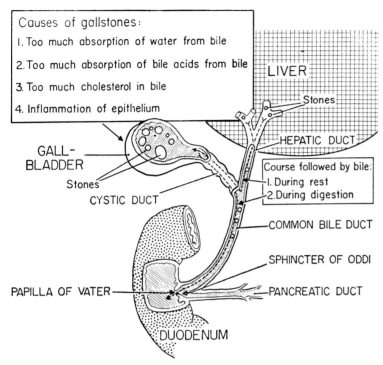

Causes of gallstones:
1. Too much absorption of water from bile
2. Too much absorption of bile acids from bile
3. Too much cholesterol in bile
4. Inflammation of epithelium

LIVER

Stones

HEPATIC DUCT

GALL-BLADDER

Stones

Course followed by bile:
1. During rest
2. During digestion

CYSTIC DUCT

COMMON BILE DUCT

SPHINCTER OF ODDI

PAPILLA OF VATER

PANCREATIC DUCT

DUODENUM

FIGURE 15–49 Formation of gallstones. (From Guyton, A. C.: Textbook of Medical Physiology. 5th ed. Philadelphia, W. B. Saunders Co., 1976.)

ROENTGENOLOGIC EXAMINATION
OF THE BILIARY TRACT

Introduction. Prior to the gallbladder examination, it is advisable to remove as much gas and fecal material from the gastrointestinal tract as possible. Cascara sagrada or enemas given at least 24 hours before the examination may be of considerable assistance. Pitressin may be employed intravenously (0.5 to 1 cc.) in those patients in whom it is not contraindicated on the basis of hypertension or arteriosclerosis.

It is also well to obtain a plain film of the entire right side of the ab-

domen in the posteroanterior projection prior to the administration of any contrast agent. The gallbladder itself is not usually delineated with accuracy on such films, but if it should contain calcareous material, this would immediately be evident from this preliminary study.

A visualization of the gallbladder requires that some form of contrast substance be introduced into it. Tetrachlorphenolphthalein had long been known as a bile secretion and had been used as a test for liver function.

In recent years new compounds such as Priodax, Telepaque, Teridax, Monophen, and Cholografin (see Table 15–2) have been introduced which accomplish the same thing without many of the undesirable side effects attributed to the earlier contrast medium. Each of the newer compounds has certain contraindications and some adverse effects. Table 15–2 lists this information for Telepaque and Cholografin.

Methods of Study. There are several possible roentgenologic techniques that can be used to study the biliary system. These are:
1. Plain film of the abdomen.
2. Oral cholecystograms (including opacification of bile duct calculi).
   a. Rectal cholecystography.
3. Intravenous cholangiography.
4. Percutaneous transhepatic cholangiography.
5. Operative and postoperative cholangiography.
6. Retrograde peroral fiber optic cholangiography (see Pancreas).
7. Biliary angiography.
   a. Liver.
   b. Gallbladder.

Plain Film of the Abdomen. The plain film of the abdomen should always precede contrast studies involving any organs contained in the abdomen.

In the case of the biliary tract, this should consist of: (1) KUB (kidney, ureter, bladder) film as described in Chapter 11, and (2) a 10 × 12 inch film of the right upper quadrant of the patient, with the patient in either the right posterior oblique or left anterior oblique projection (the same projection that is utilized subsequently in oral cholecystography). This film should extend from the iliac crest as close as possible to the right hemidiaphragm. The entire right lobe of the liver is usually included.

TABLE 15–2. Comparison of Two of the Major Compounds Employed for Gallbladder Visualization

Year of Introduction	Compound	Pharmacology	Contraindications	Accuracy and Adverse Effects
1949	Telepaque	Ethyl propanoic acid derivative Insoluble in water; soluble in alkali and 95% alcohol 66.68% iodine Excreted mostly via gastrointestinal tract	Acute nephritis Uremia Gastrointestinal diseases with disturbed absorption	Fails only in 3% of normal gallbladders or less with one dose Side reactions less than with Priodax Great opacity may obscure some gallstones
1953–1955	Cholografin	Iodipamide (triiodobenzoic acid derivative) For intravenous use (photosensitive) 64% iodine With normal liver 90% excreated in feces, 10% in urine With poor liver function: mostly excreted by kidneys (hence pyelograms)	Primary indication: Postcholecystectomy syndrome Contraindications: Iodine sensitivity Combined urinary and hepatic disease	Sensitivity high Side effects minimal with slow injection 77–85% successful biliary tree visualizations Visualization faint; usually gallbladder visualization too faint for significant accuracy Serious reactions: 2.5% Lesser reactions: 38.8%

Oral Cholecystograms. The compound most frequently employed for oral study is *Telepaque*, a moderately lipid-soluble substance that is poorly soluble in an aqueous system. (*Cholografin*, the compound used in intravenous application, is freely soluble in an aqueous solution but is not appreciably absorbed from the gastrointestinal tract. This contrast agent will be discussed under intravenous cholangiography.)

After administration of Telepaque, there is a circulating level of 1 to 16 mg. per cent within 2 hours. Some patients, particularly those with less than 4 mg. per cent at 2 hours, show a rise at the 14 hour period. Shehadi* has indicated that there are two distinct peaks in the absorption curve, one at 4 hours and a second, higher peak at 10 hours, and it is for this reason that the 10 hour interval is assumed to be the optimum time for film study for most patients.

Berk and Lasser* have demonstrated the following cycle: the Telepaque is absorbed in the gastrointestinal tract, whereupon it is delivered to the liver. It is thereafter excreted in the bile, and if the extrahepatic biliary passages are open, it finds its way to the gallbladder. In the gallbladder the contrast agent and bile are concentrated above the level of the original bile. If, however, the gallbladder is inflamed or its mucosa is otherwise pathological, the contrast medium is absorbed from the gall-

bladder, and concentration of the agent does not occur sufficiently for roentgenologic visualization. When Cholografin is used, it accumulates in the gallbladder in the same form in which it is administered in sufficient concentration usually for visualization, although it is not as opaque as Telepaque. (For an understanding of the chemistry and conjugations involved, reference should be made to the original articles.)

Although many investigators may prefer one or another of these agents, preference in recent times has generally remained with Telepaque. There are some advantages and disadvantages of Telepaque versus *Oragrafin* (White and Fischer).* The degree of opacification of the gallbladder and visualization of the biliary ducts is similar with both these oral cholecystographic agents. Calculi are more often demonstrated with Telepaque, but on the other hand, stones are not as often concealed by the lesser density of Oragrafin. The incidence of diarrhea is much higher and that of nausea and cramps slightly higher with Tele-

---

*References may be obtained in Meschan, I.: An Atlas of Anatomy Basic to Radiology. Philadelphia, W. B. Saunders Co., 1975, Chapter 14.

paque. There are also less side effects with a double dose technique of Oragrafin as compared with Telepaque.

TECHNICAL ASPECTS OF ORAL CHOLECYSTOGRAPHY

Preparation of the patient. Prior to examination, it should be determined that: (1) the patient is not sensitive to iodine-containing contrast agents, and (2) the patient has been on a diet which might reasonably have produced previous evacuation of the gallbladder by fatty stimulation.

If possible, there should be at least one fat-containing meal the day prior to the cholecystographic examination in order to empty a distended gallbladder.

On the evening prior to the examination, the meal should be fat-free and may consist of fruit or fruit juice, fresh vegetables cooked without butter, a small portion of lean meat, toast or bread with jelly, coffee or tea but no milk, cream, butter, eggs, or any foods containing fat. Nothing should be eaten after the evening meal, although water may be taken in moderate amounts.

At about 10 P.M. six Telepaque tablets (3 grams) should be swallowed, each with one or two mouthfuls of water, a total of at least one full glass of water. To avoid nausea or vomiting, an interval of 5 minutes after each tablet may elapse. If roentgen examination is scheduled for 9 A.M., the best time for administration of Telepaque is between 9 and 11 P.M. on the night preceding the examination.

On the following morning, breakfast should be omitted.

The patient may be given an enema if it is discovered that the contrast agent in the gastrointestinal tract interferes with adequate visualization of the gallbladder.

Dose considerations. It is probable that 3 grams of Telepaque are sufficient for all adults irrespective of weight (Whitehouse and Martin).* With some patients we have used doses as high as 6 grams (12 tablets) within a period of 24 hours. Different studies on the renal toxicity of contrast medium in patients with hepatorenal damage have called attention to the danger of larger doses of oral cholecystographic media (Seaman, Cosgriff, and Wells).* It has therefore been recommended that *a dose of 6 grams not be exceeded within a period of 24 hours, and if such a dose has been employed, that it not be repeated for a period of at least 1 week.*

Pediatric patients may be given proportionately smaller doses (Harris and Caffey).*

Film and fluoroscopic techniques. On the morning after the patient has taken the contrast medium, films are repeated in the left anterior oblique position (patient prone) with various degrees of obliquity. Each film should be studied until satisfactory visualization of the gallbladder is obtained. The gallbladder should be completely clear of interfering gas or other opaque shadows. Sufficient kilovoltage should be employed so that the contrast agent will not in itself obscure filling defects within the gallbladder (Fig. 15–51).

Upright or lateral decubitus films are also obtained routinely to determine possible stratification or mobility of filling defects within the gallbladder (Fig. 15–53). Fluoroscopy with compression spot-film studies may be employed for this purpose.

Following this first part of the examination, the patient is given a meal consisting of foods with a high fat content such as eggs, butter, toast or cream; or a synthetic cholagogue such as Bilevac may be employed.

After the fatty meal or fat stimulation is administered, the films of the right upper quadrant are repeated in identical positions (Fig. 15–52). Body section radiography may be employed at any time in the procedure to obtain better visualization of the gallbladder proper or of the ductal system.

When the customary dose of six tablets is used, visualization of the extrahepatic ducts can be obtained in most patients in 5 to 20 minutes after the fat meal. However, if visualization of the extrahepatic ducts is especially indicated a somewhat higher dose of Telepaque (6 grams) may be required.

Variations of this general procedure may be undertaken as follows: (1) The Telepaque may be taken earlier in the evening and castor oil may be administered five hours after the Telepaque tablets (Mauthe).* However, if the gallbladder is not visualized the morning following administration of the Telepaque, the examination is repeated in a day or so without the castor oil. Repetition of the examination under these circumstances is important. (2) In order to overcome biliary stasis (one of the

---

*References may be obtained in Meschan, I.: An Atlas of Anatomy Basic to Radiology. Philadelphia, W. B. Saunders Co., 1975, Chapter 14.

common causes of nonvisualization or delayed visualization of the gall-bladder) the use of bile acid for 5 to 30 days before repeating the cholecystographic examination has been recommended (Berg and Hamilton).*

Side effects. Whitehouse and Martin* have reported the following side effects from 3 gram doses of Telepaque in 400 patients; diarrhea, 25.3 per cent (of which 2.5 per cent were severe); dysuria, 13.7 per cent; mild nausea, 5.8 per cent; and mild vomiting 1.5 per cent. There were other side effects in 2.8 per cent of the cases and no side effects were noted in 62.5 per cent of the cases.

Patients with hepatorenal dysfunction constitute a group subject to potential hazards from oral cholecystography. Doses of Telepaque larger than those recommended earlier should be employed with caution. There are advantages and disadvantages to each of the various compounds, and a careful choice must be made with full knowledge of all aspects of the contrast agent employed as well as the importance of the clinical evaluation in the case at hand.

Visualization or nonvisualization. It is well documented also that repeat examinations of the gallbladder following initial failures of visualization, or inadequate visualization, without evidence of gallstones will be interpreted as normal. In Rosenbaum's series* of 450 consecutive patients examined by cholecystography, there were 66 visualizations in which evidence of gallstones was initially absent or inadequate. After the second dose of Telepaque and repeat roentgen study, findings were interpreted as normal in 10 per cent of those with initial nonvisualization and in 64 per cent of those with initially inadequate visualization.

THE SIGNIFICANCE OF NONVISUALIZATION OF THE GALLBLADDER IN PATIENTS WITH INTACT GALLBLADDER. ABNORMALITY OF FUNCTION. There are certain basic assumptions that must be verified as far as possible in order to interpret oral cholecystograms:

1. That the patient actually has taken the contrast agent.

2. That adequate absorption of the agent has occurred (no esophageal, gastric, or intestinal obstruction).

3. That the liver function is adequate for secretion of the test compound.

4. That the ductal system above the level of the gallbladder is not obstructed.

5. That the common bile duct is not obstructed (in which case there may be some associated gallbladder disease).

The oral cholecystogram is fundamentally a function test. It must not, however, be assumed that nonvisualization necessarily indicates abnormal function in certain rare instances. Complete absence of the gallbladder is a rare anomaly but can occur.

A surprisingly high proportion of men with cholelithiasis are asymptomatic (70 per cent of men with stones and 86 per cent of a control group have no symptoms).† Of 30 per cent of patients with gallstones, two-thirds had only the unreliable signs and symptoms of dyspepsia and epigastric pain, symptoms which are found in 10 per cent of normal controls. Also, typical biliary colic can be a misleading description, since it is found in about 3.6 per cent of those with no stones and in 0.9 per cent of normal men.

Intravenous Cholangiography (Fig. 15–50). CONTRAST MEDIUM. The contrast agent, sodium iodipamide (Biligrafin in Germany), was replaced in 1955 by iodipamide methylglucamine and introduced in the United States under the trade name of Cholografin methylglucamine. The standard dose for the adult is 20 ml. of the latter compound. This dose contains approximately 5 grams of iodine. Approximately 90 per cent of the compound is excreted by the liver and 10 per cent by the kidneys. In patients with liver damage, a greater percentage will be excreted by the kidney. Wise has reported that in 12 years of experience with over 5000 injections, there have been no fatal reactions in the Lahey Clinic. Normal reactions such as nausea, vomiting, hypotension, or urticaria have, on occasion, occurred. (A dose greater than 20 ml. is contraindicated and may be toxic.)

With these basic criteria in mind, *intravenous cholangiography is indicated in the following situations* (Fig. 15–50):

1. Nonvisualization by the oral route. According to Wise,* 12 per cent of these patients were found to have gallbladders which appeared normal and in which no calculi were visualized. Of 201 patients with intact gallbladders not visualized by the oral route, visualization was accomplished in 70 by the intravenous method, and 24 of these were considered normal. All of those whose gallbladders were not visualized by the intravenous method were found later to be diseased.

---

*References may be obtained in Meschan, I.: An Atlas of Anatomy Basic to Radiology. Philadelphia, W. B. Saunders Co., 1975, Chapter 14.

†Wilbur, R. S., and Bolt, R. J.: Incidence of gallbladder disease in "normal" men. Gastroenterology, *36*:251–255, 1959.

SITUATIONS JUSTIFYING USE OF INTRA-
VENOUS CHOLANGIOGRAPHY

1. Nonvisualization of gallbladder by oral route.
2. Need to distinguish gallbladder disease and obstructive disease of the distal common duct.
3. Evaluation of the postcholecystectomy syndrome.
4. Preoperative examination to demonstrate calculi in the common bile duct before cholecystectomy.
5. History of biliary abnormality in infants and children.
6. Emergencies in which speed is a factor.
7. Suspicion of a tumor near the porta hepatis.
8. Recent or subsiding jaundice in which bilirubin and BSP levels are appropriate to help differentiate infective hepatitis and common duct stones.
9. Functional biliary disorders in which a study of the duct system may help differentiate organic disease.

FIGURE 15–50

2. Differentiation of gallbladder disease and obstructive disease of the distal common duct. (a) If the common duct is less than 7.0 mm. in diameter, nonvisualization of the gallbladder is due to cystic duct obstruction or primary gallbladder disease. (b) If the common duct is dilated, the cause of nonopacification may be common duct obstruction alone or a combination of cystic duct obstruction and common duct obstruction.

TECHNIQUE OF INTRAVENOUS EXAMINATION. 1. Good catharsis on the night prior to the examination.

2. A plain film of the right upper quadrant in the right posterior oblique (and in some instances, left anterior oblique).

3. A preliminary subcutaneous injection of 5 mg. of parabromdylamine is given. The patient is examined in the hydrated and nonfasting state.

4. A test dose of 1 cc. of Cholografin is administered intravenously, and a 3 minute interval is allowed to elapse until the remaining 19 cc. are injected over a minimum period of 10 minutes ("minor" reactions occur in 4.3 per cent). Drip infusion may be employed.

5. The first film is obtained following the completion of the injection in the supine position with the left side elevated approximately 15 degrees. Low kilovoltage is used.

6. Repeat films are obtained at 10 to 20 minute intervals thereafter for 40 to 60 minutes.

7. If no visualization is obtained at 60 to 90 minutes in a patient in whom the gallbladder has not been removed, a film of the right upper quadrant is made at 4 hours and if possible at 24 hours for visualization of the gallbladder.

8. Once a film giving the best possible visualization is obtained, films are made at 20 minute intervals in order to evaluate radiodensity, particularly if it appears that the duct is dilated and partially obstructed. (If the density and retention of the contrast medium in the bile ducts is greater at 120 minutes than at 60 minutes, partial obstruction of the common bile duct or main biliary tract is present.) If the duct is normal in size without evidence of obstruction and good drainage is seen, the study may be terminated in 60 to 90 minutes.

9. *Body section radiography should be performed as an additional adjunct when ductal visualization is optimum* (Fig. 15–54).

10. In children with suspected anomalies of the extrahepatic biliary system, between 0.6 and 1.6 cc. of 20 per cent sodium iodipamide (Cholografin) per kilogram of body weight was injected slowly by Hays and Averbrook* and exposures made at intervals over a 4 hour period. This intravenous injection was preceded by a test dose for sensitivity of 0.5 cc. (Methylglucamine iodipamide should require half this dosage.)

Hazards of intravenous cholangiography. Accidents during gallbladder studies with Cholografin were studied by Frommhold and Braband.* They collected data on 22 deaths attributed directly or indirectly to its administration. This death rate, even including doubtful and delayed deaths, represented a figure of 0.00035 per cent. This compares favorably with the death rate due to intravenous urography reported by Pendergrass—0.0009 per cent in a review of 12,200,000 excretory urograms performed over a 27-year period.* The sensitivity tests were negative in 5 of the 22 recorded fatalities with intravenous cholangiography.

*References may be obtained in Meschan, I.: An Atlas of Anatomy Basic to Radiology. Philadelphia, W. B. Saunders Co., 1975, Chapter 14.

Oral Cholecystograms

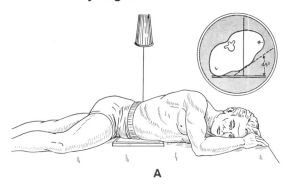

A

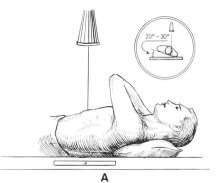

A

ALTERNATE POSITION
OF PATIENT FOR
STUDY OF GALLBLADDER

B

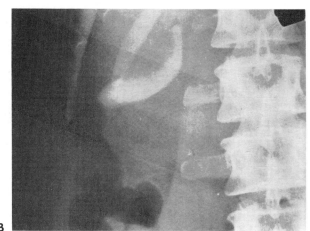

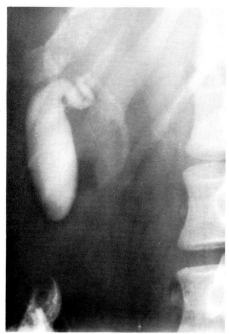

B

FIGURE 15–51 Radiograph of gallbladder following oral cholecystograms. *A*. Position of patient. (Note that the patient may be either prone or supine.) *B*. Radiograph so obtained.

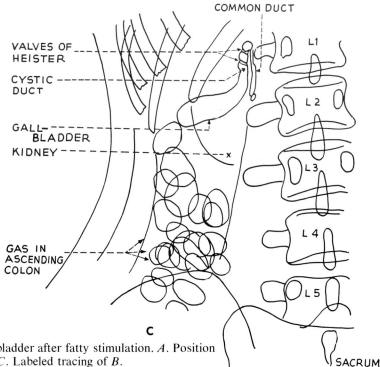

COMMON DUCT

VALVES OF
HEISTER

CYSTIC
DUCT

GALL-
BLADDER

KIDNEY

GAS IN
ASCENDING
COLON

L1

L2

L3

L4

L5

SACRUM

C

FIGURE 15–52 Gallbladder after fatty stimulation. *A*. Position of patient. *B*. Radiograph. *C*. Labeled tracing of *B*.

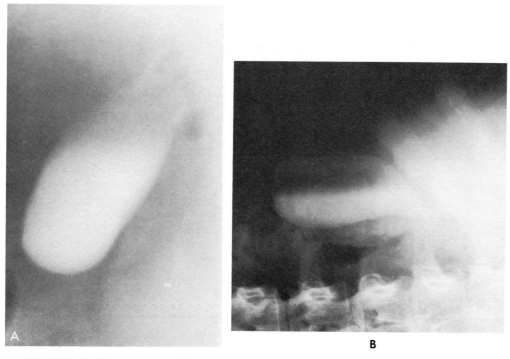

FIGURE 15–53 Layering of Telepaque that may occur normally in the gallbladder. *A.* Erect. *B.* Lateral decubitus with patient lying on left side.

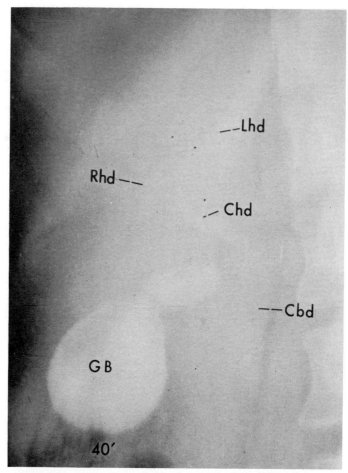

FIGURE 15–54 Visualization of the gallbladder and its ductal system made possible by tomography of the gallbladder: (GB) Gallbladder. (Cbd) Common bile duct. (Chd) Common hepatic duct. (Lhd) Left hepatic duct. (Rhd) Right hepatic duct. This film was obtained 40 minutes after the intravenous administration of Cholografin.

Direct Cholangiography. There are three types of direct cholangiography: (1) operative cholangiography (at the time of operation); (2) postoperative or T-tube cholangiography (during the postoperative period) (Fig. 15–55); (3) peroral fiberoptic cannulation and injection of the common bile duct. (See section on Pancreas, Fig. 14–58D.)

Cholangiography at the time of surgery, in the opinion of Edmunds et al.,* should be performed in all cholecystectomy patients without selection except in those with serious debility. Clinical indications for common duct exploration as presently accepted are not sufficiently accurate to reduce the number of negative explorations. There are, indeed, many reports of common duct stones revealed by operative cholangiograms when no clinical indications for exploration were present (Hight et al.).* Fully 95 per cent of all secondary operations on the biliary tract are for intraductal stones that may have been overlooked.

Also, the performance of cholangiography at the time of operation gives the surgeon an opportunity to make certain that all calculi have been removed from, or are no longer present in, the biliary tree.

Cholangiography at the time of operation provides a means of recognizing noncalculus obstruction of the common duct also (Partington and Sachs).*

The T-tube cholangiogram allows a study of the common bile duct in the postoperative period prior to removal of the T-tube. In this way, a determination of patency of the common bile duct is determined.

Technique. Twenty-five to 50 per cent methylglucamine diatrizoate or sodium diatrizoate (Renografin or Hypaque) is directly injected into the biliary tree (in approximately 5 ml. fractions) either at the time of operation by means of a polyethylene tube inserted into the common duct or through a T-tube that has been previously introduced into the common hepatic duct at surgery. The contrast agent is warmed to body temperature before use.

For the *operative cholangiogram*, the contrast agent may be injected in three or four fractions of approximately 5 cc. each, and films obtained in sequence during the injection of each fraction. The films are numbered so that the sequence can be identified at the time of viewing. Care is exercised to remove all air bubbles from the syringe and connecting tube prior to injection. A cassette tunnel placed beneath the patient prior to surgery to allow proper positioning of the cassette under sterile conditions is important. A grid-cassette (or Bucky grid) beneath the table is also necessary to enhance detail. Diaphragmatic movement is suspended by the anesthetist just prior to exposure and the exposures are made as rapidly as possible.

The films must be viewed immediately, so that additional studies may be taken as necessary.

The *postoperative cholangiogram* through the T-tube is performed as follows: a needle on the end of a long transparent catheter is carefully inserted into the end of the rubber T-tube and held vertically so that air that may not have been entirely expelled will rise to the surface. Every care must be exercised to avoid the injection of air into the biliary tree, since interpretation in respect to filling defects may thereby be complicated.

Approximately 5 cc. of the contrast agent is injected under fluoroscopic control and a spot film is obtained in the anteroposterior projection. The patient is then rotated into the left posterior oblique position and the procedure repeated with an additional 5 cc. injection. A further injection is made when the patient is placed in the right posterior oblique, and finally, a fourth exposure is made with the patient supine once again in the straight anteroposterior. Ordinarily, a total of 20 to 25 cc. of the contrast agent is sufficient to obtain these several views. During this procedure the introduction of the fluid must be done gently and the rate slowed when necessary if resistance is met or if the patient complains of right upper quadrant discomfort. After the final injection, a right lateral film may be obtained if desired.

Also, if desired, another roentgenogram may be taken 15 minutes after the injection to visualize the emptying of the biliary tract. Depending upon the degree of delay, additional films may be taken at 15 minute

---

*References may be obtained in Meschan, I.: An Atlas of Anatomy Basic to Radiology. Philadelphia, W. B. Saunders Co., 1975, Chapter 14.

or half-hour intervals until the patency of the biliary tract is determined (Hicken et al., 1959).*

If an obstruction is encountered, it is recommended that withdrawal of as much of the contrast agent as possible be attempted prior to the removal of the injection apparatus.

An effort is made to visualize both the right and left hepatic ducts as well as the common bile duct in its entirety. At times, biliary calculi make their way into one or the other of the hepatic ducts after or during surgery and these would go unrecognized were it not for this procedure.

Operative cholangiography markedly decreases the risk of overlooking stones in seemingly normal common ducts at cholecystectomy. This possibility is estimated to occur in 10 to 18 per cent of cases (Vadheim and Rigos).*

According to Chapman et al.,* normal operative cholangiographic findings are reliable evidence that the common bile duct does not contain stones or obstruction and therefore need not be explored.

Sachs* has emphasized that unnecessary common duct exploration is reduced from 45 to 50 per cent to 4 to 5 per cent, and that overlooked stones are reduced from 16 to 25 per cent to 4 per cent.

Hess (1967)* indicated an incidence of overlooked stones of 0.9 per cent in 650 cholangiograms.

COMPLICATIONS. Edmunds et al.* have reported that in 535 operative cholangiograms, there were four instances of complications which could possibly have been caused by these procedures. There were two cases of cholangitis, one case of acute hemorrhagic pancreatitis, and one case in which perforation of the common duct was thought to have occurred. All the patients survived their complications.

---

*References may be obtained in Meschan, I.: An Atlas of Anatomy Basic to Radiology. Philadelphia, W. B. Saunders Co., 1975, Chapter 14.

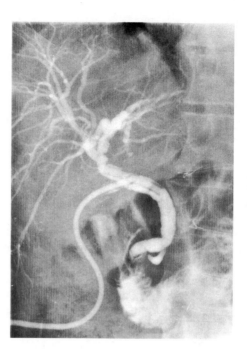

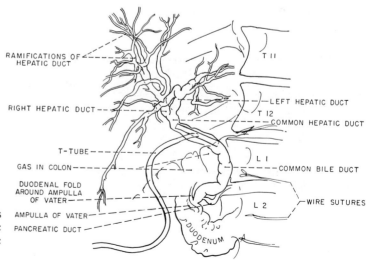

FIGURE 15–55 Thirty-five per cent Renografin T-tube cholangiogram and its tracing. This contrast medium gives a more complete visualization of all hepatic radicles. This is extremely important since stones may be concealed in the hepatic radicles only to descend later and cause a recurrence of symptoms.

Biliary Angiography (Deutsch; Farrell; Rösch et al.; Redman and Reuter).* Selective celiac and mesenteric artery angiography for visualization of the gallbladder has been utilized for the diagnosis of gallbladder diseases which cannot be made by routine roentgenologic means.

TECHNIQUE. The technique is similar to the Seldinger technique previously described for percutaneous transfemoral or brachial artery catheterization. Forty to 50 cc. of a contrast medium is injected directly into the celiac artery, or about half this quantity into the mesenteric artery. If selective catheterization of the cystic artery or hepatic artery can be accomplished, this route is desirable. Methylglucamine diatrizoate (Renografin) or sodium diatrizoate (Hypaque) is utilized. A pressure injector is employed so that the chosen volume is injected within 2 seconds, and exposures are made in rapid sequence—two per second for 4 seconds and one per second for 4 seconds thereafter. Thereafter ten exposures at 3 second intervals may be utilized. *Transjugular cholangiography* is a modification of the Seldinger technique, in which a catheter introduced via the jugular vein is directed into a hepatic vein (Weiner and Hanafee, for review).* This technique avoids percutaneous liver entry and yet accomplishes a good visualization of an obstructed hepatic venous system.

---

*References may be obtained in Meschan, I.: An Atlas of Anatomy Basic to Radiology. Philadelphia, W. B. Saunders Co., 1975, Chapter 14.

NORMAL GALLBLADDER MEASUREMENTS

The normal measurements of the gallbladder were derived angiographically by Redman and Reuter from 25 normal gallbladders as follows:

	Mean Measurement	Range	Standard Deviation
Area	21.1 sq. cm.	11.4–33 cm.	5 cm.
Width	3.6 cm.	1.9– 5 cm.	0.77 cm.

Conclusions: Gallbladders measuring more than 35 sq. cm. or having a width of more than 5 cm. may be considered distended.

FIGURE 15–56

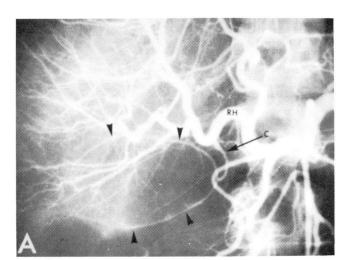

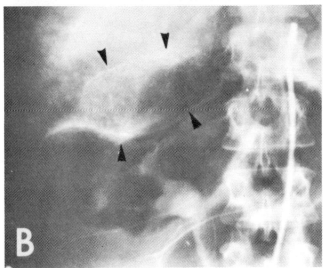

FIGURE 15–57 Celiac arteriogram. *A. (RH)* Right hepatic artery. *(C)* cystic artery. Arrowheads point out branches of cystic artery. *B.* Venous phase showing cystic veins. (From Ruzicka, F. F., Jr., and Rossi, P.: Radiol. Clin. North Am., 8:3–29, 1970.)

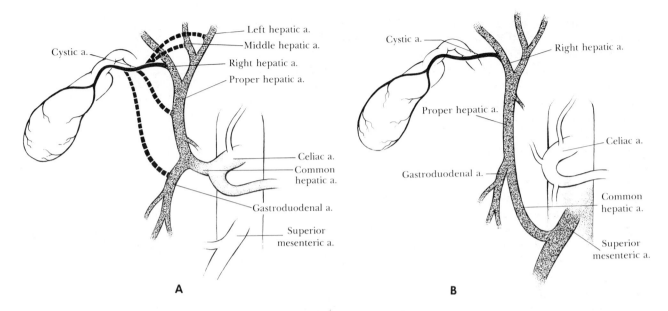

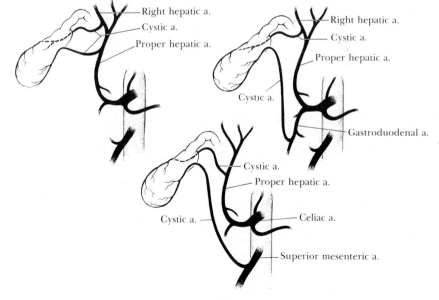

FIGURE 15–58 Cystic artery variations. In *A*, the solid vessel line indicates the most frequent site of origin of the cystic artery. The interrupted vessel lines show the more common variations. In *B*, the cystic artery arises from the right hepatic, which is a branch of the superior mesenteric artery. In *C*, three of the more common variations of double cystic arteries are shown. (From Ruzicka, F. F., Jr., and Rossi, P.: Radiol. Clin. North Am., 8:3–29, 1970.)

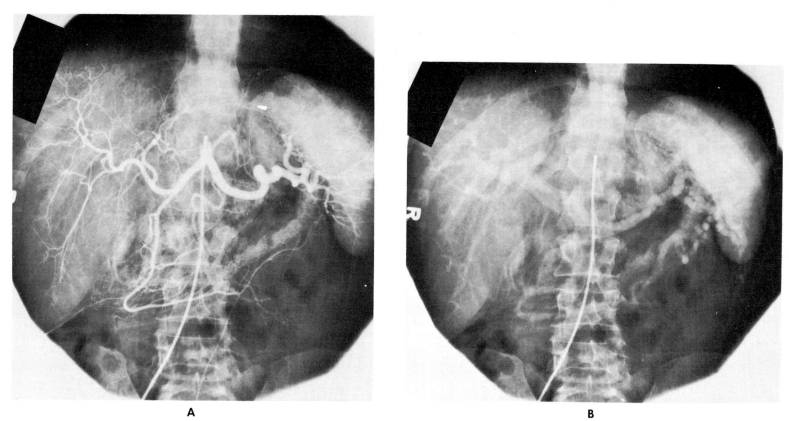

A

B

FIGURE 15–59 *A.* Normal hepatic arteriogram. *B.* Portal or splenoportal venogram following celiac arteriogram.

Portal Phlebography. The basic anatomy has been described previously. The splenic and superior mesenteric veins comprise the main tributaries of the portal vein, with the inferior mesenteric usually draining into the splenic and the coronary vein terminating at the junction of the splenic and portal veins.

TECHNIQUES FOR STUDY. Percutaneous injection of the spleen results in opacification of the splenoportal trunk (Fig. 15–61). This procedure is performed by injection directly into the splenic pulp. Ordinarily, 50 cc. of 70 per cent methylglucamine or sodium diatrizoate or its equivalent is employed. This volume is forcefully injected in 5 or 6 seconds, and exposures of one film per second for 12 to 15 seconds are usually adequate. The patient should be maintained in apnea during the injection and exposure. The following blood vessels are seen in rapid sequence: (1) the splenoportal trunk, (2) the intrahepatic portal branches, and (3) the sinusoidal system of the liver. The sinusoidal phase reaches a maximum within 16 to 24 seconds and then fades, although it may persist for as long as 60 seconds.

The injection may be made directly into a cannulated branch of the portal system at surgery, and under these circumstances, the opacification is limited mostly to the vein injected along with the portal vein.

The splenic, superior mesenteric, and portal veins usually have approximately the same diameter and are confluent in the upper lumbar or lowermost thoracic region, which is usually projected over the spine. At the porta hepatis, the portal vein bifurcates into its two main branches. The coronary vein and the inferior mesenteric vein are also visualized, especially in the presence of increased resistance to flow within the liver. Other tributaries of the portal system may also be shown, such as the gastroepiploic veins, the pancreatic veins, or even the short gastric veins. The right main branch is usually readily detected along with its main ramifications, but there is a considerable superimposition of branches, making intimate detail difficult to obtain; the left main branch may be only partially visualized. It is thought that the better visualization of the right branch is due to its posterior position, and the effect of gravity of the contrast agent within the blood. The portal branches divide 5 to 7 times and almost any angle up to 90 degrees may be encountered, but branching occurs in a symmetrical manner and tapering of vessels is gradual. Although the more proximal vessels are straight, branches of the fourth to seventh order may be somewhat curved.

In the sinusoidal phase, the density of the contrast agent is fairly uniform. A spotted appearance is usually abnormal. There may, however, be some variation in density due to varying thicknesses of different parts of the liver. Since the left lobe is usually poorly opacified in this phase it cannot be evaluated accurately.

The other basic method of visualization of the extrahepatic portal venous system is by injection into the celiac artery and obtaining sequential studies during the venous phase. The splenoportal axis is usually fairly well defined (Fig. 15–60). Some of the veins that may be identified in this type of study are the gastric veins, coronary veins, gastroepiploic veins, and even the pancreaticoduodenal veins. The rapidity of celiac injection and the volume of contrast agent employed will frequently determine the intensity of visualization. Usually the inferior mesenteric vein will not be seen unless the inferior mesenteric artery is selectively injected.*

Diagrams illustrating the main routes of blood flow through regularly appearing tributaries of the portal system are shown in Figures 15–61 and 15–62. Thus, short gastric, pancreatic, inferior mesenteric, superior mesenteric, coronary, gastric, and esophageal dilated vessels become visible. This technique is particularly useful for demonstration of esophageal varices.

SUMMARY OF CIRCULATION THROUGH THE PORTAL VENOUS SYSTEM. Venous blood, carrying materials absorbed from the alimentary tract, passes into the liver through the portal vein and branches out progressively to reach the sinusoid in the individual liver lobules. The blood then reaches the central vein of the lobule. Arterial blood enters through the hepatic artery with oxygenated blood and it too enters the sinusoids to reach the central vein. The central veins are the actual beginnings of the hepatic venous system. The central veins from several lobules unite to enter subloblular veins, and these in turn merge to form increasingly larger trunks, finally converging to form three hepatic veins, which then enter the vena cava.

---

*Ruzicka, F. F., and Rossi, P.: Normal vascular anatomy of the abdominal viscera. Radiol. Clin. North Am., *8*:3–29, 1970.

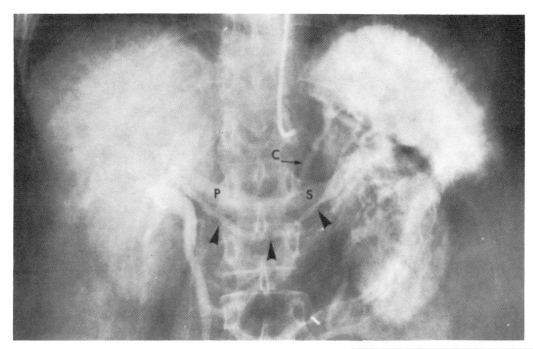

FIGURE 15–60 Venous phase of celiac artery injection. A double splenoportal axis is shown. The usual axis is made up of the splenic vein (*S*) and portal vein (*P*). Coronary vein (*C*) enters splenic vein. The anomalous axis (arrowheads) arises from a confluence of short gastric veins and splenic hilar radicles and passes parallel to the main S-P axis to enter the liver separately just below the portal vein. (From Ruzicka, F. F., Jr., and Rossi, P.: Radiol. Clin. North Am., *8:*3–29, 1970.)

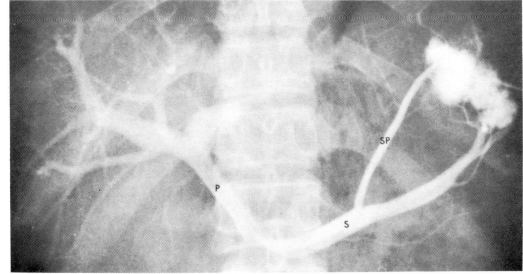

FIGURE 15–61 Normal splenoportogram. Injection into the splenic pulp results in visualization of splenoportal axis. Superior polar vein *(SP)* is part of splenoportal axis. Tributaries are not visualized normally by this technique. However, capsular veins of spleen and adjacent small vessels may fill during splenic injection in the normal patient. (*S*) Splenic vein, (*P*) portal vein. (From Ruzicka, F. F., Jr., and Rossi, P.: Radiol. Clin. North Am., *8:*3–29, 1970.)

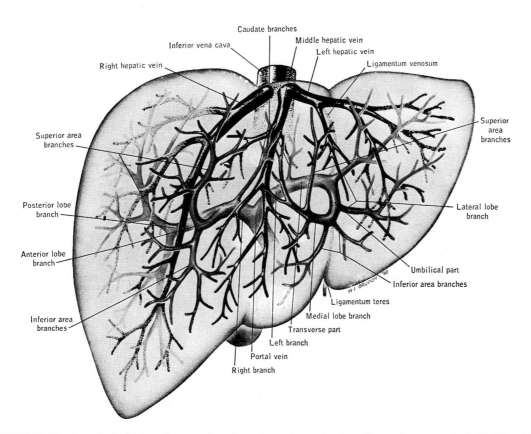

FIGURE 15–62 Intrahepatic distribution of the hepatic and portal veins. (From Anson, B. J. (ed.): Morris' Human Anatomy, 12th ed. New York, McGraw-Hill Book Company, 1966. Copyright © 1966 by McGraw-Hill, Inc. Used by permission of McGraw-Hill Book Company.)

16

COMPUTED WHOLE BODY TOMOGRAPHY

ISADORE MESCHAN, M.A., M.D.

NEIL T. WOLFMAN, M.D.

Assistant Professor, Department of Radiology, Bowman Gray School of Medicine of Wake Forest University, Winston-Salem, North Carolina

with anatomical sketches by
GEORGE C. LYNCH

Professor of Medical Illustration, Bowman Gray School of Wake Forest University, Winston-Salem, North Carolina

INTRODUCTION

Computed head tomography was introduced in 1972 by Ambrose and Hounsfield (see discussion in Chapter 7 on computed tomography of brain and skull). In February 1974, the first ACTA total body scanner went into operation at Georgetown University Medical Center. Since then, a moderate number of whole body scanners made by different manufacturers have been installed in institutions throughout the world.

Computed Tomographic Equipment

As shown in Chapter 7, the basic computed tomographic (CT) equipment consists of the following: (1) a patient table; (2) an x-ray scanning unit that moves at 1- to 10-degree intervals through a 180- to 360-degree arc; (3) an x-ray control unit that energizes the x-ray tube (or x-ray tubes), resulting in the emission of highly collimated beams of x-rays; (4) receptor devices that receive the "remnant radiation" on the far side of the patient after it has passed through the patient; (5) a computer that summates the photons of energy transmitted through the patient in each pass; (6) a computer that reconstructs the summated photons of radiation into an image that can be viewed on a cathode ray tube; and (7) a photographic unit that records the image from the face of the cathode ray tube. To assist in these basic functions there are motor generators, high-voltage generators, cooling oil pumps, and a keyboard apparatus to "instruct" the computer devices regarding scanning operations and image data manipulations. The scanning device, consisting of an x-ray tube (or x-ray tubes) on one side and scintillation or gas-filled detectors on the other, is spoken of as a "gantry."

With the early models that were designed to examine the head, the patient's head was introduced into a flexible water bag within an opening in the gantry. The water bag served to limit the dynamic range of radiation to which the detectors would be exposed. (It is electronically more difficult to maintain the calibration of the detectors over the very wide range required if the detectors are exposed to the raw x-ray beam as it scans beyond the edge of the patient's head.) The water bag also served as a reference medium for relative x-ray attenuation with respect to water.

In the newer CT systems the water bag has been abandoned; a hole through the gantry in a "doughnut" configuration permits any part of the patient's body to be introduced for CT examination. Although some units still surround the body part examined with unit density material, devices using such an approach are less than satisfactory, since they result in the loss of information-bearing photons before they reach the detectors and also result in unnecessary irradiation of the patient.

The scintillation or gas-filled detectors opposite the x-ray tube not only are more sensitive than x-ray film in discriminating fine differences in x-ray attenuation, but the collimators of these detectors also reduce the amount of scattered radiation, thus preventing further degradation of the image.

The Head Computed Tomographic Scanner (see also Chapter 7)

The first scanner was developed by Emitronics Limited of England, which published a report of its products in 1972 at the Annual Congress of the British Institute of Radiology; this scanner, however, was specifically designed for brain scanning. By mid-1973 the first *head* CT scanner was being made in the United States. The first unit with whole body scanning capability—the ACTA scanner—now being manufactured by the Pfizer Medical Systems, was introduced early in 1974. Other companies soon announced production of similar devices.

Design of Scanning Apparatus. In the years since the first commercial units were available, the time required to obtain a CT image has been required by many orders of magnitude. Scan times are now quoted in seconds, rather than minutes. The diminishing scan time is the consequence of two basic design improvements, which in turn result in more efficient data collection and less mechanical motion of the x-ray source and detectors. These two developments are the following:

1. The geometry of the x-ray beam has changed from the original

narrow beam of x-rays to a thin, fanlike beam. The fastest scanners available today employ a wide-angle fan beam and several hundred detectors in a rotational design.

2. The mechanical motion of the x-ray source and detectors has been diminished. The early CT scanners moved in 1-degree increments following the completion of each lateral translational scan until an arc of 180 degrees was completed. The most recently developed CT scanners are able to complete a scan in 1 to 20 seconds by utilizing the fan beam geometry and multiple detectors. This single motion scanning is accomplished by a bank of detectors as well as by a fan beam geometry. Stationary fan beams may impinge on stationary arcs of hundreds of detectors. Such a design permits one to "suspend" cardiac motion by the extremely rapid scan time. Electrocardiographic "gating" would also allow one to obtain an image of the heart in any selected phase of the cardiac cycle. For example, the heart could be scanned only during the peak of diastole, and by means of intravenous contrast enhancement, the chambers would be clearly visualized.

Computer Hardware and Software. Apart from the design changes in the scanning apparatus, there has been significant improvement in the computer hardware and software. Changes in the algorithms have resulted in the attainment of image reconstruction within seconds after scanning. The combination of all of these devices has made feasible extremely rapid scanning and rapid reconstruction. Moreover, new algorithms allow the reconstruction of a series of cross-sections into sagittal and even isometric thru-dimensional displays.

The detail in the reconstructed image depends, in part, on the number and size of the squares used by the computer to reconstruct the image. Each square represents a finite area in the cross section of the patient's head or body, and the computer assigns a specific average density to each square, thereby reflecting the number of x-ray photons computed to have been absorbed by that volume of tissue. It is thus apparent that the smaller and more numerous the computed boxes are, the more representative the reconstruction will be. Since each of these boxes represents not only an area of tissue but also a finite thickness of tissue,

the term *voxel* (volume element) has been applied. When the voxel is displayed on a cathode ray tube, it is referred to as a *pixel* (picture element). The dimensions (given in voxels or pixels) of the reconstructed image represent the matrix size. The early CT scanners used a matrix of 80×80 voxels, resulting in an image composed of visible and, therefore, objectionable boxes. Currently, most CT systems use a matrix of 256×256 voxels or 512×512 voxels. This yields an image in which the voxels are not readily apparent.

There is a limit to how fine a matrix one can use in image reconstruction. As the voxel gets smaller and smaller, one starts to detect the random statistical fluctuation of x-ray photons passing through each tiny volume of tissue, rather than the linear attenuation coefficient of this tiny tissue volume. To avoid this problem of the very fine matrix (512×512 or finer), one must increase the number of photons passing through the patient—that is, one must increase the radiation dosage.

The tissue volume represented by each picture element in the display matrix has been significantly reduced in the new matrices; at present, element size ranges from 1×1 mm. to 2×2 mm. in cross section. Moreover, the scan slices, when such are employed, can now become collimated from 13 mm. to 3 mm. in width so that the tissue volume represented by each picture element ranges anywhere from 3 to 68 cu. mm. These changes have increased both image resolution and detection of smaller tumors or other abnormalities in the areas scanned.

Speed is particularly important, since respiratory and peristaltic motion seriously degrade the computed tomographic image. Moreover, while rotational fan-beam scanners can collect more readings in a shorter period of time, their detectors must be very carefully calibrated with respect to each other in order to obtain good images. Any mismatches will result in undesirable artifacts. Glucagon may be used to temporarily "stop" peristaltic gastrointestinal activity, and iodinated contrast agents are used to enhance blood vessels or the gastrointestinal tract.

Radiation Exposure of Patient. Another important consideration is radiation exposure to the patient. With most of the current CT scanners, the radiation skin dose received by the patient during an abdominal examination is less than during the average barium enema. Nevertheless, one must strive to minimize the dose as much as possible, in particular by confining the examination to the anatomic region of interest or suspicion. The skin dose on the side of x-ray entry is approximately 1.25 rads, and on the exit side the dose is 0.25 rads per CT "slice."

In the reconstructed image, the computer assigns each voxel a relative density number based on an arbitrary scale of -1000 to $+1000$, called "Hounsfield units." (The original EMI units were one-half of these — going from -500 to $+500$.) This scale is mathematically related to the linear attenuation coefficient of the tissue represented by that voxel. On this scale, air is assigned a density of -1000; water, a density of 0; and compact bone, $+1000$. (Refer to Fig. 7–64.) Most CT systems provide an electronic device at the display console that permits the observer to sample any area of the image and receive a computer readout of the density number of the selected area. The console also provides a mid-range "window" attenuation coefficient and a "width" as desired around that window.

Currently Available CT Scans of the Body

The ensuing pages present examples of currently available CT scans of the body. The images were selected at segmental levels below the calvaria. Although computed tomography has made a dramatic appearance on the horizons of medical imaging, there still remains a need for the more familiar modalities previously described: angiography, pneumoencephalography, conventional radiography, ultrasonography, and radionuclide imaging. The various roles of these modalities is beyond the scope of this text.

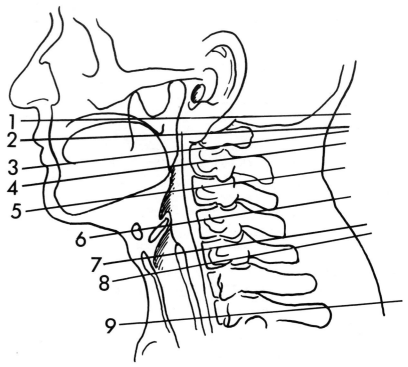

FIGURE 16–1 Line diagram showing the position of the computed tomographic cuts of the lower face and neck.

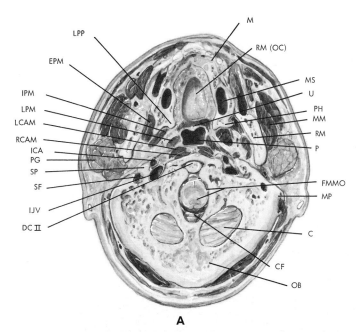

A

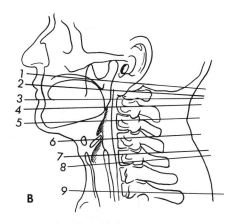

FIGURE 16–2 *A.* Diagram of lower face at level No. 1, showing anatomic parts encountered in this slice. *B.* Miniature of Figure 16–1 for orientation. *C.* Computed tomograph obtained at this level; enhanced by artist. (Courtesy of W. Martin Dinn, M.D.)

B

LPP	=	Lateral pterygoid plate
EPM	=	External pterygoid muscle
IPM	=	Internal pterygoid muscle
LPM	=	Levator palatini muscle
LCAM	=	Longus capitis anterior muscle
RCAM	=	Rectus capitis anterior muscle
ICA	=	Internal carotid artery
PG	=	Parotid gland
SP	=	Styloid process
SF	=	Stylomastoid foramen
IJV	=	Internal jugular vein
DC II	=	Dens of C II
M	=	Maxilla
RM (OC)	=	Roof of mouth (oral cavity)
MS	=	Maxillary sinus
U	=	Uvula
PH	=	Pterygoid hamulus
MM	=	Masseter muscle
RM	=	Ramus of mandible
P	=	Pharynx
FMMO	=	Foramen magnum and medulla oblongata
MP	=	Mastoid process

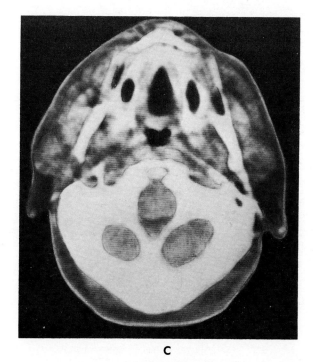

C

C	=	Cerebellum
CF	=	Cerebrospinal fluid
OB	=	Occipital bone

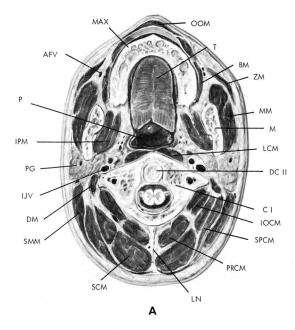

A

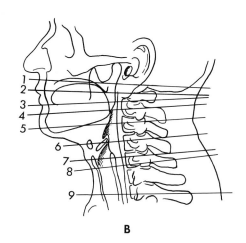

FIGURE 16–3 *A.* Diagram of lower face at level No. 2, showing anatomic parts encountered in this slice. B. Miniature of Figure 16–1 for orientation. *C.* Computed tomograph obtained; enhanced by artist. (Courtesy of W. Martin Dinn, M.D.)

B

MAX	=	Maxilla
AFV	=	Anterior facial vein
P	=	Pharynx
IPM	=	Internal pterygoid muscle
PG	=	Parotid gland
IJV	=	Internal jugular vein
DM	=	Digastric muscle
SMM	=	Sternocleidomastoid muscle
SCM	=	Semispinalis capitis muscle
OOM	=	Orbicularis oris muscle
T	=	Tongue
BM	=	Buccinator muscle
ZM	=	Zygomatic muscle
MM	=	Masseter muscle
M	=	Mandible
LCM	=	Longus capitis muscle
DC II	=	Dens of C II
CI	=	C I
IOCM	=	Inferior oblique capitis muscle
SPCM	=	Splenius capitis muscle
PRCM	=	Posterior rectus capitis muscle
LN	=	Ligamentum nuchae

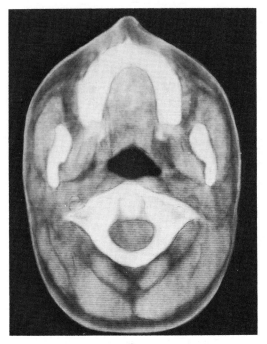

C

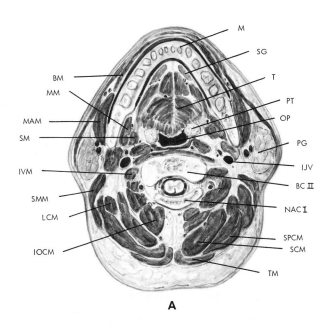

A

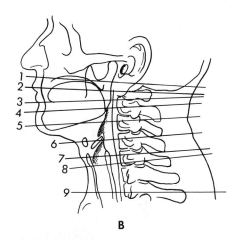

FIGURE 16–4 *A.* Diagram of lower face at level No. 3, showing anatomic parts encountered in this slice. *B.* Miniature of Figure 16–1 for orientation. *C.* Computed tomograph obtained; enhanced by artist. (Courtesy of W. Martin Dinn, M.D.)

B

BM	=	Buccinator muscle
MM	=	Mylohyoideus muscle
MAM	=	Masseter muscle
SM	=	Styloglossus muscle
IVM	=	Intertransversarius muscle
SMM	=	Sternocleidomastoid muscle
LCM	=	Longissimus capitis muscle
IOCM	=	Inferior oblique capitis muscle
M	=	Mandible
SG	=	Sublingual gland
T	=	Tongue
PT	=	Palatine tonsil
OP	=	Oropharynx
PG	=	Parotid gland
IJV	=	Internal jugular vein
BC II	=	Body of C II
NAC I	=	Neural arch C I
SPCM	=	Splenius capitis muscle
SCM	=	Semispinalis capitis muscle
TM	=	Trapezius muscle

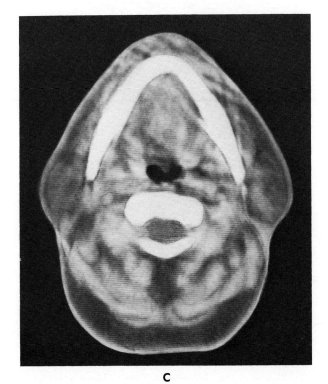

C

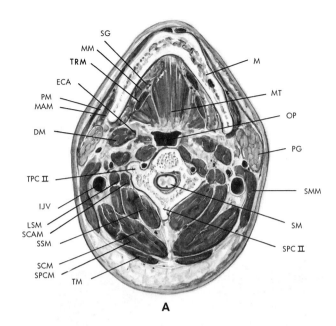

A

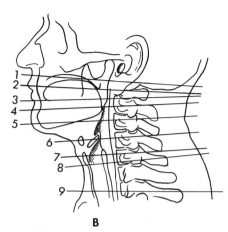

FIGURE 16–5 *A.* Diagram of lower face at level No. 4, showing anatomic parts encountered in this slice. *B.* Miniature of Figure 16–1 for orientation. *C.* Computed tomograph obtained; enhanced by artist. (Courtesy of W. Martin Dinn, M.D.)

B

SG	=	Sublingual gland
MM	=	Mylohyoideus muscle
TRM	=	Triangularis muscle
ECA	=	External carotid artery
PM	=	Platysma muscle
MAM	=	Masseter muscle
DM	=	Digastric muscle
TPC II	=	Transverse process C II
IJV	=	Internal jugular vein
LSM	=	Levator scapulae muscle
SCAM	=	Scalenus medius muscle
SSM	=	Semispinalis cervicis muscle
SCM	=	Semispinalis capitis muscle
SPCM	=	Splenius capitis muscle
TM	=	Trapezius muscle
M	=	Mandible
MT	=	Muscle of tongue
OP	=	Oropharynx
PG	=	Parotid gland
SMM	=	Sternocleidomastoid muscle
SM	=	Spinal medulla
SPC II	=	Spinous process C II

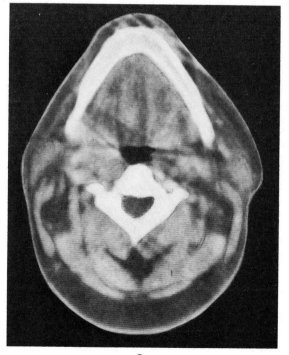

C

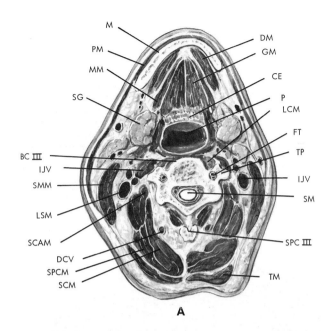

A

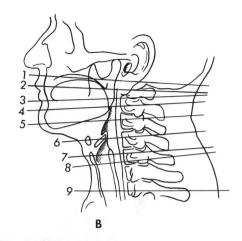

FIGURE 16–6 *A.* Diagram of lower face at level No. 5, showing anatomic parts encountered in this slice. *B.* Miniature of Figure 16–1 for orientation. *C.* Computed tomograph obtained; enhanced by artist. (Courtesy of W. Martin Dinn, M.D.)

B

M	=	Mandible
PM	=	Platysma muscle
MM	=	Mylohyoideus muscle
SG	=	Submaxillary gland
BC III	=	Body of C III
LSM	=	Levator scapulae muscle
SMM	=	Sternocleidomastoid muscle
IJV	=	Internal jugular vein
SCAM	=	Scalenus medius muscle
DCV	=	Deep cervical vein
SPCM	=	Splenius capitis muscle
SCM	=	Semispinalis capitis muscle
DM	=	Digastric muscle
GM	=	Geniohyoid muscle
CE	=	Cartilage of epiglottis
P	=	Pharynx
LCM	=	Longus colli muscle
FT	=	Foramen transversarium
TP	=	Transverse process
SM	=	Spinal medulla
SPC III	=	Spinous process C III
TM	=	Trapezius muscle

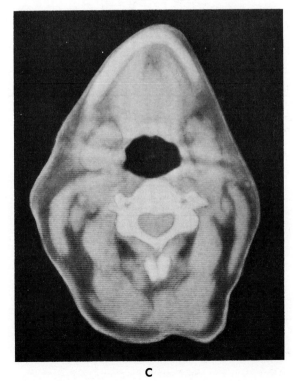

C

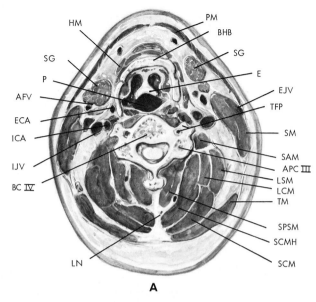

A

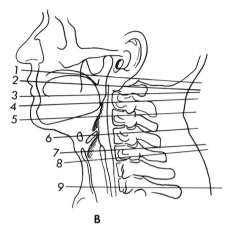

FIGURE 16–7 *A*. Diagram of neck at level No. 6, showing anatomic parts encountered in this slice. *B*. Miniature of Figure 16–1 for orientation. *C*. Computed tomograph obtained; enhanced by artist. (Courtesy of W. Martin Dinn, M.D.)

B

HM	=	Hyoglossus muscle
SG	=	Submaxillary gland
P	=	Pharynx
AFV	=	Anterior facial vein
ECA	=	External carotid artery
IJV	=	Internal jugular vein
ICA	=	Internal carotid artery
BC IV	=	Body of C IV
LN	=	Ligamentum nuchae
PM	=	Platysma muscle
BHB	=	Body of hyoid bone
E	=	Epiglottis
EJV	=	External jugular vein
TFP	=	Transverse foramen and process
SM	=	Sternocleidomastoid muscle
SAM	=	Scalenus anterior muscle
APC III	=	Anterior process C III
LSM	=	Levator scapulae muscle
LCM	=	Longissimus capitis muscle
TM	=	Trapezius muscle
SPSM	=	Semispinalis cervicis muscle
SCM	=	Semispinalis capitis muscle
SPCM	=	Splenius capitis muscle

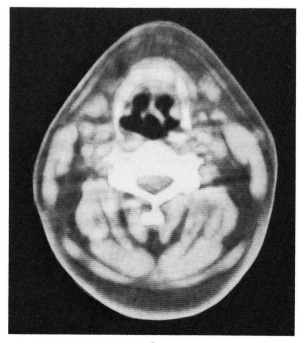

C

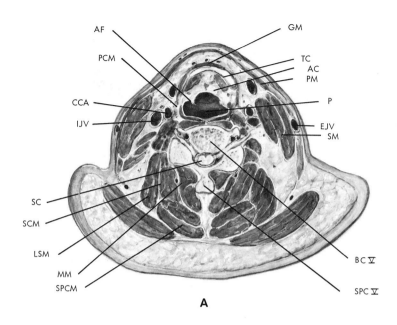

A

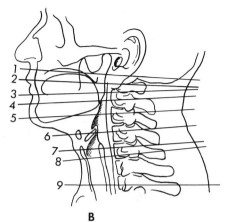

B

FIGURE 16–8 *A*. Diagram of neck at level No. 7, showing anatomic parts encountered in this slice. *B*. Miniature of Figure 16–1 for orientation. *C*. Computed tomograph obtained; enhanced by artist. (Courtesy of W. Martin Dinn, M.D.)

AF	=	Aryepiglottic fold
PCM	=	Pharyngeal constrictor muscle
CCA	=	Common carotid artery
IJV	=	Internal jugular vein
SC	=	Spinal cord
SCM	=	Semispinalis capitis muscle
LSM	=	Levator scapulae muscle
MM	=	Multifidus muscle
SPCM	=	Splenius capitis muscle
GM	=	Geniohyoid muscle
TC	=	Thyroid cartilage
AC	=	Arytenoid cartilage
PM	=	Platysma muscle
P	=	Pharynx
EJV	=	External jugular vein
SM	=	Sternocleidomastoid muscle
BC V	=	Body of C V
SPC V	=	Spinous process C V

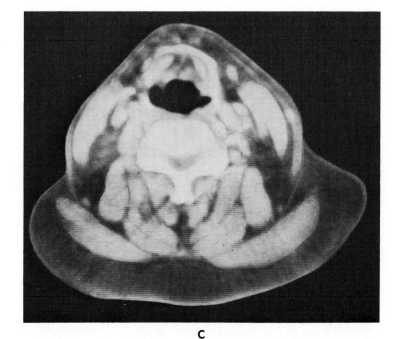

C

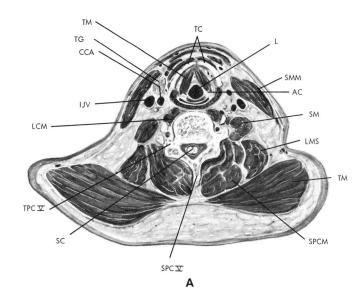

A

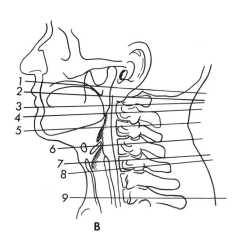

FIGURE 16–9 *A.* Diagram of neck at level No. 8, showing anatomic parts encountered in this slice. *B.* Miniature of Figure 16–1 for orientation. *C.* Computed tomograph obtained; enhanced by artist. (Courtesy of W. Martin Dinn, M.D.)

B

TC	=	Thyroid cartilages
TM	=	Trapezius muscle
TG	=	Thyroid gland
CCA	=	Common carotid artery
IJV	=	Internal jugular vein
LCM	=	Longus colli muscle
TPC V	=	Transverse process C V
SC	=	Spinal cord
SPC V	=	Spinous process C V
L	=	Larynx
SMM	=	Sternocleidomastoid muscle
AC	=	Arytenoid cartilage
SM	=	Scalenus muscles
LMS	=	Levator muscle of scapula
SPCM	=	Splenius capitis muscle

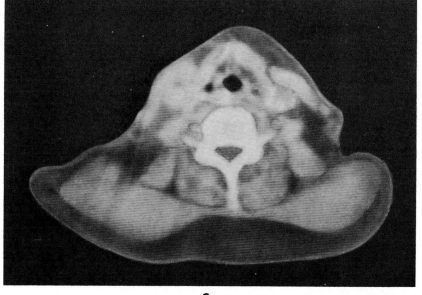

C

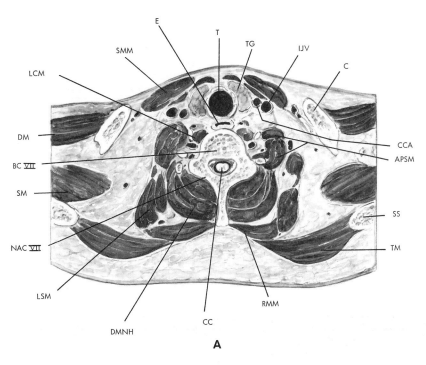

A

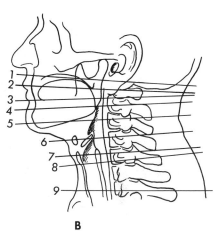

FIGURE 16–10 *A*. Diagram of neck at level No. 9, showing anatomic parts encountered in this slice. *B*. Miniature of Figure 16–1 for orientation. *C*. Computed tomograph obtained; enhanced by artist. (Courtesy of W. Martin Dinn, M.D.)

B

E	=	Esophagus
SMM	=	Sternocleidomastoid muscle
LCM	=	Longus colli muscle
DM	=	Deltoid muscle
BC VII	=	Body of C VII
SM	=	Supraspinatus muscle
NAC VII	=	Neural arch C–VII
LSM	=	Levator scapulae muscle
DMNH	=	Deep muscles of neck and head
CC	=	Cervical cord
T	=	Trachea
TG	=	Thyroid gland
IJV	=	Internal jugular vein
C	=	Clavicle
APSM	=	Anterior and posterior scalene muscle
SS	=	Spine of scapula
TM	=	Trapezius muscle
RMM	=	Rhomboid minor muscle

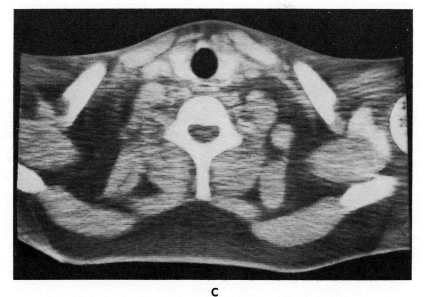

C

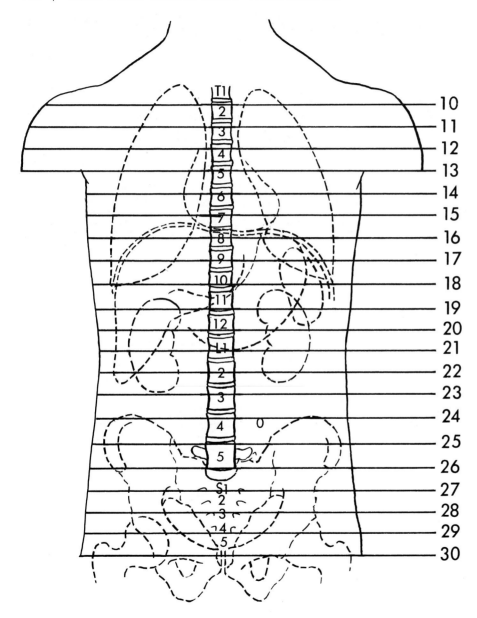

FIGURE 16–11 Line drawing showing the position of the computed tomographic cuts of the thorax and abdomen.

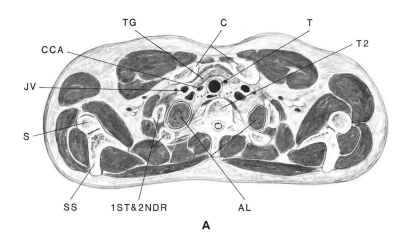

A

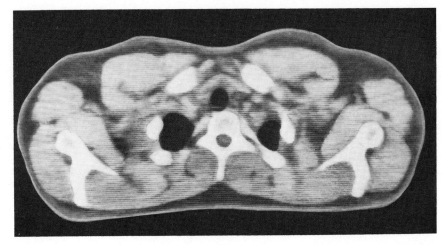

C

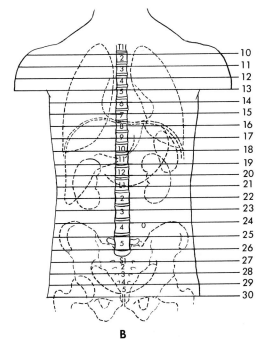

B

FIGURE 16–12 *A*. Diagram at shoulder level (T2) at cut No. 10, showing anatomic parts encountered in this slice. *B*. Miniature of Figure 16–11 for orientation. *C*. Computed tomograph obtained; enhanced by arist. (Courtesy of W. Martin Dinn, M.D.)

C	=	Clavicles
TG	=	Right lobe of thyroid gland
CCA	=	Common carotid artery
JV	=	Jugular vein
S	=	Scapula
SS	=	Spine of scapula
1st and 2nd R	=	First and second ribs
T	=	Trachea
T2	=	T2 level
AL	=	Apices of lung

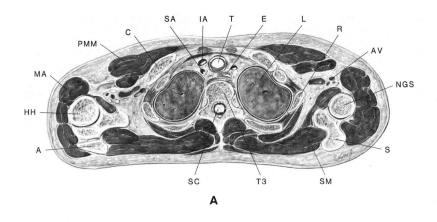

A

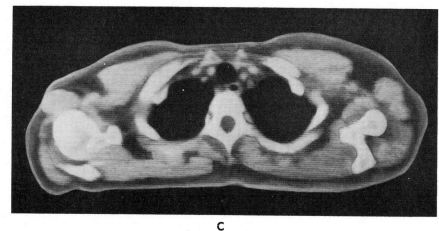

C

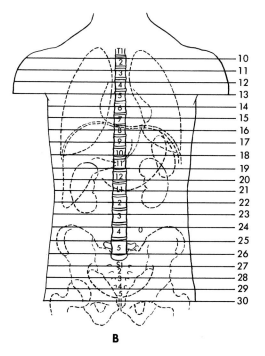

B

FIGURE 16–13 *A*. Diagram at thoracic level (T3) at cut No. 11, showing anatomic parts encountered in this slice. *B*. Miniature of Figure 16–11 for orientation. *C*. Computed tomograph obtained; enhanced by artist. (Courtesy of W. Martin Dinn, M.D.)

IA	=	Innominate artery
SA	=	Subclavian artery
C	=	Clavicle
PMM	=	Pectoralis major muscle
MA	=	Muscles of arm
HH	=	Head of humerus
A	=	Acromion
SC	=	Spinal cord
T	=	Trachea
E	=	Esophagus
L	=	Lung
R	=	Rib
AV	=	Axillary vessels
NGS	=	Neck and glenoid of scapula
S	=	Scapula
SM	=	Supraspinatus muscle
T3	=	T3 level

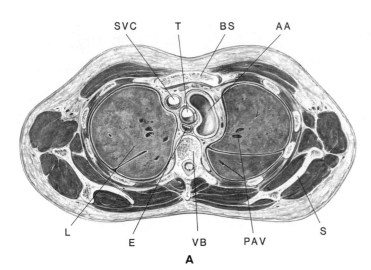

A

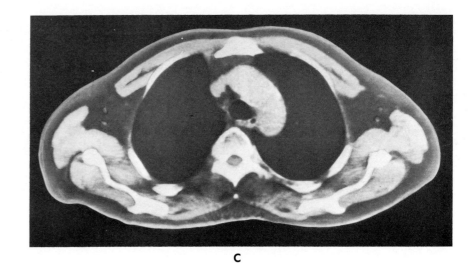

C

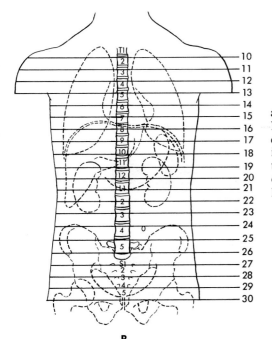

B

FIGURE 16–14 *A.* Diagram at aortic arch level (T4) at cut No. 12, showing anatomic parts encountered in this slice. *B.* Miniature of Figure 16–11 for orientation. *C.* Computed tomograph obtained approximately at this level.

T	=	Trachea
SVC	=	Superior vena cava
L	=	Lung
E	=	Esophagus
BS	=	Body of sternum
AA	=	Aortic arch
S	=	Scapula
PAV	=	Pulmonary arteries and veins
VB	=	Vertebral body

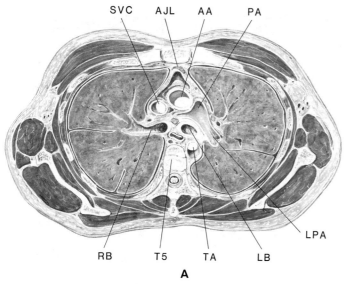

A

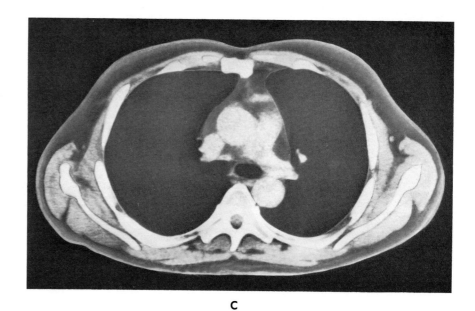

C

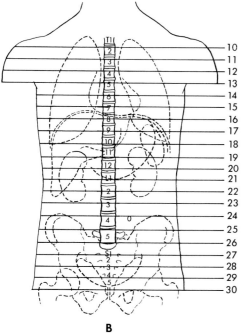

B

FIGURE 16–15 *A*. Diagram at thoracic level (T5) at cut No. 13, showing anatomic parts encountered in this slice. *B*. Miniature of Figure 16–11 for orientation. *C*. Computed tomograph obtained approximately at this level.

AJL	=	Anterior junction line
SVC	=	Superior vena cava
RB	=	Right bronchus
T5	=	T5 level
AA	=	Ascending aorta
PA	=	Undivided pulmonary artery
LPA	=	Left pulmonary artery
LB	=	Left bronchus
TA	=	Thoracic (descending) aorta

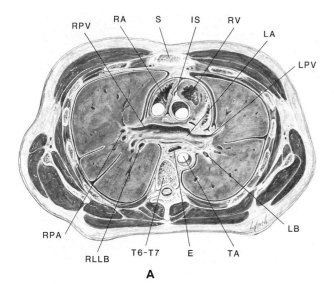

A

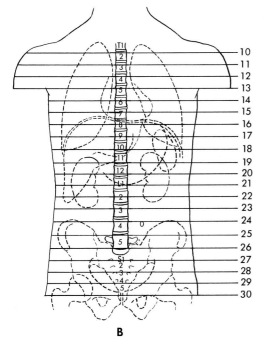

B

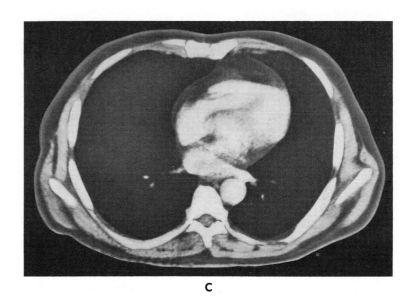

C

FIGURE 16–16 *A*. Diagram at thoracic level (T6–T7) at cut No. 14, showing anatomic parts encountered in this slice. *B*. Miniature of Figure 16–11 for orientation. *C*. Computed tomograph obtained approximately at this level.

S	=	Sternum
RA	=	Right atrium
RPV	=	Right pulmonary vein
RPA	=	Right pulmonary artery
RLLB	=	Right lower lobe bronchus
T6 – T7	=	T6 – T7 level
IS	=	Interventricular septum
RV	=	Right ventricle
LA	=	Left atrium
LPV	=	Left pulmonary vein
LB	=	Left bronchus
TA	=	Thoracic aorta
E	=	Esophagus

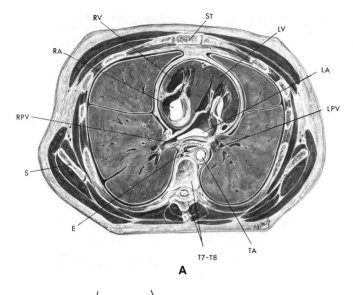

A

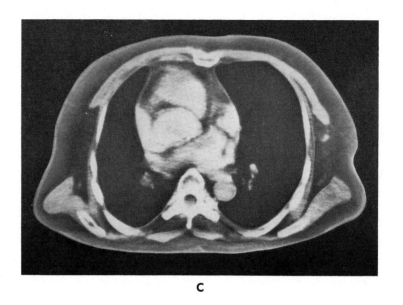

C

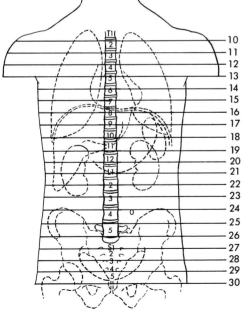

B

FIGURE 16–17 *A*. Diagram at thoracic level (T7–T8) at cut No. 15, showing anatomic parts encountered in this slice. *B*. Miniature of Figure 16–11 for orientation. *C*. Computed tomograph obtained approximately at this level.

RV	=	Right ventricle
RA	=	Right atrium
RPV	=	Right pulmonary vein
S	=	Scapula
E	=	Esophagus
ST	=	Sternum
LV	=	Left ventricle
LA	=	Left atrium
LPV	=	Left pulmonary vein
TA	=	Thoracic aorta
T7 – T8	=	T7 – T8 level

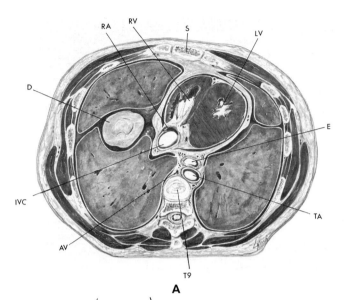

A

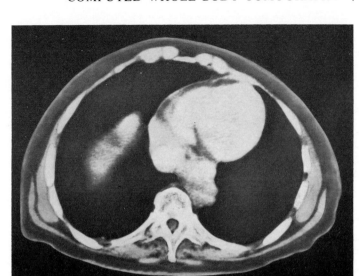

C

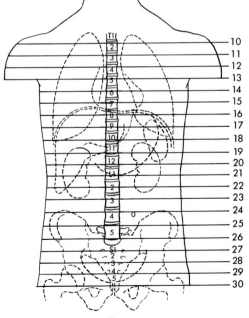

B

FIGURE 16–18 *A*. Diagram at thoracic level (T9) at cut No. 16, showing anatomic parts encountered in this slice. *B*. Miniature of Figure 16–11 for orientation. *C*. Computed tomograph obtained approximately at this level.

RV	=	Right ventricle
RA	=	Right atrium
D	=	Diaphragm
IVC	=	Inferior vena cava
AV	=	Azygos vein
S	=	Sternum
LV	=	Left ventricle
E	=	Esophagus
TA	=	Thoracic aorta
T9	=	T9 level

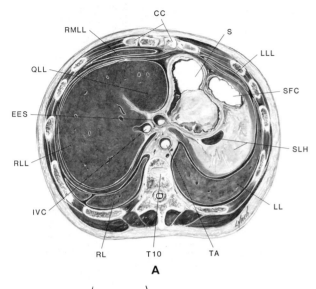

A

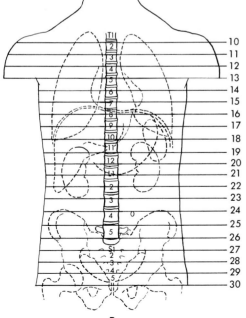

B

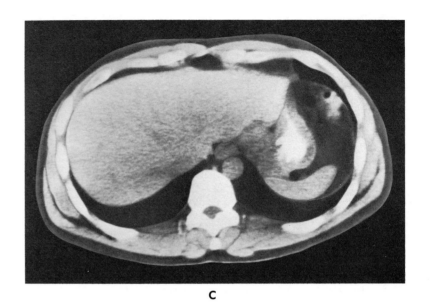

C

FIGURE 16–19 *A*. Diagram at junction of thorax and abdomen (T10) at cut No. 17, showing anatomic parts encountered in this slice. *B*. Miniature of Figure 16–11 for orientation. *C*. Computed tomograph obtained approximately at this level.

CC	=	Costal cartilages
RMLL	=	Right middle lobe of lung
QLL	=	Quadrate lobe of liver
EES	=	Esophagus entry to stomach
RLL	=	Right lobe of liver
IVC	=	Inferior vena cava
RL	=	Right lung (lower lobe)
T10	=	T10 level
S	=	Stomach
LLL	=	Lingula of left lung
SFC	=	Splenic flexure of colon
SLH	=	Spleen and left hemidiaphragm
LL	=	Left lung
TA	=	Thoracic aorta

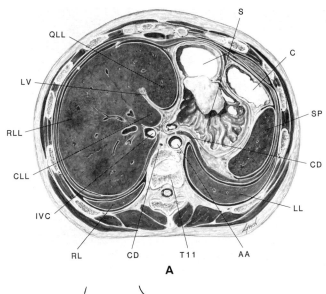

A

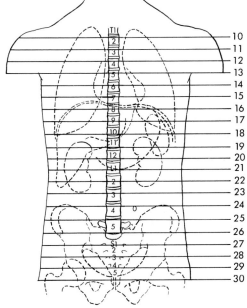

B

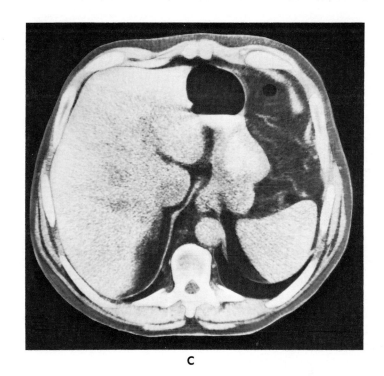

C

FIGURE 16–20 *A*. Diagram at junction of thorax and abdomen (T11) at cut No. 18, showing anatomic parts encountered in this slice. *B*. Miniature of Figure 16–11 for orientation. *C*. Computed tomograph obtained approximately at this level.

QLL	=	Quadrate lobe of liver
LV	=	Ligamentum venosum
RLL	=	Right lobe of liver
CLL	=	Caudate lobe of liver
IVC	=	Inferior vena cava
RL	=	Right lung
CD	=	Crus of diaphragm
S	=	Stomach
C	=	Colon
SP	=	Spleen
LL	=	Left lung
AA	=	Abdominal aorta
T11	=	T11 level

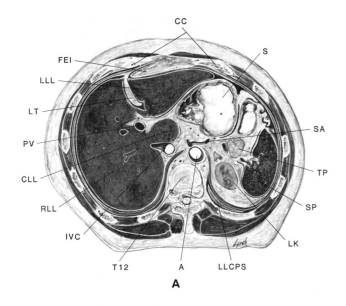

A

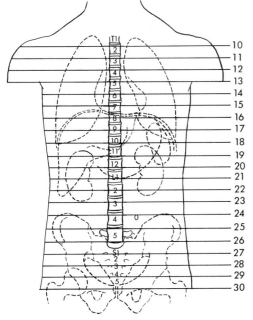

B

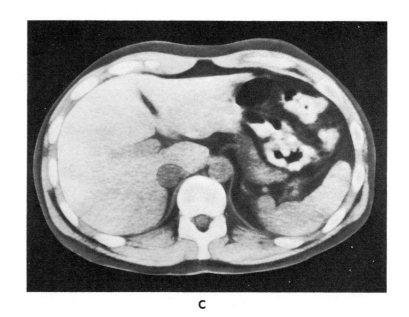

C

FIGURE 16–21 *A*. Diagram at upper abdomen level (T12) at cut No. 19, showing anatomic parts encountered in this slice. *B*. Miniature of Figure 16–11 for orientation. *C*. Computed tomograph obtained approximately at this level.

CC	=	Costal cartilages
FEI	=	Fat, extraperitoneal and intraperitoneal
LLL	=	Left lobe of liver
LT	=	Ligamentum teres
PV	=	Portal vein
CLL	=	Caudate lobe of liver
RLL	=	Right lobe of liver
IVC	=	Inferior vena cava
T12	=	T12 level
A	=	Aorta
S	=	Stomach
SA	=	Splenic artery
TP	=	Tail of pancreas
SP	=	Spleen
LK	=	Upper pole of left kidney
LLCPS	=	Left lung in costophrenic sulcus

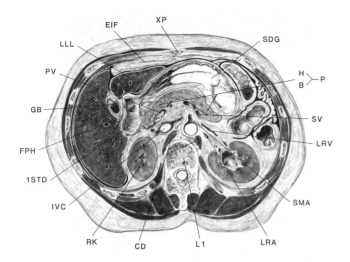

A

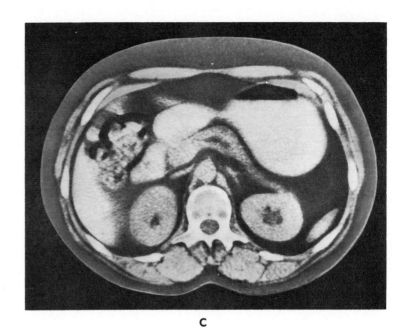

C

B

FIGURE 16–22 *A*. Diagram at upper abdomen level (L1) at cut No. 20, showing anatomic parts encountered in this slice. *B*. Miniature of Figure 16–11 for orientation. *C*. Computed tomograph obtained approximately at this level.

XP	=	Xiphoid process
EIF	=	Extraperitoneal and intraperitoneal fat along falciform ligament
LLL	=	Left lobe of liver
PV	=	Portal vein
GB	=	Gallbladder
FPH	=	Fat in porta hepatis
1st D	=	First part of duodenum
IVC	=	Inferior vena cava
RK	=	Right kidney
CD	=	Crura of diaphragms
SDG	=	Stomach with dilute gastrografin
H ⟍ P B ⟋	=	Head, body of pancreas
SV	=	Splenic vein
LRV	=	Left renal vein
SMA	=	Superior mesenteric artery
LRA	=	Left renal artery
L1	=	L1 level

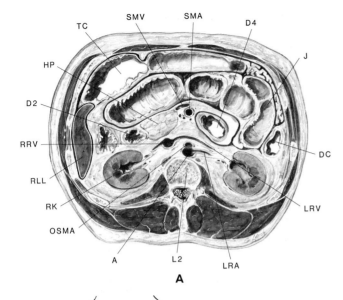

A

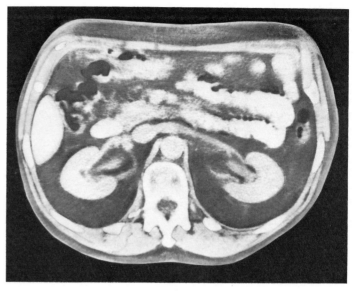

C

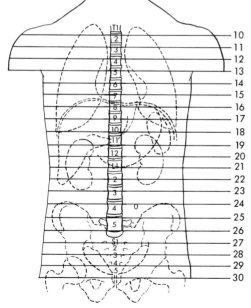

B

FIGURE 16–23 *A*. Diagram at upper abdomen level (L2) at cut No. 21, showing anatomic parts encountered in this slice. *B*. Miniature of Figure 16–11 for orientation. *C*. Computed tomograph obtained approximately at this level.

SMV	=	Superior mesenteric vein
TC	=	Transverse colon
HP	=	Head of pancreas
D2	=	Second portion of duodenum
RRV	=	Right renal vein
RLL	=	Right lobe of liver
RK	=	Right kidney
OSMA	=	Origin of superior mesenteric artery
A	=	Aorta
L2	=	L2 level
SMA	=	Superior mesenteric artery (more distal)
D4	=	Fourth portion of duodenum
J	=	Jejunum
DC	=	Descending colon
LRV	=	Left renal vein
LRA	=	Left renal artery

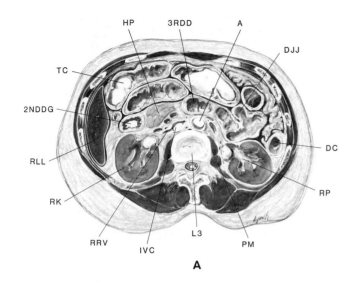

A

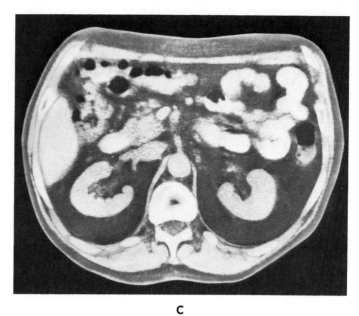

C

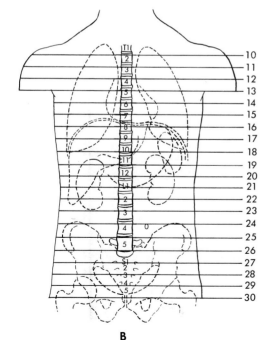

B

FIGURE 16–24 *A*. Diagram at midabdomen level (L3) at cut No. 22, showing anatomic parts encountered in this slice. *B*. Miniature of Figure 16–11 for orientation. *C*. Computed tomograph obtained approximately at this level.

3rd D	=	Third portion of duodenum
HP	=	Head of pancreas
TC	=	Transverse colon
2nd DG	=	Second portion of duodenum with gastrografin
RLL	=	Right lobe of liver
RK	=	Right kidney
RRV	=	Right renal vein
IVC	=	Inferior vena cava
A	=	Aorta
DJJ	=	Duodenojejunal junction
DC	=	Descending colon
RP	=	Renal pelvis
PM	=	Psoas muscle
L3	=	L3 level

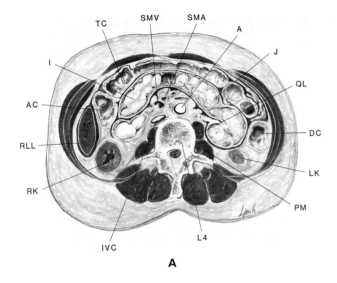

A

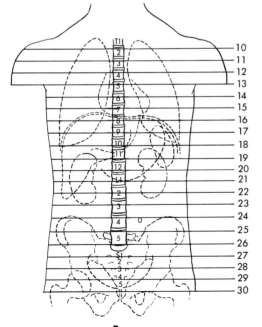

B

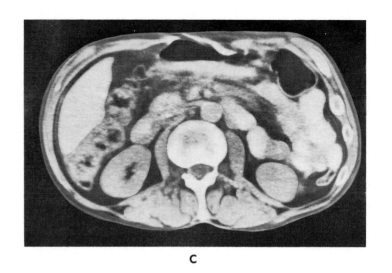

C

FIGURE 16–25 *A.* Diagram at midabdomen level (L4) at cut No. 23, showing anatomic parts encountered in this slice. *B.* Miniature of Figure 16–11 for orientation. *C.* Computed tomograph obtained approximately at this level.

SMV	=	Superior mesenteric vein
TC	=	Transverse colon
I	=	Ileum
AC	=	Ascending colon
RLL	=	Right lobe of liver
RK	=	Lower pole of right kidney
IVC	=	Inferior vena cava
SMA	=	Superior mesenteric artery
A	=	Aorta
J	=	Jejunum
QL	=	Quadratus lumborum muscle
DC	=	Descending colon
LK	=	Left kidney (lower pole)
PM	=	Psoas muscle
L 4	=	L 4 level

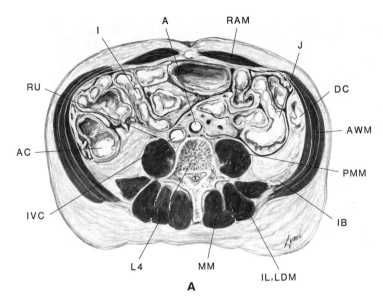

A

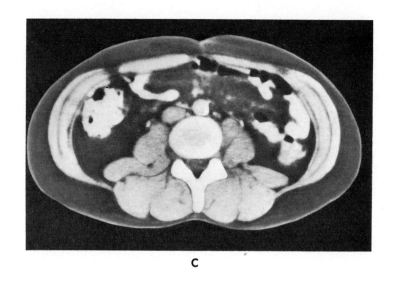

C

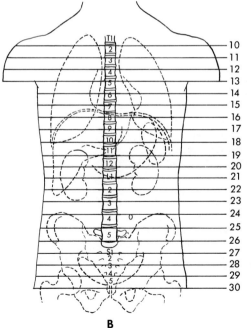

B

FIGURE 16–26 *A*. Diagram at umbilicus level (L4) at cut No. 24, showing anatomic parts encountered in this slice. *B*. Miniature of Figure 16–11 for orientation. *C*. Computed tomograph obtained approximately at this level.

A	=	Aorta
I	=	Ileum
RU	=	Right ureter
AC	=	Ascending colon
IVC	=	Inferior vena cava
L4	=	L4 vertebra
RAM	=	Rectus abdominis muscle
J	=	Jejunum
DC	=	Descending colon
AWM	=	Abdominal wall muscles (external and internal oblique muscles and transverse abdominal muscle)
PMM	=	Psoas major muscle
IB	=	Iliac bone
IL, LDM	=	Iliocostalis lumborum and longissimus dorsi muscles

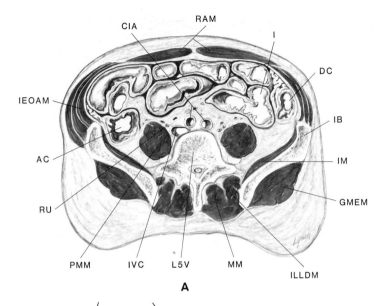

A

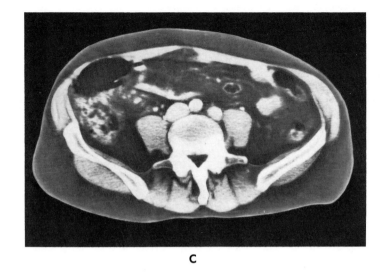

C

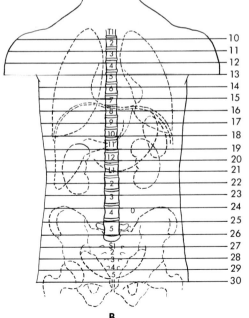

B

FIGURE 16–27 *A.* Diagram at lumbar level (L5) at cut No. 25, showing anatomic parts encountered in this slice. *B.* Miniature of Figure 16–11 for orientation. *C.* Computed tomograph obtained approximately at this level.

RAM	=	Rectus abdominis muscles
CIA	=	Common iliac arteries
IEOAM	=	Internal and external oblique abdominal muscles
AC	=	Ascending colon
RU	=	Right ureter
PMM	=	Psoas major muscle
IVC	=	Inferior vena cava
L5 V	=	L5 vertebra
I	=	Ileum
DC	=	Descending colon
IB	=	Iliac bone
IM	=	Iliacus muscle
GMEM	=	Gluteus medius muscle
ILLDM	=	Iliocostalis lumborum and longissimus dorsi muscles
MM	=	Multifidis muscle

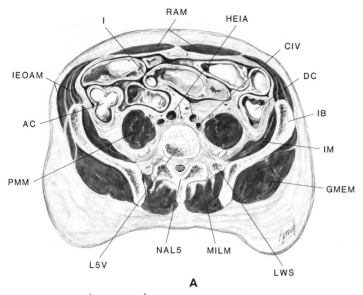

A

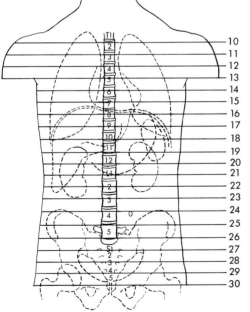

B

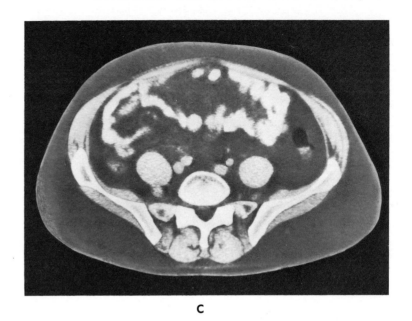

C

FIGURE 16–28 *A*. Diagram at lumbar level (L5) at cut No. 26, showing anatomic parts encountered in this slice. *B*. Miniature of Figure 16–11 for orientation. *C*. Computed tomograph obtained approximately at this level.

RAM	=	Rectus abdominis muscles
I	=	Ileum
IEOAM	=	Internal and external oblique abdominal muscles
AC	=	Ascending colon
PMM	=	Psoas major muscle
L5 V	=	L5 vertebra
NA L5	=	Neural arch L5
HEIA	=	Hypogastric and external iliac arteries
CIV	=	Common iliac vein
DC	=	Descending colon
IB	=	Iliac bone
IM	=	Iliacus muscle
GMEM	=	Gluteus medius muscle
LWS	=	Lateral wing of sacrum
MILM	=	Multifidis and iliocostalis lumborum muscle

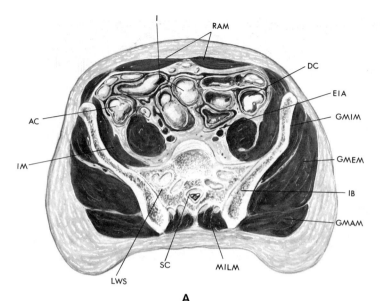

A

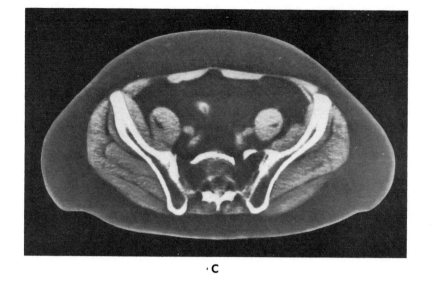

C

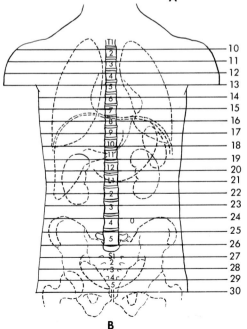

B

FIGURE 16–29 *A*. Diagram at sacral level (S1) at cut No. 27, showing anatomic parts encountered in this slice. *B*. Miniature of Figure 16–11 for orientation. *C*. Computed tomograph obtained approximately at this level.

RAM	=	Rectus abdominis muscle
I	=	Ileum
AC	=	Ascending colon
IM	=	Iliopsoas muscle
LWS	=	Lateral wing of sacrum
SC	=	Sacral canal
DC	=	Descending colon
EIA	=	External iliac artery
GMIM	=	Gluteus minimus muscle
GMEM	=	Gluteus medius muscle
IB	=	Iliac bone
GMAM	=	Gluteus maximus muscle
MILM	=	Multifidis and iliocostalis lumborum muscles

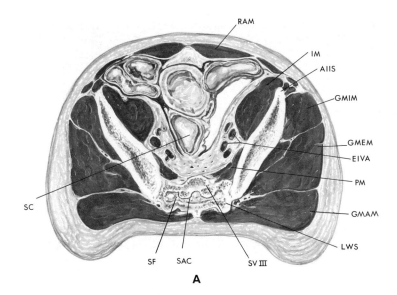

A

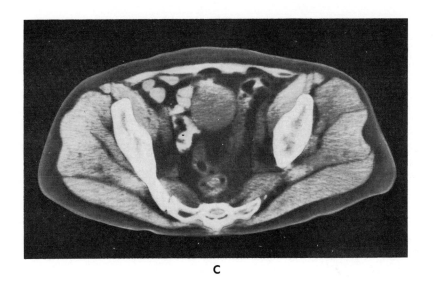

C

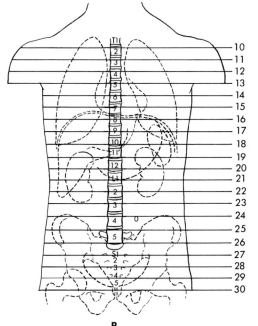

B

FIGURE 16–30 *A*. Diagram at sacral level (S3) at cut No. 28, showing anatomic parts encountered in this slice. *B*. Miniature of Figure 16–11 for orientation. *C*. Computed tomograph obtained approximately at this level. (CT is slightly oblique and includes obturator internus muscle.)

SC	=	Sigmoid colon
SF	=	Sacral foramen
SAC	=	Sacral canal
RAM	=	Rectus abdominis muscle
IM	=	Iliopsoas muscle
AIIS	=	Anterior inferior iliac spine
GMIM	=	Gluteus minimus muscle
GMEM	=	Gluteus medius muscle
EIVA	=	External iliac vein and artery
PM	=	Piriformis muscle
GMAM	=	Gluteus maximus muscle
LWS	=	Lateral wing of sacrum
SV III	=	Sacral vertebra III

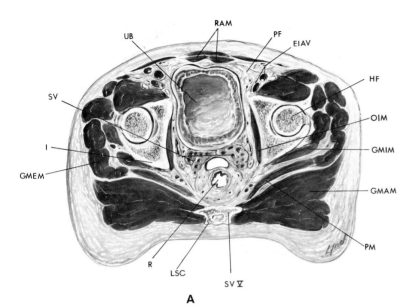

A

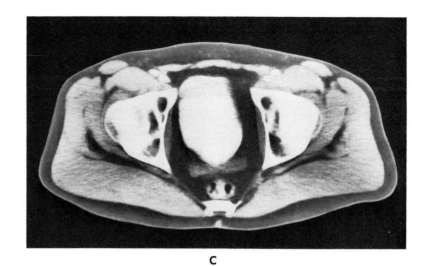

C

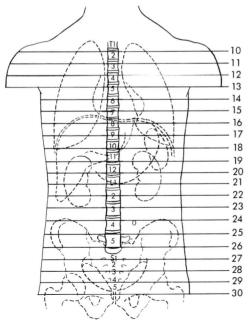

B

FIGURE 16–31 *A.* Diagram at sacral level (S4) at cut No. 29, showing anatomic parts encountered in this slice. *B.* Miniature of Figure 16–11 for orientation. *C.* Computed tomograph obtained approximately at this level.

RAM	=	Rectus abdominis muscles
UB	=	Urinary bladder
SV	=	Seminal vesicles
I	=	Ischium
GMEM	=	Gluteus medius muscle
R	=	Rectum
LSC	=	Lateral sacral crest
PF	=	Perivesical fat
EIAV	=	External iliac artery and vein
HF	=	Head of femur
OIM	=	Obturator internus muscle
GMIM	=	Gluteus minimus muscle
GMAM	=	Gluteus maximus muscle
PM	=	Piriform muscle
SV V	=	Sacral vertebra V

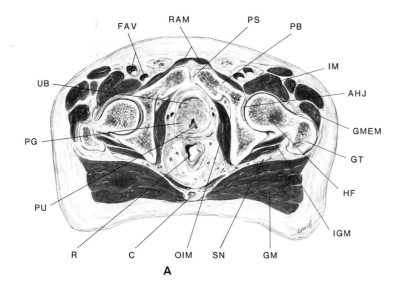

A

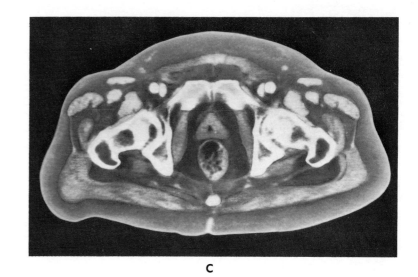

C

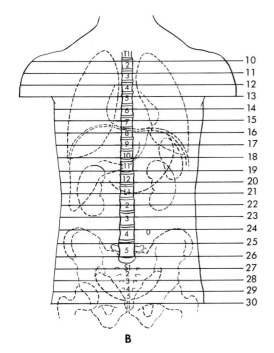

B

FIGURE 16–32 *A.* Diagram at coccygeal level (S5) at cut No. 30, showing anatomic parts encountered in this slice. *B.* Miniature of Figure 16–11 for orientation. *C.* Computed tomograph obtained approximately at this level.

RAM	=	Rectus abdominis muscles
FAV	=	Femoral artery and vein
UB	=	Urinary bladder
PG	=	Prostate gland
PU	=	Prostatic urethra
R	=	Rectum
C	=	Coccyx
PS	=	Pubic symphysis
PB	=	Pubic bone
IM	=	Iliopsoas muscle
AHJ	=	Acetabulum and hip joint
GMEM	=	Gluteus medius muscle
GT	=	Greater trochanter
HF	=	Head of femur
IGM	=	Inferior gemellus muscle
GM	=	Gluteus maximus
SN	=	Sciatic nerve
OIM	=	Obturator internus muscle

REFERENCES*

Ambrose, J.: Computerized X-ray scanning of the brain. J. Neurosurgery, *40*:679–695, 1974.

Ambrose, J., and Hounsfield, G.: Computerized transverse axial tomography. Br. J. Radiol., *46*:148–149, 1973.

Eycleshymer, A. C., and Schoemaker, D. M.: A Cross-Section Anatomy. New York, Appleton-Century-Crofts, 1970.

Gonzalez, C. F., Grossman, C. B., and Palacios, E.: Computed Brain and Orbital Tomography. Technique and Interpretation. New York, John Wiley & Sons, 1976.

J. Lloyd Johnson Associates: The effect of computed tomography on hospital practice. Northfield, Ill., J. Lloyd Johnson Associates, 1976.

Meyers, M. A.: Dynamic Radiology of the Abdomen: Normal and Pathologic Anatomy. New York, Springer-Verlag, 1976.

New, P. F. J., and Scott, W. R.: Computed Tomography of the Brain and Orbit. Baltimore, The Williams & Wilkins Co., 1975.

Ter-Pogossian, M. (ed.): Workshop on Reconstruction Tomography in Diagnostic Radiology and Nuclear Medicine: Proceedings. Baltimore, University Park Press, 1977.

Whalen, J. P.: Radiology of the Abdomen: Anatomic Basis. Philadelphia, Lea & Febiger, 1976.

---

*Only a few of the major references are listed here, since the student may find more extensive bibliographies within these major publications.

INDEX

Note: Page numbers in *italics* refer to illustrations. Page numbers followed by the letter "t" refer to tables.